Functional Imaging

Functional Imaging

Editors

Gustav K. von Schulthess, MD, PhD
Professor and Director, Nuclear Medicine
Department of Medical Radiology, Nuclear Medicine
University Hospital
Zurich, Switzerland

Jürgen Hennig, PhD
Professor, Department of Radiology-MR
University Hospital
Freiburg, Germany

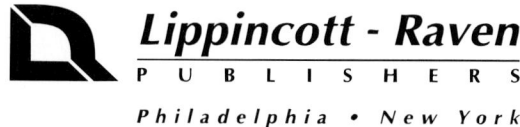

Lippincott - Raven
PUBLISHERS

Philadelphia • New York

Acquisitions Editor: James D. Ryan/Joyce-Rachel John
Manufacturing Manager: Dennis Teston
Associate Managing Editor: Kathleen Bubbeo
Production Service: Textbook Writers Associates, Inc.
Cover Designer: David Levy
Indexer: Sandi J. Schroeder
Compositor: Maryland Composition
Printer: Kingsport Press

Printed in the United States of America

9 8 7 6 5 4 3 2 1

Library of Congress Cataloging-in-Publication Data

Functional imaging : principles and methodology / edited by Gustav von
  Schulthess and Jürgen Hennig
     p. cm.
  Includes bibliographical references and index.
  ISBN 0-397-51606-1
  1. Diagnostic imaging. I. Schulthess, Gustav Konrad von.
II. Hennig, Jürgen.
  [DNLM: 1. Diagnostic Imaging—methods. WN 180 F979 1997]
RC78.7.D53F86 1997
616.07′54—dc21
DNLM/DLC
for Library of Congress   97-27805
                                           CIP

For Alexandre, Patrick, and Benjamin
—GKvS

To my wife, Annemarie,
and my children, Julian and Olivia
—JH

Contents

Contributing Authors

Michael Bach, PhD
*Division of Neuroophthalmology, University Hospital, 5 Killianstr, D 79106
Freiburg, Germany*

R. Beisteiner, PhD
*University Clinic of Neurology and Ludwig Boltzman Institute for Functional Brain
Topography, Währinger Gürtel 18-20, A-1090 Vienna, Austria*

Alfred Buck, MD
*Senior Staff, Department of Medical Radiology, Nuclear Medicine, University
Hospital, Ramistr 100, CH-8091 Zurich, Switzerland*

Cyrill Burger, PhD
*Head, Imaging Analysis Group, Department of Medical Radiology, Nuclear
Medicine, University Hospital, Ramistr 100, CH-8091 Zurich, Switzerland*

Luder Deecke, MD
*Professor of Neurology, University Clinic of Neurology and Ludwig Boltzman
Institute for Functional Brain Topography, Währinger Gürtel 18-20, A-1090
Vienna, Austria*

Johannes M. Fröhlich, PhD
*Free Consultant and Scientific Affairs Manager, Guerbet AG, Winterthurerstrasse
92, CH-8006 Zurich, Switzerland*

Guido Gerig, PhD
*Assistant Professor of Image Data Analysis, Swiss Federal Institute of Technology,
Gloriastr 35, CH-8092 Zurich, Switzerland*

Jürgen Hennig, PhD
Professor, Department of Radiology-MR, University Hospital, Hugstetterstr 55, 79106 Freiburg, Germany

Willi A. Kalender, PhD
Professor of Medical Physics, Institute for Medicine and Physics, University of Erlangen-Nürnberg, Krankenhausstraße 12, D-91054 Erlangen, Germany

August P. Schubiger, PhD
Director, Institute of Radiopharmacy, Paul Scherrer Institute, 5232 Villigen-PSI, Switzerland

Christoph Suess, MD
Institute for Medicine and Physics, University of Erlangen-Nürnberg, Krankenhausstraße 12, D-91054 Erlangen, Germany

Gábor Székely, PhD
Department of Electrical Engineering, Swiss Federal Institute of Technology, Gloriastr 35, CH-8092 Zurich, Switzerland

Arno Villringer, MD
Division of Neuroimaging, Neurological Clinic, Charité, Humboldt University, Schumannstrasse 20-21, 10098 Berlin, Germany

Gustav K. von Schulthess, MD, PhD
Professor and Director, Nuclear Medicine, Department of Medical Radiology, Nuclear Medicine, University Hospital, Ramistr 100, CH-8091 Zurich, Switzerland

J. Vrba, PhD
CTF Systems, Inc., 15-1750 McLean Avenue, Port Coquitlam, British Columbia V3C 1M9, Canada

Peter N.T. Wells, PhD
Professor and Chief Physicist, Department of Medical Physics and Bioengineering, Bristol General Hospital, Guinea Street, Bristol BS1 6SY, United Kingdom

Foreword

During the past decades, medicine has developed from an empirical art into a rational science. It became obvious that physiologic function is the result of an exceedingly complex and almost miraculous interplay between a multitude of chemical reactions. Medicine serves the purpose of maintaining and restoring biologic functions under adverse circumstances. However, no progress in medical procedures and no goal-oriented and properly adapted treatment are possible unless tools are available for visualizing functional processes at various levels from macroscopic localization to a detailed study of the underlying chemical reactions. Here perhaps more than anywhere else, the proverb "One picture is worth ten thousand words" applies.

Indeed, the visualization of physiologic function is one of the clues for further progress in the understanding of biomedical processes, in the design of new therapeutic procedures, and in their clinical application. Fortunately, techniques in biomedical imaging have advanced during the past decade. Today, many techniques of visualization are available, providing a wealth of information inconceivable 10 years ago. Their importance in clinical and research-oriented medicine is growing daily. The appearance of this book on functional imaging is thus very timely, filling a gap that needs to be closed.

Medical imaging has reached a level of sophistication that can no longer be mastered by a single individual, so it is not astonishing that a team of scientists and medical practitioners with diverse fields of expertise stands behind this book. For the practicing medical doctor, knowing the principal features of all available techniques is essential to allow for proper decisions to be made in critical situations. This book provides the necessary information in an authoritative but still easily understandable form. Specialists, on the other hand, can find here a wealth of in-depth knowledge on "their own" technique. In addition, it is important that specialists also broaden their scope by an occasional study of alternative or complementary imaging procedures. This will, at the same time, stimulate their inspiration and facilitate a fruitful interaction between practitioners and researchers in different fields.

A closer look at the various imaging techniques reveals that the basic concepts are invariably the same in all disciplines of functional imaging from nuclear medicine to x-ray imaging, magnetic resonance, magnetoencephalography, and ultrasound. Similar data-processing procedures are used, although the sources of the data may be radically different. Also, the image-presentation techniques are virtually identical in all fields. And finally, the data reduction and interpretation serve the same goal: to enhance the utility and the reliability of medical treatments.

In the hands of clinical practitioners and biomedical researchers, this book will undoubtedly have a significant and positive impact on the quality of medical treatments in the future. It will allow for an optimal usage of a large arsenal of fascinating and powerful functional imaging techniques and may lead to further improvements of the underlying methodology.

Richard R. Ernst, PhD
Physikalische Chemie
Eidgenössisch Technische
Hoch schule (ETHZ)
CH-8092 Zurich, Switzerland

Preface

This textbook covers the imaging of organ function in humans. The approach is multidisciplinary; thus the text does not just provide information on a particular technique but rather discusses functional imaging by keeping a broad view on the different modalities, "contrast agents," and postprocessing techniques available. Clinicians and scientists alike will find useful information on the other imaging techniques with which they are not familiar.

Function imaging and *functional imaging* are terms that are freely applied to many medical imaging procedures. We like to define the terms in the widest sense. By function or functional imaging we mean all imaging procedures that provide information beyond the mere morphologic representation of a structure. It is true in many instances that the depiction of morphology already yields some information on organ function; a morphologically altered organ may imply that its function is impaired. Hence it is sometimes quite difficult to draw the line between what is functional imaging and what is morphologic imaging. In this book we work with the definition that function imaging gives information that cannot be inferred directly from looking at the anatomic features in the image. The Renaissance anatomists already could depict the cardiovascular system in detail, but it took 100 years until William Harvey in the seventeenth century discovered the circulation. Hence, while morphology sometimes may suggest function, it is often difficult or impossible to infer function from anatomic features imaged. Because of the limitations of current-day imaging devices, we also focus on function that can be observed macroscopically, although all function has a microscopic correlate. Furthermore, this book also includes some information on methods that cannot strictly be called imaging methods, such as electric or magnetic source "imaging." The reason for including these techniques is that, combined with imaging techniques, they are capable of giving information with a very high spatial resolution.

Although one could probably trace the origin of functional imaging to the early days after the discovery of x rays and certainly to the time when radiologists started to use contrast agents, functional imaging proper is only a few decades old and started to show some clinical relevance with the advent of nuclear medicine. Specifically, the use of iodine-131 to identify the regional distribution of thyroid hormone production and thus differentiate between "hot" and "cold" nodules as well as disseminated thyroid hyperfunction could be labeled as the beginning of clinical functional imaging. The imaging techniques to assess function have quickly multiplied and become so complex by now that it is even difficult to keep track of the developments in the field of one's expertise. Highly relevant information from related fields may therefore often go unnoticed. In fact, one often observes some factionalism that "actively" ignores developments in related fields. Furthermore, techniques long ago developed and explored in one field are being "rediscovered" and "sold" as new techniques in a second field. This factionalism is a result of funding pressures, where researchers have to overstate that the methodology they propose to study a given problem is unique, and also a result of political pressures, as expensive imaging equipment—and this is what much modern function imaging is all about—is often distributed among different departments in the same institution. Otherwise, not all equipment is available at a given institution, and the result may be "blindness" toward the equipment not available. The rather independent development of different disciplines working on different aspects of—at least in the light of current research—the same problem has led to very specific and idiosyncratic schools of thought, which makes communication difficult even for those willing to "jump over the fences of their own scientific biotopes." We sincerely hope that this book on methodology of functional imaging can serve to find a common basis and thus to further communication and the exchange of ideas.

The contents of a book on functional imaging can be based on either the various imaging modalities with the clinical applications as subchapters or vice versa. Both approaches have their advantages and drawbacks. A modality-oriented order would probably contain a lot of irrelevant information for a reader whose main interest will be, for example, brain activator studies and who will not necessarily be interested in the intricacies of, for example, measuring myocardial performance. It also would put a totally wrong emphasis on the tools compared with the applications for which these tools were created. We have decided to use a mixed approach. This text will describe the basics of the various imaging techniques with a strong emphasis on their use for functional studies.

Our intention is to be useful to those who might be well versed in the application of a particular technique but might have only rudimentary knowledge of most of the others. The book therefore tries to keep at a level to be not only understandable but also interesting to those without any prior knowledge in the various specialities, knowing that interest is a prerequisite to understanding. At the same time, we want to give information that goes beyond the "as if" state of knowledge transmitted by many texts aimed at nonspecialists. Our goal is to give information at a level profound enough to be useful for scientists working in the field. This can only be reached if we are successful in not merely describing the fundamentals of each technique but also in creating some real understanding of its potential, which remains of use, even when the fast proliferation of the various techniques makes many specific details obsolete in a short period of time.

We have chosen a two-leveled approach in order to make this text of interest for both the uninitiated and the specialist. The plain text sticks to the basics and relays the fundamental concepts with a minimum of formal notation. Boxes are used with additional information in formal notation.

Finally, it would be overambitious if we would attempt to raze all fences and bridge all gaps between the different disciplines working on functional imaging. We will be highly satisfied if this book serves as a friendly tour guide helping to understand the "natives" of each field and be understood by those who visit ours.

Functional Imaging

Functional Imaging, edited by
Gustav von Schulthess and Jürgen Hennig.
Lippincott–Raven Publishers, Philadelphia, © 1998.

1

Basic Principles of Image Formation

Jürgen Hennig

The *Dictionary of Science and Technology* (Academic Press, 1992) defines an *image* as ''a likeness or representation of a person or object.'' If we take the terms *representation* and *object* in their most general form, images can be produced not only from visible entities like sunsets, beaches, and boy/girlfriends or from things that we could see, if we could see them, like the inside of Jupiter or the chromosomes of a fruitfly, but images also can be made from abstract concepts like the temperature over the Himalayas, the population density of Southern China, or the income tax revenue per square meter across Geneva. Even totally immaterial ideas can be presented in image form. Fractal curves or the pictures by Maurice Escher are examples of the fact that images are powerful tools to communicate ideas without words. Images are thus of a much more general nature compared with pictures, which confine themselves to be flat somethings that can be seen. Since images are normally presented as pictures, the two are often confused. A colored representation of a Mandelbrot curve can be conceived as the image of a fractal or just as a pretty picture, and its fascination probably lies in the fact that it is both. Pictures can thus be regarded as the vessel, whereas the image constitutes the content. An artist paints a picture in order to create an image. Well, at least some artists do.

Why this semantic discourse? Mainly in order to emphasize that there is always some degree of abstraction involved in an image. This is good to keep in mind when looking at the images created by some of the imaging modalities discussed in this book, which deceptively look like pictures of cross sections of the body but really are pictorial representations of images created by some more or less indirect measurement process. No matter how realistic they look, they can thus easily show something that is not really there. For the purpose of this book, this is extremely fortunate, since it allows us to measure functions that are not necessarily related to any changes in the visual appearance

J Hennig: Department of Radiology, University Hospital, Freiburg, Germany.

of the tissues under study. Diffusion, perfusion, brain activity, and even metabolic changes are some examples of functional measurements that will be covered in the following chapters.

Images in the general sense can be formed directly in the mind of, for example, the reader of a book or the mathematician looking at the formula for a graph. For image-measurement techniques, however, a physical correlate is needed for the various image-formation steps. Most important is the carrier, which constitutes the link between the observed object—the patient or volunteer—and the observer represented by some kind of receiver of the imaging modality.

Physics offers (currently) two kinds of carriers useful for transmission of information: electromagnetic radiation, covering the frequency range from very long radiowaves up to radioactive radiation, and pressure waves below and—more important—beyond the frequency spectrum of audible sound.

The last decades brought a tremendous proliferation of multiple methods that allow us to look into the human body. The huge repertoire of imaging techniques developed within this century, including x-ray, ultrasound, scintigraphy, positron emission tomography (PET), single photon emission computed tomography (SPECT), magnetic resonance imaging (MRI), to name just a few, is based entirely on the interaction of radiation with matter. In fact, if ultrasound is excluded, all the others use electromagnetic radiation.

In order for an image to be formed, it is necessary that the radiation used interacts in some way with the observed object. Basic interactions are absorption, emission, scattering, and reflection. In the most basic ways to form an image, which we also use heavily in our visual perception, the observed object is opaque for the radiation used. An image of the surface of the object can then be formed either by use of reflected radiation or—even simpler—as a projection image if the spatial distribution of the absorbed radiation is received, forming the shadow of the object.

The development of clinical imaging techniques started with the discovery of x-rays by C. W. Roentgen in 1895. His first image of the bones of the hand of his wife was—like the millions of conventional x-ray images taken every year—acquired as a projection image, taking advantage of the much higher opacity of bones to x-rays compared with soft tissues. This way of forming an image is still used very successfully and constitutes the backbone of radiologic diagnosis. The fast development of medical imaging techniques within the last two to three decades is, however, based on a—conceptually and technically—much more demanding image-formation process that creates images from inside of the body, most often in the form of two-dimensional cross-sectional images called *tomograms* after the first such cross-sectional x-ray technique.

If we contemplate the conditions necessary for forming such images from within, we find that these are so special and even contradictory that it is nearly a miracle that any one method has been found to produce them, let alone the great variety of different methods using different measurement principles.

In our daily experience we very rarely encounter a situation where we perceive the inside of an object, which is exactly what these modern imaging techniques are doing. The reason is very simple: Materials tend to be either translucent, in which case we see through them, or opaque, in which case we see only their surface. In order to see inside a material, it has to be sufficiently translucent to look into but at the same time reflect or attenuate light such that local variations of the signal intensity arise in order to form an image. The balance between translucence and opaqueness is extremely precarious and very seldom fulfilled. Examples of things we can ''look into'' in daily life are in fact hard to find. Fire or colored ink dropped into water might qualify, but even here we perceive the surface more than the inside.

From the preceding it is clear that the body has to be somewhat but not quite translucent for the radiation used for any such imaging technique. In the following chapters it will be demonstrated that the interaction of matter with radiation depends very heavily on the wavelength used or, in other words, the frequency spectrum.

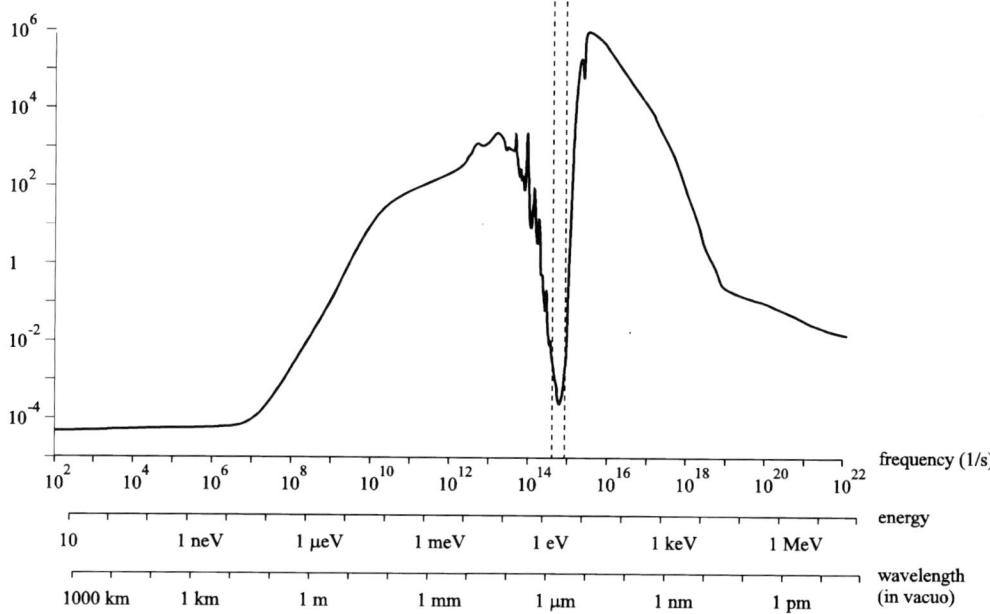

Figure 1. Absorption spectrum of water over the frequency spectrum from long-range radio waves up to high-enery radiation. The range of the visible spectrum is indicated by the two dotted vertical lines. The horizontal axis is given in frequency and energy units as well as in the wavelength of the radiation. Note that both axes are logarithmic in scale; the ratio of the frequencies at both ends of the spectrum thus is 10^{20} : 1, or 100,000,000,000,000,000,000 : 1!

For electromagnetic radiation, a large part of the spectrum is very efficiently absorbed via various mechanisms (Fig. 1). The corresponding range consequently cannot be used for tomographic imaging. Windows exist either at very short wavelengths (x-rays and beyond) or in the band of longer wavelengths starting in the near-infrared and extending via microwave and radiofrequency bands to the low-frequency end of the spectrum. This limitation of the electromagnetic spectrum as the carrier of the image information limits, of course, the range of possible mechanisms that can interact with the carrier. Optical absorbance and reflectance, the basis of our direct visual perception, are ruled out, since light simply does not penetrate into tissue.

Given our knowledge about bodily absorbance over the electromagnetic spectrum, and also given the fact that it appears to be unlikely that fundamental new mechanisms by which waves interact with matter will be discovered, there is a general feeling that there will be no new imaging techniques in the future and developments in the field will be improvements in quality rather than true innovations. This I do not expect, however. There are a great number of physical mechanisms that could in principle be the basis of an imaging experiment but which have not yet been used, either because no feasible measurement technique for such use has been found or because state-of-the-art technical equipment is inadequate for that purpose.

In this book the various imaging techniques have been sorted according to the frequency (or its companion by inversion, the wavelength) of the radiation used for the interaction. It is apparent that the physical nature of the interaction is very different for the different modalities, leading to a vast range of mechanisms (and functions) that can be examined. The common use of (predominantly electromagnetic) waves as a carrier makes it nevertheless possible to state some basic principles that connect all these modalities and which define the boundary conditions for each technique.

In the following, the fundamentals of wave optics will be presented as a common basis for all imaging techniques. Together with a chapter on basic signal theory, this will serve as the common ground for the discussion of the various imaging modalities.

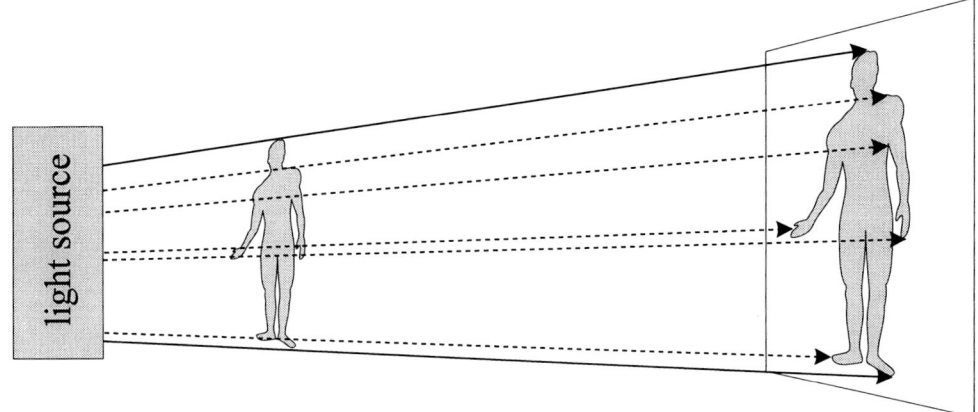

Figure 2. Basics of projection imaging: Light is regarded as a straight line. The projection image then simply is the shadow cast by the object blocking the way of the light rays.

WAVE PROPAGATION

The Huygens Principle and the Inverse Problem: Diffraction and Interference

When the imaging properties of some visual imaging device such as a photographic camera are discussed, this can be done by representing the light rays as straight lines. Projection imaging as the most simple imaging technique can thus be explained very simply (Fig. 2). Unfortunately, this representation of a light beam as a straight line is wrong in principle, although this model seems to work very well in practice. One hint that a better model might be needed to describe the behavior of light is given by the fact that it does not explain why light changes its course when it goes from one material (say air) to another (say water or glass). Even if it is known that light changes its velocity from one material to another, this can never introduce a lateral deflection as long as a light beam is regarded as a one-dimensional longitudinal "arrow."

The solution to this apparent disparity lies in the fact that light consists of electromagnetic waves with a wavelength that is so small compared with everything that is "measured" (seen) with it that a straight-line approach is justified for most purposes. This is not necessarily true when very small structures are being studied or if electromagnetic waves with a longer wavelength are being used. Both cases are exactly equivalent: Wave propagation is determined by the ratio of the wavelength to the size of the object; the absolute scale is negligible.

The rule that has to be followed for the description of waves is known as the *Huygens principle,* and it states that each point along a wave can be regarded as the origin of a spherically expanding wavefront. The actual direction in which a packet of waves will travel is then given by the interference of the wavefronts from different points along the beam (Fig. 3). Once the basic consequences of this principle are understood, it need not be applied at each and every point, but some simple rules can be used:

1. As long as the beam of light is thick compared with the wavelength, it can be assumed that it goes along a straight line.
2. In order to understand the propagation of waves around some obstacle, the Huygens principle thus must be applied only at points along the obstacle.
3. The same applies when light enters one medium from another.

Some exercises will be used to allow the reader to achieve some basic understanding of the behavior of waves: First, wave propagation through a screen with one hole is discussed (Fig. 4). The imaging device used is a simple flat screen on which the incoming waves are registered. Applying the Huygens principle, it can be seen that the image of the hole (= intensity distribution on the screen) is only similar in diameter to the hole if the wavelength used is small compared with the diameter of the hole. For larger wavelengths, the image becomes much larger than the hole itself.

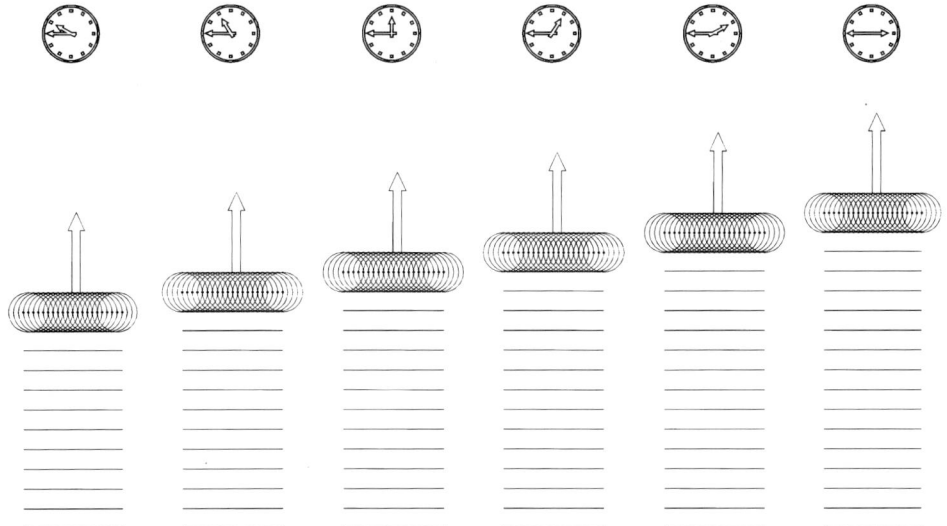

Figure 3. Huygens principle: Each point on a wavefront can be regarded as the source of a circular wave. The direction of the propagating wave is then orthogonal to the line of positive interference of the (in principle, infinite) Huygens centers. The progress of the wavefront over time is given by repetitive application of this procedure.

SOME BASICS ABOUT WAVES

The wavelength λ of a propagating wave is connected to the propagation velocity v_p and the frequency ν by

$$v_p = \lambda \nu, \qquad \lambda = \frac{v_p}{\nu}, \qquad \nu = \frac{v_p}{\lambda} \qquad (1)$$

For electromagnetic waves, v_p is identical to the velocity of light c ($=299\ 792$ km/s in vacuo). For pressure waves, as used by ultrasound and earthquakes, v_p is on the order of a few hundred meters per second for gases and up to several kilometers per second for solids. From the preceding equations it is immediately apparent that λ will be dramatically longer for electromagnetic waves compared with sound at identical frequencies and ν will be considerably lower for sound for a given λ.

One of the fundamentals of quantum theory is the fact that the energy of electromagnetic radiation always comes in integral multiples of the quantum energy given by

$$E = h\nu \qquad (2)$$

where h is the Planck constant corresponding to 6.626×10^{-34} J $\cdot$ s.

Electromagnetic radiation can thus be characterized by its wavelength, frequency, or quantum energy. In order to avoid numbers with awkward exponents, E is commonly expressed not in joules (J), but in electronvolts (eV), where 1 eV is defined as the energy gained by an electron after passing an electrical potential difference of 1 V. Table 1 lists the conversion factors between the various units. Since λ is inversely proportional to the other units, the wavenumber $1/\lambda$ is given rather than λ itself.

Table 2 is very useful because the various disciplines dealing with electromagnetic waves have adopted their own nomenclature according to the units that yield the least awkward numbers for the wavelengths used. Some examples are listed in Table 2.

Table 1.

	$1/\lambda$ (1/m)	ν (1/s)	E (J)	E (eV)
$1/\lambda$ (1/m)	1	3.344×10^{-9}	5.034×10^{24}	8.065×10^{5}
ν (1/s)	2.998×10^{8}	1	1.509×10^{33}	2.418×10^{14}
E (J)	1.986×10^{-25}	6.626×10^{-34}	1	6.242×10^{18}
E (eV)	1.240×10^{-6}	4.136×10^{-15}	1.602×10^{-19}	1

DIFFRACTION

Let us start with the simplest case first: We assume that coherent light of a certain wavelength λ goes through a narrow hole with diameter a (see Fig. 4). We observe the intensity of the light beam on a screen that is placed at a distance d from the hole. As a matter of simplicity, we assume that the distance d is very large compared with the wavelength λ as well as with a. The signal intensity at a given spot on the screen will then be a superposition of the light waves' origin from all points across the slit.

For any angle $\theta <> 0$, the light waves arriving at any point x will have a different phase according to the different path lengths. The phase dispersion will be determined by the relative phase of light originating at the edges of the slit. The observed signal intensity will be reduced with increasing x until it reaches 0 for an angle θ, which is given by $\sin \theta = \lambda/a$. At this angle, the phases of the different contributions will be evenly distributed in all directions. For larger θ, the signal intensity will grow again until it reaches a maximum at $\sin \theta = 3/2\lambda/a$. The second and all further zero points are determined by $\sin \theta = m\lambda/a$, with $m = 2, 3, 4, \ldots$.

The signal intensity as a function of x will be determined by vector addition of the various contributions (Fig. 5). Let us take the wave coming from the center of the slit as reference. We already know that the phase difference Φ between the beams from the edges will be 2π if $a \sin \theta = \lambda$. For any other beam angle θ, Φ will then be given by proportion as

$$\Phi = \frac{2\pi}{\lambda} \cdot a \cdot \sin \theta \tag{3}$$

Vector addition shows that only the cosine part of each wave will contribute to the total signal intensity as a function of the phase difference φ of each Huygens wave to the reference signal. Since the number of Huygens waves within a given range of ϑ will decrease with increasing Φ, the amplitude of each contribution as a function of φ will be given by

$$A = \frac{C}{\Phi} \cos \varphi \tag{4}$$

where C is an (as yet) unspecified scaling constant.

The total signal amplitude will then be

$$A = \frac{C}{\Phi} \int_{-\Phi/2}^{\Phi/2} \cos \varphi \, d\varphi = \frac{C}{\Phi/2} \sin \frac{\Phi}{2} \tag{5}$$

The signal intensity I is defined as the square of the signal amplitude. By $I = I_0$ for $\Phi = 0$, we finally get

$$I = I_0 \left(\frac{\sin \dfrac{\Phi}{2}}{\dfrac{\Phi}{2}} \right)^2 \tag{6}$$

This diffraction pattern is known as *Fraunhofer diffraction.*

Table 2.

	Frequency range	Common units
Electrophysiology (EEG, MEG)	Hz	
Telecommunications	Very low frequency (AM)	kHz
	Low frequency (AM)	kHz-MHz
	High frequency (AM)	MHz
	Very high frequency (FM)	MHz
	Ultra high frequency (TV)	GHz
Magnetic resonance (radiofrequency)	MHz	
Radioastronomy (microwave)		cm
Infrared spectroscopy		nm
Optical imaging		nm
Ultraviolet spectroscopy		nm
X-ray		Å, nm
Nuclear medicine		

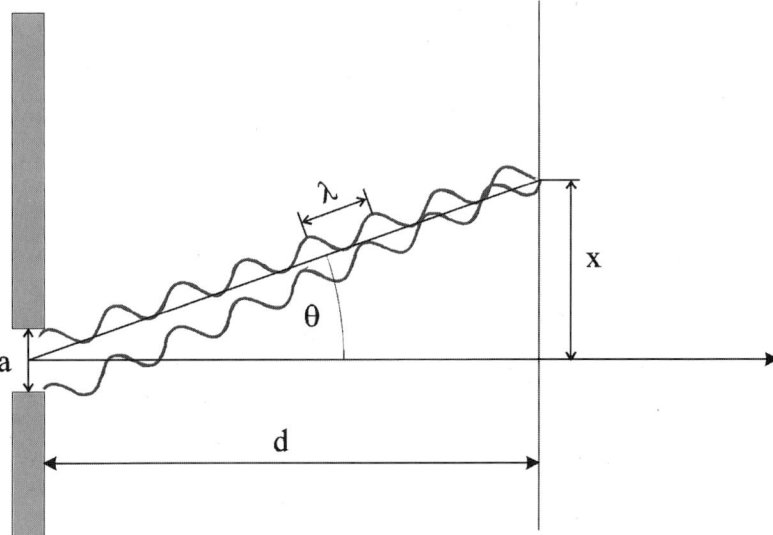

Figure 4. Diffraction at a hole. Waves with a wavelength λ pass through a hole with diameter a. Each point across the hole can be regarded as the source of a circular wavefront according to the Huygens principle. Shown are two waves from both edges of the hole falling onto a screen at a point with distance x from the center of the screen. If $a \ll d$, the angle θ of both waves with respect to the horizontal can be regarded as equal.

More interesting and complex cases can be derived by superposition. For the case of two holes, it can be seen immediately that their "images" melt together when their distance approaches the dimension of the wavelength used (Fig. 6). It can thus be stated:

The maximum attainable resolution for any imaging technique is determined by the wavelength of the radiation used.

This is a basic axiom of wave-propagation theory and has nothing to do with the nature of the waves or the kinds of interactions of waves with matter. It is thus valid for all imaging techniques and for all kinds of waves. If a resolution of 1 to 10 mm is assumed as a minimum requirement for any medical imaging technique, a limit can be defined as to which kind of radiation might be used for an "optical" imaging technique based on wave propagation. The wave-propagation speed determines the ratio between the frequency and the wavelength. For pressure waves with sound velocities on the order of 1000 to 2000 m/s, the useful frequency range thus extends to frequencies that are several orders of magnitude lower compared with electromagnetic waves. These simple arguments show that a number of techniques discussed in this book cannot form an image

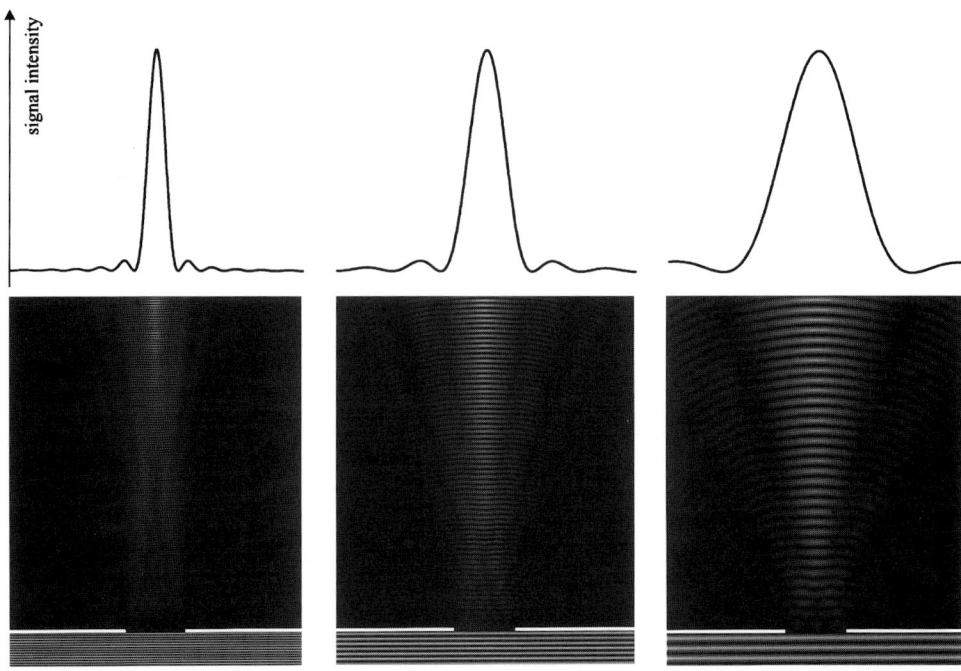

Figure 5. Intensity of the diffraction pattern as a function of the wavelength. In the diagrams at the bottom, the diffracting waves are shown as gray-scale images: A parallel wavefront going through the holes at the center will give rise to the intensity variations on the screen plotted above the images. Note that the intensity distribution directly behind the hole (Fresnel diffraction) differs from the distribution shown at larger distances (Fraunhofer diffraction).

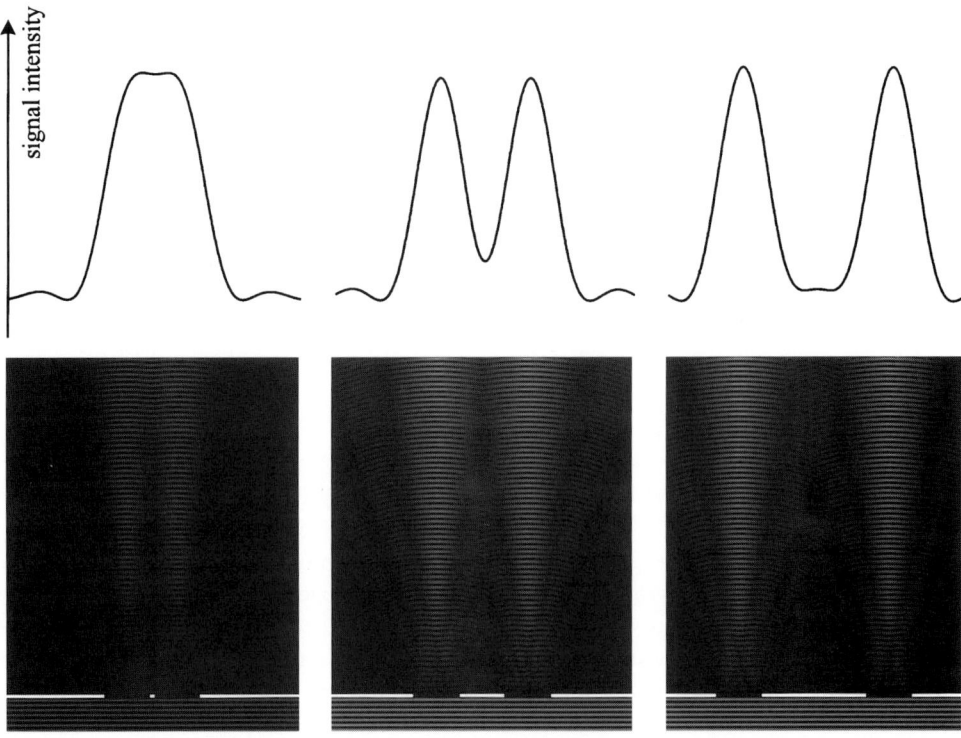

Figure 6. Diffraction at two holes as a function of the distance between the holes. It can be seen that the images of the holes start to melt together when the two holes approach each other. The distance at which the two images become unseparable depends on the wavelength according to Fig. 5.

directly (although all properties of waves discussed in this chapter are, of course, applicable and often very relevant).

If the screen contains two holes at a distance b, then the intensity at a given point on the screen will be given by superposition of the diffraction patterns of each hole:

$$I = 4I_0 \left(\frac{\sin \frac{\Phi}{2}}{\frac{\Phi}{2}} \right)^2 \cos^2 \delta/2 \tag{7}$$

where δ corresponds to the phase difference of the two waves, which is given by

$$\delta = \frac{2\pi}{\lambda} \cdot d \cdot \sin \theta + \delta_0 \tag{8}$$

The first term corresponds to the phase difference arising from the different path lengths of the two wavefronts to the screen; the second term corresponds to any initial phase difference δ_0 at the position of the holes.

It should be noted that the intensity at the central maximum is four times that of each single interference pattern due to the fact that the intensity is proportional to the square of the amplitude. This is a consequence of the coherent superposition of the two wavefronts. In daily life, when we switch on two (incoherent) light sources, the two light waves at any arbitrary point will have a random phase relation. The total intensity will thus be reduced by a factor of 2 compared with coherent superposition, and we get the familiar result that two lights are twice as bright as one.

The images of the two holes will melt into each other when the distance between the holes gets smaller. We can define a critical phase angle α at which the two images can just be distinguished. This so-called *Rayleigh criterion* is defined by

$$\alpha = 1.22\frac{\lambda}{b} \tag{9}$$

It defines the ultimate resolution that can be obtained for imaging with light of a given wavelength λ.

We can use the Rayleigh criterion to calculate the resolving power of any optical instrument. If we want to distinguish two objects that are 1 mm apart from a distance of 1 km, α can be calculated as

$$\alpha = \arctan(10^{-3} \text{ m}/10^3 \text{ m}) \approx 10^{-6}$$

For a wavelength of 500 nm (blue-green), b is then calculated as $b = 1.22 \cdot 5 \cdot 10^{-7}/10^{-6} = 61$ cm. This means that we need a telescope with an aperture of at least 61 cm to obtain this kind of resolution.

For the human eye, the relevant size for b is given by the diameter of the pupil, which is around 5 mm. For light with a wavelength of 500 nm (blue-green), a can then be calculated as 1.22×10^{-4} rad. We can therefore resolve two objects at a distance of 10 m if their distance is larger than 1.22 mm.

In order to make use of this resolving power, the light-sensitive cones have to be spaced appropriately densely. For a distance of 2.5 cm between the lense and the retina, this distance d is then given by $d = \alpha \cdot 2.5$ cm $= 3.05$ μm.

Physiologically, the cones are spaced between 1 μm at the center and 3 to 5 μm in the outer regions of the visual field, which demonstrates that the eye is a very well designed optical instrument. As another example, let us take radiowaves with a frequency of 10^7 Hz $= 100$ MHz, corresponding to a wavelength of 3 m

continued

continued

(in vacuo). We want to make images with a very modest resolution given by $\alpha = 10^{-2}$, corresponding to the ability to achieve a spatial resolution of 1 cm for a distance of 1 m or 10 cm for 10 m. The minimum aperture b of an imaging device with these specifications is then calculated as

$$b = 3 \text{ m}/10^{-2} = 300 \text{ m}$$

This is clearly far beyond any feasibility for a clinical instrument, emphasizing the point that imaging at long wavelengths cannot be based on optical principles.

One further consideration should be made regarding interference of two wavefronts: As is seen from Eqs. (1) and (8), the observed intensity also will depend on any phase difference between the two wavefronts at the respective holes. A shift of one of the waves by one-half wavelength will shift the interference pattern by one-half the distance between adjacent maxima. By setting $\delta_0 = 0$ and $\delta = 2\pi$ in Eq. (8), we calculate for two adjacent maxima

$$\delta \sin \theta = \lambda \tag{10}$$

The distance y on the screen is given by

$$y = d \tan \theta$$

where d is the distance to the screen. For small θ, we can set $\tan \theta = \sin \theta$, and we get from Eq. (10),

$$y = \frac{d}{b} \lambda \tag{11}$$

The distance between the maxima of the interference pattern is thus amplified by a factor of d/b compared with the wavelength. Any small shift of one beam with respect to the other will thus translate into a much larger shift on the screen. This is the principle of *interferometry,* which allows one to measure exceedingly small shifts by interference.

One might argue that the location of the two holes in our last example can be derived from the interference pattern visible on the screen. Finally, the Huygens principle is known, and a simple formula can be given that relates the distance of the observed intensity maxima to the distance of the holes. The calculation of the image from the source is called the *forward problem;* calculating the shape of the source from the image is thus the *inverse problem.* Even if the image of the holes does not look at all like its source, this inverse problem appears to be solvable. In fact, such algorithms are extremely useful in astronomy to enhance the resolution of images from stars or star clusters. Unfortunately, the solution of the inverse problem even for this very simple case depends on the knowledge that we are looking at a distribution of discrete point sources. This is, of course, a good assumption for looking at celestial bodies in the sky but not necessarily for medical imaging. If no such assumptions are made, it can be easily demonstrated that one and the same image can be created by vastly different sources, as demonstrated in Fig. 7. Thus a second important axiom of wave-propagation theory can be stated:

The inverse problem has no unambiguous solution by principle.

Since solving the inverse problem is equivalent to deriving the shape of an object from its image, this axiom seems to state that images are ambiguous by nature (and by watching TV or the illustrated press one tends to agree). Of course, this would be a disaster for diagnostic imaging. Luckily, this statement can be modified in practice. As has been shown, the ambiguity occurs from the interference of waves, which is important whenever

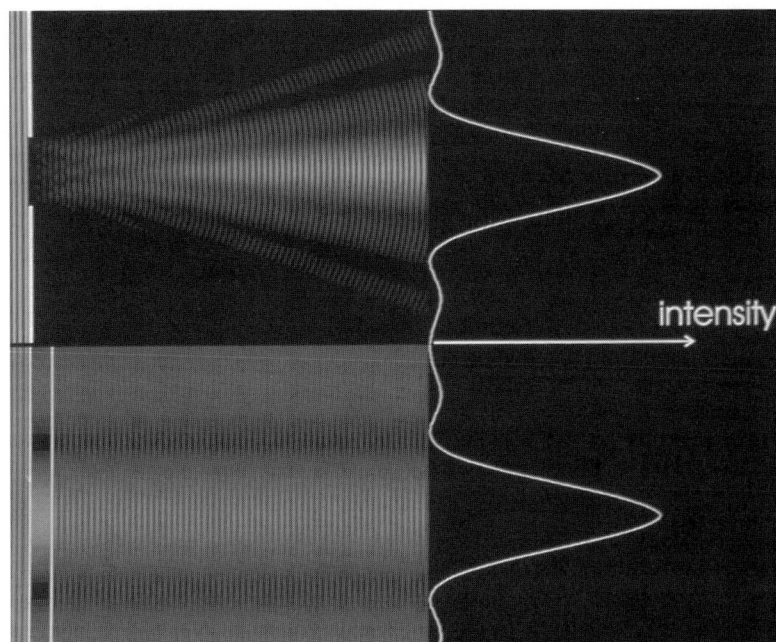

Figure 7. Ambiguity of wave propagation. The image of a hole (*top*) will be identical to the image of a semitransparent screen with appropriately varying translucency (*bottom*).

the wavelength is not negligible compared with the size of the object. For looking at larger objects or, in other words, whenever the "straight line" approach of geometric optics is applicable, the inverse problem is solvable unambiguously, and images become "true" (at least as far as physics is concerned). Of course, even in geometric optics ambiguities can arise if circumstances allow more than one way by which light can reach its destination. Mirrors, fog, and rippled glass are examples from everyday experience that can pose problems in recognition of objects from their images.

A second and very important consequence of interference relates to the intensity of interfering waves. Physics tells us that the intensity of two combined coherent waves is four times that of each single wave, whereas in our practical experience switching on another light only doubles the brightness in the room. The discrepancy is explained by the fact that by superposition of two incoherent waves, on average, only half will be in phase and thus interfere constructively, whereas the other half will be out of phase and thus cancel each other. Bringing two waves to constructive interference thus dramatically increases the observed intensity. The best-known example of this effect is laser light; other and possibly less obvious consequences are, however, crucial to many aspects of functional imaging. Magnetic resonance imaging and Doppler ultrasound are two examples of modalities that make use of coherent waves in order to achieve a sufficient signal-to-noise ratio.

Reflection and Refraction

As yet only waves propagating through a homogeneous medium have been discussed, where the velocity of wave propagation is constant throughout. In the following, waves traveling through various media with different propagation velocities are considered. If the wave-propagation velocity changes, then the wavelength also will change according to

$$\lambda = C\nu$$

where C is the wave velocity and ν is the frequency. For electromagnetic waves in vacuo, C will be the vacuum speed of light, but the equation, of course, applies equally to any kind of waves with any velocity.

The wavelength of electromagnetic radiation in matter is given by

$$I = \frac{I_0}{\epsilon} \tag{12}$$

where ϵ is the dielectric constant of the medium and I_0 is the wavelength in vacuum. For vacuum, ϵ is by definition equal to 1. Typical values for ϵ are

Air	1.00059
Water	79
Cellulose	5–6
Polyacryl	2–3
Glass	4–6

ϵ strongly depends on the wavelength of radiation and also on temperature. The values given refer to the megahertz range and room temperature.

Figure 8 demonstrates what happens when waves travel from one medium into one with lower C. According to the basic rules above, the Huygens principle is applied at the interface between the two media, taking into account that the wavelength in the denser medium will be shorter. It immediately follows that coherence is formed along a wavefront that travels at some angle to the incident beam. The angle is determined by the ratio of the wave velocities C_1 and C_2 in both media: Larger C_2/C_1 will lead to larger deflection. The refraction indices n_1 and n_2 can be defined from the angles of incidence and refraction, and it can be shown that $C_1/C_2 = n_1/n_2$.

The ratio of the intensity of reflected versus refracted waves also depends on the refraction indices and thus on the relationship between C_1 and C_2. It is important to note that this dependency is strongly nonlinear. This means that waves will penetrate much easier into a denser medium through an interface of one or several layers with intermediate n. A practical example for this nonlinear behavior is the use of a transmitter gel in ultrasound imaging. The ultrasound propagation velocity of the gel lies between that in tissue and air. By this two-step approach, fewer of the incident sound waves are reflected at the surface of the body. Another example is semireflective mirrors, where transmission from the nonreflecting side is enabled by adding a layer of material with an intermediate refraction index.

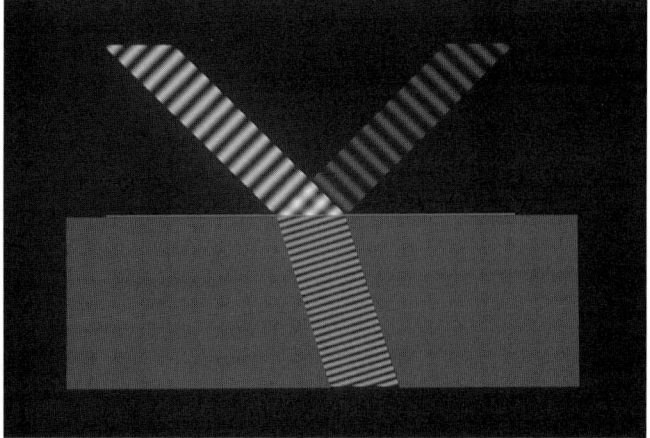

Figure 8. Refraction at a surface. Applying the Huygens principle at the surface between two substances with different refraction indices (and therefore different propagation velocities) leads to a deflection of the wavefront entering the denser medium at the bottom and reflection of parts of the waves. The image shown corresponds to refraction at the interface between air and diamond.

As yet the mechanisms that are responsible for changes in the propagation velocity in different media have not been discussed. Clearly, C must depend on the efficiency by which the wave is passed on through matter. For pressure waves, it is intuitively easy to imagine that this depends on the compressibility of the material as well as on its density; soft and heavy materials will transmit pressure less efficiently than rigid and light ones.

For electromagnetic waves it is less easy to see which kind of interaction will be important, since electromagnetic waves do not need matter as a carrier. In contrast to sound, they are transmitted even in vacuum. In general, matter will serve as some kind of an obstacle and thus slow the propagating waves down.

In classic electrodynamics, the propagation of electromagnetic radiation is described by the Maxwell equations. The differences in propagation velocities are taken into account heuristically by the dielectricity constant ϵ such that the velocity v in matter is given as c (in vacuum) divided by the square root of ϵ.

The application of the Huygens principle described above, which links the refraction index n to the velocity of light, leads to the surprising identity

$$n = \sqrt{\epsilon}$$

The dielectric constant of water, as measured, for example, by the electrical field in a capacitor, is 81. The fact that this value does not at all agree with the optical refraction index, which is 1.33 rather than 9, is only seemingly in contradiction to the Maxwell equations. The observation that white light is separated into a colorful spectrum already demonstrates that the refraction index and thus the dielectric constant strongly depends on the wavelength of the radiation. This is due to the fact that water (like many other media) is not at all homogeneous when looked at on the scale of the wavelength of light. The refraction index of water is thus a quite complex function of the wavelength (Fig. 9). For frequencies below 10^{10} Hz, n really corresponds to about 9, in agreement with the measured dielectric constant. The prediction of the Maxwell equations, which connect the previously unrelated fields of optics and electromagnetism, is thus exactly correct. It is worth noting that the wavelength of electromagnetic radiation in water (and in organic tissue) can be nearly one order of magnitude smaller than one would assume from calculations based on the speed of light in vacuo. This can be quite important, since it has already been shown for simple transmission through a hole that waves start to interfere appreciably when the observed object approaches the wavelength.

Interference is also important for reflection and refraction. One example is a wavelength-selective constructive interference when waves pass through several surfaces such

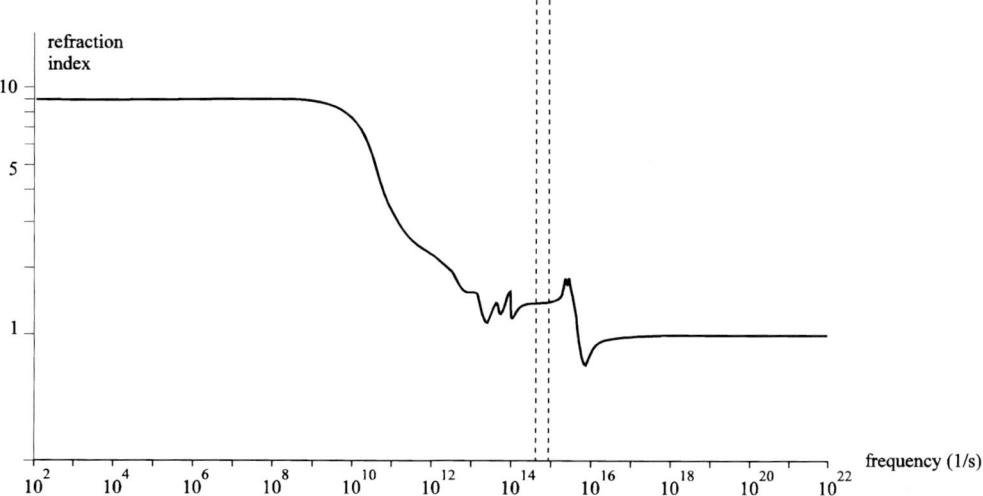

Figure 9. Refraction index of water as a function of frequency. The intensity spread is identical to that for the absorption spectrum shown in Fig. 1.

as the front and back of a flat sheet of translucent material. This leads to the rainbow-colored appearance of a thin soup bubble or a film of oil on a flat surface.

Positive interference also occurs on multiple reflections inside of a body with reflective parallel surfaces. If the dimension of the body is an exact multiple of the wavelength, this leads to constructive interference. This principle is used for lasers, as well as to build resonators for electromagnetic waves in the mega- to gigahertz range. A side effect of this use of interference to amplify waves is, of course, that the spatial distribution of the waves inside the medium will have valleys and troughs and thus be extremely nonhomogeneous.

Scattering, Absorption, and Emission

Scattering, absorption, and emission are very closely related phenomena. Since absorption of radiation and thus energy causes a transition into a nonequilibrium state of higher energy, it will always be followed by some kind of emission process in order to reinstate thermal equilibrium. If the frequencies of the incoming and outgoing wave are identical, the process is called *scattering*. Alternatively, all or part of the incoming radiation can be absorbed and finally converted into thermal energy.

The nature of possible interactions depends on the kind and wavelength of the radiation used and the specific properties of the matter under investigation. Apart from more gradual changes in the frequency dependence, several sharp lines appear in the absorption spectrum of even simple molecules like water (Fig. 10). These indicate specific interactions, where the incoming radiation is in resonance with some intrinsic vibration node of the molecule.

In order to understand the nature of these interactions, a crude understanding of the molecular structure is necessary. Although for quantitative calculations quite intricate quantum mechanical computations are required in order to predict the various interactions, a basic understanding can be afforded using a quite simple model with only a few ingredients.

Molecules are built from nuclei, which carry a positive charge, and negatively charged electrons. Practically all mass is concentrated in the nucleus; the electrons serve as an elastic glue that binds the atom together. The final structure of the molecule will be

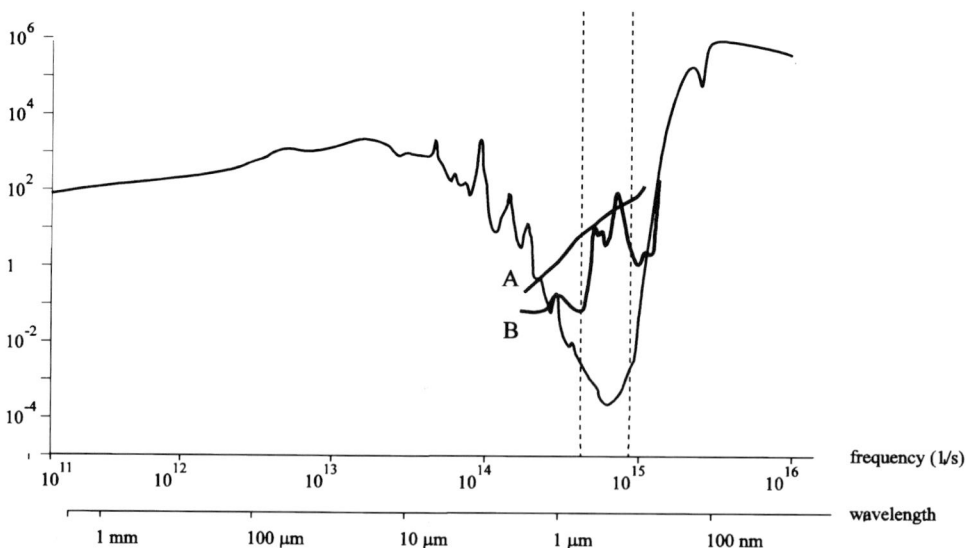

Figure 10. Absorption spectrum of water in the range from microwave frequencies to ultraviolet. The spectrum shows the enlarged central part of the spectrum in Fig. 1. Distinct absorption peaks, especially in the infrared region (5×10^{13} to 5×10^{14}) are clearly visible. In addition to water, the relevant parts of the spectrum covering the visual range for the biologic chromophores melanin (**A**) and hemoglobin (**B**) are also shown.

determined by the interaction of the attractive and repellent forces between the electric charges of these basic particles. Quantum mechanics tells us that the electrons will not orbit the nucleus along any arbitrary trajectory but that they will be organized in well-defined, discrete states. Any transition between these states will correspond to an energy change, which will be accompanied by the absorption or emission of electromagnetic radiation with a frequency that follows the very basic equation

$$E = h\nu$$

Such discrete states exist not only for the orbits of the electrons but also for any degree of freedom of the molecule. The various modes of mechanical vibrations and rotations are quantized as well as the various possible rotation modes of the nucleus and electrons called *spin*. The total number of energy transitions for a given molecule will therefore be quite high, with a few high-energy transitions for lifting an electron into a higher orbit and an increasing number of possible transitions when going to lower and lower energies, finally reaching a quasi-continuum for which some transition can be found for any small increment of the wavelength.

From this simple model, a number of possible basic interactions can be derived. The following list is roughly ordered according to the energies involved:

Elastic scattering: This describes the interaction of radiation as an alternating electromagnetic field with the electrical field formed by the electrons and nucleus. No radiation is absorbed in this process; the direction of the outgoing radiation is, however, changed. Gases normally form an electrical dipole; the incoherent scattering for this case is known as *Rayleigh scattering,* which beautifully explains why the sky is blue and the sunset is red but is of little consequence for medical imaging.

Inelastic scattering: This is distinguished from elastic scattering such that parts of the energy of the incoming radiation will be converted to any of the possible transitions mentioned above. The energy and thus the frequency of the outgoing radiation will be lowered compared with the incident beam. For the special case of motional transitions of molecules, this type of scattering is known as *Raman scattering* after the physicist C. V. Raman, who first described this phenomenon.

Resonance absorption: If the energy of the incoming radiation is exactly equal to one of the possible transitions, resonance absorption will occur. Radiation of the same frequency can be reemitted either by spontaneous or by stimulated emission induced by the following radiation. This process can be repeated several times, until the radiation leaves the substance again.

Fluorescence: Fluorescence occurs when the excited molecule goes to a longer-lived intermediate state prior to radiative return to the ground state. The reemitted radiation will thus be delayed in time and have a lower frequency. The lifetime very strongly depends on the energy of the transition: The higher the energy, the shorter will be the lifetime. As shown by Einstein, the ratio of the spontaneous emission rate to the absorption rate scales with the third power of the transition frequency. For optical light, it is on the order of 10^{-8} s, and a room thus becomes immediately bright when we switch on the light. In contrast, for transitions in the radiofrequency range, the spontaneous response time lies on the order of many years! In working with radiofrequency waves (as in MRI), additional so-called relaxation mechanisms are thus required to reestablish equilibrium.

Photo effect: If the energy of the incoming light is high enough, it can eject an electron out of the molecule. The energy difference between the incoming radiation and the ionizing energy of the electron goes into kinetic energy of the ejected electron.

Compton scattering: If the energy of the incoming radiation is much higher than the ionizing energy, then radiation will be emitted apart from ejection of the electron.

All these processes will lead to modifications of the intensity, direction, and wavelength of the outgoing radiation as a complex function of the incoming waves. Since the interactions happen on a molecular scale, these processes happen even in macroscopically homogeneous materials.

Looking at these basic interactions, it becomes apparent that the border between scattering, absorption, and emission is not very well defined and somewhat depends on which model is used in order to understand some experimental observation.

Elastic scattering can be well described using the Maxwell equations for the interaction of electromagnetic waves with molecular electric dipoles without involving absorption and emission. It can thus be regarded as a scattering-only process, although a quantum mechanical model involving absorption and reemission of photons with identical energy gives an equally valid description. In all other preceding processes the total energy of the outgoing radiation is lower than that of the incident wave. Therefore, some kind of absorption process has to be taken into account. Since the relevant interactions are very specific to each wavelength, they will therefore be discussed in the respective chapters on the various modalities that make use of some of these processes.

Wave-propagation theory becomes important whenever the scattering medium starts to become inhomogeneous on a scale that is on the order of the wavelength. It has already been demonstrated that the signal intensity arising from coherent interference of waves coming from two closely spaced holes is double that of incoherent superposition of two light sources. Similarly, interference will significantly influence scattering processes if the scattering centers start to lump together. A look at the sky serves as an impressive demonstration for this effect: As long as all components of the atmosphere are homogeneously distributed, light from the sun will be scattered elastically. The air is translucent, and the sky is blue due to the strong $1/\lambda^4$ dependence of the scattering intensity. When water molecules start to condense, their separation gets smaller than the wavelength of light, and coherent interference, as discussed earlier, starts to occur. As a first consequence, the scattering efficiency will grow tremendously, since it now scales with the square of the number of scattering centers within the range of one wavelength as compared with a linear increase for the former homogeneous distribution. The average scattering length will thus be reduced from several tens of kilometers to a few meters or even centimeters: Opaque clouds begin to form.

The number of scattering centers within a given wavelength is, of course, much larger for longer wavelengths. This counters the $1/\lambda^4$ dependence of the scattering intensity at each scattering center: Clouds are white rather than blue.

Another demonstration of the drastic influence of interference on the scattering intensity is the fact that both oil and water are clear liquids, whereas milk as a spatially nonhomogeneous mixture of both is opaque. Adding detergent to milk removes this inhomogeneity and reestablishes the translucency of the mixture, although the scattering at each molecule remains the same.

Organic tissues display structure, and thus inhomogeneities occur at practically all scales: No matter which wavelength is used, there will always be some structure in the body on a similar scale, and scattering will occur. Therefore, scattering processes have to be reckoned with to some degree at practically all wavelengths ranging from radio-frequency waves in the meter range down to x-rays with wavelengths on the atomic scale. All the imaging techniques described in this book are therefore, in principle, more complicated than taking a photograph on a clear day.

Conclusions

It has been demonstrated that imaging becomes simple whenever the wavelength is negligibly small compared with the dimension of the structures under observation. For longer wavelengths, interference effects will arise that lead to increasingly severe disparities between the objects and their images and eventually set a limit to the achievable resolution.

For imaging of the human body, the relevant range of wavelengths where such phenomena can occur lies on the order of 1 mm to 1 m, corresponding to a frequency of 3×10^7 to 10^{11} Hz. (Note that the range of frequencies does not coincide with the range of wavelengths due to the change in the refraction index of water over that range according to Fig. 9.) It will thus be mainly imaging techniques using radiowaves (Chap.

8) as well as ultrasound (Chap. 11) where these considerations become important. With typical propagation velocities for pressure waves in tissue, which are on the order of 1500 m/s, a useful frequency range in the range above 1 MHz corresponding to a wavelength of 1.5 mm appears to be indicated for ultrasound in order to minimize interference effects at least within larger structures.

Even if shorter wavelengths are being used, interference due to coherent scattering at inhomogeneous tissue structures will lead to scattering. The macroscopic imaging properties can, however, be described by geometric optics, where the imaging properties can be defined by the propagation of linear rays of radiation. Scattering is then taken into account as a stochastic change in the direction of the rays.

At the other end of the scale, at the low-frequency range relevant for EEG and MEG, such a geometric model becomes totally meaningless. When the physical dimensions of the experiment become much smaller compared with the wavelength, the Huygens principle will tell us that waves will be isotropically radiated in all directions, and the concept of spatially varying fields appears to be much more adequate for our understanding.

It is nevertheless useful to note that both extremes, linear propagation of a sharp ray as well as space isotropically filled with a slowly varying electromagnetic field, are manifestations of one and the same basic process, which can be visualized by using the Huygens principle and—for the case of electromagnetic radiation—be exactly described by the Maxwell equations.

HOW AN IMAGE IS FORMED

Forming an image requires some kind of interaction between the carrier waves and the object under study. Any of the mechanisms discussed earlier by which waves interact with the medium in which they travel can be used as a basis of image formation. Emission of waves is at the basis of imaging methods in nuclear medicine, tissue-dependent absorption is the key process for x-ray techniques, and refraction and reflection is used for ultrasound. Scattering is the "bad guy" in this list, since it makes it awfully difficult to trace the received waves back to their origin. It is nevertheless an essential factor to be taken into account in most imaging techniques.

The "oddball" among the imaging techniques is MRI. It uses radiofrequency (rf) waves with wavelengths on the order of several meters, which precludes the formation of images with a resolution necessary for medical imaging. MRI thus requires a totally different approach to image formation, which will be discussed in Chap. 8. The general rules of wave propagation nevertheless apply to the rf waves used in MRI and can strongly influence the outcome of a measurement, especially in frequency ranges achieved on a field systems, where the wavelengths are on the order of the dimensions of the observed structures.

Apart from the method of interaction of waves with matter, imaging techniques also can be categorized according to the various ways by which the signals are detected and finally be brought into an image format. The easiest way to form an image is to cast a shadow (Fig. 11A). This was the principle used by C. W. Roentgen for his first x-ray image and still forms the backbone of diagnostic imaging. Hundreds of millions of such conventional projection x-ray images are produced every year using this simple approach.

The next step to sophistication is optical imaging, by which light coming from the source of radiation is focused onto the image plane and thus forms one pixel of the final image (Fig. 11B). Compared with projection imaging, optical imaging offers a significantly improved signal-to-noise ratio, since each pixel collects many rays, which go out from their source in different directions.

Unfortunately, the range of wavelengths for which such an optical approach can be used is quite narrow: For wavelengths considerably longer than the visible band, the propagation of waves in matter becomes too complex for simple focusing by a lens. It is also clear that at longer wavelengths very soon the resolution attainable by optical principles becomes insufficient. At much shorter wavelengths, radiation can be regarded more and more as linear rays, which is the ideal condition for optical imaging. The index

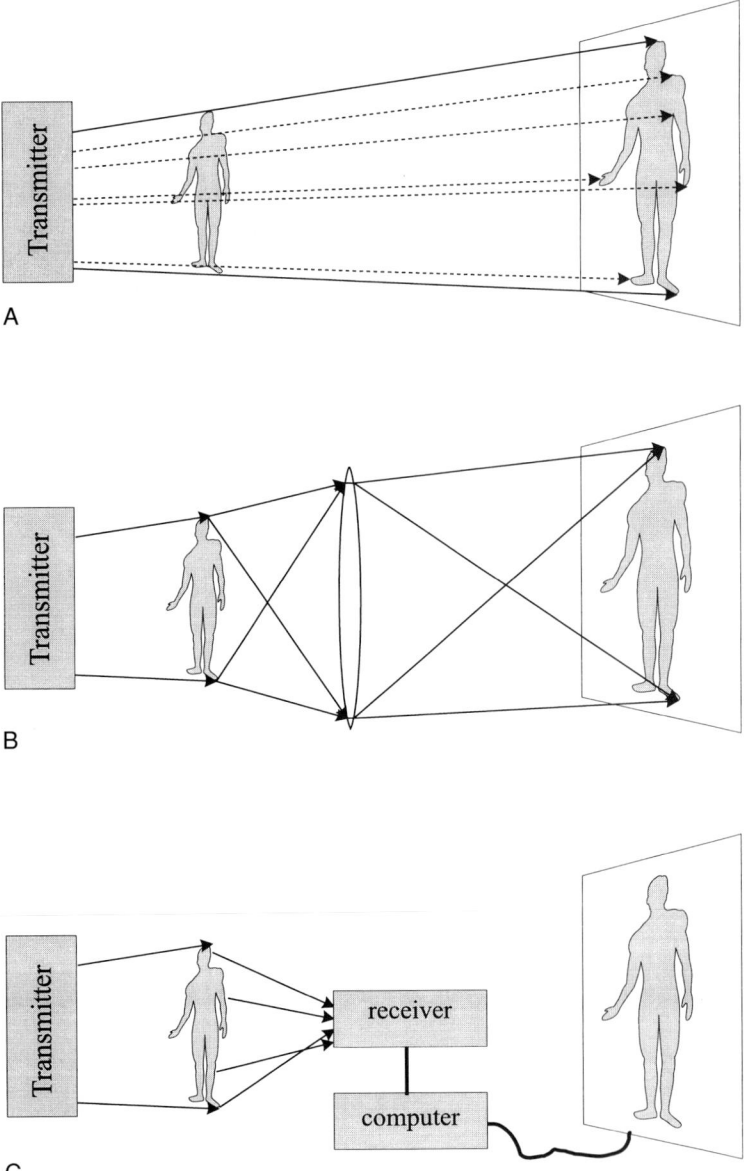

Figure 11. Principles of image formation. Projection imaging (**A**) has already been mentioned (see Fig. 2). Optical imaging (**B**) relies on the refocusing of light wavefronts originating at the surface of the object onto a screen by an appropriate refocusing device such as an optical lens. Indirect imaging techniques (**C**) produce images from the received signals by appropriate postprocessing techniques using a computer.

of refraction between different materials becomes, however, more and more similar. Therefore, at wavelengths beyond the ultraviolet range, there are simply no materials available that can be used to build a lens for, let's say, x-rays. The range of wavelengths for the use of optical imaging principles is thus restricted to the close surroundings of the visible band.

The final step of abstraction is to use indirect imaging techniques, in which the incoming waves are not immediately arranged in order to form an image but simply recorded by some appropriate detector (Fig. 11C). The image is then formed using some appropriate postprocessing method. An important prerequisite for this indirect approach to image formation is the availability of detectors that transform the incoming waves into a digital signal, which is a string of numbers, that can then be transferred to a computer for image reconstruction. The fast proliferation of techniques for medical imaging is thus closely linked to the development of appropriate detectors and of powerful computers that can be used to perform the complex algorithms for image reconstruction in reasonable execution times.

Image Quality

For any imaging method, the image quality will depend on the performance of each component of the imaging process. Imperfections can occur as a result of technical problems in the transmitter or receiver system or be more fundamental in nature such as scattering or interference. For digital imaging methods, the translation of the signal into numbers (digitization) and the reconstruction algorithms used also will have some intrinsic influence on the image properties.

The basic criteria to assess the image quality are

Geometric distortions
Resolution
Signal-to-noise ratio

A true and undistorted image is one in which an object always appears the same, no matter at which position of the image field it occurs. Overall geometric distortions are in general not seen as a severe problem in medical imaging so long as they stay within reasonable limits. Exceptions, of course, occur in applications where some exact geometric measures are meant to be taken, as in planning of radiotherapeutical treatment.

Resolution

The image resolution defines the size of the smallest structure that can be distinguished. The intrinsic resolution determined by the properties of wave propagation has been discussed in the preceding section. The receiver system should be designed such that it transfers this intrinsic resolution to the final image. In terms of resolution, it is thus quite meaningless to use receivers with a nominal resolution that is higher than that of the measurement process itself. Such a resolution overkill, nevertheless, can be useful to overcome other experimental imperfections and is thus frequently being used (EEG, MEG) (Fig. 12).

In analogue imaging techniques, the image resolution is normally defined using the *modulation transfer function* (MTF). The MTF measures the ratio of the inherent contrast of a sinusoidal grid to the contrast of the image as a function of the spatial variation of the grid. If the variation of the grid approaches the resolution limit of the imaging system, its image will become more and more blurred, and the MTF will thus approach zero.

In digital imaging techniques, each image point is represented as a discrete pixel. A more common parameter to define the image resolution in this case is the *point-spread function* (PSF). The PSF shows how the image of a pointlike object looks. The equivalence of the PSF and the MTF can be derived from the insight that a point can be defined as a superposition of an infinite number of sinusoidal waves with frequencies ranging from zero to infinity. The MTF can then be calculated as the amplitude of the frequency spectrum of the PSF. Vice versa, the PSF can be derived by superposition of sinusoids with intensities given by the MTF. The algorithm used for going from the image domain, in which the PSF is expressed, to the domain of spatial frequencies, where the MTF resides, is called *Fourier transformation.* One of its many miraculous properties is the fact that the algorithm used for frequency analysis is identical to that of frequency synthesis except for some scaling factor. Fourier transformation is discussed extensively in Chap. 8 on MRI, where it is of fundamental importance.

The resolution in digital imaging is, of course, determined by the pixel size of the digital image. This is obvious for direct digital imaging techniques, where the analogue screen (photographic plate) is replaced by a two-dimensional array of detectors. It is also true for indirect imaging methods, where the final image is derived by some more or

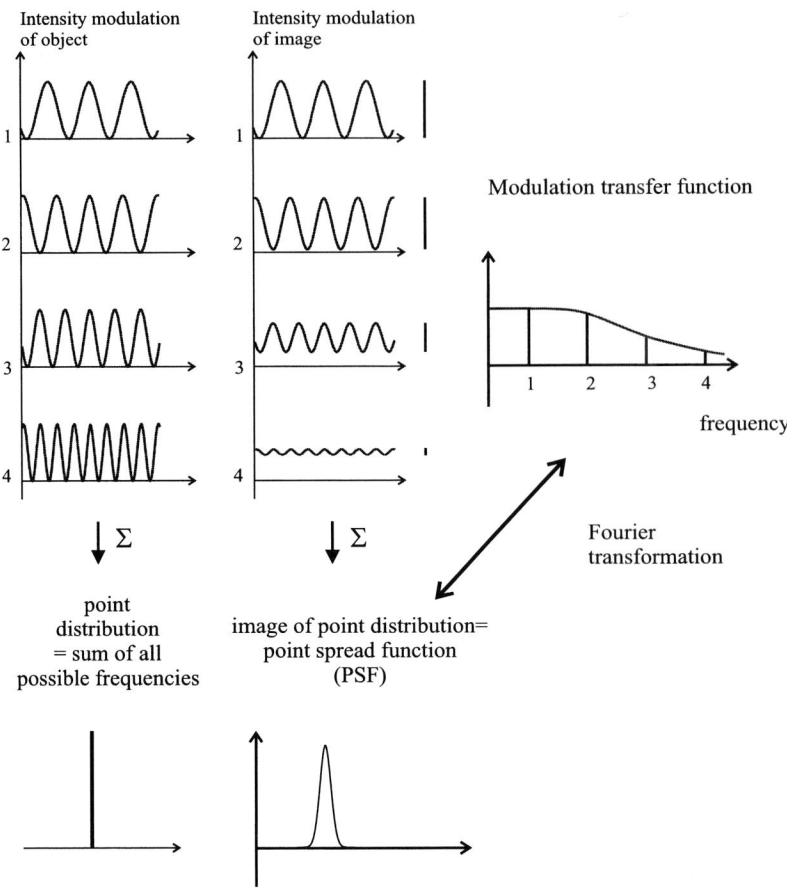

Figure 12. Equivalence of the modulation transfer function (MTF) and the point-spread function (PSF). The MTF measures the intensity variation of the image of a grid with periodic intensity modulation as a function of the modulation frequency. The observed modulation amplitude will start to drop when the distance between two maxima approaches the minimal resolution of the imaging device. The PSF represents the image of a pointlike image. The equivalence of the MTF and the PSF follows from the insight that a discrete point distribution can be expressed mathematically as a sum of sinusoids over an infinite frequency range. The MTF then must be equal to the frequency spectrum of the PSF. The algorithm used for frequency analysis is called *Fourier transformation.* Note that in practice a rectangular grid of black and white stripes is used to measure the MTF.

less complex reconstruction algorithm from a series of measurement data. Mathematically, the number of uniquely defined image points cannot be greater than the number of measurement points irrespective of the actual algorithm that is used for reconstruction. Thus a simple rule can be stated:

For any digital imaging process, the maximum attainable resolution is defined by the field of view and the number of acquired data points if the resolution is isotropic over the field of view.

Although this rule seems to set a very strict limitation to any digital imaging process, it needs to be read carefully in order to avoid misunderstanding. The key word is *isotropic.* Basically, image resolution needs only to be isotropic if nothing is known beforehand about those locations in the image where high resolution is needed. If—in the other extreme—the basic structure of the image is known before the measurement, one could at least theoretically design an image-reconstruction algorithm that has high resolution only at the locations corresponding to sharp edges and lower resolution where the intensity profile is flat. One can thus get away with a vastly lower number of measurement points in order to reconstruct the same high-resolution image. It is therefore preferable to use a more general rule:

For any digital imaging process, the number of acquired data points defines the number of image elements that can be measured independently.

In this definition, the term *resolution* has vanished. A simple example that demonstrates the power of this generalized rule is an image that is made up of simple image elements such as a superposition of squares with variable size. Such an image can be defined using very few data points (the size and location for each square), whereas its definition in terms of an isotropic resolution requires on the order of 100,000 pixel elements. A "Mondrian imager," which is sensitive to the detection of the size and location of squares, would thus allow reconstruction of a true image from a few measurement points, whereas its detection by a conventional system would take considerably more effort.

In practice, such approaches to breaking down images into a reduced set of elements are very important for data compression in order to save storage space and to speed up transmission of digital images. The power of this approach for making image acquisition more efficient has only just begun to be exploited for a number of modalities. The problem is first to find an appropriate set of classifying image elements. Medical images are no Mondriaans, and much more sophisticated approaches have to be used to break down an image into a smaller set of elements that are still sufficiently descriptive. The second and even more challenging task is then to transform the thus defined reconstruction algorithm into a physical measurement process. First approaches based on wavelet transforms or singular value decomposition have been published for several of the imaging modalities discussed in this book. Such more intelligent sampling strategies are expected to lead to considerable improvements in digital imaging compared with the dumb (but robust) pixel-by-pixel sampling common in current imagers. Especially in those functional applications where changes are to be observed inside certain parts of the body, adaptive approaches are expected to lead to tremendous improvements in the acquisition efficiency, where a pixel-by-pixel high-resolution image is acquired only once or at an appropriate time interval; the functional information about the change that is occurring is then, however, determined using much more efficient algorithms. One such approach, which has already been gained widespread acceptance, is the keyhole imaging technique in MRI.

Signal-to-Noise Ratio

The signal-to-noise (S/N) ratio of an image is determined by two components: The ratio of the intensity of the effective signal to that of radiation at the same wavelength that is present during the measurement gives the extrinsic signal-to-noise ratio. The efficiency of the receiver for detecting the radiation and the noise produced by the imaging process determines the intrinsic signal-to-noise ratio of the measuring system. Of course, all imaging systems are designed such that the observed signal-to-noise ratio should be determined by the intrinsic S/N ratio. Extrinsic noise sources are excluded (or at least minimized) by appropriate shielding measures.

In principle, all components in the measurement chain transmitter–object (patient)–receiver–image processor are liable to give rise to intrinsic noise (Fig. 13). It is worthwhile to keep in mind that the image noise will be dominated by the worst link along the chain. It is thus rather useless to improve the receiver system if the signal-to-noise ratio is dominated by patient noise or by transmitter fluctuations. It is also worth noting that the highest signal attained by the most sensitive receiver does not necessarily optimize the signal-to-noise ratio. Using receiver designs that can discriminate the proper signal from ambient noise is often better than using those which are very sensitive but "dumb." In analogue receiver designs, a distinction between signal and ambient noise

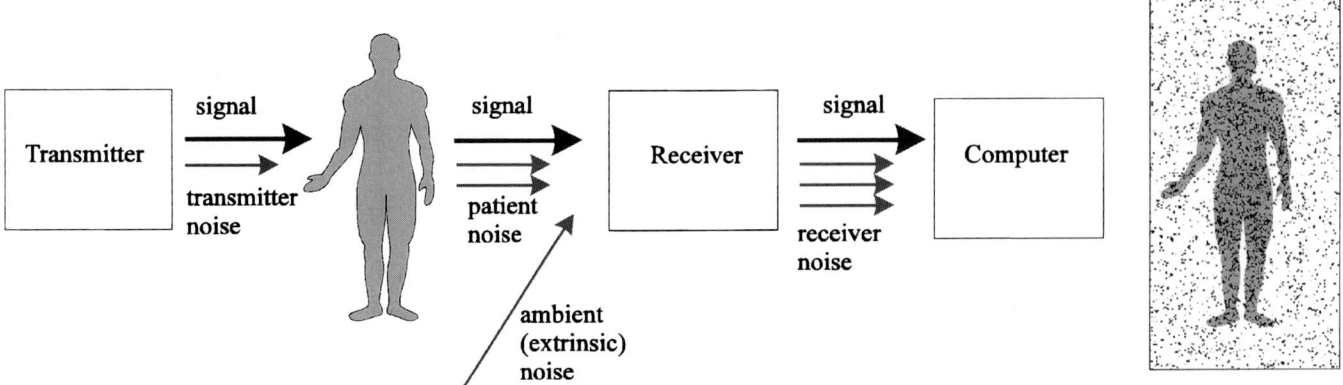

Figure 13. Potential noise sources. The observed image noise will be a sum of the contributions from transmitter noise, noise coming from the patient, ambient noise, and receiver noise. The main source of noise will vary considerably among different imaging modalities.

can be made using appropriate geometric designs. One of the major advantages of digital techniques is the possibility for using advanced noise-reduction techniques, especially when the transmitter signal can be locked to the receiver as in phase-sensitive detection.

Principles of Digital Image Formation

Replacing a plain-film or another such analogue device by a two-dimensional array of digital detectors leads to a very simple image-reconstruction algorithm by which the pixel intensities are given as some appropriate representation of the recorded data. Nevertheless, this conceptionally straightforward approach already yields some substantial improvements. Most important is the possibility to adjust the attribution of intensity values to each data point such that the apparent image contrast can be maximized either manually or automatically. In addition to this look-up table adjustment, filtering algorithms can be used to increase the image quality. Common filters are low-pass filters, which increase the S/N ratio at the cost of somewhat lower resolution, and edge-enhancement or high-pass filters, which lead to better edge detection.

A problem for such direct digital imaging techniques is the high spatial resolution of the previous analogue devices, which requires a huge amount of detectors if it is to be achieved by direct pixel-by-pixel digitization. Consequently, hybrid approaches are often used, by which the image is first registered on an analogue device such as electrostatic foil and then digitized line by line by scanning with an appropriate one-dimensional detector.

Indirect Methods of Digital Imaging: Backprojection

Direct or hybrid digital imaging techniques constitute an improvement over purely analogue systems if the technical problems are solved. The kinds of images that can be formed, however, are restricted by the possibilities of the particular radiation used to directly produce a two-dimensional image. Cross-sectional images require indirect approaches, since the image plane is virtual and thus cannot interact with the measurement waves to directly form an image.

It is clear that the reconstruction of an image from the measured signal intensities in a receiver is equivalent to solving the inverse problem for the particular application. The approaches and algorithms used for this task depend on the particular wavelength and the receiver system. This is most often highly idiosyncratic for each imaging modality and will therefore be discussed in the respective chapters. There is, however, one digital reconstruction algorithm that is common to a wide variety of imaging techniques and

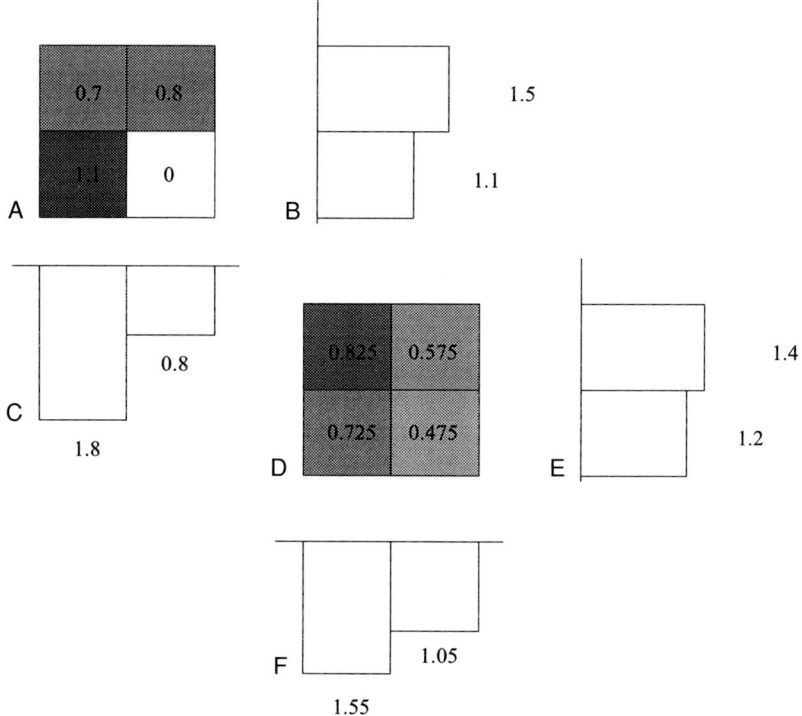

Figure 14. Demonstration of the inconsistency resulting from straightforward application of the backprojection algorithm. The original 4-pixel object (**A**) yields the projection intensities shown in (**B**) and (**C**). Backprojection leads to an image (**D**) that is different from the original object. In addition, the projection intensities of images (**E**) and (**F**) are different from those of the original object. Repetitive application of projection and backprojection will lead to an image with a homogeneous intensity distribution.

which will therefore be discussed in this introductory chapter. This is the *backprojection algorithm,* the mathematics of which were published in 1917 by Radon and whose first widespread application in medical imaging was in x-ray computed tomography. The basic idea of backprojection is to reconstruct an image from one-dimensional projections taken at various angles (Fig. 14).

Let us start with a very simple case that serves to illustrate this approach and also demonstrates some of its inherent problems. The object consists of four squares with different inherent intensities. Two projections are measured at right angles to each other. This yields four data points for four pixel intensities. Apparently, this constitutes a well-defined problem, and only the right algorithm needs to be found in order to reconstruct the image from the data. This is, however, fallacious. The sum of the intensities over each projection must, of course, be equal and identical to the total integral over the four pixels. The problem is consequently underdefined. This can be easily verified by finding other pixel intensities that yield the same projections. This lack of linear independence of the measurement points can be easily generalized to larger matrices, where linear-dependent terms exist not only for the total integral but also for any arbitrary subset.

The first insight about backprojection can be thus stated as follows:

The number of linearly independent image elements will always be lower than the number of measurement points.

Rather than trying to reconstruct the maximum number of independent measures by consecutive removal of redundant data points, common backprojection algorithms try to find the distribution of pixel intensities that represents the true image with the highest likelihood. The easiest approach, which has given this problem its name, can be derived as follows: If it is not known from which point along the projection direction the measured intensity arises, it appears to be reasonable to distribute the signal evenly on all pixels along the projection path. The pixel intensities will then be given by the sum of the contribution of each projection ray. Performing this algorithm on the simple example demonstrates two problems: First, signal intensity will be projected into pixels, which are known not to contain any signal. Second, backprojection will be inconsistent in the sense that the projection intensities from the backprojected image are different from the originally measured projection intensities. Repetitive projection and backprojection will in fact very rapidly lead to an image with equal distribution of all signal intensities across all pixels. This demonstrates that the backprojection algorithm tends to smear out the intensities across the image.

For a 2 × 2 matrix, the number of independent solutions is infinite. The signal intensity in any pixel can indeed be set to zero, and there will still be a solution that yields the intensities of the measured projections. For larger matrices and more projections, the situation does improve, however. It can be shown that the region of uncertainty limits itself to the starlike region of intersection of the projection rays. The blurring effect can then be corrected for if the image is filtered by an edge-enhancement filter such that the (mathematically predictable smearing) is just canceled. Filtered backprojection will thus deliver a reasonably well-defined image if projections are being acquired at a sufficient number of projection angles. Depending on the basic quality of the acquisition data, different filters can be used to trade off some image resolution in order to gain signal-to-noise ratio. Even some basic properties describing the physics of the measurement can be incorporated into an appropriate filter. The decay of the signal intensity with the distance from the source due to absorption, which affects the measured intensities in imaging techniques in nuclear medicine, can be taken into account by applying a ramp filter to the projection rays. Similarly, the signal attenuation by absorption of x-rays can be accounted for by an appropriate filter.

These linear filters affect the signal intensities in all pixels in the same way. They are therefore adequate when the interaction of the measurement radiation with matter is more or less homogeneous all over the image. They are, however, not very well suited to take care of any local interactions such as scattering at bone structures in x-ray tomography or reabsorption of emitted photons in nuclear medicine.

Iterative algorithms that take such local interactions into account have to be used in order to improve the reconstruction. They use a model of the image that describes the particular absorption, scattering, emission, etc. characteristic of each pixel. A backprojection data set is then calculated from this model and compared with the measured data. From the difference between calculated and measured data, an improved model is derived, and the procedure is repeated until the projections from the model agree with the experimental data. This type of approach lends itself to very accurate solutions and can incorporate any arbitrary and nonlinear behavior of the imaging process. Compared with filtered backprojection, which can be performed very fast on appropriate processors, this algebraic approach is, however, very computer-intensive and currently too time-consuming for clinical routine. With the advance of faster computer systems, these techniques will, however, become more and more available and eventually will replace filtered backprojection.

Further discussions of various refinements of projection reconstruction algorithms will be given in Chap. 6.

REFERENCES

1. Jackson JD. *Classical electrodynamics.* New York: John Wiley and Sons (1975).
2. Krestel E. *Imaging systems for medical diagnostics.* Berlin: Siemens (1990).
3. Tipler PA. *Physics for scientists and engineers.* New York: Worth Publishers (1991).
4. Webb S. *The physics of medical imaging.* Adam Hilger England: Bristol (1988).

Functional Imaging, edited by
Gustav von Schulthess and Jürgen Hennig.
Lippincott–Raven Publishers, Philadelphia, © 1998.

2

Contrast Agents and Radiopharmaceuticals

Johannes M. Fröhlich, August P. Schubiger, and Gustav K. von Schulthess

INTRODUCTION AND OVERVIEW

Functional imaging defines regional function and thereby physiology in relation to anatomy. While some physiologic processes, such as the pulsatile motions induced by the heart, can be seen using fluoroscopy, magnetic resonance imaging (MRI), or ultrasound directly and without external interventions, many processes require the introduction of marker molecules to make various physiologic processes visible. By far the most frequent application route of such markers is the intravenous route. In nuclear medicine (NM), imaging is not possible without the introduction of radiopharmaceuticals emitting the radiation necessary for adequate visualization. This has the great advantage that the signal-to-noise (S/N) ratio is exceedingly high in such studies, even if minute amounts of substances are used. It is only determined by how specifically a compound is accumulated in the region of interest over the surroundings. In all other imaging modalities, substantial contrast is already present without the introduction of extrinsic markers; hence enhancement of contrast has to be marked enough to be noticeable in the presence of existing signal.

There is a wide spectrum of agents used to enhance various processes during imaging. Initially, the intention was obviously to enhance contrast to improve morphologic delineation of an organ or a structure. This approach was introduced into x-ray diagnosis early in the twentieth century and has been further developed constantly since then. Typically, radiopaque contrast agents have been used to improve morphologic diagnosis in bowel

JM Frölich: Scientific Affairs Manager, Guerbet AG, Zurich, Switzerland.
AP Schubiger: Institute of Radiopharmacy, Paul Scherrer Institute, Villigen-PSI, Switzerland.
GK von Schulthess: Department of Medical Radiology, University Hospital, Zurich, Switzerland.

Table 1. *Concentration range and suitability of methods and contrast-enhancing compounds for various function studies**

	Conc. range	NM	X-ray	MRI	US
Flow[†]	≤mmol	+	+	+ +	+ +
Perfusion	≤mmol	+ +	+	+ (+)	+
Elimination	≤mmol	+ +	+	+	−
Metabolism	≤μmol	+ +	−	+	−
Messenger system					
High conc., low affinity	≤μmol	+ +	−	+ (+)	−
Low conc., high affinity	≤nmol	+ +	−	−	−

* Quantitative information, + +; qualitative information only, +.
[†] Contrast-enhancing agents not mandatory in MRI and US.

disease, vascular disease, cerebral disease, and urinary tract disease. However, already the application of such agents often yields minimal functional information. Except for bowel contrast agents, the other agents mentioned have to get to the organs of interest, and in the cases cited, this requires vascular blood flow, cerebrospinal fluid (CSF) circulation, and renal function, respectively. Thus it is difficult to classify contrast media as strictly serving morphologic versus partly functional examination purposes. Nevertheless, as a general rule, marker molecules used in high concentration are mainly used to enhance morphology and support morphology-related diagnoses, whereas markers that can be used in lower concentrations will tend to be more useful in imaging function. One convenient way to classify agents is according to the concentration at which they are needed to produce an easy-to-visualize effect on a medical image (Table 1). While in x-ray diagnosis the concentration of radiopaque agents has to be in the molar range to produce adequate contrast, and the same is true for echopharmaceuticals, magneto-pharmaceuticals are effective in 10 to 100 mM concentrations and NM radiopharmaceuticals can depict substances down to concentrations in the pico- and nanomolar ranges. From the preceding statement it is clear that NM procedures are very suitable for functional imaging, whereas x-ray imaging has severe limitations in this domain. In fact, in almost all situations, a radiopharmaceutical will be used at concentrations where it has neither pharmacologic nor physiologic effects, as is to be expected in the pico- to nanomolar concentration ranges. On the other hand, injection of an intravenous contrast agent in x-ray diagnosis has substantial pharmacologic effects.

A good overview of the potentials of contrast media and their respective imaging methods to depict function is gained when classifying physiologic processes and asking oneself which ones can be imaged using a given combination of imaging method and contrast-enhancing marker. A convenient classification is given in Table 1, where we have divided physiologic processes into five categories. The dominant process pervading many aspects of physiology is perfusion, which can be subdivided into *blood flow* and tissue perfusion proper and related to the circulation, *blood volume;* it is at the basis of most substance transport of the organs of interest. A second physiologic process is *elimination* of substances, be it by the renal or hepatic route. Substances reaching an organ—if not passing by it—will be taken up by the cells, and *metabolism* occurs. Alternatively, the substance of interest is a *molecular messenger* and is somehow associated with a ligand-receptor type of interaction. Classifying contrast-enhancing markers according to the classes underlined above gives a good overview of their ability to yield information on a physiologic process. As expected from Table 1, the list of substances available to evaluate function with NM is long, while it is short for x-ray contrast agents (Table 2).

In this chapter some basic aspects and properties of radiopharmaceuticals and contrast agents will be discussed. However, it has to be kept in mind that there are physiologic processes and ''imaging'' mechanisms that do not require extrinsic contrast agents. One large group of methods is based on electrophysiology, as discussed in Chap. 10. Furthermore, contrast mechanisms exist in various imaging methods that permit functional evaluation. Obviously, motion of all sorts can be identified if the image-acquisition rate is substantially faster than the time constants involved in that motion. While infrared

Table 2. *Compounds used for obtaining functional information**

		NM	X-ray	MRI	US
Perfusion	Brain		(ivCA)	Gd-chelates	Microbubbles
	Tc-HMPAO			Gd-macromol.	or
	Tc-ECD			USPIO	particles
	Xenon				
	Water (PET)				
	Lung		(ivCA)	Gd-chelates	—
	Microspheres				
	Heart		(ivCA)	Gd-/Dy-chelates	Microbubbles
	Tc-MIBI etc.			Mn-DPDP?	
	Tl				
	NH3/Rb (PET)				
	Kidney		(ivCA)	Gd-chelates	—
	Tc-chelates				
	Hippuran anal.				
	Tc-DMSA				
Blood volume	Brain		(ivCA)	Gd-/Dy-chelates	
	Co, Tc-Ery				
Elimination	Kidney		(ivCA)	Gd-chelates	—
	Tc-chelates				
	Hippuran anal.				
	Tc-DMSA				
	Liver			Gd-EOB-DTPA	
	Tc-HIDA			(cholegraphic CA)	
				Mn-DPDP	
				SPIO (endocytosis)	
Metabolism	Brain			C-13 labeled	
	Glucose			compounds	
	Oxygen				
	Heart				
	Glucose (PET)				
	Fatty acids				
	Acetate (PET)				
	Tumors			Metalloporphyrins	
	Glucose (PET)				
	Amino acids				
Messenger system	Markers of receptor systems oligopeptides for most important systems			Glycoprot. markers (liver)	

* In parens: minimal information only, or only PET marker available.

imaging is highly temperature sensitive, the most notable intrinsic contrast mechanisms that yield functional information are found in MRI. Specifically, MRI is very flow, motion, and temperature sensitive (which for the former two is also the case for ultrasound). Hemoglobin itself acts as an intrinsic contrast agent because deoxygenated hemoglobin is strongly paramagnetic, and much of functional brain imaging is based on this so-called BOLD (blood oxygen level–dependent) contrast-enhancing effect. Furthermore, there are various ways for in vivo and in vitro spin labeling in MRI as well as magnetic resonance spectroscopy (MRS), and finally, MRS is able to measure metabolite concentrations of various compounds present in the low millimolar range. Hence not all functional imaging procedures are in need of the extrinsic application of physiologic "spy" molecules. However, since the effects observed are very modality specific, they are discussed in the chapters dealing with specific modalities.

FUNDAMENTALS OF RADIOPHARMACEUTICALS

Radiopharmaceuticals are chemical substances containing radioactive nuclides. Unlike sealed radioactive sources, they can undergo distribution and metabolic processing prior to excretion from the body. Some characteristics are unique to radiopharmaceuticals. As trace amounts of radiopharmaceuticals are administered, they do not elicit a physiologic response and are therefore considered to be subpharmacologic (see Table 1). Although their chemical toxicity is nil, a minimal radiation risk is associated with their use.

Radiopharmaceuticals may be used for diagnostic but also therapeutic applications (22), although in this series only diagnostic uses are considered. Diagnostic radiopharmaceuticals ideally trace or mimic certain physiologic processes without altering the process in any way so that a true measure of function can be obtained. One important aspect of such studies, therefore, is that the integrity and biologic behavior of the chosen substance are not altered by the radionuclide used or by the radiolabeling procedure.

Radionuclides

Due to their absorption characteristics, electromagnetic radiations (gamma and x-rays) are most suitable forms for external detection. Particulate radiation, being efficiently absorbed by tissue, leads to a high radiation burden, and external quantification is problematic. One exception is the β^+ (positron radiation), which annihilates immediately with an electron to yield two 511-keV gamma rays that are emitted in opposite directions. Coincidence counting then allows direct quantification to be performed (see Chap. 5). The nuclides clinically employed in this way are generally referred to as *positron emission tomographic* (PET) *radionuclides,* whereas the former are called *single photon emission computed tomographic* (SPECT) *radionuclides.* For a more detailed account of the nature and application of gamma and positron radiations, refer to Chap. 6.

A radionuclide useful for diagnostic application is characterized by a number of properties. In terms of its decay mode, electron capture, and isomeric transition from metastable states, gamma- and x-ray emissions are appropriate, with no particulate radiation except in the case of the positron emitters. For the SPECT radionuclides, photon energies are ideally in the range of 100 to 200 keV. Below 100 keV tissue adsorption and scatter become significant, whereas above 200 keV there is low detection efficiency. The two 511-keV gamma rays associated with all positron emitters display very low absorption in tissue and allow easy quantification by virtue of their coincidence. In all cases the effective half-life of the radionuclide should be equal to one to two times the duration of imaging. Chemical reactivity is also a prerequisite, preferably allowing the nuclide to be compounded into several chemical forms. Figure 1 lists a selection of radionuclides used in NM studies.

Nuclide	$T_{1/2 phys.}$		γ-Energie(keV)	
^{99m}Tc	6	h	140	
^{123}I	13	h	159	
^{127}Xe (gas)	36	d	200	SPECT
^{201}Tl	3.1	d	80 + 167	+
^{67}Ga	3.2	d	92 + 185 + 296	γ-camera
^{111}In	2.8	d	173 + 247	
^{15}O	2.1	min	$\beta^+ \rightarrow 511$	
^{13}N	10	min	$\beta^+ \rightarrow 511$	PET
^{11}C	20	min	$\beta^+ \rightarrow 511$	
^{18}F	110	min	$\beta^+ \rightarrow 511$	
^{131}I	8	d	364 + β^-	γ-camera

Figure 1. Radionuclides often used for diagnostic (and functional) nuclear medicine applications.

Radiopharmaceuticals

A rational approach to designing a suitable radiopharmaceutical or radiotracer is to combine knowledge of both physiology and biochemistry of various organ systems and the properties of certain compounds. The desire for tissue-specific localization of radiotracers has placed more emphasis on the development of agents based on the receptor-specific approach. This approach is based on the well-known structure-activity relationship concept, whereby a drug molecule reacts with a specific biologic receptor or enzyme because of their complementary chemical structures. A useful classification of radiopharmaceuticals has been suggested based on their mechanism of localization that categorizes them into two groups: substrate nonspecific and substrate specific (8).

Accordingly, substrate-nonspecific agents do not participate in a specific chemical reaction. Radiopharmaceuticals that localize by diffusion, compartmental confinement, capillary blockage, cell sequestration, and phagocytosis are examples (Table 3). Substrate-specific agents must participate in a definite chemical reaction or take part in a specific ligand-substrate interaction. Examples are radiotracers that localize by entering into biochemical or metabolic processes involving enzyme systems (15, 21), protein receptors (Fig. 2 and Color Plate 1), or antigen-antibody reactions. Some broadly used examples are given in Table 3.

Ideally, for any radiopharmaceutical that should participate as a tracer in physiologic or biochemical processes, the radionuclide should be an isotope of an atom commonly

Table 3. *Some typical radiopharmaceuticals with a description of the alterations introduced by the radionuclide and its use in nuclear medicine*

Radiopharmaceutical	Alteration	Application
L-[Methyl-^{11}C]methionine	None, ^{12}C replaced by ^{11}C	Amino acid transport and incorporation
[2-^{18}F] FDG	^{18}F is "mimicking" an OH group, metabolism stops at ^{18}F-desoxyglucose-6-phosphate	Glucose metabolism
[ω-^{123}I]Iodoheptadecanic acid	^{123}I is "mimicking" a CH_3 group	Fatty acid metabolism in the heart
^{99m}Tc-L,L-ECD	No physiologic analogue, new development of a ^{99m}Tc kit	Brain perfusion

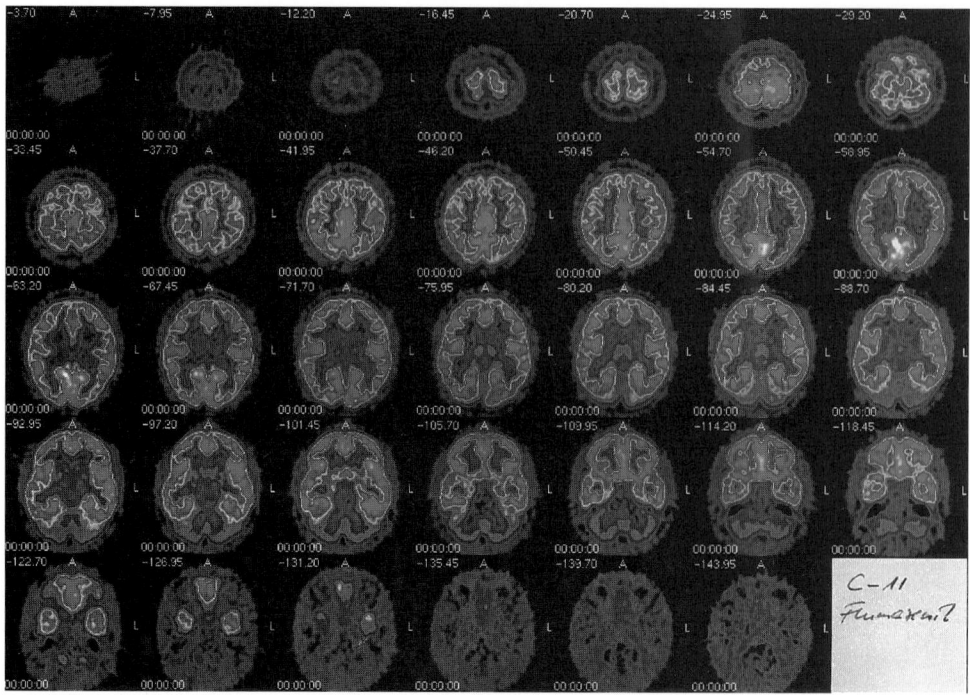

Figure 2. [¹¹C]Flumazenil distribution 30 to 60 minutes following injection. Note that the pattern matches the known distribution of the benzodiazepine receptors, with the highest concentration in the occipital and frontal cortex and lower values in cerebellum, basal ganglia, thalamus, cerebellum, and pons. See also Color Plate 1.

found in the parent biologically active material, such as ^{11}C for ^{12}C, ^{13}N for ^{14}N, or ^{15}O for ^{16}O, since the risk of disturbing normal behavior is correspondingly reduced. In such cases, the behavior of the radiopharmaceutical should be identical to that of the "cold" physiologic molecule (e.g., [^{11}C] methionine). However, the half-lives of ^{11}C, ^{13}N, and ^{15}O are so short that these radiopharmaceuticals have to be produced on site immediately prior to application. This requires the establishment of a cyclotron facility together with a full radiochemistry service, with accompanying demands on resources, materials, and personnel.

Na ^{123}I AND Na ^{131}I FOR THYROID FUNCTIONAL IMAGING

The thyroid gland is the site for the production and storage of the thyroid hormones thyroxine (T_4) and triiodothyronine (T_3). The base of the production of T_3 and T_4 is thyroglobulin, with tyrosine residues that react with iodide. This trapping of iodide is the rate-limiting step in the transport process.

By administering $^{123}I^-$ or $^{131}I^-$ to the body, these radioactive iodides are undergoing the same metabolic pathways as inactive I^-. The amount of the radioiodide injected (nanogram range) is negligible compared with the daily dietary intake of iodine (~100-μg range). Therefore, the radioiodide does not alter in any way the physiologic behavior of the thyroid.

Radioiodine is the perfect substrate-specific metabolic radiotracer to image the function of the thyroid gland. The uptake study of iodine allows the assessment of thyroid function, and imaging studies yield diagnostic images of the thyroid gland or metastatic lesions.

Radioiodide can be considered the paradigm of a radiopharmaceutical and exemplifies the virtues of the functional imaging of a metabolic process.

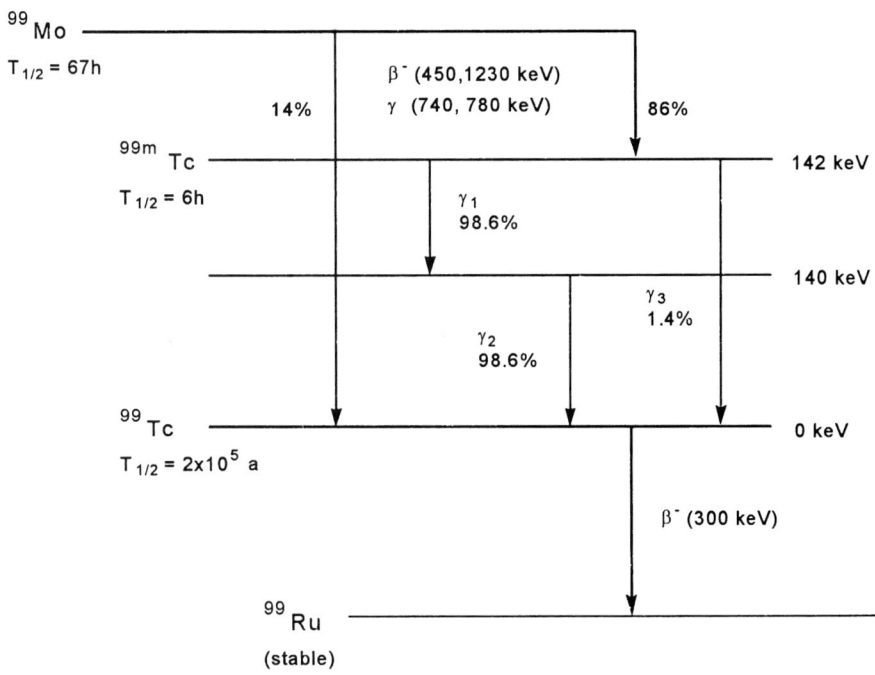

Figure 3. The radioactive decay scheme of ^{99}Mo and ^{99m}Tc.

If no appropriate radionuclide is available, or if the molecule does not allow such labeling techniques to be used, one has to resort to the application of alternative radionuclides. In some cases, functional groups in the pharmaceutical to be labeled can be replaced with radionuclides with similar physiologic characteristics such as lipophilicity or space volume. For example, in 2-[^{18}F]deoxyglucose, the hydroxyl group on carbon 2 in the glucose is replaced by fluoride, and in ω-[^{123}I]heptadecanoic acid, the final methyl group is replaced by iodide (Table 3).

It must be emphasized, however, that any potential alteration in the physiologic behavior of such radiopharmaceutical has to be considered carefully because the risk exists that the function to be measured is influenced. This is, of course, most important for completely novel radiopharmaceuticals (e.g., ^{99m}Tc compounds), where physiology and metabolism are basically unknown. Table 3 outlines the advantages and disadvantages of the use of some typical radionuclides.

The most widely available radionuclide for NM application is ^{99m}Tc (27). Its uniqueness is due to the mother nuclide ^{99}Mo, which decays to the daughter ^{99m}Tc (Fig. 3). In 1957, Powell developed and refined a generator system at the Brookhaven National Laboratories in the United States. The commercially available ^{99}Mo/^{99m}Tc generator yields technetium in the form of pertechnetate $TcO_4{}^-$. As pertechnetate, technetium will not bind to other chemical species; however, it can be reduced to a positively charged form that will complex with a variety of molecules (Fig. 4). Its use ultimately led to the introduction of "instant" kits for the preparation of ^{99m}Tc radiopharmaceuticals. The main advantages of ^{99m}Tc are its suitable half-life of 6 hours, its high photon yield of 88% at 140 keV that has good tissue penetration, and its lack of associated beta radiation, which results in a low radiation dose.

The radiochemistry needed to synthesize the various types of radiopharmaceuticals is not the subject of this book and is a speciality in itself. The choice of appropriate chemistry depends on the nature of the radionuclide and pharmaceutical chosen to be applied. For example, the synthesis of a ^{11}C compound needs fast synthetic organic chemistry, whereas the formulation of a ^{99m}Tc complex requires coordination chemistry and the preparation of an ^{123}I antibody protein chemistry.

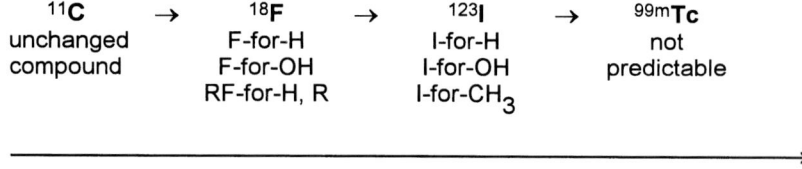

^{11}C	→	^{18}F	→	^{123}I	→	^{99m}Tc
unchanged		F-for-H		I-for-H		not
compound		F-for-OH		I-for-OH		predictable
		RF-for-H, R		I-for-CH_3		

increasing physiological changes

increasing availability

Figure 4. The problem of analogue tracer. From Stšcklin G. Tracers for metabolic imaging of brain and heart-radiochemistry and radiopharmacology. *Eur J Nucl Med*, 19, 527 (1992).

Several ideas presented in this chapter have been outlined in more detail in ''Radio-pharmaceuticals in Nuclear Medicine Practice,'' by Kowalsky and Perry (1987), to which the interested reader is referred (13).

RADIOPAQUE CONTRAST AGENTS

General Principles

The gray-scale or contrast on an x-ray film depends on the varying absorption of x-rays by the tissue or mass irradiated (Fig. 5). Thicker slices, material with a higher density, and molecules with a higher atomic mass increase x-ray absorption and thus reduce the film irradiation. Since the imaging of different body tissues depends on contrast differences (signal differences toward noise) and, consequently, on absorption differences, certain organs and compartments must be made visible with the help of contrast agents (CAs). Principally, one can introduce either substances with a lower density (negative CAs) compared with the surrounding tissues, such as gases (xenon, CO_2), or substances with a higher density (positive CAs), such as iodine-containing molecules (see Table 4), barium-sulfate suspensions, or just any heavy metal.

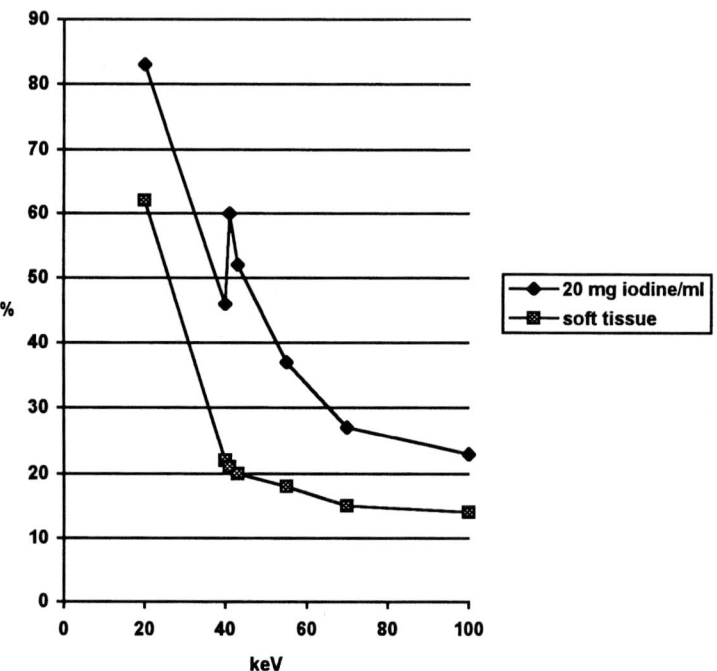

Figure 5. Absorption rate of x-rays in percent in relation to irradiation energy (*K* edge for iodine at 33 keV). Courtesy of Laboratoire Guerbet, Aulnay-sous-Bois, France.

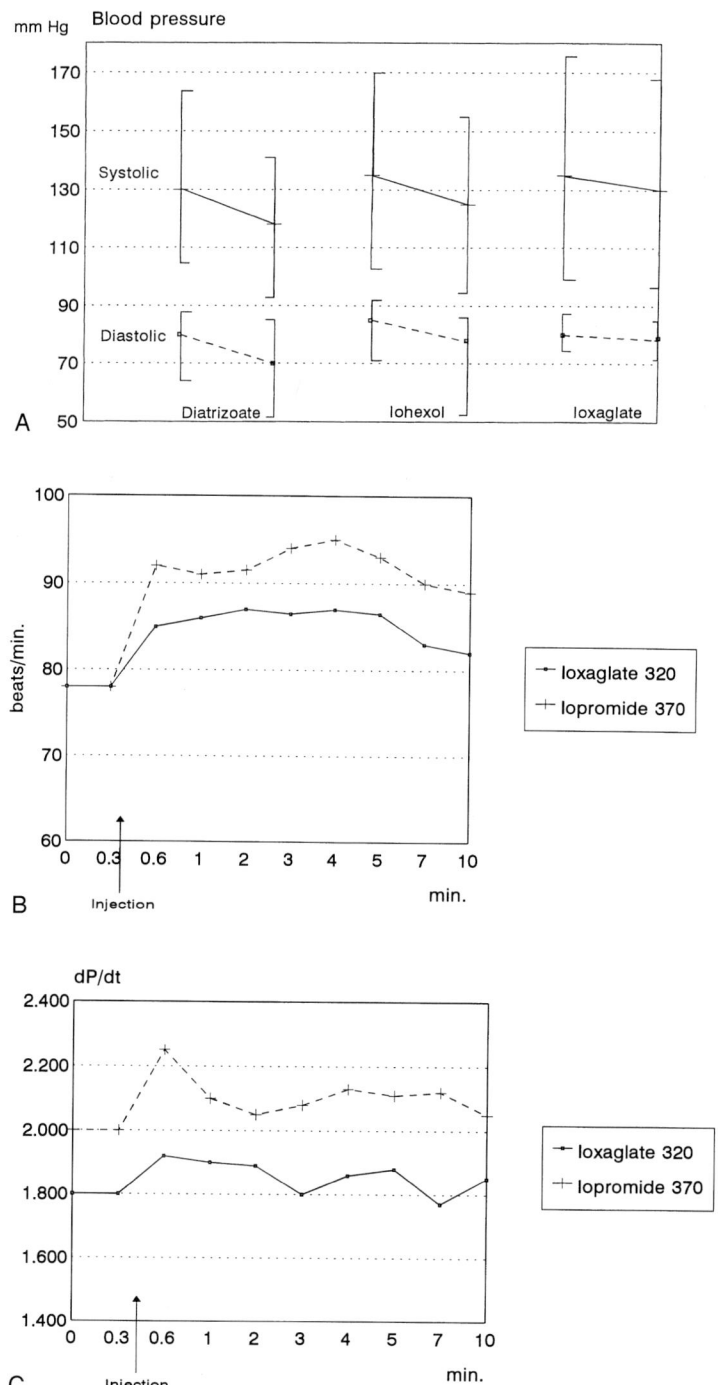

Figure 6. Interference of iodinated contrast medium on cardiac function. (**A**) Blood pressure. (From Cumberland DC. Low-osmolality contrast media in cardiac radiology. *Invest Radiol* 1984;19:S301–S305.) (**B**) Heart rate. (From Neiss AC et al. Comparison of sodium-meglumine ioxaglate and iopromide in coronary angiography. *Ann Radiol* 1989;32:49–53.) (**C**) Variations in *dP/dt*. (From Neiss AC et al. Comparison of sodium-meglumine ioxaglate and iopromide in coronary angiography. *Ann Radiol* 1989;32:49–53.) Courtesy of Laboratoire Guerbet, Aulnay-sous-Bois, France.

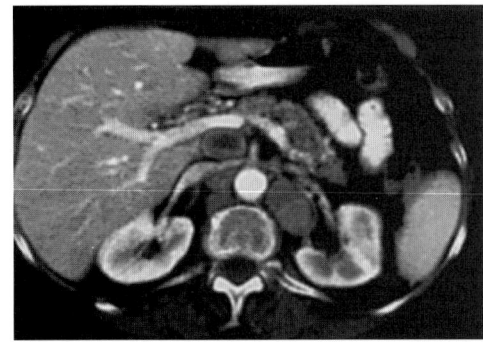 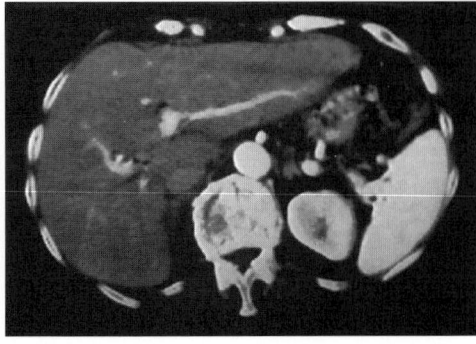

A   B

Figure 7. Computed tomography of the abdomen with contrast enhancement: early vascular phase. Courtesy of Laboratoire Guerbet, Aulnay-sous-Bois, France.

The main CAs in use nowadays are water-insoluble barium sulfate for gastrointestinal (GI) tract diagnosis and water-soluble iodinated CAs for intravascular applications (Figs. 7 to 9) as well as some GI examinations (Tables 4 and 5).

Physicochemical Properties

The ideal CA should have many, if not all, of the following properties: ease of use, high water solubility, high heat and chemical stability, pharmacologic inertness, low viscosity (especially at high concentrations), low or isoosmolality with plasma, no metabolization and a selective excretion (i.e., renally), and a high safety margin (low chemotoxicity, nonantigenic) allowing high and repeated dosing, all at a reasonable cost. The pharmacologic development and choice of a CA are always a compromise between the need to improve safety, to improve contrast quality, and to exploit interactions (clotting, thrombocyte activation) according to the chosen imaging technique. This balance depends on the following parameters:

- Iodine concentration
- Osmolality
- Hydrophilicity
- Viscosity
- Ionic or nonionic character

Chemical Structure/Iodine Concentration

Besides the GI barium sulfates, all currently available radiopaque CAs are triiodinated benzoic acid derivatives, allowing the safe injection of large amounts of iodinated compounds into the bloodstream. The choice of iodine as the ideal high-atomic-number x-ray absorber was probably in part due to the high biocompatibility of solutions of covalent attached iodine to the benzene ring. The currently available CAs can be subdivided into four main groups with fundamental physicochemical differences (Table 6).

The units for measuring iodine concentration and hence the contrast potency of a contrast agent are as follows:

Omnipaque 350: with 350 mg of iodine per milliliter of solution

- Corresponding to 35 g of iodine per 100 ml of solution
- Corresponding in the case of Omnipaque 350 to 75.5 g of iohexol (DCI-ICN) per 100 ml of aqueous solution

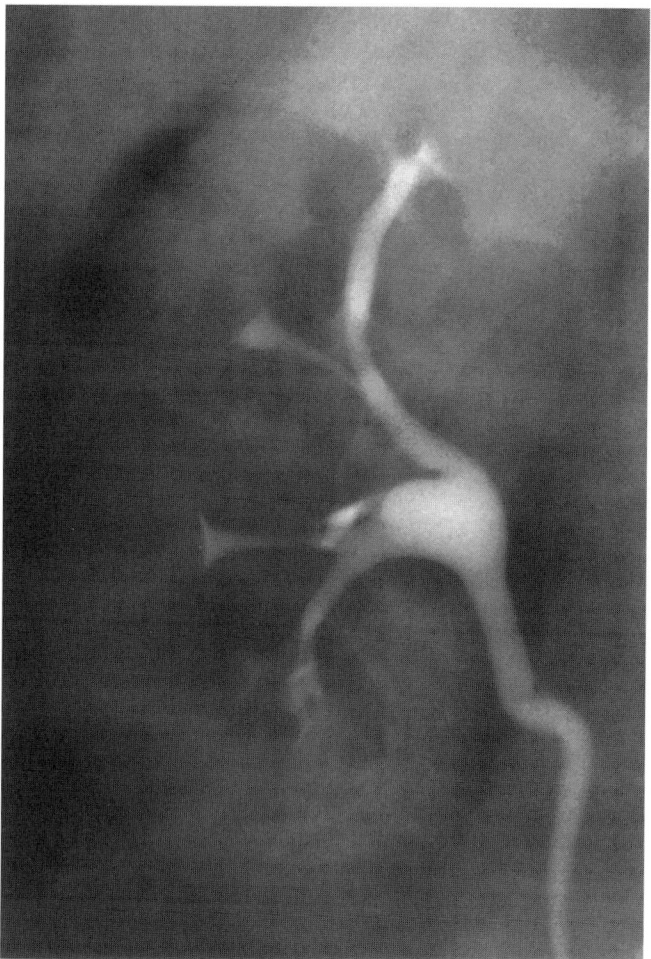

Figure 8. Pyelogram phase obtained at 8 minutes following injection of a urographic contrast agent. Courtesy of Laboratoire Guerbet, Aulnay-sous-Bois, France.

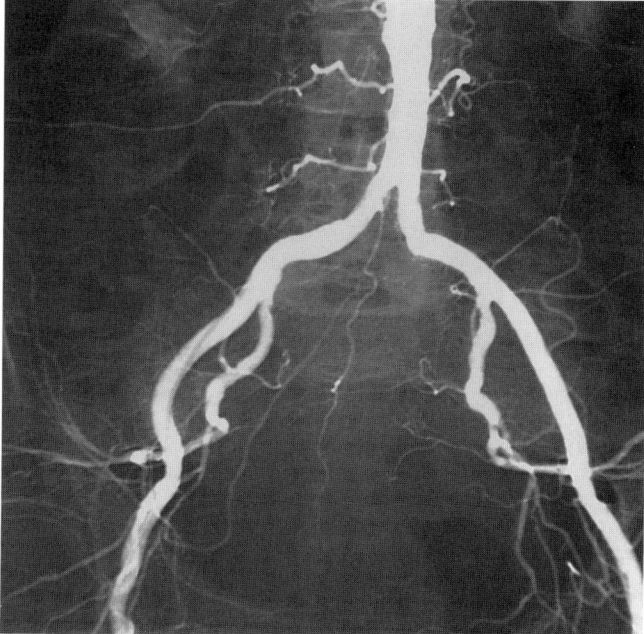

Figure 9. Digital subtraction angiogram of the superior mesenteric arteries with iobitridol 350. Courtesy of Laboratoire Guerbet, Aulnay-sous-Bois, France.

Table 4. *Classification of x-ray contrast agents (CAs) in relation to their chemical structure*

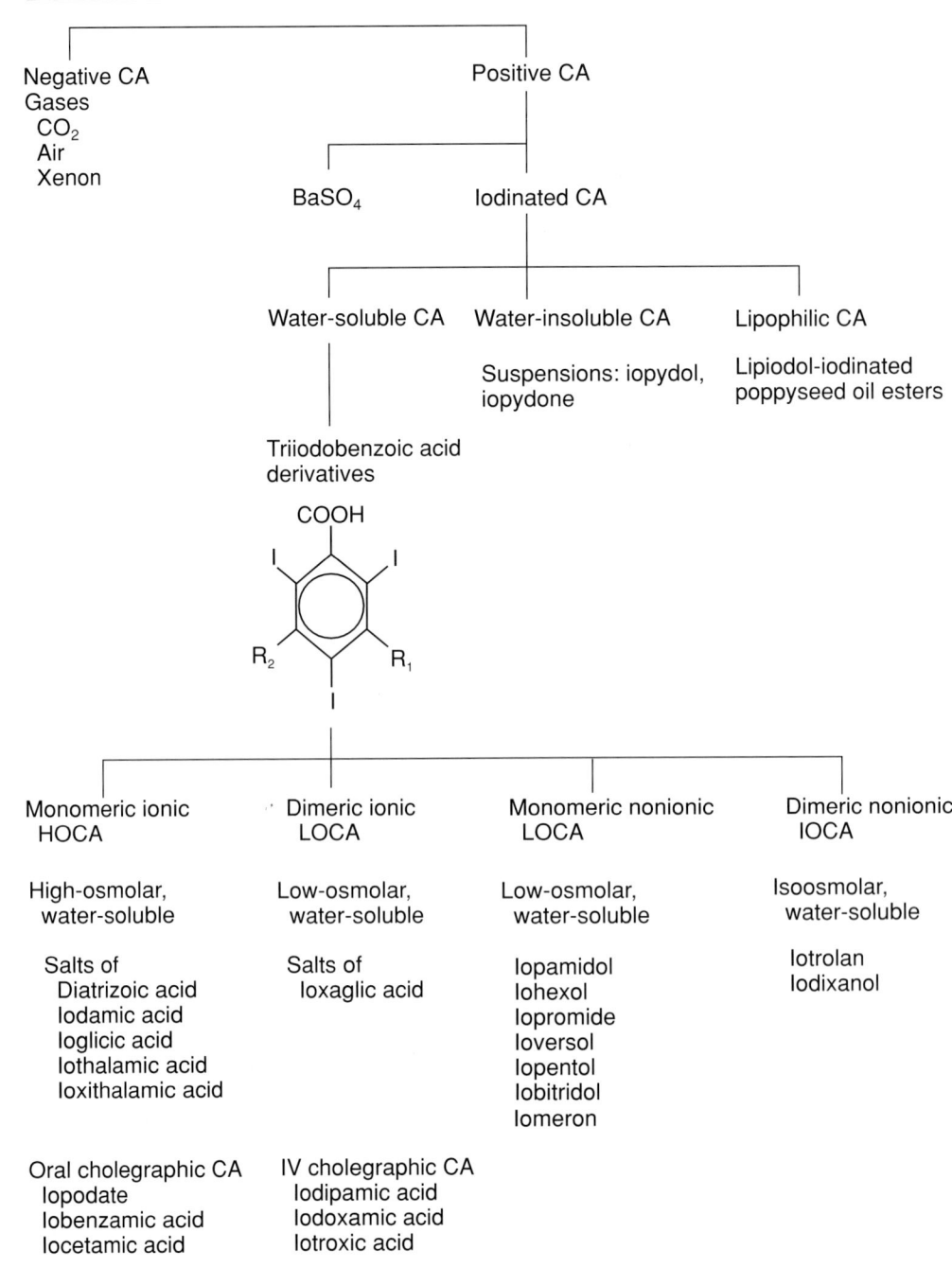

Negative CA
Gases
  CO_2
  Air
  Xenon

Positive CA

BaSO$_4$ Iodinated CA

Water-soluble CA   Water-insoluble CA   Lipophilic CA

Suspensions: iopydol, iopydone

Lipiodol-iodinated poppyseed oil esters

Triiodobenzoic acid derivatives

Monomeric ionic HOCA	Dimeric ionic LOCA	Monomeric nonionic LOCA	Dimeric nonionic IOCA
High-osmolar, water-soluble	Low-osmolar, water-soluble	Low-osmolar, water-soluble	Isoosmolar, water-soluble
Salts of Diatrizoic acid Iodamic acid Ioglicic acid Iothalamic acid Ioxithalamic acid	Salts of Ioxaglic acid	Iopamidol Iohexol Iopromide Ioversol Iopentol Iobitridol Iomeron	Iotrolan Iodixanol
Oral cholegraphic CA Iopodate Iobenzamic acid Iocetamic acid	IV cholegraphic CA Iodipamic acid Iodoxamic acid Iotroxic acid		

Table 5. *Classification of radiopaque contrast agents (CAs) in relation to their usage*

Indication/technique	Purpose	Type

Angiography/DSA
  Occlusive processes
  Vascular diseases
  Mass lesions (trauma, infection, neoplasia)
	Opacification of the vessel	Water-soluble CA with preference of LOCA or IOCA due to less pain → IA/IV → selective

Urography
  Nephrogram: masses (tumors and cysts), renal functioning
  Pyelogram: GFR, postrenal obstruction
  Excretory urography: hematuria, obstructions, infections, trauma, prostatic hypertrophy
  Direct urography or retrograde pyelography: better visualization of ureters and calyces, urinary tract laceration, fistula, renal insufficiency
	Opacification and delineation of the kidneys and the collecting systems of the urinary tract	Water-soluble CA

Computed tomography
  Vascular phase: hypo- or hypervascular areas, infarction, ischemia
  Parenchymal phase (capillar integrity, interstitial volume, tissue blood volume)
  Accumulatory and eliminatory phase (pathologies)
  Urinary tract and elimination
	Increase the degree of contrast between normal body structures and to improve the differentiation of pathologic processes from normal tissue	Intravascular, water-soluble CA
		Radiopaque media
		  Into the gastrointestinal tract
		  Into the cerebrospinal fluid space: CT cisternography
		  Into the urinary tract
		  Xenon (quantification of local cerebral blood flow, xenon extraction fraction)
		  Iodinated esters of poppyseed oil (liver, HCC), RES agents

Myelography	Depiction of diseases or abnormalities of the spinal column, spinal canal, and central nervous system	Nonionic LOCA or IOCA

Radiologic examination of the alimentary tract (segment-specific)
  Digestive disorders
  Distinct changes in bowel habit
  Abdominal pain
  Bleeding
  Inflammatory diseases
  Tumors, masses (polyps)
	Adequate delineation and depiction of the lumen or mucosal surface from the surrounding soft tissues	Oral or rectal application of barium sulfate (for mucosal details) or water-soluble iodinated agents (full-column opacification)

Cholecystographic and cholangiographic studies
  Cholelithiasis (gallstones)
  Cholecystitis
  Anatomical abnormalities
  Abnormal gallbladder functioning
	Opacification of the gallbladder and of the hepatobiliary system (bile ducts) due to their hepatobiliary excretion	Cholecystographic medium (oral administration), cholangiographic medium (slow intravenous, drip infusion)

Arthrography Congenital, posttraumatic, or degenerative joint disorders (ruptures, tears of ligaments, loose bodies, cysts, masses)	Radiologic examination of the joint cavity, articulations, and surrounding tissues	Negative or positive CA into the joint space, water-soluble CA (LOCA, IOCA)
Hysterosalpingography	Radiographic demonstration of intrauterine abnormalities and Fallopian tube patency (fertility)	Direct instillation of a radiopaque CA into the uterine cavity, oil-soluble CA, water-soluble CA (high viscous solutions, dimers)
Lymphography	Visualization of the lymphatic system	Indirect: subcutaneous injection Direct: into isolated and cannulated lymph vessel or lymph node Oil-soluble CM (Ethiodol, Lipiodol) Water-soluble CA (Iotrolan)
Bronchography	Radiographic examination of the bronchial tree	Direct instillation of water-soluble CA or aqueous suspensions of iodinated agents

Table 6. *Main groups of water-soluble contrast agents*

Chemical structure	Compound (brand)	Electric charge dissociation	Osmolality for 300–350 mg/ml in mOsm/kg H_2O	Viscosity 350 mg/ml 37°C in mPa · s	Hydrophilicity log p octanol/water
Monomeric high-osmolar CA (HOCA)	Diatrizoate (Angiografin, Urografin) Iothalamate (Conray) Ioxithalamate (Telebrix) Ioglicate (Rayvist)	Anions + sodium and/or meglumine	1500–2400	5.2–9.5	−4.10
Dimeric low-osmolar CA (LOCA)	Ioxaglate (Hexabrix)	Anion + sodium and meglumine	550–600	7.5	−2.4
Monomeric low-osmolar, nonionic CA (NI-LOCA)	Iopamidol (Iopamiro, Solutrast, Niopam, Isovue) Iohexol (Omnipaque) Iopromide (Ultravist) Ioversol (Optiray) Iopentol (Imagopaque) Iobitridol (Xenetix) Iomeprol (Iomeron)	Nonionic	520–900	8–12	−2.35 to −3.57
Dimeric isoosmolar CA (IOCA)	Iotrolan (Isovist) Iodixanol (Visipaque)	Nonionic	300	8.1–17.7	−3.65 to −4.81

From Krause W et al. Physiochemical parameters of x-ray contrast media. *Invest Radiol* 29(1), 72–80 (1994).

The higher the iodine concentration, the better is the opacification and hence contrast toward tissues without CA uptake. This depends also to a large extent on tissue diffusibility and distribution of the CA (osmolality, viscosity, hydrophilicity).

The side groups on C1 of the benzene ring define if the agent is ionic (dissociating acid group COOH forming a salt solution) or nonionic (with a nondissociating amide group). Side groups on C3 and C5 serve to protect and stabilize the iodine on the benzene ring and to increase hydrophilicity of the molecule (see Tables 4 and 6). Thus water solubility is increased while the hydrophobic interactions with proteinaceous or tissue-binding sites are reduced in order to improve clinical tolerance. The cleavage of iodine from the aromate leads to the presence of inorganic iodide in the solution. Even though this is limited to less than 130 ppm, one must consider it when performing a radionuclide iodine uptake test of the thyroid, which after the use of water-soluble CA is blocked for 2 to 6 weeks.

Osmolality

The osmotic pressure of a solution is determined by the number of dissolved particles (or freely mobile particles), whether ions, molecules, or aggregates, it contains per unit of volume that exercise a kind of pressure on surrounding semipermeable membranes. Osmolality, which usually is expressed in milliosmoles per kilogram of water (mOsm/kg H_2O), allows us to define three of the four important CA categories (see Table 6):

1. High-osmolar contrast agents (HOCA), with 5 to 8 times the osmolality of human serum
2. Low-osmolar contrast agents (LOCA), with 1 to 3 times the osmolality of human serum
3. Isoosmolar contrast agents (IOCA), with a hypo- or isoosmolar status compared with human plasma

Osmolality depends mostly on iodine concentration and less on temperature.

When injecting a CA (usually hyperosmolar) into a blood vessel, osmotic equilibrium is upset and water flows from the extravascular space and out of the blood cells into the vessel. Simultaneously, the low-molecular-weight particles (not protein-bound CA) pass through the fenestrated endothelium of the vessels. The result is an increase in intravascular volume, a fall in hematocrit, hypervolemia with vasodilatation, a reduction in peripheral resistance, a decrease in blood pressure, extracellular dehydration, and in some cases bradycardia besides local pain-intensive reactions (pain and warmth) near the injection site.

For urography and, to some extent, for CT scanning, the resulting osmotic diuresis is preferred in order to optimize the distension of the urinary tract.

Reduction of osmolality resulting from the introduction of new chemical entities has allowed considerable progress (7):

- Decreasing the influx of water into the vascular compartment (less pain, less extracellular dehydration)
- Reducing the dose-dependent disturbances of cardiac function (hemodynamic effects)
- Improving renal safety
- Ensuring low local endothelial toxicity

Viscosity

Viscosity is a measure of the flow properties of the solutions and depends strongly on the concentration of iodine, is inversely proportional to temperature, and increases with larger molecules (dimers, long side chains). Viscosity affects the maximum injection speed and the passage through thin needles or catheters and also determines intravenous contrast flow (distribution, tailoring effects along the vessel wall near the injection site). Local tolerance also may depend on viscosity, since pain and warmth seem to increase with higher viscosity.

Hydrophilicity and Water Solubility

The presence of charged groups as in ionic CAs increases their water solubility but also changes blood electrical conductivity and the overall electrolyte balance. Nonionic compounds, because of the absence of any charged group, are made water soluble by increasing the hydrophilic groups and especially the hydroxyl groups on the side chains.

Hydrophilia, quantitatively measured as the distribution of a substance between a solvent (octanol, butanol) and an aqueous buffer, correlates with the binding to plasma proteins, the neurotoxicity, the diffusion through the blood-brain barrier, and certain allergic (idiosyncratic) side effects of CAs.

The lipophilicity of cholegraphic CAs must be relatively high so that they are excreted by the liver into the biliary system.

Electric Charge

Ionic CAs in solution dissociate into cations (e.g., sodium, meglumine) and anions (acid), affecting the electrical potential on cell membranes and the electrical conductivity of body fluids and changing the overall electrolyte balance. Especially when injected into the cerebrospinal fluid (CSF), their use is associated with violent tonic and clonic spasms, convulsions, and epileptogenic activity due to neurotoxicity (contraindicated for myelography). On the other hand, they seem to have a positive effect on inhibition of blood coagulation and thrombocyte activation.

Highly concentrated nonionic CAs can cause, due to their lack of charged groups, a temporary decrease in the plasma concentration of physiologic electrolytes, which might cause ventricular fibrillation in patients at risk.

Effects on myocardial contractility seem to depend on osmolality and electric charge. Using standard HOCAs, one can observe a profound drop in systolic blood pressure after coronary angiography. Low-osmolar agents produce fewer hemodynamic alterations than do standard contrast media but still have transient positive inotropic and negative inotropic effects (compare with Fig. 6).

Possible Use of Contrast Media (see Figs. 7 to 9)

The multiple possibilities of application of CAs coincide with the wide range of x-ray imaging techniques (see Table 5). In addition to the simple mechanical filling of cavities and lumina, CAs opacify organs in a function-depending manner. In many instances, the qualitative functioning of an organ or metabolic pathway is depicted (compare the renal elimination and hepatic uptake of hepatobiliary agents).

In conventional plain-film radiography, luminal filling mainly serves to recognize the morphologic structure of a certain lumen and its mural pathologies (GI mucosa with barium and CO_2). In certain cases, qualitative functional information might result, e.g., assessment of tone or peristaltic effects in cavities (GI tract, vessels, ureters with retrograde filling).

In CT scanning, the main indication for CAs is the delineation of vessels and the opacification of well-vascularized tissue. The demonstration of pathologic structures may depend on differences of enhancement within a single organ. It is occasionally possible to differentiate a certain structure as a result of flow patterns (hemangioma: slow concentric inflow; see Fig. 12 from Chap. 3).

New software and hardware techniques allow us to follow the CA bolus, its exact inflow, its distribution pattern, and its outflow. Distribution volume, perfusion, and other pharmacokinetic constants can in principle be defined and measured for an imaged section (see Chap. 3).

Pharmacokinetics of Intravascular Contrast Agents

The intravascular contrast agents distribute according to a two-compartment model (see Chap. 4) as iodinated contrast agents are rapidly distributed from the vascular space (compartment 1) into the interstitial compartment (compartment 2). Penetration into the intracellular compartment is of no clinical importance, since only very little quantities can be detected (Fig. 10).

CAs are therefore markers of the extracellular fluid space and are eliminated by renal glomerular filtration without being metabolized (see Fig. 8). The pharmacokinetics of an intravenous CA are shown in Fig. 11 and are essentially characterized by

- A short distribution half-life on the order of 4 to 10 minutes ($t_{1/2\alpha}$, mainly vascular and interstitial)
- An elimination half-life on the order of 1.5 to 2 hours ($t_{1/2\beta}$)
- A distribution volume of 0.25 liter/kg = 14 to 20 liters per adult
- A percentage of protein binding, which is generally below 5% for a water-soluble CA (but strongly dependent on the measuring technique)
- A total clearance of 1 to 2 ml per minute per kilogram of body weight

At normal dosages, a water-soluble CA does not cross the intact blood-brain barrier (BBB) or the placenta (into the fetus).

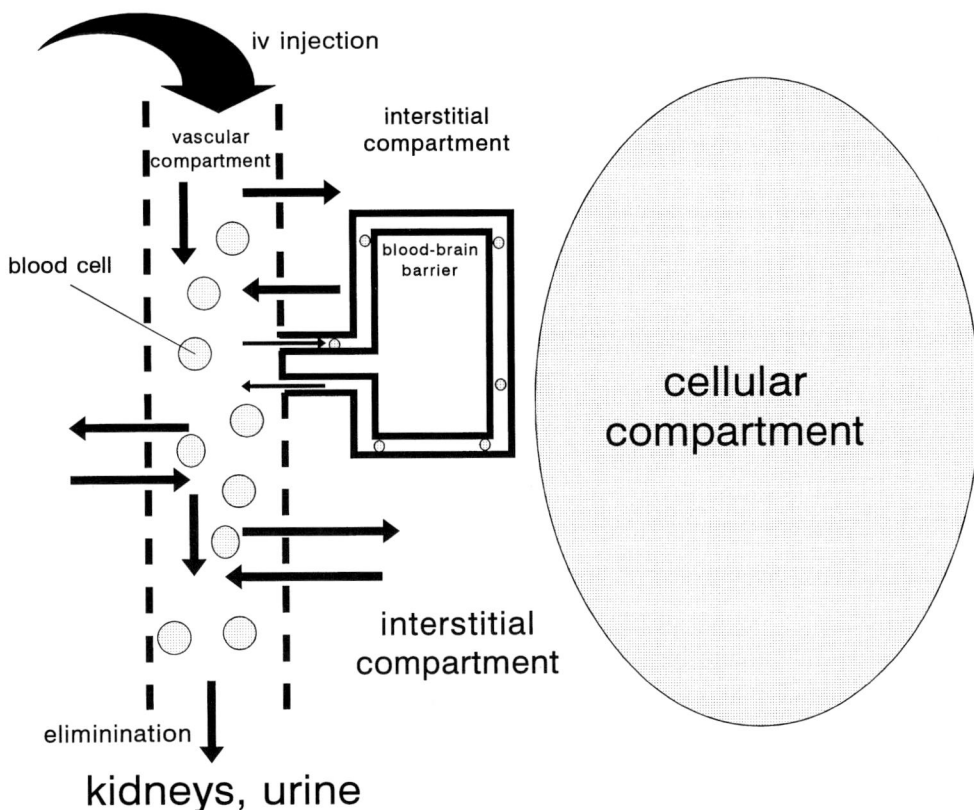

Figure 10. Pharmacokinetics of iodinated contrast agents: A two-compartment model.

Application, Flow, and Distribution

From the diagnostic and imaging point of view, distribution kinetics, compactness of the contrast bolus, and flow profile including persistence are important features of CAs for the interpretation of clinical images. The vascular phase is utilized in angiography for visualizing the vascular system. Due to the rapid onset of diffusion into the extra-vascular space, the radiologic technique must be adapted for short-term imaging. For example CO_2 angiography often demonstrates an inhomogeneous bubble-like tailoring effect that in certain cases prevents its use due to these uneven flow profiles.

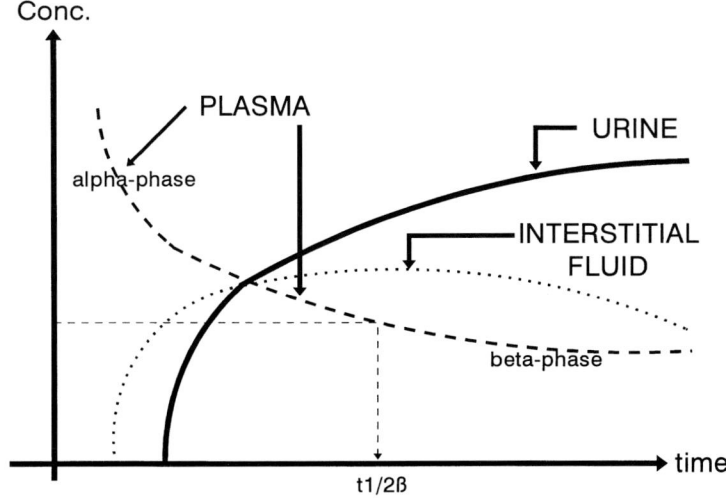

Figure 11. Concentrations of iodinated CAs in plasma, interstitial fluid, and urine after injection.

The interstitial phase is visualized only after a few minutes and often depicted with tomodensitometric techniques or with CT scanning. With faster imaging techniques, particularly CT scanning, the vascular distribution phase (α phase) of CAs that precedes the interstitial diffusion allows the differentiation of lesions with a high vascularization from those with lower or poor vascularization. Imaging with a certain time delay depicts lesions with a slower washout of the CA.

In cerebral applications, the BBB permeation of CAs provides important diagnostic clues. In general, the visualization and characterization of a pathologic mass depend essentially on its histopathologic structure, predominance of a deep vascular area, and the access and diffusibility (hemodynamics) of the regional blood flow. Further, the rheologic properties and interactions of CAs and blood play an important role in governing flow dynamics and circulatory transport through the capillary bed.

Flow and distribution of water-soluble contrast agents depend on many extrinsic and intrinsic factors:

- Injection rate and pressure
- Needle gauge diameter, length of tubes
- Physicochemical properties of the CA (viscosity, osmolality, chemotoxicity, water solubility)
- Protein binding
- Concentration and temperature
- Injection site
- Vascularization (IV, IA, capillaries)
- Distribution volume and interstitial volume (two-compartment model)
- Permeability of membranes and compartments
- Heart frequency and stroke volume
- Endothelial activation with strong hemodynamic activation
- Elimination (clearance rate, three-compartment model, renal uptake)
- Local blood flow (ml/min) and hemodynamics, especially in peripheral vascular disease or infarction

High-osmolar CAs (HOCAs) generally generate a strong water inflow into the vascular compartment with a certain vasodilatation distal to the injection site, an increase of the vascular volume leading to an increased cardiac load (hypervolemia), and an increase in renal diuresis (sometimes increasing the tubular distension).

Low-osmolar CAs (LOCAs) have less strong vasodilution and vasodilatation effects, induce less diuresis, and reach higher concentrations in the renal tubuli. Dimers diffuse less rapidly into the extravascular space or out of compartments (perilymphatic region, arthrographic compartments, fallopian tubes), but they nevertheless induce a quite strong hemodynamic activation when injected intravascularly (19).

Elimination and Renal Nephrogram

Due to their low molecular weight, low protein-binding capacity, and high water solubility, CAs are mainly eliminated through the kidneys by glomerular filtration. This defines their elimination rate. Renal flow dynamics, blood rheology, and the Donnan balance have an important impact on the primary filtration rate. Most water-soluble CAs induce a short cortical blood flow increase, while the medullary rate is reduced (vasoconstriction). These effects vary depending on osmolality and chemical structure (e.g., the dimeric ioxaglate has a higher medullary blood flow rate in comparison with nonionic LOCAs). Since the tissue oxygen concentration depends on these hemodynamic effects, they might contribute to renal compatibility (17).

Due to the high water reuptake in the nephrons (and sodium for certain ionic CAs), osmotic pressure might reach 1500 mOsm/kg H_2O in the collecting tubules, thus increasing the concentration of the urinary CA dramatically.

After the intravascular application of a CA, one can differentiate two main phases of renal excretion (see Fig. 8):

1. Nephrographic phase (10 to 120 s after injection)
   a. Cortical arteriogram (10 to 15 s after injection, vascular phase)
   b. Cortical nephrogram (20 to 45 s after injection, vascular-tubular phase)
   c. General nephrogram (45 to 120 s after injection, tubular phase)
2. Urographic phase with CA in the descending urinary collecting system (120 to 180 s after injection)

Imaging time and diagnostic goals must thus be coordinated. Since the elimination rate of water-soluble CAs resembles that of creatinine or mannitol, they are a marker of renal function and especially of glomerular filtration. In cases of renal impairment, the nephrogram gives differential information on

- The perfusion rate
- The elimination rate

by showing an abnormal density curve over the kidneys. Increasing density with time reflects obstruction; a persisting nephrogram without any density reduction reflects either acute tubular necrosis or an acute bacterial infection (nephritis). A reduced and persistent density reflects an acute pre-, intra-, or postrenal complication.

With increased dosage and dehydration of the patient, the risk of renal impairment or nephrotoxic reactions increases dramatically (see ''Tolerance'' below).

Despite the almost complete renal (>90%) elimination, CAs are eliminated to a certain degree via feces, skin, and saliva and can induce late allergic reactions (rushes, skin reactions) after a couple of days. Extrarenal elimination routes may take on greater importance in certain pathologic circumstances with the kidneys. Small amounts of inorganic iodide, which has been liberated (catalyzed) from the central benzoic ring structure and that contaminates the solution, cause the specific thyroid uptake or blockage (for water-soluble CAs, between 7 and 15 days).

Due to their free C5 group on the benzene ring, hepatotropic CAs have a strong albumin binding, are taken up through the anionic receptor system of the hepatocytes, and are eliminated via a saturable transport mechanism into the bile ducts and finally appear in the bile.

Full control of the pharmacokinetics and elimination rate of new compounds in development seem to conduct to innovative applications. Blood pool iodinated CAs whose extravascular diffusion is slowed down by increased molecular size have allowed compartmental and perfusion imaging in preclinical settings. The diagnostic contribution in cases of tumors and ischemia has yet to be confirmed.

Tolerance

The ideal CA would be an agent without any untoward physiologic effects. In fact, there exist some pharmacologic effects that are of a certain practical importance and thus desirable. The inhibitory effect on blood clotting, the inhibition of thrombocyte activation, and certain erythrocyte interactions give the ionic CA an advantage over nonionic CAs when performing interventional procedures. Further, the rapid shift of fluid from the extravascular and cellular compartments into the blood induces a certain increase in blood flow and vascular distension, allowing for better visualization of vessels in angiography or of the renal tubuli.

Due to the high amounts of substance injected in a short time period, CAs usually produce a myriad of physiologic effects as a result of their pseudoallergic potential, hyperosmolarity, or direct chemotoxicity (molecular toxicity). Adverse reactions to CAs can be classified according to their severity (Table 7), according to their reaction predictability (Table 8), or according to their appearance (acute or delayed). An important distinction should be made between dose-response or toxic effects and hypersensitive or idiosyncratic reaction forms.

Anaphylactoid or pseudoallergic reactions may be seen alone or in combination in any severity up to life-threatening responses and often are accompanied by manifestations induced by chemotoxic effects (nausea, vomiting, hypotension, cardiac effects). It is often

Table 7. *Classification of adverse reactions to contrast agents due to severity*

Minor	Intermediate	Severe
Sensation of heat	Vomiting	Syncope, convulsion
Nausea	Faintness	Pulmonary edema
Injection-site pain	Bronchospasm	Shock, hypotension
Pruritus	Edema	Life-threatening cardiac
Mild pallor	Dyspnea	Arrhythmia
Diaphoresis	Chills	Cardiac or respiratory arrest
Local urticaria or hives	Extensive urticaria	
Transient arrhythmia		

impossible to define the exact mechanism of complication, its pathophysiology, or its etiology. Different strategies have been chosen to reduce clinical complications. For example, it is widely held that certain risk factors cause a higher incidence of contrast-related complications (Table 9), thus underlining the importance of an efficient anamnesis for prevention. Further studies must be undertaken to focus the context of different organ systems (cardiac, renal, cerebral, vascular), their interrelationship, and different complicating variables, such as underlying cardiac disease, altered vascular function due to atherosclerosis, altered BBB, and underlying renal failure (Table 10). Better understanding of these variables will automatically lead to better prevention and treatment of complications. Another approach consists of the development of newer CAs with less interactions with body tissues (stabilized hydrophilicity, isotonicity) and metabolic functions and of a higher specificity in order to reduce the dosage (3).

The clinical experience with an increased incidence of late reactions (occurring 2 to 3 days after the diagnostic procedure) due to the intravascular application of dimeric isoosmolar CAs (iotrolan, iodixanol) teaches one that further investigations are necessary to understand the molecular pharmacology beyond the simple improvement in comfort achieved by lowering the osmolality.

Functional Interactions

Even though a CA should be inert and without any pharmacologic potential, the clinical reality shows that there are numerous effects following injection. Most reactions are unpredictable, and some are dose dependent, with higher risks when increasing the dosage. The goal of this section is to outline the predictable effects of CAs, which can be classified into three groups:

1. Release of biologically active mediators or cell-specific effects
2. Hemocompatibility or blood interactions
3. Organ-specific effects

Cell-Specific Effects and Release of Biologically Active Mediators

The facts that information on local concentrations of mediators is very limited, that mediator responsiveness varies between individuals, and that different cell types (and

Table 8. *Classification of adverse reactions to contrast agents due to reaction predictability*

Predictable	Unpredictable	Intercurrent complications
Dose-dependent reactions	Pseudoallergic (anaphylactoid)	Myocardial reactions
Osmolality-dependent reactions	Mediator-dependent reactions	Pulmonary embolism
Chemotoxic reactions	Vagal reactions	Convulsions
Drug-CA interactions		Septicemia

Table 9. *Risk factors conducting to a higher incidence of undesired contrast agent–dependent reactions*

Allergy/asthma	Multiple myeloma (dysproteinemia)
Previous reactions to contrast media	Dehydration
High dosages or frequent application	Higher age ($>$65–70)
Diabetes	Newborns
Preexisting renal failure	Seizure history
Hepatic insufficiency	Pheochromocytoma

hormone-like chemical messengers) are almost always involved with complex regulatory mechanisms make it extremely difficult to interpret cellular compatibility.

Histamine. It has been proposed that the release of histamine and serotonin from both mast cells and basophils and/or the peripheral acetylcholinesterase effect could in part explain the etiology of anaphylactoid reactions. In vitro studies have proved that the release of histamine by radiographic CAs is dose, and to a certain extent molecule, dependent. In vivo studies have demonstrated that histamine release occurs in both patients with and without anaphylactic reactions. Release could be mediated by a still unknown receptor, could be secondary to the generation of anaphylatoxins from activation

Table 10. *Organ-specific reactions*

Organ	Type of impairment	Pathophysiology
Lungs, respiration	Edema, epiglottitis	Pseudoallergic
	Bronchospasm	Pseudoallergic
	Increased bronchial secretion	Pseudoallergic
Heart	Cardiac arrhythmia, fibrillation	Chemotoxicity, electrophysiologic balance, pseudoallergic
	Hypotension	Osmolality, pseudoallergic
	Shock	Osmolality, dosage, pseudoallergic
	Cardiac arrest	Osmolality, dosage, pseudoallergic
Gastrointestinal tract	Nausea	Chemotoxicity, pseudoallergic
	Vomiting	Chemotoxicity, pseudoallergic
	Diarrhea	Osmolality
	Intestinal cramping	Pseudoallergic
Kidneys	Functional impairment	Dosage, chemotoxicity
	Renal failure	
Brain (BBB)	Convulsions	Osmolality, chemotoxicity
	Vomiting	Vomiting center
Skin	Pruritus	Pseudoallergic
	Urticaria, hives	Histamine release
	Angioedema	
Blood and endothelium	Blood coagulation	Chemotoxicity
	Activation of the complement system with mediators (bradykinin, serotonin)	Calcium-binding anaphylactic
	Thrombocytopenia	
Thyroid gland	Blockage of iodide clearance	Increased iodide supply
	Hyperthyroidism	Autonomous regulation
	Thyreotoxic crisis	T_4 metabolization increased, r-T_3 secretion increased
Genitourinary	Uterine cramps	Pseudoallergic
	Urgency to urinate	Dosage, diuresis (osmolality)

of the complement system, and/or could be due to hyperosmolarity. The cellular diuretic effect of hyperosmolar CAs causes an increase in intracellular calcium concentration that sets in motion the secretory response. The action of histamine can only be considered to provide a partial explanation for the spectrum of side effects occurring with CAs, since antihistamines block anaphylactoid reactions only to a certain extent and since there is no correlation between the strength of reaction and plasma histamine concentration. A lower degranulation of mast cells in the lungs and reduced histamine release due to lower CA concentrations could explain why CAs are better tolerated when injected intraarterially.

Complement. Substantial clinical data demonstrate activation of the complement system by radiographic CAs (probably over the alternative pathway). The wide interrelationship of the complement system with other systems (immune-host-defense, coagulation, kinin-bradykinin system) explains the further activation of other mediators with their specific pharmacologic effects: such as the lysosomal enzymes, increase in vascular permeability, contraction of smooth muscles, chemotaxis of leukocytes, hypotension due to bradykinin, consumptive coagulopathy with activation of coagulation. The effects are obviously determined by the balance between activation and inhibition when the patient is exposed to CAs.

There are several other factors in the plasma that should be analyzed: the interactions with the blood coagulation cascade, the impairment of the fibrinolytic system as fibrin breakdown products can be found after the application of a CA in the blood, the release of prostaglandins and arachidonate pathways, the rapid secretion of serotonin through thrombocytes, and CA-endothelium interactions (BBB as a specific mode).

Hemocompatibility and Blood Interactions

In addition to the vascular compartment with its wide variety of blood cells, hemocompatability also involves the endothelium and to a certain extent vascular flow dynamics. Thus even isoosmolar CAs induce in general a strong increase in blood flow so that factors other than hypertonicity must be implicated in the vasodilatory effect of CAs (19). Blood that comes into contact with CA-containing syringes or other foreign bodies such as catheters or guidewires shows an increased red cell aggregation, blood clotting, and conglomerate formation. This effect is increased with nonionic CAs and strongly reduced with ionic, dimeric low-osmolar agents (ioxaglate).

Ionic CAs are stronger coagulation inhibitors with a prolongation of blood coagulation time and reduction in fibrin formation. Conversely, nonionic CAs have a much weaker anticoagulant effect with a higher impairment of fibrinolysis (Fig. 12).

New results (5, 11, 12) have revealed that there is likely an agent-related difference in the risk of platelet activation and aggregation where high concentrations of CAs are known to exist (see Table 11).

Clinical results from the EPIC trial seem to confirm that the type of CA used during invasive interventional procedures might reduce thromboembolic complications and myocardial infarction, thus influencing survival (1).

Organ-Specific Effects

Heart. Contractility of the myocardium, electrophysiology, and the myocardial perfusion rate are altered. The osmolarity-dependent vasodilatation (hemodynamic effect) induces a systemic blood pressure decrease and consequently a tachycardia. Usually, the injection of a CA induces a short positive inotropic effect that is followed by a negative inotropic effect. Other effects include an increase in the heart rate, a prolongation of the QT interval in ECG, and an increase in coronary perfusion. This last effect seems to be more important in the normal vascular bed and decreased in ischemic regions, thus inducing a "steal effect." The physiologic effects of CAs on the myocardium, on impulse

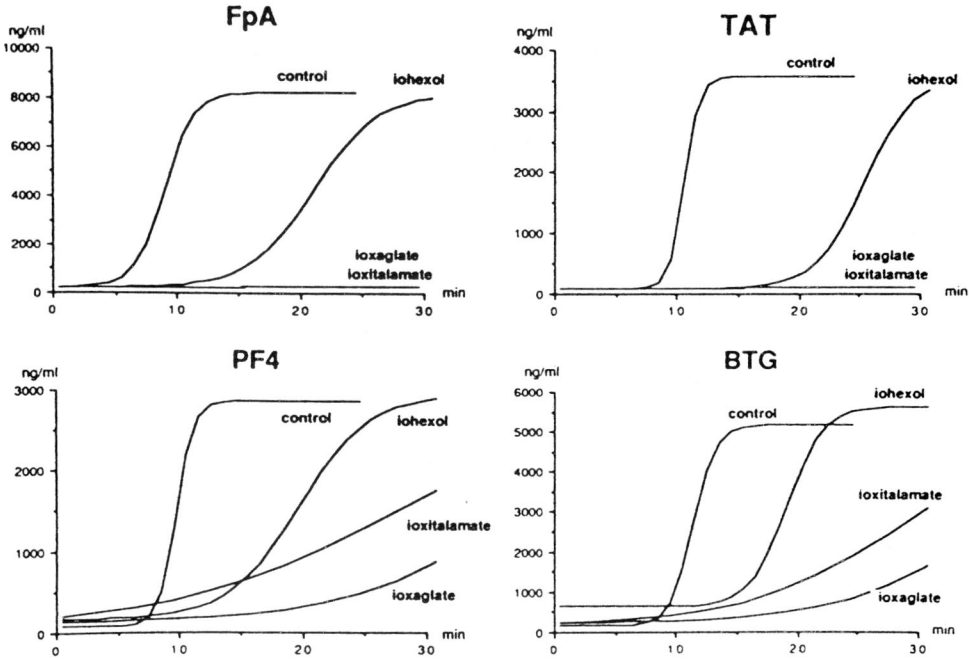

Figure 12. Theoretical sigmoid curves of the kinetics of the in vitro generation of nonanticoagulated human whole blood clotting parameters in the presence of 10% v/v CA. Courtesy of Laboratoire Guerbet, Aulnay-sous-Bois, France. Ionic CAs inhibit blood coagulation activation induced by artificial surfaces shown by the absence of fibrinopeptide A (*FpA*) and generation of thrombin-antithrombin complexes (*TAT*). Nonionic CAs delay the appearance of these parameters. Delay and impairment of platelet activation are expressed through extracellular release of platelet factor 4 (*PF4*) and/or beta-thromboglobulin (*BTG*). From Eloy R, Corot C, Belleville J: Contrast media for angiography: Physicochemical properties, pharmacokinetics and biocompatability. *Clin Mat*, 7, 89–197 (1991).

generation, conductivity, and contractility, are of primary importance in coronary angiography but also when CAs are injected into the cardiac chambers or greater vessels.

Kidneys. Since CAs are mainly excreted by the renal route, both morphologic and functional effects must be studied for any agent. Hyperosmolar CAs induce an increase in diuresis and are thus diuretic. With higher dosages and in the case of a preexisting renal impairment, the incidence of nephrotoxic reactions is strongly increased (in prospective studies from 12% to 89%). Since these consequences develop over several days, the maximum of an acute nephrotoxic reaction is reached after 4 to 7 days. The most sensible indicators of early renal damage are a reduction in creatinine clearance (functional assay), α_1-microglobuline in the plasma, and the excretion of tubular brush border enzymes in the urine.

Thyroid Gland. Iodine containing CAs do not have a direct effect on the thyroid gland, but since they always contain free iodide that enters iodine metabolism, they have an influence on thyroid function. Either the supplemental iodine induces a reduction in

Table 11. *Risk of platelet activation and aggregation*

Nonionic LOCM	90% platelet activation	Quick aggregation,
	Profound platelet degranulation (80%)	somewhat reversible
Ionic HOCM	Activation, but at a slower rate (70%)	No platelet aggregation
	25% degranulation	
Ionic LOCM,	No activation	No aggregation
ioxaglate	No degranulation	
	Inhibits the thrombin-induced in vitro	
	activation of platelets	

hormone synthesis (Wolff-Chaikoff effect) or it induces a hyperthyroidism in patients with iodine deficiency–induced goiters (incidence of 1 in 50,000). Only the increased amount of available iodide results in a perceptible pathology. The risk of a thyreotoxic reaction is higher for elder patients but cannot be assessed prior to performing the diagnostic procedure with the CA. A reduction in thyroid function is mainly a risk for newborns and small children. These latter effects are transient.

MRI CONTRAST AGENTS: MAGNETOPHARMACEUTICALS

Introduction

Due to its high intrinsic soft-tissue resolution, inherent contrast, and noninvasive nature (nonionizing radiation), the need for a contrast-enhancing agent in MRI was strongly debated at the beginning. The uncertain diagnostic gain in MRI due to contrast media enhancement coupled with the need for injection of large quantities of metals, whose toxicity profiles were unknown, raised severe doubts as to the benefits of MRI extrinsic contrast enhancement. On the other hand, most pathologic lesions produce regions with increased T1 and T2 relaxation times regardless of their nature: tumor, edema, hemorrhage, inflammation, or necrosis.

It was soon recognized with the clinical development of water-soluble, unspecific gadolinium complexes (NMG2-Gd-DTPA, NMG-Gd-DOTA) that additional pathologies could be detected and better delineated, thus permitting an increase in diagnostic sensitivity and specificity with an enhancement of anatomic detail (Fig. 13). These first unspecific extracellular MRI contrast agents resulted in an extension of the clinical indications of MRI. Furthermore, considerable effort was directed toward specific, target-oriented paramagnetic derivatives and, second, toward the development of particulate magnetopharmaceuticals. Due to their high relaxation efficacy especially, superparamagnetic iron oxide particles promise a high clinical effectiveness.

More important for the future, MRI CAs will permit the extension of imaging conditions into regions with poor tissue contrast and signal. Agents such as the gadolinium complexes, which increase the tissue signal, will permit an image aquisition in regions

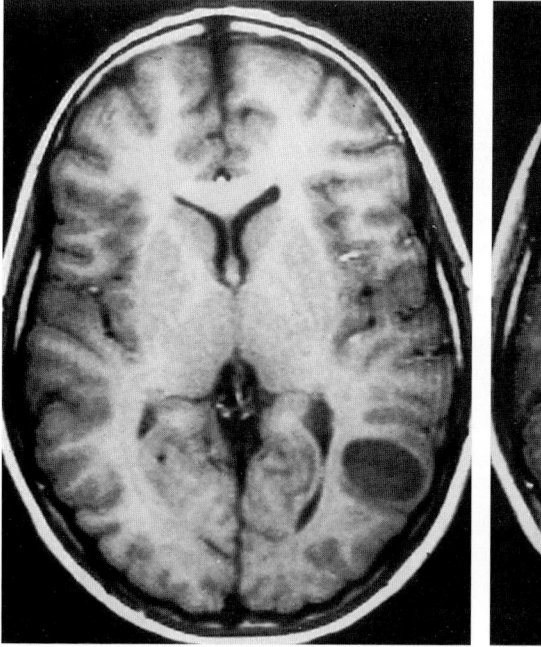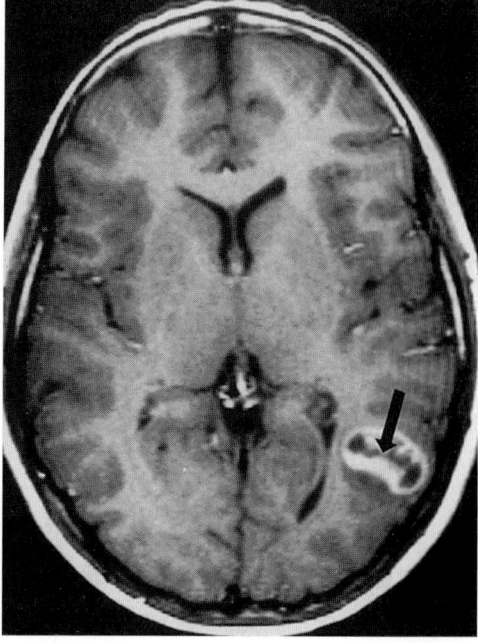

Figure 13. Left parieto-occipital tumor on a T1-weighted sequence: subependymal astrocytoma before and after Gd-DOTA administration. (From D. Balériaux Erasme, ULB, Belgium with the courtesy of Laboratoire Guerbet, Aulnay-sous-Bois, France.)

Table 12. *Classification of MRI CAs*

Signal enhancement	Central moiety	Distribution	Examples
Positive enhancement Paramagnetic chelates Predominant T1-effect Solute in solution	Gadolinium 3+	Extracellular	Gd-DTPA, Gd-DOTA, Gd-HP-DO3A, Gd-DOTA-BMA Gd-BOPTA
	Nitroxide radicals		Nitroxides
	Gadolinium 3+ Fatty water immiscible liquids	Gastrointestinal	Gd-DTPA buffer sol, vegetable oils, fatty emulsions, sucrose polyesters
	Gadolinium 3+	Vascular/blood pool agents	Albumines, dextranes, polylysines, PEGs, liposomes, short moieties like amino acid chains or sugar rests
	Gadolinium 3+ Iron 3+ Manganese 2+	Hepatocyte Anionic receptor	Gd-BOPTA, Gd-EOB-DTPA, Fe-HBed, Fe-EHPD Mn-DPDP
	Gadolinium 3+	RES-directed	Paramagnetic liposomes
	Gadolinium 3+	Lymph node	Polylysine-(Gd-DTPA)$_x$-dextrane
	Gadolinium 3+, various	Tumor directed	Metalloporphyrins Antibody-PEG-(Gd-DTPA)
Negative enhancement High magnetic moment Superparamagnetic particle suspensions Predominant T2 and susceptibility effect	Dysprosium 3+	Extracellular	Dy-DTPA, Dy-DTPA-BMA
	Iron oxides	Gastrointestinal	Iron oxide nanoparticles SPIO (Lumirem, Abdoscan)
	Water miscible		Barium sulfate suspensions, clays
	Water-immiscible liquids		PFOB, gas producing pellets
	Dysprosium 3+	Vascular/blood pool agents	Albumin-(Dy-DTPA)$_x$
	Iron oxides		MION, USPIO
	Iron oxides	Hepatocyte	AG-USPIO, MION-ASF
	Iron oxides	RES-directed	SPIO, USPIO, MION, superparamagnetic liposomes
	Iron oxides	Lymph node	USPIO, MION-46
	Iron oxides	Tumor	Antibody (Fab) carrying MIONs

with a low magnetization, rapid pulsing sequences, and/or small flip angles, thus improving discrimination and image-aquisition times. The ability to perform dynamic imaging with contrast agents also will enable potential assessment of organ function parameters, including perfusion studies and functional MRI studies (see Chap. 7).

Therefore, one of the goals of MRI CAs is to add functional information to the generally remarkable morphologic information available from the unenhanced images. Table 12 gives an overview over the different strategies of CA development, even though several of them still must prove to be efficacious and safe in the future.

Contrast Enhancement, Relaxivity, Susceptibility

Signal intensity on MRI images is primarily determined by proton relaxation times (T1 and T2) and by proton density (Table 13). The presence of a pharmaceutical can be imaged if it alters one of these parameters. The simplest strategy is to displace water, e.g., by filling the GI tract with a fatty emulsion or perfluorooctylbromide (PFOB, Imagent) and thus changing intraluminal signal intensity (modification of proton density).

However, the majority of MRI CAs are chosen for their ability to modify tissue relaxivity (T1 and T2 times of tissues). Thus a proton in vacuum relaxes in 10^{16} years, in an aqueous solution in about 1 second, and near magnetopharmaceuticals or MRI CAs in some milliseconds. In opposition to x-ray CAs, where the incident beam is scattered or blocked, MRI CAs have an indirect effect and "catalyze" the relaxivity of surrounding protons.

MRI CAs can be classified into four categories based on their effect on the nuclear magnetic resonance (NMR) behavior of nearby nuclei (Table 13). Relaxation enhancement of a certain complex can be characterized by its relaxivities R1 (longitudinal

Table 13. *Physicochemical strategies reflecting the different interactions between an MRI CA and the surrounding protons*

Shift reagents	Ni^{2+} Dy^{3+} Lanthanide shift reagents	Cause large changes in the resonant frequency, by up to hundreds of ppm Small changes in the relaxation rate Short electron spin relaxation time (short period of time for energetic interactions)
Relaxation agents	Gd^{3+}, Mn^{2+}, Cu^{2+}, Fe^{3+} (half-filled *f* or *d* electron shells)	Little shift in resonant frequency Large enhancement of nuclear relaxation rate Long electron spin relaxation time
Susceptibility agents	Superparamagnetic iron oxide particles, high concentrations of paramagnetic agents	High magnetic moment induces a strong local magnetic field (inhomogeneity) and thus increases dephasing and T2* relaxation
Displacement of protons	Fatty liquids and emulsions Perfluorooctylbromides (PFOBs)	Displacement of water by filling the compartment, of interest

relaxivity/spin-lattice) and R2 (transverse relaxivity/spin-spin), usually expressed in units of millimoles per second (molar relaxivity). If the resulting signal intensity (SI) is plotted versus concentration, a linear relationship exists for certain concentrations, as shown in Fig. 14.

Relaxation depends on resonance frequency and temperature, which must be specified. The linear relationship between relaxation rate and concentration of a complex is only valid for a certain concentration range, thus expressing in terms of a model the functioning rapid exchange between the bulk solvent environment and the coordination sites of the metal complex. The relaxation rate of protons in a water molecule coordinated to a paramagnetic ion is given by the *Salomon-Bloembergen equation,* which expresses the relaxation rate as the sum of dipolar (through space) and scalar (through bonds) contri-

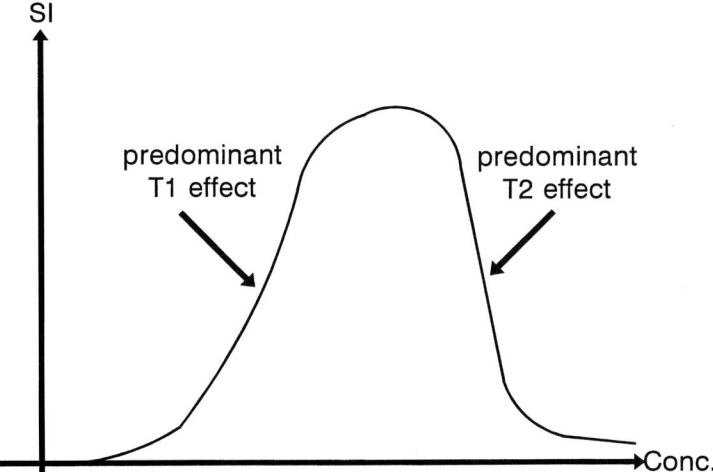

Figure 14. Plot of the signal intensity (SI) for an aqueous solution of a paramagnetic complex as a function of concentration. At low doses, paramagnetic chelates have a negligible effect on T2 relaxivity (ascending branch). At higher doses, T2 relaxation time shortening becomes large enough to overcome T1 effects (descending branch). Superparamagnetic ferrites usually have a predominant T2 relaxation time shortening, thus decreasing tissue signal intensity. In the case of USPIO or at low concentrations (without aggregates), a certain T1 effect can be noticed.

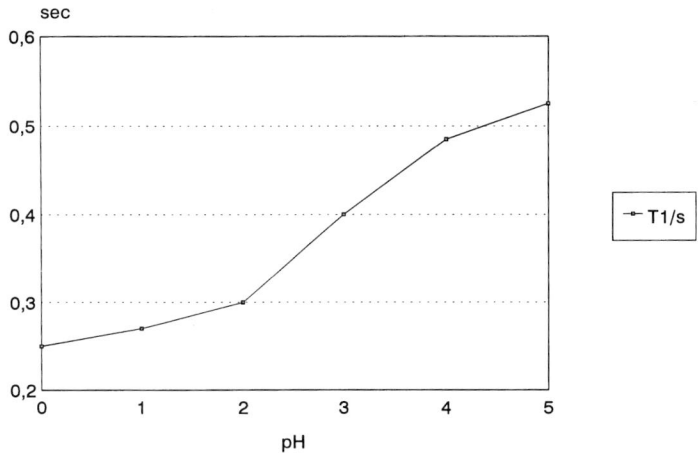

Figure 15. Dependence of the longitudinal relaxation time (T1) of the water protons of an 8 m*M* Cu-EDTA solution on the pH value of the solution.

butions (mainly inner sphere) to spin relaxation. Large molecules or more rigid ones rotate much more slowly and have longer rotational correlation times. This can cause a large increase in relaxivity.

Furthermore, the wide spectrum of interactions must be extended to the molecular interactions between the central metal ion with the surrounding protons where inner- and outer-sphere coordination and diffusibility of water molecules influence the relaxivity and energy exchange rate. Thus barium sulfate–gadolinium suspensions show a reduced T1 relaxivity compared with the free gadolinium solutions due to a reduced inner-sphere interaction because the free protons cannot get as close to the gadolinium central atom as in the free solutions. The predominant T2 effect of dysprosium depends on its large magnetic moment but very short electronic relaxation time, thus not allowing any inner-sphere interaction.

These fundamental concepts, which are valid for substances and especially complexes that can influence the NMR properties of water at high dilutions, can be controlled by varying either their chemical or magnetic properties. Thus these substances might be used as visual amplifiers and MRI-sensitive chemical indicators depicting the changed molecular environment in relation to certain functions: the spatial distribution of pH (Fig. 15) and the mapping of redox potential and reducing agents and of mass transport diffusion.

From the practical point of view, it is useful to divide these different relaxation mechanisms into two subclasses: (a) *paramagnetic positive enhancers* (see Fig. 13) and (b) *susceptibility effect, signal-suppressing negative CAs* (Fig. 16). In reality, this separation is arbitrary because they are often present together, and predominance depends on concentration, distribution, and pulse sequence. In order to classify the MRI CAs in development, one must consider as well their pharmacokinetics and their distribution volume (see Table 12).

The mathematical basis that predicts signal intensity (SI) in a tissue with known relaxation times for a spin-echo pulse sequence can be extracted from the Bloch equation:

$$\text{SI (SE)} = K(1 - e^{-TR/T1})\,(e^{-TE/T2})$$

where K is a constant. When TR $\gg$ T1, the first term $e^{-TR/T1}$ reaches 0, making signal intensity independent of T1. If TE $\ll$ T2, the second term approaches 1, making signal intensity independent of T2. Thus the image weighting defines the predominant relaxation and signal effect of an MRI CA. Since MRI CAs in general decrease both T1 and T2 relaxation times, one might expect the two effects to cancel each other. Fortunately, this does not occur because the effect of MRI CAs on relaxation times T1 and T2 is not equal. In the case of Gd complexes, only higher dosages exert a certain T2-dependent

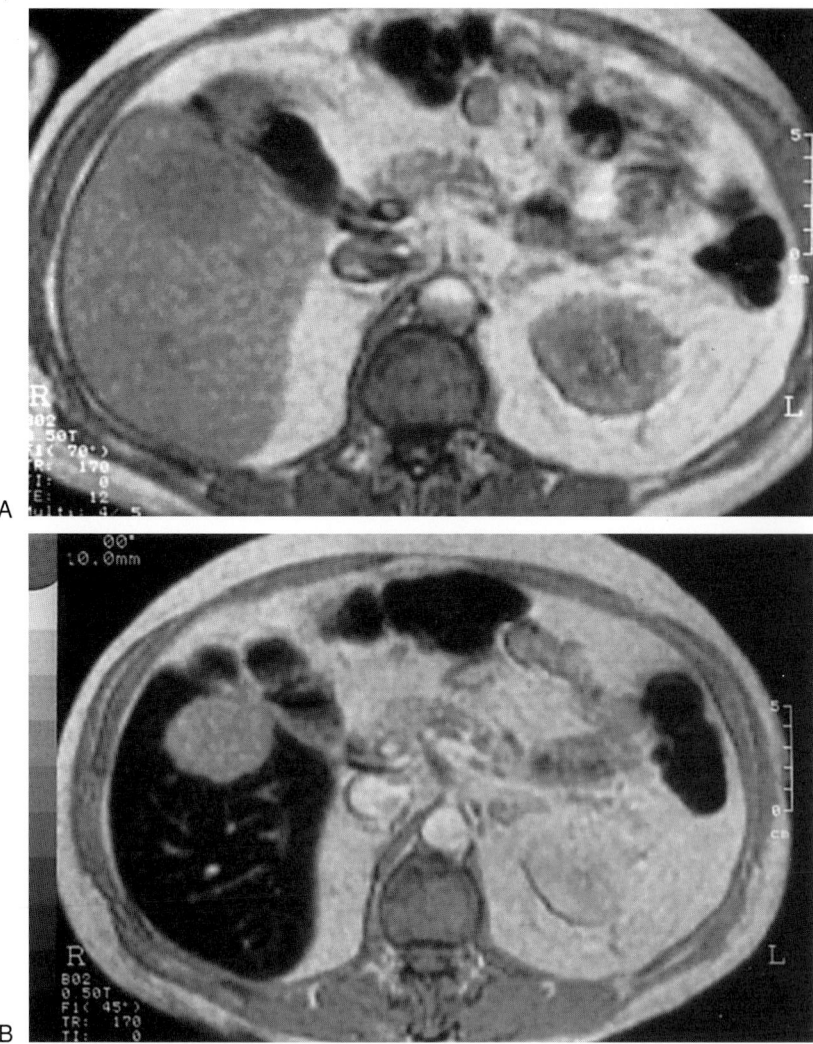

Figure 16. Liver metastasis from a colorectal cancer. Courtesy of Laboratoire Guerbet, Aulnay-sous-Bois, France. (**A**) Pre-Endorem section, T1-weighted gradient-echo (GE) sequence at 0.5 T (GE 170/70°/12). (**B**) Post-Endorem section, T2*-weighted gradient-echo (GE) sequence (GE 170/45°/12), demonstrating the better contrast-to-noise ratio. The strong decrease in signal intensity in the liver parenchyma depends on the endocytotic activity of Kupffer cells, which take up the superparamagnetic nanoparticles of iron oxide given intravenously. Focal liver lesions without such an uptake are better visualized.

SI decrease (e.g., concentrated Gd complexes in the renal collecting system and the urine of the bladder; Fig. 17). In general, a T1-weighted pulse sequence is the preferred image weighting to demonstrate the signal-enhancing effect of Gd complexes (Figs. 13 and 18).

Positive enhancers (paramagnetic) with unpaired electrons in the core interact with the relaxation of nearby water protons and predominantly affect T1 shortening at lower dosages, thus producing an SI increase.

Negative CAs (superparamagnetic, high magnetic moments) produce a strong localized disturbance of magnetic field homogeneity. Due to a cooperative alignment of the electronic spins of the individual paramagnetic atoms they contain, a high magnetic moment is created. The effect on water proton relaxation depends on the compartmentalization and arrangement of these negative MRI CAs. Nearby protons will experience this field inhomogeneity as a susceptibility effect (outer sphere) causing rapid dephasing of the spins (strong T2 and T2* effect). This effect is best seen on T2-weighted and gradient-echo pulse sequences (Figs. 16 and 19).

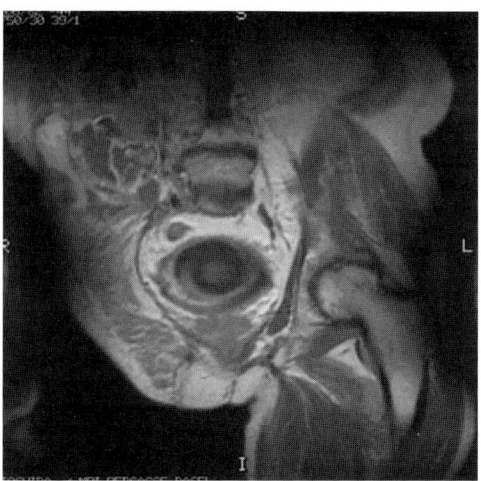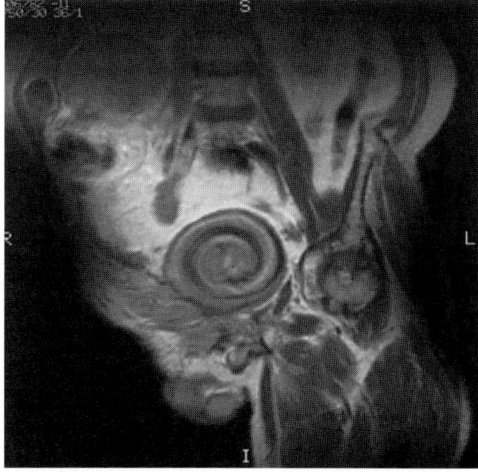

Figure 17. Coronal Gd-DOTA–enhanced T1-weighted sequences (SE 750/30) through the urinary bladder of a patient who had undergone hemipelvectomy. The spiral pattern is presumed to be caused by laminar flow of contrast containing urine causing a predominant T2 effect (SI decrease).

This can be exploited, for example, by increasing the intravascular magnetic susceptibility by injecting high amounts of paramagnetic or superparamagnetic compounds into the vessels. With the aid of imaging sequences of the gradient-echo type, these effects can be maximized.

T1 or inner-sphere interactions depend on the accessibility of the central core to water protons and thus on the size and compartmentalization of the iron oxide particles. Certain smaller nanoparticles have a high R1 relaxivity, thus increasing the signal in the vascular space when injected intravascularly (see Fig. 14).

Physicochemical Properties

The two basic requirements for an MRI CA are (a) that it has a favorable safety profile and (b) that it sufficiently enhances the relaxivity of surrounding tissue water protons. Biocompatibility is governed mainly by the interrelated properties of complex chemistry of the paramagnetic chelates: thermodynamic stability, pH-dependent or protonation equilibrium, entropy and enthalpy of chelate formation, stability with respect to release of the metal ion, and low affinity for competing ions (Ca^{2+}, Cu^{2+}, Zn^{2+}, Fe^{3+}) present physiologically (Table 14).

While the biocompatibilty is optimized due to the strong captation and shielding of the central metal ion with the aid of a chelating ligand, the number of exchanging water molecules with the complex is reduced compared with a plain gadolinium chloride

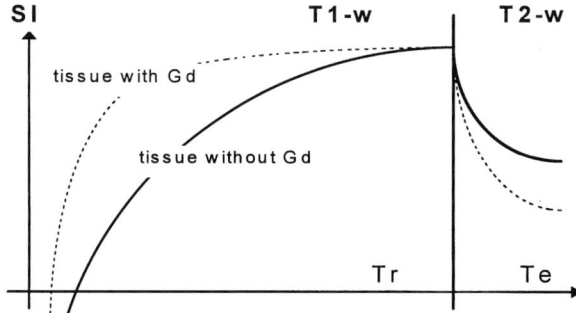

Figure 18. Pharmaceutical alteration of MRI signal intensity due to T1 or T2 weighting (compare with Fig. 17).

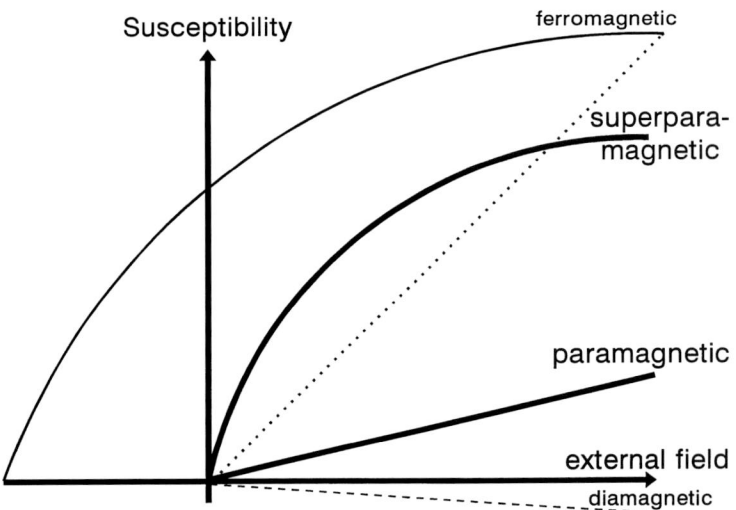

Figure 19. Magnetic susceptibility in relation to the magnetic property of the central atom.

solution, thus reducing molar relaxivity. From a practical point of view, a solution for GI use preferably should be stabilized with the aid of a buffer in order to maintain thermodynamic stability and reduce eventual release of gadolinium at a low pH (Fig. 20).

Pharmacokinetics

The pharmacokinetic behavior of the extracellular agents is analogous to that of water-soluble iodine contrast agents. Once applied intravascularly, they have a distribution half-life of about 2.5 minutes, have a rapid plasma clearance, and are distributed into the extracellular space, enhancing the tissue in proportion to tissue perfusion (at equilibrium state). In the CNS they normally do not cross the blood-brain barrier but enhance tissue lacking this barrier (pituitary glands, tumors, inflammatory foci). Elimination is mainly governed by glomerular filtration without metabolization ($t_{1/2\beta}$ = 90 min). The usual clinical dose of the 0.5 M concentrated commercialized solutions is 0.1 to 0.2 mmol/kg of body weight or 0.2 to 0.4 ml/kg of body weight. The distribution volumes depict the interstitial distribution, with 17 liters for an adult.

Initially, perfusion and later blood pool differences of organs can be compared when they equilibrate during various distribution phases after injection. Since the contrast of a tissue or a lesion to surrounding tissue depends on signal-intensity differences, the kinetic profile in relation to the imaging protocol and the resulting temporal signal change determine diagnostic sensitivity and conspicuity. Thus a microadenoma in the pituitary gland might only be depicted during the early vascular distribution phase, while it will become isointense on delayed scans.

Table 14. *Main physicochemical properties of the extracellular gadolinium complexes in clinical use*

	Gd-DOTA	Gd-DTPA	Gd-DTPA-BMA	Gd-HP-DO3A
DCI	Meglumine gadoterate	Dimeglumine gadopentetate	Gadodiamide	Gadoteridol
Structure	Macrocycle ionic	Linear ionic	Linear nonionic (neutral)	Macrocycle nonionic (neutral)
Thermodynamic stability at pH = 7.4 (log K)	18.8	17.7	14.9	17.1
Kinetic stability: half-life in HCl 0.1 M	>1 month	10 min	30 seconds	3 hours
Transmetallization with Zn^{2+}	1%	21%	25%	1%
Osmolality, mOsm/kg H_2O	1350	1940	790	630
Additional stabilization	0	0.2% meglumine-DTPA	5% NaCa-DTPA-BMA	0.1% Ca-HP-DO3A

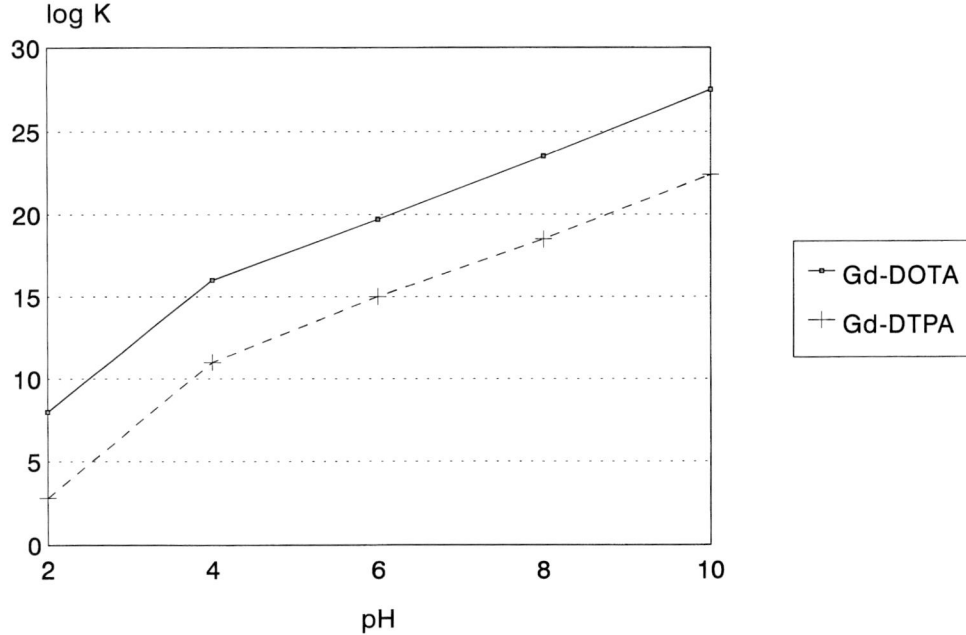

log K

Figure 20. Plot of the conditional thermodynamic stabilities of Gd-DOTA and Gd-DTPA as a function of pH.

Reticulo-endothelial-system (RES)-directed superparamagnetic contrast agents, a new class of MRI CAs with selective uptake in the liver, spleen, bone marrow, and other RES-containing organs show a longer, controllable vascular persistence (vascular distribution half-life = 15 minutes to 24 hours) and a highly variable ferrite degradation. Their pharmacokinetics depend on the particle size (50 to 150 nm) and the coating (particle charge, repulsion). Due to their long intracellular persistence (when endocytosed in the liver) and their potent magnetic properties, the imaging windows are prolonged to at least 6 hours, with signal decrease even lasting for several days. Doses range between 10 and 20 μmol Fe per kilogram of body weight. Eventually, the metabolized iron becomes part of the normal body iron stores and is thus innocuous.

Tolerance and Toxicity

The safety profile of the water-soluble gadolinium complexes Gd-DTPA, GD-DOTA, Gd-DTPA-BMA, and Gd-HP-DO3A seems to be excellent for a dose range of 0.1 to 0.3 mmol/kg and with an incidence of reactions quite similar to that of saline solutions. Postmarketing surveys (Table 15) and clinical studies reveal that the range of adverse events (AEs) is quite similar to that for iodinated CAs but with a much lower incidence

Table 15. *Adverse events (AEs) in postmarketing studies with Gd-DOTA*

Type of AE	No. AEs	Incidence (%) in 4169 cases
Nausea/vomiting	13	0.31
Local warmth/coldness	7	0.16
Headache	4	0.10
Dizziness	5	0.12
Urticaria	2	0.05
Paresthesia/mouth sensations	3	0.07
Respiratory problems	1	0.02
Others	8	0.19

From Neiss AC et al: Efficacité et tolérance du DOTA-Gd lors d'une enquête multicentrique européenne. Résultats préliminaires sur 4169 cas. *Rev Im Med*, 3, 383–387 (1991).

Table 16. *Influence of Gd complexes on signal intensity*

Influence: none or very little	Moderate	Significant
Cerebrospinal liquid	Liver	Kidney/urine
Healthy brain parenchyma	Pancreas	Nasal mucosa
Muscle	Gastrointestinal mucosa	Tumors, metastases
Fat	Infarctions (time window)	Inflammations
Bone (disk)	Ischemia	MS: active lesions
Bile, gall bladder	Synovial liquids	Infections
Cysts		Postoperative scars
Necrosis		Vessel display (venous)
Fibrous tissue		Hemangioma
Organ epithelium		Synovial proliferation
Some benign or devitalized tumors		

and a dose-dependent predominance of idiosyncratic reactions. The most common noted AEs are headache, injection-site coldness or warmth, nausea, localized pain, paresthesia, dizziness, and in rare cases, allergy-like reactions. Stronger anaphylactoid reactions with shock, glottic edema, and dyspnea are extremely rare but may arise more frequently in the case of known allergies. Injection rate does not influence tolerability. With linear complexes, a transient serum iron and bilirubin rise can be observed in about 10% to 20% of the patients, which is probably due to a hemolytic effect.

Even in patients with renal failure or impairment, a good renal tolerance has been demonstrated. The elimination through the kidneys is prolonged, but in patients with a glomerular filtration rate of 20 ml/min, no effect on electrolytes, serum creatinine, or distribution volume can be demonstrated. The faster removal by hemodialysis should be considered.

In the case of the liver-specific superparamagnetic nanoparticles of iron oxide (SPIO, ferumoxides-USAN, Endorem, Feridex), their pharmaceutical stabilization and specific application form seem to define tolerance. Thus, initially, when used as a bolus injection, hypotension was reported, while the slow infusion of the diluted suspension is well tolerated with some transient AEs reported. Lumbar pain, which is well known from iron injections in general, is the most frequent AE (4.7% in the clinical studies). Probably the exhaustion of opsonization is at the origin of this effect. The injected iron is incorporated into the body iron pool but degraded at a slow rate, thus allowing a long imaging window (6 to 24 hours) (see Fig. 16).

Clinical Use

In addition to the issue of disease detection, there is the objective of characterizing (tissue typing) abnormal tissues detected. The pharmaceutical manipulation of tissue signal intensity has been recognized as a possible solution to improve sensitivity, specificity, and accuracy by improving the detection rate and the delineation and characterization of lesions.

The general dosage is 0.1 mmol Gd per kilogram of body weight or 0.2 ml/kg. In certain cases, the dosage may be increased in order to depict more CNS lesions (sensitivity). In contrast to CT, no MRI CAs are required to delineate the vessels. For very fast three-dimensional (3D) angiography techniques using extremely short TRs, gadolinium might be necessary to increase the blood signal. In the CNS, all areas of increased permeability of the blood-brain barrier without necrosis are prone to signal increase through the administration of gadolinium (see Fig. 13). In the rest of the body, areas with a high proportion of interstitial fluid (mucosa, inflammation), with a rapid perfusion and long intrinsic relaxation times show the highest increase in signal intensity (Table 16). Functional information that potentially can be obtained includes organ and lesion perfusion, blood pool, renal function, and monitoring of therapy.

The most promising area for using current MRI CAs to quantitatively assess function is brain perfusion as the blood-brain barrier prevents interstitial leakage (see Chap. 3).

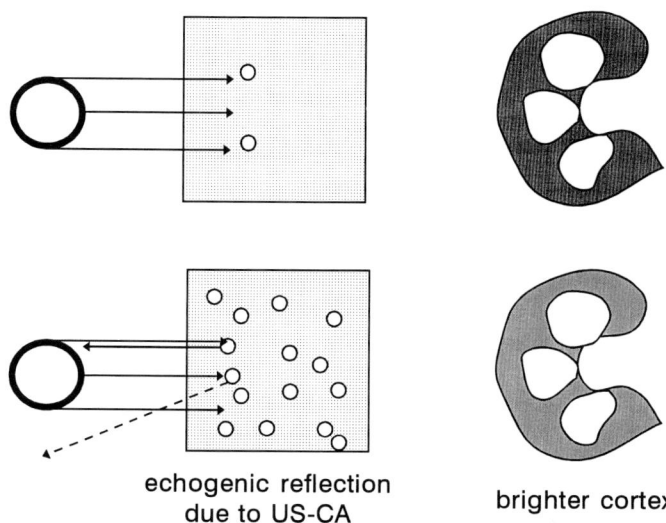

echogenic reflection
due to US-CA

brighter cortex

Figure 21. Effects of US CAs on gray-scale images: more echogenic reflection from the vascular bed, thus making the renal cortex brighter on the image.

This allows one to measure quantitatively the blood volume–dependent dilution effect of different parts of the brain.

In addition to reducing significantly the size threshold for MRI detection of liver lesions, the SPIO-based liver MRI CAs allow one to improve characterization of these lesions (hemangioma with signal increase in T1-weighted pulse sequences, benign lesions with a T2*-dependent signal decrease due to active endocytosis) and to depict diffuse endocytotic functioning of RES containing tissue (liver, spleen, bone marrow, pathologies) (see Fig. 16).

ULTRASOUND CONTRAST AGENTS: ECHOPHARMACEUTICALS

Similar to x-rays, sound waves pass through the various tissues and are attenuated by either scattering (reflection or refraction) or energy absorption. However, unlike x-ray imaging, the production of ultrasound images is based on detecting the reflected portion (echo) of the attenuated sound waves (Fig. 21). Whether or not a sound wave will be reflected at a given tissue component is primarily dependent on the acoustic impedance properties, which are defined by its density and the velocity of sound in the medium. Spatial resolution is also dependent on the sound frequency, where high frequencies have a good resolution but small penetration depth and low frequencies are the opposite. Since the acoustic impedance values between the various soft tissues are small, echopharmaceuticals (US CAs) have been proposed to increase acoustic impedance differences at tissue interfaces and secondly to increase the respective echo intensity, thus depicting directly filled compartments or moving agents (Table 17) (see Chap. 10).

Further applications that have increased the clinical importance of ultrasound are the possibility to measure blood flow velocities through the *Doppler effect,* thus integrating functional information into a morphologic image (see Chap. 10).

The investigation of echogenicity of US CAs was based mainly on their substantial acoustic impedance differences relative to soft tissue. The most effective principle by far that has emerged is the diffraction of ultrasonic waves on gas bubbles (microbubble-containing solutions and emulsions) and colloidal, sometimes temperature-dependent diphasic systems (Table 17) (pharmaceuticals). Microbubbles must be smaller than 8 μm in diameter to cross the lung capillary bed.

Blood pool imaging seems to be the most important clinical feature, even though tissue-targeted agents are under development and several GI approaches may succeed.

Table 17. *Potential ultrasound contrast agents: echopharmaceuticals*

Form	Substances	Properties, indications

Solutions	Shaken saline
	Indocyanin green
	0.5 *M* sodium citrate
	0.2 *M* calcium
	  gluconate
		Gas bubbles: short half-life, difficult
		  reproducibility, cavitation and shaking
		  effects

Colloidal
  emulsions
  (foams)
	Perfluorooctylbromide
	  (PFOB)
	Lipid emulsions
	Dodecafluoropentane
	  (EchoGen) liquid-
	  liquid dispersion
		High density, low acoustic velocity,
		  accumulation in the RES
		Narrow size distribution (0, 1–2 μm)
		Converts to a gas at body temperature
		  (phase shifting)
		Droplets 0.3 μm; as a gas they have a
		  substantial decrease in density: diameter
		  of 2 to 5 μm
		Lower solubility in blood, thus a longer
		  persistence, prolonged Doppler
		  enhancement (15 min)

Colloidal
  suspensions
	Iodipamide
	  ethyl ester
	  microparticles	

Suspensions
  with gas
  microbubbles
	Galactose
	  microparticle
	  suspension
	  (Echovist)
		10-ml portion of an aqueous microparticle
		  suspension (99% < 12 μm) with very
		  fine gas bubbles (3 μm/97% < 7 μm);
		  viscosity 11.4 mPa · s (25°C); can't
		  pass the lung capillary bed
		Right heart disease diagnostics
		Septum defects
		Hysterosalpingography
		Phlebography

	Levovist: galactose
	  microparticle
	  suspension
	  forming
	  microbubbles
	  contains 0.1%
	  palmitic acid as a
	  flexible monolayer
	  stabilizer
		Crosses the lungs
		Withstands the intracardiac systolic
		  pressure
		Bubbles: 1–8 μm, mean 2–3 μm

	Gas-filled albumin
	  capsules (Albunex)
		Systemic vascular enhancement due to a
		  higher longevity
		Limited echogenicity: B mode
		Diameter 4–10 μm
		  Left wall motion assessment
		  Transpulmonary transit time
		  Left ventricular washout

The indications can be summarized to

Blood vessels	→	detection of weak signals and slow flow
Body cavities	→	delineation and communications
Functional, vascular	→	transit time for hemodynamics
Functional, targeted	→	to highlight metabolic properties
With microbubbles	→	for remote pressure measurements
Intraluminal	→	endothelial damage or plaque characterization

The ability to track the passage of a bolus of an injected echo enhancer through an organ or region of interest opens up the possibility for functional studies. Measurements are obtained by generating a time-reflectivity curve, the reflectivity being obtained either directly, by digital capture of the ultrasound signals (B mode, spectral, or color Doppler), or indirectly, by measuring the loudness of the spectral Doppler audio output or the density on film of the B-mode or color changes (video densitometry).

Echo enhancers further provide an increase in the diagnostic confidence of Doppler sonography by increasing the signal-to-noise ratio and thus increasing the diagnostic certainty.

If the in vivo acoustic properties of these different systems are known, it should be possible to quantify the contrast concentration in blood and measure tissue blood volume and blood flow. This should lead to the direct imaging of ischemia and other disorders exhibiting abnormal flow and perfusion (tumors, reflux in the bladder) and offer new perspectives for the diagnosis of vascular pathologies (stenosis, thrombosis), especially in the cranium with the help of transcranial duplex sonography. Due to the improvement in signal (25 dB), currently difficult examinations may become useful as an increase in the level of confidence for most ultrasound examinations can be expected. Future prospects include the direct measurement of pressure changes within the heart and vessels (size variation of the gaseous phase due to pressure changes).

REFERENCES

1. Aguirre FV et al. Impact of ionic and non-ionic contrast media on post-PTCA ischemic complications: Results from the EPIC trial. *J Am Coll Cardiol,* February (Suppl), 901–914 (1995).
2. Beer H-F, Bläuenstein PA, Hasler PH et al. In vitro and in vivo evaluation of iodine-123-RO 16-0154: A new imaging agent for SPECT investigations of benzodiazepine receptors. *J Nucl Med,* 31, 1007 (1990).
3. Bettmann MA. Intravascular contrast agents: Current problems and future solutions: A review. *Acta Radiol,* 37(Suppl. 400), 3–7 (1996).
4. Bull BS, Smith DC. Effects of contrast agents on blood clotting. *J Invasive Cardiol,* 3, 24–30 (1991).
5. Chronos NAF et al. Profound platelet degranulation is an important side effect of some types of contrast media used in interventional cardiology. *Circulation,* 88, 2035–2044 (1993).
6. Cosgrove D (Ed.). Ultrasonographic echo-enhancing agents. *Clin Radiol,* 51(Suppl 1), (1996).
7. Dawson P, Clauss W. *Kontrastmittel in der Praxis.* Berlin: Springer-Verlag (1993).
8. Eckelmann WC, Reba RC. The classification of radiotracers. *J Nucl Med,* 19, 1179 (1987).
9. Elke M. (Ed.). *Kontrastmittel in der radiologischen Diagnostik. Eigenschaften-Nebenwirkungen-Behandlung.* Stuttgart: Thieme (1992).
10. Fischer AE, Hall LD. Roles for paramagnetic substances in MRI: Contrast agents, molecular amplifiers, and indicators for redox and pH mapping. *MAGMA,* 2, 203–210 (1994).
11. Hardeman MR et al. Activation of platelets by low-osmolar contrast media: Differential effects of ionic and nonionic agents. *Radiology,* 192, 563 (1994).
12. Hay KL, Bull BS. Analysis of platelet activation and aggregation produced by three classes of contrast media. *JVIR,* 6, 211 (1995).
13. Kowalsky RJ, Perry JR. Radiopharmaceuticals in nuclear medicine practice. In: S Baum (Ed.). Series: *Current Practice in Nuclear Medicine.* Stamford CT: Appleton & Lange (1987).
14. Krause W et al. Physicochemical parameters of x-ray contrast media. *Invest Radiol,* 29(1), 72–80 (1994).
15. Mazière B, Mazière M. Where have we got to with neuroreceptor mapping of human brain? *Eur J Nucl Med,* 16, 817–835 (1990).
16. Neiss AC et al. Efficacité et tolérance du DOTA-Gd lors d'une enquête multicentrique européenne. Résultats préliminaires sur 4169 cas. *Rev Im Med,* 3, 383–387 (1991).
17. Nygren A et al. Effects of intravenous contrast media on cortical and medullary blood flow in the rat kidney. *Invest Radiol,* 23, 753–761 (1989).
18. Peters PE, Zeitler E. *Röntgenkontrastmittel-Nebenwirkungen-Prophylaxe-Therapie.* Berlin: Springer-Verlag (1991).
19. Pugh ND, Sissons GRJ, Ruttley M. The effect of iodixanol, a new isotonic contrast agent, on femoral blood flow in man. *Clin Radiol,* 45, 243–245 (1992).
20. Richards P. Nuclide generators. In: GA Andrews, RM Knisely, HN Wagner Jr (Eds.). *Radioactive pharmaceuticals.* Oak Ridge, TN: U.S. Atomic Energy Commission, 155 (1965).
21. Schelbot HR. Current status and prospect of new radionuclides and radiopharmaceuticals for cardiovascular nuclear medicine. *Semin Nucl Med,* XVII, 145–181 (1987).
22. Schubiger PA, Alberto R, Smith A. Vehicles, chelators, and radionuclides: Choosing the ''building blocks'' of an effective therapeutic radioimmunoconjugate. *Bioconjug Chem,* 7, 165–179 (1996).
23. Schubiger PA, Hasler P-H et al. Evaluation of a multicentre study with Iomazenil a benzodiazepine receptor ligand. *Nucl Med Commun,* 12, 569–582 (1991).
24. Steinbrich W, Gross-Fengels W (Eds.). *Interventional radiology. Adjunctive medication and monitoring.* Berlin: Springer-Verlag (1993).
25. Stöcklin G. Tracers for metabolic imaging of brain and heart-radiochemistry and radiopharmacology. *Eur J Nucl Med,* 19, 527 (1992).
26. Swanson DP, Chilton HM, Thrall JH. *Pharmaceuticals in medical imaging.* New York: Macmillan (1990).
27. Verbruggen AM. Radiopharmaceuticals: State of the art. *Eur J Nucl Med,* 17, 346–364 (1990).

Functional Imaging, edited by
Gustav von Schulthess and Jürgen Hennig.
Lippincott–Raven Publishers, Philadelphia, © 1998.

3

Principles of Quantitative Function Analysis: Physiologic Modeling

Gustav K. von Schulthess, Cyrill Burger, and Alfred Buck

INTRODUCTION

Understanding a physiologic process implies that we make ourselves a model of this process. This model may help us to understand the process qualitatively but also to analyze the process quantitatively using mathematical methods. In this chapter we examine some of the basic assumptions involved in understanding physiologic processes in general. Very notably, tissue perfusion is an important physiologic process in most organs. Therefore, a substantial fraction of this chapter is devoted to tissue perfusion and its analysis. A second quantity that is important for quantitative analysis of many processes, including perfusion, is blood volume, and therefore, this chapter also will discuss some basic aspects involving the determination of blood volume. The remainder of the chapter is devoted to other important physiologic parameters, namely, tissue oxygenation and the general analysis of kinetics of metabolism and receptor-ligand kinetics as encountered in the analysis of cerebral receptor systems. The aim of this chapter is to emphasize the principles common to the methods used to analyze function, while specific procedures particular to an imaging modality are discussed in Chaps. 6, 7, 9, and 11. Thus the general principles of function analysis are discussed here, and the specific applications are discussed in the respective chapters on the imaging modalities.

Quantitative analysis of a physiologic process requires a model. The great ''art'' of modeling is to choose the ''right'' model, that is, to identify a model that adequately

GK von Schulthess, C Burger, and A Buck: Department of Medical Radiology, Nuclear Medicine, University Hospital, Zurich, Switzerland.

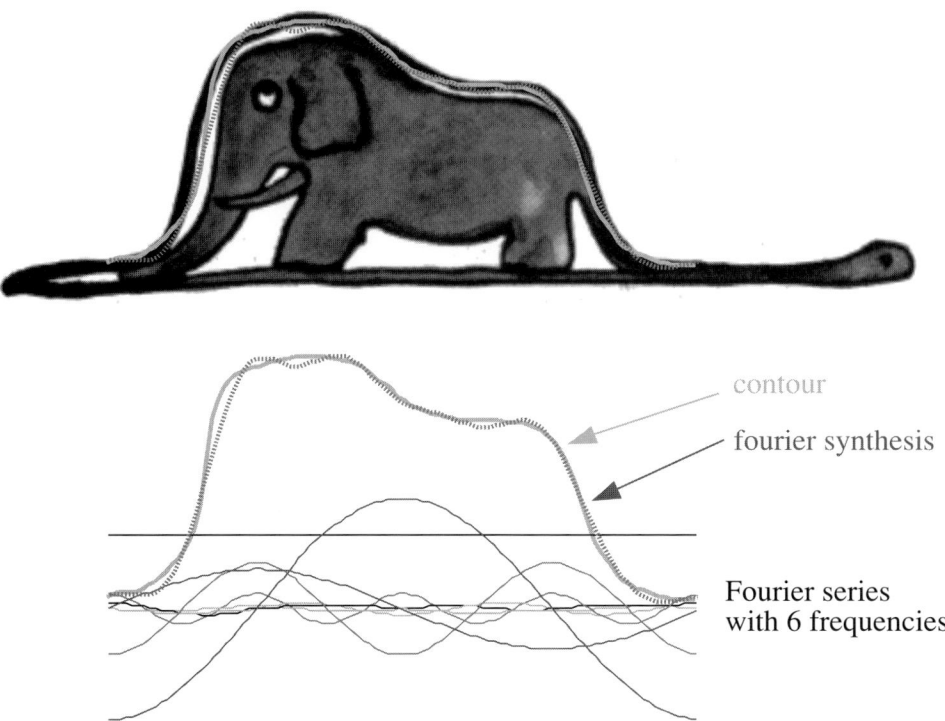

Figure 1. This famous illustration taken from St. Exupéry's "The Little Prince" shows how simple it is to fit even an elephant, here eaten by a snake and as seen by the little prince, with a quite limited number of parameters. The fits using an increasing number of Fourier harmonics are shown up to the choice of six free parameters, where the fit is already quite adequate. The use of Fourier harmonics is a standard procedure in curve fitting; sine waves of increasing frequency covering a fixed spatial interval are used to approximate the desired function, which in our case is the outline of the elephant.

describes the process under evaluation with a minimum of free parameters. This is very important because usually the data to be analyzed are not very accurate. Hence the use of too many free parameters—introduced by too complex a model to analyze the data—will result in arbitrary predictions. It is common knowledge taught to physics students in the first years that "with four parameters you can fit an elephant and with six also his trunk," as illustrated in Fig. 1, where the outline of the famous elephant eaten by a snake as drawn by St. Exupéry in his "Little Prince" is fitted with consecutive Fourier harmonics: the Fourier elephant!

On the other hand, if the model oversimplifies matters, it will be unable to describe the experimental data appropriately and therefore provide no insight. Then the model will fail to yield a good mathematical fit to the data. A simple model is also useless except for telling us that the process studied is more complex than we thought it was. It was Einstein who once said, "A model should be as simple as possible, but not simpler."

When trying to understand physiologic or pathophysiologic interactions of biomolecules in the human body, the physicochemical equilibrium or dynamic processes in which these molecules are involved have to be studied in order to derive a model. Equilibrium processes are easier to study because of the virtually unlimited measurement time available. In the human body, such processes are usually just in a "quasi-equilibrium." Such quasi-equilibrium states exist due to some homeostatic control system that maintains the concentration of a given substance constant, and they do not approximate an equilibrium process in the true physical sense. Examples of such quasi-equilibria are the tight control of body electrolyte concentrations, blood glucose level, even blood cell counts, and most conceivable other substances or cell populations.

Studying dynamic processes is usually much more interesting but more difficult, since measurements have to be obtained frequently enough to not miss the essential temporal

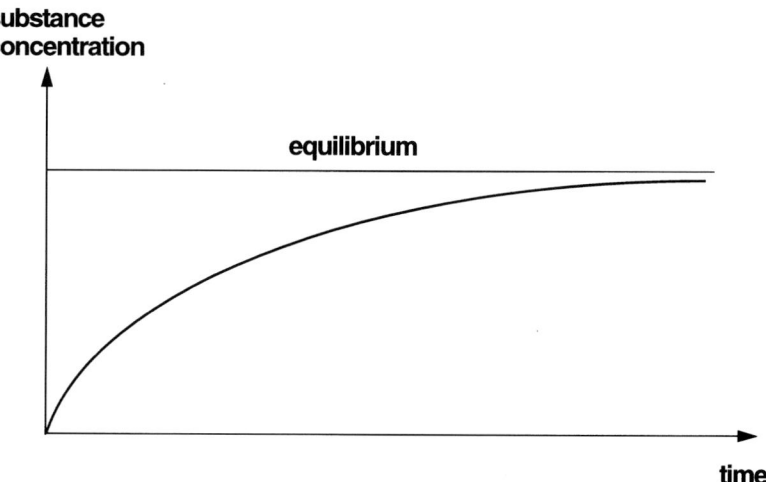

Figure 2. A simple example of the behavior of a system as a function of time is the monoexponential approach of a "concentration" to a final value. Mathematically, this curve is given by the function $C(t) = C(0)(1 - e^{t/T})$. Various processes are modeled with this expression, e.g., the concentration of bound ligand molecules to receptor sites as a function of time provided that the receptor sites are present in much larger quantities than the ligand and that the ligand binds slowly to the receptor after injection. MR experts among the readers will recognize immediately that this is the function describing the behavior of the z magnetization in an MR experiment; the final concentration is here the "concentration of magnetization." Notice that this curve requires the fitting of two parameters, $C(0)$ and T, and also notice that measuring the system under equilibrium conditions will only give us $C(0)$; determination also of T requires several data points along the entire curve.

features of the process. When a system is disturbed and one observes it as it approaches the equilibrium again, one can determine important constants that characterize the system, such as kinetic uptake constants, kinetic receptor affinity constants, etc. In fact, chemists have long used instant variations in temperature, pressure, and other physical variables (temperature, pressure, etc. "jump" experiments) to disturb the equilibrium of a system and observe how it approaches equilibrium again. Such an approach permits one to quantify chemical reaction rate constants using relatively simple mathematical formalisms. In fact, magnetic resonance (MR) experiments are also such experiments, since the spins are disturbed in their magnetization equilibrium and then observations are made of how the system approaches equilibrium magnetization again. An illustration of the simple behavior of a disturbed system in its approach to equilibrium is given in Fig. 2.

While this approach is useful to study reaction processes in vitro, it also can be used to study physiologic processes in vivo. Concentration jump experiments are used to study dynamic physiologic process whenever marker substances are introduced into the body by intravenous injection or inhalation, rarely by arterial or intrathecal injection. As the bolus passes through the cardiovascular system, perfusion can be studied, and if the reaction is slow enough so that a ligand can distribute itself in the body, the reaction of this ligand with a "receptor" or whatever binding site can be evaluated. This type of experiment has indeed become the mainstay in the study of physiologic and pathophysiologic processes in vivo. The principle is the same, whether various types of x-ray, MRI, or ultrasound contrast media are injected, and certainly applies to nuclear medicine (NM) procedures including positron emission tomography (PET), where the latter represents the paradigmatic methodology for quantification of human biochemical processes in vivo, but it also applies to spin-labeling procedures in MR spectroscopy. Of all the tracer substances used, only radiopharmaceuticals in NM have been successful to the point where clinically relevant data are extracted routinely from the temporal course of radioactivity in an organ after injection of the radiopharmaceutical. In CT, contrast media are almost exclusively used for contrast enhancement (see Chap. 2), although some work has demonstrated that in principle standard contrast media transit (2) and xenon (13, 22) can be used to determine perfusion in the brain. In MRI, the combination of ultrafast image-acquisition techniques (14, 36, 38) and contrast media bolus injections might become useful to determine some functional parameters. This is due to the facts that no unacceptable radiation burden is incurred when imaging the same section multiple times and that MRI contrast agents are effective at doses typically a factor 10 smaller than x-ray contrast agents (see Chap. 2). In MR spectroscopy (MRS), pharmacology can be studied when injecting marker substances such as ^{13}C-labeled compounds in ^{13}C spectroscopy or by specifically saturating the spins of a certain compound and assessing how this saturation affects related metabolites. To understand such experiments, modeling is also relevant. MRS also can be used to study dynamic processes if metabolites are measured as a function of various physiologic states, i.e., before and after exercise. Nevertheless, MRS most often measures actual concentrations of biomolecules rather than the turnover of these substances. The major drawback of MRS is currently its very limited spatial resolution and low sensitivity, making many important processes in the body unaccessible to in vivo analysis by MRS techniques. Ultrasound contrast media are used mainly to enhance the vasculature (see Chap. 2). Their effects also occur at high concentrations comparable with those used in x-ray diagnosis. In summary, NM procedures can be used to evaluate a wide range of physiologic processes. MRI and MRS show great promise to yield functional information in physiologic processes involving relatively large concentrations of molecules. What kind of processes are accessible to MR studies is yet to be seen, but it is clear that MR methods are at best able to detect concentrations of molecules in the micromolar range. Sonographic and x-ray contrast agents are used in millimolar to molar quantities and can be used to characterize processes such as perfusion, blood volume, and renal, hepatobiliary, and reticuloendothelial clearance.

Since in most imaging experiments that make use of contrast media or radiopharmaceuticals a substance is injected, the first key problem we have to analyze to understand measurements of physiologic processes in vivo is perfusion. Perfusion as the main mechanism to supply various organs with oxygen and nutrients is an important process to be studied in itself, and many methods have been developed to assess tissue perfusion. Often it is also extremely relevant to incorporate perfusion into a model to be used for the quantitative analysis of a metabolic or receptor system. If the reaction in such a system occurs with similar time constants as the passage of a bolus through the organ studied, the system behavior cannot be understood if perfusion effects are ignored. Even in a biochemical process such as receptor binding, the perfusion effect (i.e., getting the receptor marker to the site of action, like the brain cells) can dominate the entire process. Hence one can find oneself in a situation where even though one attempts to measure a receptor density in a given tissue, a tracer with ''bad'' characteristics will—while binding to the receptor—not demonstrate this receptor binding but, in the final analysis, serve merely as a tracer to quantify perfusion.

Modeling is of major relevance in physiologic studies for two reasons. First, a quantitative understanding of a process is possible only by defining a model of how a substance injected into the body will behave as it distributes itself among different compartments and as it interacts with various binding sites. Once the model has been defined and computed predictions of the model have been derived, they can be compared with the data measured. This applies to modeling of data obtained with imaging methods in general. Second and more specific to NM data, the substances used to study biochemical processes often are not inert biochemically; they undergo metabolic changes. Since in NM one only detects the decay of the radioactive isotopes but not the entire molecule, one has to quantitatively understand how the tracer distributes itself during the time course after injection and in what biochemical forms it will appear. Forcibly, there will be some emphasis on radioactive tracer methods because they are most sensitive to study biochemical systems and can evaluate processes such as receptor binding, which involves reactions of substances present merely in nano- and picomolar concentrations. A vast array of biochemical processes can thus be studied with NM with little or no interference with the process by the injection of the tracer.

Modeling has therefore a particular relevance in NM examinations, but as stated, attempts are being made to also use MR contrast agents to evaluate processes other than perfusion and blood pool distribution. While the concepts are formulated in words such that the interested reader can understand them without any substantial mathematical background, some quantitative analyses are also given.

TISSUE PERFUSION

General Considerations

As stated, the measurement of tissue perfusion is probably the single most important undertaking in quantitative function imaging. This is not only due to the fact that substrates have to get to the various tissues by perfusion but that many organs respond to certain stimuli by an increase in perfusion. This perfusion increase may be altered by physiologic interventions or by disease. Notable examples are the increased coronary perfusion during exercise and the increased splanchnic perfusion under caloric stimulation but also the observation that neural activation by various tasks leads to increased perfusion of the involved cerebral territories. This effect has been used in PET and more recently in functional MRI experiments to understand cerebral function as a response to various stimuli.

Various degrees of model complexity are needed to quantify tissue perfusion depending on the question asked, the substance used, and the experimental setup. We shall explore here the various models and their complexity so as to understand the approaches taken in measuring perfusion with the different imaging modalities. At the basis of any quantitative perfusion measurement is the conservation of mass principle, which simply states that the amount of substance in a volume of interest, also called the *central volume,* must equal the amount that has flowed into that region minus the amount that has left it. Quite obviously, an inert substance (one that does not undergo chemical transformation) neither can be created nor can it disappear in the central volume. If we use the concentration of the substance, which is equal to mass per unit volume, the principle states that the rate of change of the concentration of a substance in a tissue region is proportional to the difference of the inflow to that region and the removal of substance from the same region (Fig. 3). Differently stated, the substance traverses the central volume differently depending on the size of this central volume; given a fixed input, the substance is diluted more strongly in a large central volume than in a small one. This observation is called the *central volume theorem,* and we will discuss this in detail later.

When applying this principle to various organ systems, four considerations are of prime importance.

- Entry and exit routes of the substance have to be known. For the brain and the heart, an inert substance can only get into a tissue region by entering via the arteries carrying blood to it, and it can only be removed from the tissue by venous drainage. Obviously, in the kidney, the liver, and the lung, urinary and biliary excretion and exhalation,

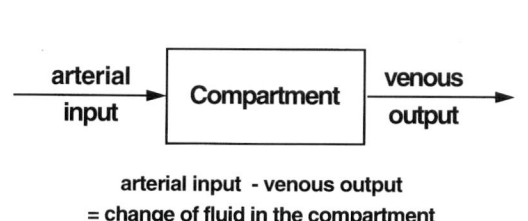

arterial input - venous output
= change of fluid in the compartment

Figure 3. The conservation of mass principle is simple. What flows into an area has to leave it again or else it accumulates in that region. In a steady state or equilibrium state, anything that enters has to leave as well. One example is the blood flow through the lungs; the right and left ventricles have to pump equally. If the left ventricle is impaired, the imbalance leads to accumulation of fluid in the lungs, and pulmonary edema ensues that eventually impairs right ventricular function; a new steady state is established.

respectively, are alternative exit routes to the venous removal of a substance. In addition, in the lung, input also can come via inhalation.

• One has to understand what happens with the substance within the perfused tissue. Whether one intends to measure tissue perfusion or use the substance merely as marker or contrast agent, one notes that it will behave differently depending on which organ it is perfusing; i.e., it will remain intravascularly, diffuse throughout the tissue studied, be captured by some binding sites, etc.

• The tracer material has to mix with the perfusate before entering the organ so that its motions are truly representative of the fluid motions themselves.

• The amount of tracer added to the fluid is small enough so as not to disturb the fluid flow.

All these assumptions may seem trivial and satisfied easily, but this is often not the case, and one has to check their validity carefully for each substance for which a quantitative model is to be established. Examples of substances which—in principle—can be used as perfusion markers are iodinated contrast media, chelates of gadolinium or technetium (Gd-DTPA, Tc-DTPA, Gd-DOTA, etc.), xenon, and the oxy/deoxyhemoglobin system in the blood, which can serve as intrinsic MR ''contrast agent.'' Furthermore, there exists a large number of organ-specific NM perfusion markers—such as macroaggregates of albumin for the lung; thallium, technetium sestamibi, ammonia, and rubidium for the heart; technetium-HMPAO, technetium-ECD, carbon dioxide, and water for the brain; and technetium-DMSA for the kidney—that all stick to the organ in relation to perfusion.

Perfusion experiments can be classified as follows:

• Wash-in experiments
• Wash-out experiments
• Equilibrium experiments
• Bolus experiments

Various agents suitable for perfusion measurements were discussed in Chap. 2 and are classified in Table 1. The classic tracers to validate perfusion experiments are radioactively labeled microspheres (Fig. 4), which are washed into the tissue under study in proportion to the regional perfusion. Microspheres cannot be used in clinical practice except in the lung because arterial injections into the feeding arteries are necessary. In the lung, rather than microspheres made of latex, macroaggregates of albumin are used because of their biodegradability. The perfusion agents used in clinical NM, except for xenon, carbon dioxide and water, fully or partly emulate the microsphere principle; that is, they flow into the organ of interest and are ''trapped'' there. Microspheres proper and macroaggregates of albumin accumulate quantitatively in the organ studied because they get stuck mechanically, while the other substances, often called *chemical microspheres,* are transformed chemically by the cells in the organ of interest and cannot leave them again (Fig. 5). The model for such substances is only a wash-in model in almost ideal situations, as in the case of [^{13}N]ammonia in the heart. Usually the model has to account for the fact that only part of the substance remains in the central volume during its first pass, while the other part is removed by venous drainage.

The other perfusion agents do not use the wash-in type of experiment described above; they serve as first-pass agents, and in essence, bolus tracking has to be done to derive quantitative flow information, unless the substance can somehow be brought into the tissue almost instantly. In this case, we are dealing with a so-called wash-out experiment, whose quantitative analysis is also relatively simple. In clinical practice, wash-out experiments are only possible with injections into the feeding arteries of the various organs or by steady-state breathing of, for example, xenon gas. Regarding bolus perfusion agents, there are two fundamentally different classes of substances: the freely diffusible agents such as water and xenon on the one hand and the chelate or iodinated contrast agents on the other. Xenon and carbon dioxide and water are freely diffusible tracers in all organ systems because they permeate the tissues including the intracellular compart-

Table 1. *Perfusion agents in use and of potential utility (in brackets)*

Methodology	Wash-in	Wash-out	"Equilibrium"	Bolus
NM				
General (arterial)	Microspheres*	Xenon (into feeding art.)		H_2O (PET)
Brain	*Tc-HMPAO†*		H_2O (PET)	
	Tc-ECD†			Xenon
Heart	*Tc-MIBI†*			
	Thallium†			
	Rhubidium (PET)†			
	Ammonia (PET)†			
Lung	Macroaggregates of albumin*			
Kidney	*Tc-DMSA†*			
	Tc-MAG3			
	I-Hippuran			
X ray				
General				*[Iodinated CA]*
Brain		Xenon		Xenon
				Iodinated CA
RES	*Lipiodol*			
MRI			*[Gd chelates]*	
General	*Spin-labeling*	*Spin-labeling*		
Brain				Gd chelates
				Dy chelates
Heart	*[Mn-DPDP]*			*Gd chelates*
Lung	*[Hyperpol., xenon]*	*[Hyperpol., xenon]*		
RES	*Ferrite part.*			
Ultrasound				
General				*Microbubbles*

Note: ( ) = for qualitative assessment only; *italics* = semiquantitative assessment.
* "Mechanical" microspheres.
† "Chemical" microspheres.

ments quickly (Fig. 6). Due to their complete tissue permeation, freely diffusible tracers remain relatively long in the central volume. The chelates and iodinated contrast agents remain in the intravascular space in the brain because of the blood-brain barrier and have a very rapid transit there (Fig. 7). This requires very rapid data taking for perfusion measurements. In organs other than the brain, such as the heart, these agents quickly diffuse into the extravascular space. A strictly intravascular substance is ^{11}C-labeled

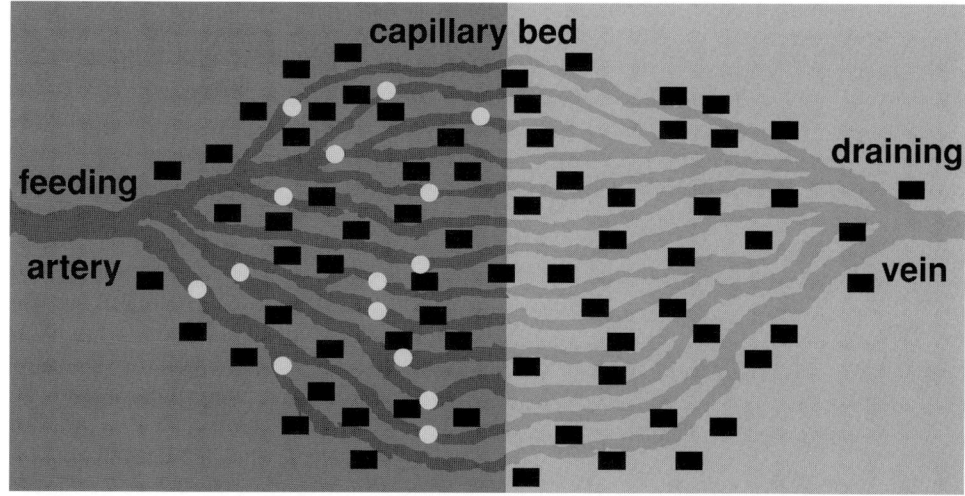

Figure 4. Microspheres enter the capillary bed but physically get trapped as the vessels narrow. Hence the microspheres and macroaggregates of albumin are only found on the arterial side of the vascular tree in the arterioles or capillaries.

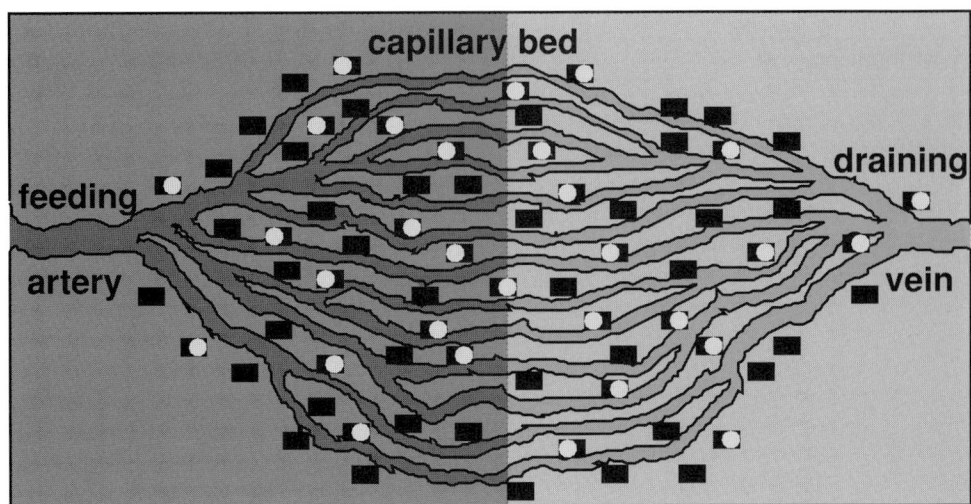

Figure 5. "Chemical" microspheres stay in the organ under examination because they undergo intracellular reactions. The extraction process and other elimination mechanisms clear the substance from the vascular and extracellular compartments. The remaining substance resides in the cells in proportion to the tissue perfusion, but in contrast to the situation depicted in Fig. 4, the substance is intracellular and not intravascular.

carbon monoxide, which is tighty bound to the red blood cells, and there are now reports on gadolinium macrocompounds and very small ferrite particles that remain intravascular in any organ. Extravasation has important consequences for perfusion model calculations, because when extravasation of the substance occurs, multicompartment modeling is necessary to account for the substance behavior (Fig. 8). In the brain, the chelates are so-called nondiffusible tracers; they do not diffuse throughout the tissue, while in other organs they are partly diffusible, and partition considerations between the intra- and extravascular compartments have to be made.

The agent for equilibrium-type blood flow measurements is [^{15}O] water. The methodology for quantitative flow measurements used in such experiments is unique to this short-lived radioactive tracer, and the use of this method is mainly discussed in Chap. 5. The intrinsic oxy/deoxyhemoglobin concentration marker would, if anything, be a wash-out marker; one substance (oxyhemoglobin) that produces no contrast effect flows

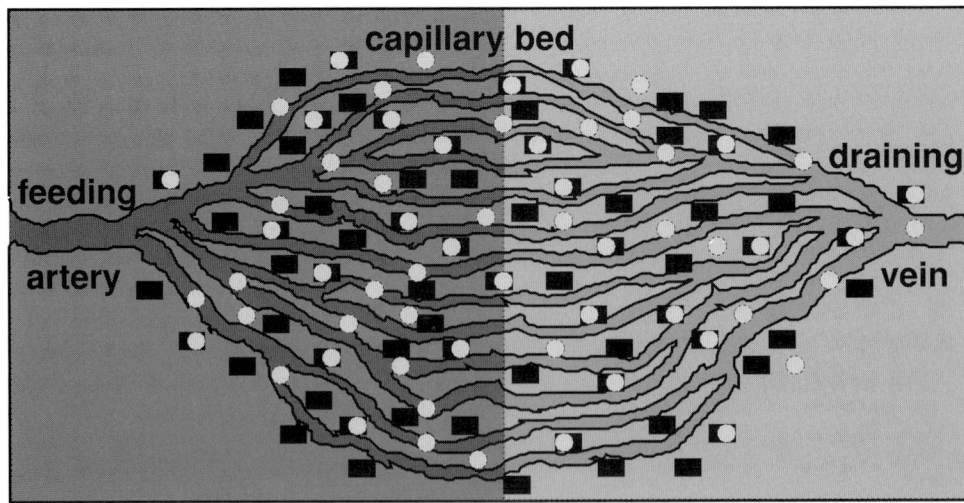

Figure 6. A freely diffusible substance distributes throughout the various compartments of an organ; hence molecules of it are found intravascularly, in the extracellular fluid, and also inside the cells.

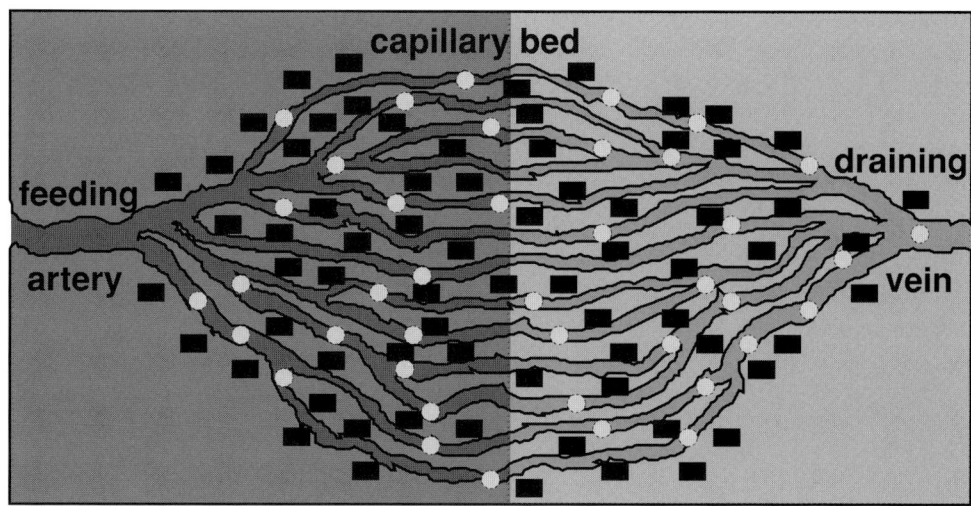

Figure 7. Intravascular space marker. The substance stays strictly inside the vessels, enters the central volume on the arterial side, and exits on the venous side. Substances satisfying these conditions are carbon monoxide, the Gd chelates, and most iodinated contrast agents in the brain, and there are some experimental intravascular MRI contrast agents such as Gd macromolecules and small ferrite particles. In other organs, the Tc and Gd chelates as well as most iodinated x-ray contrast agents are extracellular fluid markers that distribute between the vascular compartment and the extracellular compartment but do not enter the cell.

into the organ, while deoxyhemoglobin, producing a paramagnetic contrast effect (see Chap. 8), is washed out of it. Use of this effect to measure flow would, however, require that the production of deoxyhemoglobin be constant over brain and throughout brain tissue, which we know is not the case.

After this introductory overview, we now proceed to analyze the perfusion problem in general, specifying it then for the various types of measurements listed above. Depending on the imaging method chosen to evaluate perfusion, the conservation of mass principle, which is at the base of any quantitative measurement of tissue perfusion, is adapted to simplify analysis. The simplest quantitative analyses apply for the wash-in, steady-state (equilibrium), and wash-out methods, where it is assumed either that the substance gets into the tissue but is not removed (microsphere principle) or that by some equilibrium process or a perfect bolus a substance is present in the tissue of interest at time zero of the experiments and is then washed out by perfusion. In the latter case it is assumed that the gas is evenly distributed throughout the brain initially or distributes itself virtually instantly and evenly throughout the corresponding cerebral hemisphere to be washed out of the brain and completely removed in the lungs; hence recirculation of substance has not to be accounted for. In fact, recirculation complicates matters very much, and in all perfusion experiments where it occurs, the experiments are done such that one can correct for it. Mathematically, the most complex analysis is required when using the bolus methods.

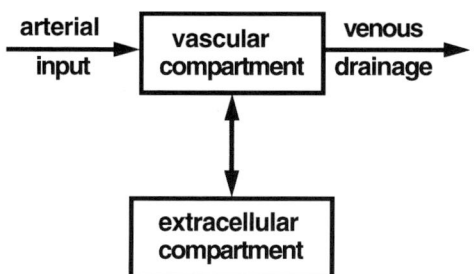

Figure 8. A model for a substance that exchanges between intravascular and extracellular fluid compartments. The exchange of substance between these two compartments has to be taken into account for proper modeling using a two-compartment model. This is the case when wanting to use Gd-DTPA for quantitative perfusion measurements in the heart.

Quantitative Description of Tissue Perfusion

Our point of departure to quantitatively describe tissue perfusion is Fick's principle, derived from conservation of mass considerations, which states that the tracer substance accumulated in a tissue region (central volume) over time equals the amount of substance brought into that region minus the substance removed from the region during that time (see Fig. 3).

We shall call the concentration in the tissue of interest C_t, the concentration in arterial blood C_a, and the concentration in venous blood C_v. The tissue concentration C_t is an average of substance in the arteries, veins, and capillaries, the extracellular fluid, and/or the cellular compartments. Obviously, for a substance not crossing the blood-brain barrier such as a Gd-chelate or carbon monoxide, C_t will be the concentration of the substance present inside the vessels multiplied with the ratio of the vascular space to the total tissue volume: rBV, the relative regional blood volume (see below). This is on the order of 3% to 5% in the brain but closer to 15% in the kidney. Concentrations are measured in grams per milliliter, but when radioactivity is used for a measurement, it is equally reasonable to use units of megabecquerel per milliliter because a simple measurement of the activity in arterial or venous blood downstream of the injection site permits one to calculate how many megabecquerels there are in a gram of substance.

Since in any physiologic steady state there is no fluid accumulation in the tissue under consideration, the arterial input has to equal the venous outflow (provided that there are no other exit or entry routes, as noted above), and this regional flow f is measured in milliliters of fluid per minute and per milliliter of tissue. Hence it has the dimensions of inverse time (1/min). The quantitative description of Fick's principle is

$$dC_t/dt = f(C_a - C_v) \tag{1}$$

where all the concentrations are functions of time. Note that in a steady state there can be no change in the tissue concentration of substance. Thus dC_t/dt has to be zero, which simply means that what flows into the tissue will flow out; in a steady state, inflow and outflow of substance are equal. If flow is high, much substance is brought into but also much is removed from the tissue, while with low flow, little is brought in and little is moved out, and this occurs independently of the amount of substance present in the tissue. We can make a simple analogy to our bank account. By knowing the average balance on our bank account (the tissue concentration), we have no way to deduce what our average earnings (inflow) and spendings (outflow) on the account are! A clinical example in nuclear medicine is lung ventilation scanning. Patients with chronic obstructive pulmonary disease have lung regions that are poorly ventilated; ''inflow'' and ''outflow'' of xenon gas into and out of the region are slower than in normally ventilated lung areas. These areas are detected during the so-called wash-in and wash-out phases but not during the steady-state phase of the pulmonary ventilation scan; eventually the xenon concentration in these regions is similar to that in the normal lung tissue, but the turnover of gas is slower, which can only be seen when a dynamic experiment is performed.

If the substance can freely diffuse, its concentrations in venous blood and in the perfused tissue are in equilibrium. Their relative concentrations depend on the relative solubility of the substance in the tissue and in the venous blood. The ratio between C_t and C_v is called the *partition coefficient P*. For a substance with high water solubility, such as water itself, P can be safely assumed to be 1. For an intravascular substance strictly speaking, P would be 0; however, in an imaging experiment that images a mixture of small blood vessels and tissue, we can equal P to the fraction of the blood vessel volume to the total amount of tissue volume. This quantity is important in itself and is known as the *regional blood volume (rBV)*. For normal brain it is known from the literature and is on the order of 0.03 to 0.05, but in general, rBV has to be measured.

Introducing P as defined above into Eq. (1) yields

$$dC_t/dt = f(C_a - C_t/P) = f/P(PC_a - C_t) \tag{2}$$
$$\text{(g/ml tissue/min)} \qquad \text{(ml g/ml/ml tissue/min)}$$

Equation (2) is a first-order linear differential equation that can be integrated using standard methods (6):

$$C_t(t) = C_t(0) \exp(-ft/P) + f \exp(-ft/P) \int_0^t C_a(t') \exp(f - t'/P)dt' \quad (3)$$

This equation will be used when analyzing the various methods for perfusion imaging and was developed originally and used extensively to study the principles of inert gas exchange between blood and tissues (24). The second term on the right side is a so-called convolution operation and is abbreviated as $\exp(-kt)*C_a(t)$.

The time-integrated form of Eq. (1) is given by

$$C_t(t) = C_t(0) \exp(-kt) + f \exp(-kt)*C_a(t) \quad (4)$$

where $k = f/P$ is called the *wash-out constant,* and the asterisk is the abbreviation for the convolution operation. This general equation can be used to quantitatively describe all the approaches to the measurement of tissue perfusion and adapted to the kind of experiment and tracer substance used, as will be done in the course of this chapter. We note here that if the initial concentration in the tissue is zero, the first term of the preceding equation is zero, and the second term represents the system response to an arterial input bolus, which is a monoexponentially decaying tissue concentration if the input is an idealized "instant" input bolus. If the arterial input is "nonideal," the arterial input curve has to be "convolved" with this decaying exponential function.

As noted earlier, the various types of perfusion measurements can be categorized into four large groups: wash-in (microsphere), wash-out, equilibrium, and bolus injection perfusion measurements. Equilibrium experiments cannot yield tissue perfusion information directly, as seen by looking at Eq. (1); if the left-hand side is zero, the equation will not yield an expression for the tissue perfusion f. In the ensuing sections we will quantitatively discuss the various types of perfusion measurements.

Mechanical and Biochemical Microspheres

Mechanical microspheres are particles with a diameter larger than that of capillaries, hence larger than about 8 μm. If injected into the feeding arteries—or a vein if the organ of interest is the lung—the microspheres will produce microemboli in the vascular bed of the organ of interest and are thereby extracted completely from the bloodstream, provided that there are no arteriovenous shunts present. Understanding the microsphere principle to measure perfusion is very important for several reasons.

1. Microsphere-type perfusion measurements (mechanical and chemical) have been implemented in various clinical examinations to qualitatively and quantitatively assess organ perfusion. While these clinical examinations are currently all based on isotope techniques and hence are NM imaging procedures, it is not completely excluded that MR agents eventually can be used in analogous fashion.
2. Many new tracers presumed to be of interest to investigate cellular metabolism or cellular receptor systems act in fact like microspheres and end up simply being "new" perfusion markers rather than something else. A simple example would be a ligand binding instantly and tightly to an organ receptor present in high concentration. The receptors would then extract the ligand quite effectively and remove it from the bloodstream. Like microspheres, the ligand would be completely removed during first pass, and a wash-in perfusion experiment would result. Consequently, no information on the receptor-ligand system could be obtained, but we would learn something about tissue perfusion.
3. Microspheres are *the* "gold standard" used to validate any new marker with regard to its suitability as a perfusion marker.

As stated and as a matter of routine, the microsphere method is used in lung perfusion scanning for the detection of pulmonary emboli. In this case, the microspheres are macroaggregates of human serum albumin. Available as ''kits,'' these aggregates are technetium (^{99m}Tc)–labeled prior to injection into the patient, and when imaging with a gamma camera, areas of poor perfusion appear as areas of decreased radioactivity. Because microspheres are efficiently removed by the pulmonary capillary filter, perfusion of organs other than the lungs cannot be assessed with this method unless the aggregates are injected into the feeding artery of the organ under study. This is obviously impractical in a clinical setting.

Radioactively labeled microspheres are used as quantitative perfusion markers in animal experiments and are available commercially for this purpose. Injected at the appropriate place (i.e., into the left cardiac ventricle or atrium, where good mixing occurs), they can be used to quantitatively measure flow in any organ. They serve as the standard method against which any new perfusion tracer is validated (21). Once the microspheres have been injected and have lodged in the organ, the distribution of radioactivity can be measured quantitatively by PET, or the organs of interest are excised and tissue slices are counted in counters or with quantitative autoradiography. The quantitative measurement of tissue flow with this method additionally requires sampling of the arterial input of microspheres. In fact, the total concentration of microspheres in the tissue at the end of the experiment has to equal the flow times the arterial microsphere concentration summed up over the measurement time. Since microsphere accumulation is strictly proportional to tissue flow, any other tracer that has similarly ideal characteristics for flow measurements will show a linear relationship on a graph where microsphere perfusion at various flows is plotted against perfusion as measured with the other tracer (Fig. 9). Whether the substance used is suitable as a quantitative tracer of perfusion depends on this graphic relation.

Many clinically used tracer substances are *chemical* microspheres; that is, they are biochemically extracted by the organ of interest in proportion to tissue perfusion. Any biochemical system that has a rapid and large binding capacity for a substance acts like a ''sink'' for it. Thus the substance is removed from the circulation in the organ examined and has the same properties regarding flow as microspheres themselves, hence the term

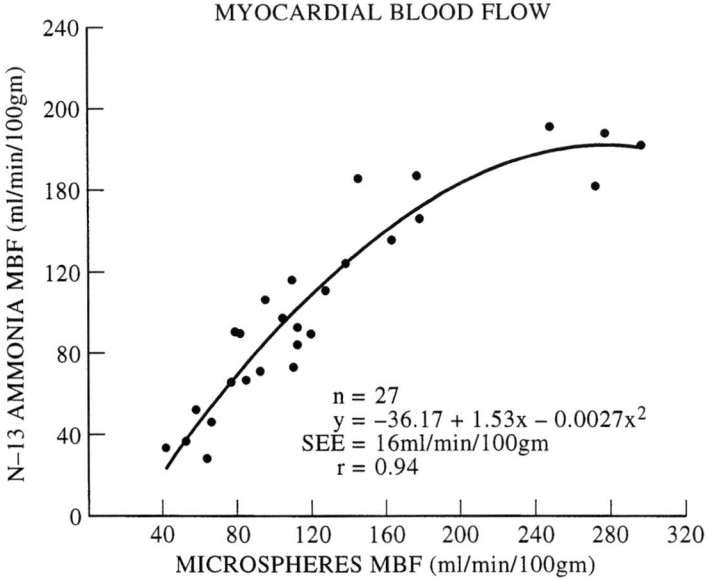

Figure 9. Graph showing microsphere flow versus flow as measured by ammonia. While over a large range of flow rates there is a straight-line relation between the two markers, at higher flow a deviation from the linear relation suggests that there is saturation of the ammonia "uptake" system. Nevertheless, the range of the linear relation is such that ammonia is seen to be an excellent perfusion marker in the heart, except for the very highest flow rates, which are at best attained with maximum vasodilatation. From Shah A, Schelbert HR, Schwaiger M et al. Measurement of regional myocardial blood flow with N-13 ammonia and positron-emission tomography in intact dogs. *J Am Coll Cardiol,* 5(1), 92–100 (1985).

chemical microsphere. We will examine this issue here and later when discussing multi-compartment modeling of metabolic and receptor binding processes. Clinical quantitative perfusion measurements using this approach are implemented with ammonia (^{13}NH$_3$) and PET (33) for the heart. Ammonia acts like a microsphere in the heart because—catalyzed by glutamine synthetase—it rapidly reacts with glutamate to form glutamine in the myocardial cells and is thereby quantitatively removed from the circulating ammonia pool. Due to the high myocardial capillary density, the reaction is essentially complete over a wide range of tissue perfusion, hence satisfying the conditions for a quantitative perfusion tracer. In the brain, ammonia is unsuitable as a perfusion marker because the lower capillary density does not in general permit a quantitative extraction of the tracer. Extraction thus becomes flow dependent, which for quantitative analysis is undesirable.

Most substances used for perfusion assessment in NM have nonideal microsphere characteristics and are used for the *qualitative* assessment of perfusion only, partly because of their characteristics and partly because of the difficulty to extract quantitative data from single photon emission computed tomographic (SPECT) studies. Methods in clinical use include ^{99m}Tc-labeled HMPAO and ECD for cerebral perfusion; ^{99m}Tc-MIBI, thallium-201, and rubidium-82 for myocardial perfusion; and ^{99m}Tc-DMSA for renal perfusion. Thallium-201 has additional properties. Thallium is taken up very efficiently by the myocytes through Na-K-ATPase and therefore acts as a potassium analog. It also leaves the myocytes again through the potassium channels during recurrent myocardial depolarization. As a result, thallium is also marker of myocardial viability, and so would rubidium-82, were it not for its short half-life, which prevents observation of the viability

---

The method to quantify tissue perfusion with microspheres uses the fact that the concentration of the substance in the organ is zero initially [$C_t(0) = 0$], and therefore, only the second term in Eq. (3) has to be considered (wash-in experiment). Since there is no organ wash-out in microsphere experiments, all the microspheres will eventually lodge in the tissue, while their concentration in venous blood remains zero. The wash-out constant $k = f/P$ is thus equal to zero, and the partition coefficient P becomes infinitely large. Extraction occurs fast because all microspheres are removed during their first pass through the organ, provided there is no shunt. The tissue concentration C_t thus quickly approaches a constant concentration $C_t(\infty)$, which can then be measured at leisure in vitro by counting the radioactivity of tissue slices or in vivo using PET with microspheres labeled with a positron-emitting label. With $k = f/P = 0$, Eq. (3) reduces to

$$C_t(\infty) = f \int_0^\infty C_a(t')\, dt' \tag{5}$$

This equation simply states that the total tissue concentration of the substance is equal to the tissue flow f (ml/min/ml tissue) times the amount of substance present in the arterial blood summed up over time.

For perfusion quantification, the integral term in Eq. (5) has to be measured in order to determine the tissue flow f in addition to $C_t(\infty)$. This is accomplished by drawing blood from a peripheral artery during the entire experiment at a constant flow F (ml/min) with a pump. The volume V drawn increases in proportion to the time t: $V(t) = Ft$, or $dt = dV/F$. Determining the amount of substance m in this volume [i.e., the total number of counts when $C_t(\infty)$ is also measured as counts] is equivalent to integrating over the time course of the concentration $C_a(t)$ during the experiment. As noted above, $C_a(t)$ goes to zero quickly; hence, in practice, drawing of blood can be stopped after a few minutes.

$$\int_0^\infty C_a(V)\, dV/F = m/F \tag{6}$$

Substituting this expression in Eq. (5) and solving for f yields the tissue flow.

effects, which are longer-term effects with a characteristic time constant in the range of hours. The extraction fractions for all the substances mentioned in this paragraph are on the order of 50% to 80% under normal perfusion conditions during the first pass and decrease when tissue perfusion is augmented (see Fig. 9) (39). Hence tissue perfusion can be assessed qualitatively, but it is difficult to quantitate it with these agents.

A unique property of all quantitative and qualitative microsphere-type perfusion experiments is that after injection of the substance, its distribution can be measured at leisure. In essence, a dynamic process has been ''frozen,'' and this results in high signal-to-noise ratio images. So far only NM procedures are suitable for this type of perfusion assessment because contrast agents other than radiotracers and behaving in this fashion have toxic side effects at concentrations where they affect image intensities visibly. Nevertheless, some MRI contrast agents such as the superparamagnetic particles, when extracted by the reticuloendothelial system (RES), might approach the behavior of microspheres. Furthermore, it is conceivable that compounds truly suited for perfusion assessment using the microsphere principle will become available as new MRI contrast agents are developed.

The quantitative expression for the measurement of the flow f is obtained as

$$f = C_t(\infty)F/m \tag{7}$$

where F is the flow rate at which blood is drawn from a peripheral artery during the entire experiment of a few minutes and m is the total amount of marker substance found in the total volume of blood obtained in this fashion.

In sum, microsphere experiments are truly quantitative and simple to carry out. A measurement of the tissue concentration of substance is needed and carried out with a tomographic imaging device in vivo after all particles have lodged in the tissue. This yields the quantity $C_t(\infty)$ above. Furthermore, continuous arterial sampling at a known flow rate F is done, and the amount m of tracer in the sample is determined at the end of the experiment.

When perfusion data of substances not completely and nonlinearly extracted on first pass are analyzed quantitatively, the problem becomes more difficult because of a perfusion-dependent extraction coefficient $E(f)$ and the recirculation of the nonextracted substance.

$$C_t(\infty) = E(f)f \int_0^t C_a(t')\, dt'$$

$$\text{or} \quad f = \frac{C_t(\infty)}{E(f) \int C_a(t')\, dt'} \tag{8}$$

If the $E(f)$ curve is known, which can be obtained from calibration measurements against microspheres, and the integral is determined by arterial sampling, as described above, f can be computed. An example of such a calibration experiment for ammonia is shown in Fig. 9.

Equilibrium Model of Constant Tracer Inhalation

A second simple quantitative approach to tissue perfusion measurements uses steady-state conditions with the inhalation of a gas. When recalling the discussion of Eq. (1), we note a contradiction. There it was shown that in a steady state, flow in the tissue of interest is independent of the concentration of a flow tracer measured. The ''trick'' to still obtain perfusion information in a steady-state situation is to use a short-lived radioactive substance with a half-life comparable with the time it takes the blood to flow from the arterial input into the capillaries of the organ of interest. Perfusion assessment becomes possible because now the activity measured in an organ is dependent on how fast it got there from the arteries, and this obviously depends on flow. The slower the substance percolates through the organ, the more of it has decayed between the arterial input and the time when the tissue activity is measured. We thus understand qualitatively why the substance half-life has to be comparable with the time for it to get from the arteries to the capillaries: If the decay time of the substance is much longer than this transit time, the tissue counts measured become again independent of the tissue flow, and the method cannot be used.

The only short-lived tracers available for such experiments are PET radiopharmaceuticals, and the method uses PET in conjunction with [^{15}O]carbon dioxide. Clinical applications have been limited to the brain, and while application to other organ systems for research or clinical purposes is conceivable, for the heart, the microsphere methods described later are used. Since the equilibrium method is only of relevance for NM studies, the method is detailed in Chap. 5.

Dynamic Measurements of Perfusion: Wash-out Techniques

The simplest dynamic measurements of perfusion are the so-called wash-out techniques. The technique is applicable for all substances that are in a rapid exchange equilibrium with the perfused tissue. All imaging techniques can be used in principle to extract perfusion data with this method with an appropriate tracer substance. NM and PET examinations using the wash-out or indicator dilution technique have been implemented using radiotracers such as radioactive xenon gases (^{133}Xenon, ^{127}Xenon) and ^{15}O compounds. Computed tomographic (CT) cerebral perfusion measurements have been performed with inert xenon gas, while appropriate tracers have yet to be developed for MRI. Hyperpolarized xenon seems to offer intriguing possibilities for this purpose, although there are serious issues concerning its short half-life (1). The quantitative analysis of the wash-out problem yields a relation between tissue flow, concentration of the tracer substance in the arterial input, and concentration in the tissue. However, while radioactive counts and substance concentration can be related relatively easily for CT and MRI examinations, the relation between the contrast medium concentration and the signal changes induced by it is more complicated. Furthermore, the imaging systems used have very different properties regarding spatial and temporal resolution, and this also leads to specific adaptations of the method. The general quantitative principle, however, is valid for all techniques and will be discussed here.

Intuitively, the wash-out of a substance out of a tissue has to be proportional to tissue flow, since with large flows the substance wash-out is fast and with small flows slow. Hence a rapid concentration decrease of the substance in the tissue is consistent with high flow and a slow decrease with slow flow. This is indeed what Eq. (4) describes quantitatively. High flow results in a high wash-out constant k and thus a fast exponential decay of the concentration versus time curve, and low flow results in the opposite. Assume that by some means we have been able to instill an agent in the tissue of interest. After this initial point, the agent is washed out of the tissue. In a sense, this is the reverse situation of that which we have encountered with microspheres. While in the latter case all the substance has been washed into the tissue and none is leaving it, in the wash-out experiments, all the substance is initially in the tissue and has left it at the end of the experiment.

Intracarotid injection of radioactive xenon is closest to the idealized wash-out experiment. With intracarotid injection, the xenon bolus can be made so narrow (Fig. 10) and it mixes so rapidly throughout the cerebral hemisphere receiving the input that the experiment looks like one has added the substance to the brain at the beginning of the experiment, whereafter it is only washed out and quantitatively removed by the lung. Hence no recirculation occurs, which, as noted, complicates data analysis. The ''instant input of substance'' makes input deconvolution techniques unnecessary to analyze the data, as with other bolus injections. However, this technique, while most simple to

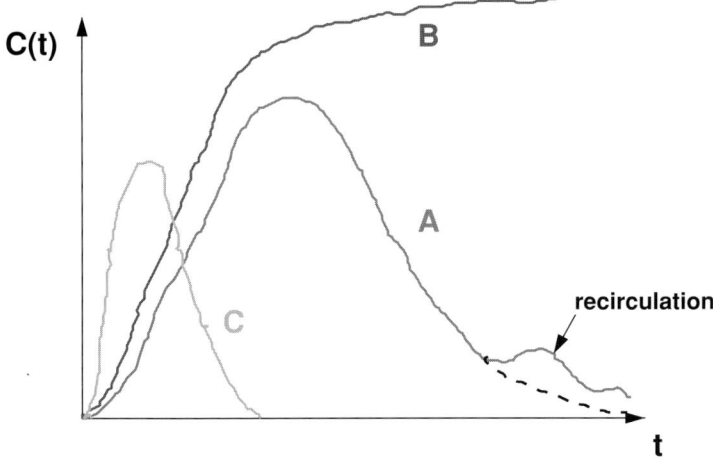

Figure 10. Tissue concentration curve after instantaneous injection of a bolus into the feeding artery. Curve *A* represents the situation where the substance enters the tissue and then is washed out again. The little second peak represents recirculation, with the dashed line being an extrapolation for the "no recirculation" situation. Curve *B* represents the tissue concentration when a constant infusion of the tracer is used, and it also represents the integral of curve *A*. From Meier P, Zierler KL. On the theory of the indicator-dilution method for measurement of blood flow and volume. *J Appl Physiol,* 6, 731–744 (1954). Curve *C* represents a short injection bolus, whose mean duration is substantially shorter than the transit of the substance through the tissue.

understand, is obviously no longer used clinically due to its invasiveness (27). Alternatively, a freely diffusible tracer is given continuously to the patient by inhalation until an equilibrium is reached in the organ of interest and then is abruptly discontinued to observe substance wash-out. This approach works with radioactive xenon gas in SPECT (40) perfusion, carbon dioxide in PET perfusion (23), and inert xenon gas in CT (13). After abruptly discontinuing the substance supply, the decrease of the substance in the tissue of interest is observed with the imaging device as a function of time. Since xenon and carbon dioxide are completely eliminated as they pass the pulmonary circulation, no recirculation of substance occurs. This simplifies quantitative analysis, particularly if it is assumed that the discontinuation of tracer occurs virtually instantaneously also in the perfused organ and not only at the level of gas application in the lung. In practice, this discontinuation is not instant; differing path lengths of the pulmonary vessels will make the indicator drop less than instantaneous in the tissue of interest. If the drop can be considered steep enough that the second part of Eq. (4) is small compared with the first part, the quantitative analysis given below also can be used for data obtained with this "discontinuation of a steady state" method.

The quantitative description of the wash-out method starts again with the principle of conservation of substance, and Fick's equation (Eq. 1) can serve as the point of departure. In the case of xenon wash-out after carotid injection or equilibrium discontinuation, the rate of change of the substance in tissue is simply proportional to the tissue concentration itself. Furthermore, the characteristic time over which the wash-out occurs is inversely proportional to the tissue flow. Mathematical analysis of this problem readily yields the result that the wash-out occurs exponentially because the second term in Eq. (4) is zero, since first the arterial concentration of substance goes to zero immediately after the beginning of the experiment and second the exponential decay constant k, the wash-out constant in Eq. (4), is proportional to tissue flow. Wash-out data therefore can be plotted semilogarithmically, and tissue flow can be extracted from the slope of the straight line or, alternatively, from the maximum tissue concentration and the area under the tissue concentration curve (height-over-area method; see below). Which method is to be applied depends on the temporal resolution of the imaging system used; high temporal resolution permits one to measure points on the wash-out curve, while low temporal resolution requires the use of the height-over-area method. One noteworthy conclusion from the quantitative analysis given below is that the dynamic methods for the determination of tissue flow require that the fractional regional blood volume *rBV* be known, while this quantity does not have to be determined in microsphere experiments. Hence absolute flow measurements with the dynamic techniques discussed in this and the next section always require the determination of blood flow and regional blood volume, although for freely diffusible tracers such as xenon the partition coefficient is nearly one. For intravascular tracers the *rBV* is equal to the fraction of vascular space to total tissue space including the vessels.

Quantitative analysis of the wash-out method is as follows: With an initial concentration $C_{t\,max}(0)$ of the substance present in the tissue, the second term on the right in Eq. (4) represents the correction for arterial input and substance recirculation. If the arterial substance concentration $C_a(t)$ goes to zero very fast and virtually no recirculation occurs, as is approximately the case if an inert radioactive gas such as xenon is injected into the carotid or breathing is discontinued, the second term approaches zero or is negligible compared with the first term, and Eq. (4) simplifies to

$$C_t(t) = C_t(0) \exp(-kt) \qquad (9)$$

This demonstrates the exponential wash-out as stated above. If Eq. (9) applies, the wash-out constant k and thus $f = kP$ can be determined from a semilogarithmic plot of the wash-out curve if the imaging system is fast enough (substantially faster than $1/k$).

Alternatively, one can integrate Eq. (9) to permit the use of the wash-out methods also for slower imaging systems. This yields the so-called height-over-area method. By integrating over the time course of the experiment and calling the area under the concentration curve A, we find

$$A = \int_0^\infty C_t(t)\, dt = C_t(0) \int_0^\infty \exp(-kt)\, dt$$

$$= -C_t(0) \exp(-kt)/k \,\Big|_0^\infty = C_t(0)/k \qquad (10)$$

or, solving for k and using $f = kP$,

$$f = kP = \frac{PC_t(0)}{\displaystyle\int_0^\infty C_t(t)\, dt} = \frac{PC_t(0)}{A} \qquad (11)$$

As stated above, P corresponds to the relative regional blood volume *rBV* for an intravascular agent, where *rBV* is a number.

The integrated form represents the expression known as the height $[C_t(0)]$ over area (A) method:

$$\frac{f}{rBV} = \frac{C_t(0)}{A} \qquad (12)$$

If the fractional regional blood volume *rBV* is known, measuring the maximum concentration $C_t(0)$ that occurs at the onset of data taking and the area under the concentration curve A, f can be determined, hence the expression *height-over-area method*. This relation also can be used in the nonideal situation, where the input bolus is of finite length. In this case, however, arterial input has to be convolved into the wash-out (Eq. 4); in other words, input deconvolution analysis is necessary.

Dynamic Measurements of Perfusion: Bolus Techniques

The wash-out techniques can be applied only if the wash-out of tracer from an organ is substantially longer than the time over which a bolus reaches the brain. Examples discussed are the intracarotid xenon injections or the discontinuation of gas inhalation. In both cases the temporal dispersion in substance arrival and discontinuation is small compared with the transit time of the substance through the tissue. Note that the experimental conditions for the wash-out techniques are only met for freely diffusible tracers because they have a relatively long tissue transit time. In essence, this means that (a) the characteristic time it takes to inject the bolus of tracer is less than a second, which is small compared with the transit time through the tissue of interest (3 to 5 s in the brain; see Fig. 10), and (b) recirculation must not occur. While these conditions are met using xenon or CO_2 intracarotid injection or inhalation, they are not met with the most conveniently used tracer or contrast substances. All completely or partly intravascular agents are not removed from the circulation fast enough so that a steady state can be reached where discontinuation would then yield a situation suitable for wash-out analysis. When using intravascular agents, physiologic necessity dictates that perfusion information can only be derived from dynamic measurements. Even with radioactive water, where the equilibrium method or the wash-out technique can be applied (see "Equilibrium Model of Constant Tracer Inhalation" and "Dynamic Measurements of Perfusion: Wash-out Techniques" above and Chap. 6), the use of bolus techniques is preferable because steady-state experiments result in a higher radiation dose compared with experiments where a single bolus of radioactive tracer is used. Hence, in the most general situation, no attempt is made to reach a steady state with a substance to perform a subsequent wash-out experiment either because of convenience or out of shear physiologic necessity. Rather, the measurements are done by observing what happens to a bolus of substance injected as it enters, perfuses, and leaves the tissue under study.

As a result, bolus techniques have become the method of choice to measure cerebral perfusion using PET with freely diffusible tracers such as $C[^{15}O]_2$ or $H_2[^{15}O]$ (20, 35). Bolus techniques are also the only methods by which standard iodinated contrast agents in CT (2) and Gd-chelate contrast agents in MRI (14, 36) can be used to measure organ perfusion. These agents remain intravascular in the intact brain but diffuse into the interstitium in other organs such as the heart (45). Hence a multitude of implementations of the fundamental principles of the bolus technique to measure tissue perfusion exist. With CT and MRI, several problems have to be considered when implementing bolus techniques, as enumerated below. We will elaborate on the general principles and identify aspects of the methodology common to all imaging systems. The quantitative physiologic foundations of the technique are of general significance.

The first problem that is only relevant in CT is the radiation burden to the patient associated with obtaining sequential images at the same level. Xenon wash-out techniques (see "Dynamic Measurements of Perfusion: Wash-out Techniques" above) are more acceptable when using CT because fewer imaging slices are needed to interpret the results. A second problem relevant for both CT and MRI is that the contrast agents currently available remain strictly intravascular only in the brain but partly extravasate into the extracellular space in other organs. This makes the bolus technique difficult to use in organs other than the brain in conjunction with these imaging methods. A third major technical problem with the bolus injection technique in this setting is that the fully or partly intravascular substances—while washed out of the tissue—are not quickly and quantitatively removed, and thus they will recirculate and reappear in the organ of interest, although at a lower concentration (see Fig. 10). This can be seen readily in many experimental contrast versus time curves. Quantitative data analysis requires that the injected bolus be so narrow in time that the first pass of the bolus through the tissue is clearly distinguishable from the passage of tracer in recirculation, that is, typically a few seconds, while recirculation time is on the order of 10 to 20 seconds. If this condition is met, wash-out of the tissue occurs again in exponential fashion until the moment where

A mathematical investigation of the problem of tissue perfusion with a bolus permits one to derive the so-called central volume theorem, which also can be used as a point of departure when quantitatively analyzing perfusion data. The central volume theorem states that the mean transit time of a substance through the tissue region equals its volume (central volume) divided by the venous outflow from that region.

Again, the principle of conservation of mass can be used as a starting point in the quantitative analysis. Equations (2) and (3) were derived by assuming that there was instant mixing between the tissue compartment and the draining veins. While this assumption will be maintained for the time being (i.e., we assume that we can measure either tissue concentration or the concentration in the draining veins), this assumption is much better for the freely diffusible tracers than for the intravascular tracers, and a critique of this assumption will have to be presented.

The first step to quantitatively analyze tissue perfusion using the bolus technique is to derive a relation between the amount of tracer substance injected, the tissue concentration, the flow, and the perfused volume. The amount of flow f out of the tissue in an infinitesimal time dt is the volume dV leaving the tissue during that time. The volume dV is the tissue flow f normalized per milliliter of tissue, multiplied by the regional blood volume rBV, V_t, and the time dt. Since concentration is defined as mass per unit volume, the total mass m leaving the tissue during the time dt is equal to the volume dV times the substance concentration in the fluid leaving the tissue $C_t(t)$.

$$dm = dV \bullet C_t(t) = f \bullet rBV \bullet V_t \bullet C_t(t)\, dt$$

Integrating this expression over the entire time of the experiment from 0 to infinity yields the total mass (or counts) of tracer substance injected, provided there is no recirculation:

$$m = f \bullet rBV \bullet V_t \int_0^\infty C_t(t)\, dt \tag{13}$$

Since the amount of injected tracer substance is known and $C_t(t)$ or a quantity reflecting it is measured with the imaging device, tissue perfusion can be determined from the preceding equation by solving for f:

$$f = \frac{m}{rBV \bullet V_t \int C_t(t)\, dt} \tag{14}$$

which is a generalized equivalent to Eq. (12). Equation (14) is known as the *Stewart-Hamilton equation* (41) and forms the clinical base for measuring the cardiac output with thermal dilution techniques, although when measuring cardiac output, integration occurs over the venous drainage of tracer rather than the tissue concentration. This equation, in fact, only measures cardiac output and not the flow through a specific artery or tissue under study because the mass m is the total amount of tracer injected, and we cannot deduce from Eq. (14) which fraction of the mass went into the tissue that interests us.

The central volume theorem can be derived as follows: Let us introduce the first moment of the concentration versus time curve, which corresponds to the mean transit time t_m of the bolus and is defined like any moment of a distribution function as

continued

continued

$$t_m = \frac{\int_0^\infty tC_t(t)\,dt}{\int_0^\infty C_t(t)\,dt} \tag{15}$$

The first moment corresponds to the center of gravity of the concentration versus time curve and thus does not coincide necessarily with the peak of the curve (Fig. 11).

If a bolus of tracer (contrast material) is injected at time $t = 0$, there is a range of times at which the tracer molecules leave the tissue studied. The distribution function of these tracer molecules $h(t)$, which have taken differing paths through the tissue and therefore have taken different times, is the mass of molecules flowing out of the volume $m(t) = f \bullet rBV \bullet V_t \bullet C_t(t)$ normalized by the total mass of molecules injected:

$$h(t) = \frac{f \bullet rBV \bullet V_t \bullet C_t(t)}{m} \tag{16}$$

which if integrated over time is equal to 1 according to Eq. (13). If we insert the expression for m from Eq. (13) into Eq. (16), we obtain

$$h(t) = \frac{C_t(t)}{\int_0^\infty C_t(t)\,dt} \tag{17}$$

$h(t)$ has the same shape as the tissue concentration curve but has units of one over time. An essential assumption made is that all particles of the perfusate move in the same manner as the tracer particles; thus $h(t)$ also gives the distribution of the time durations during which the particles of the perfusate traverse the tissue. In other words, the particles that remain in the system for a total time between t and $t + dt$ amount to $h(t)\,dt$. Since the perfusate enters and leaves the tissue at a flow rate f, the volume occupied by fluid particles traversing the tissue between times t and $t + dt$ is the tissue flow rate f times the time t it takes the particles to traverse those paths which have a given equal length. Since f is assumed to be equal for all paths, all paths of equal length take a given time t to be traversed:

$$d(rBV) = fth(t)\,dt$$

which upon integration over the duration of the entire bolus yields

$$rBV = f \int_0^\infty th(t)\,dt \tag{18}$$

Using the definition of Eq. (17) and comparing the expression thus obtained with Eq. (15), we derive the central volume theorem:

$$rBV = \frac{f \int_0^\infty tC_t(t)\,dt}{\int_0^\infty C_t(t)\,dt}$$

where the integral in the numerator equals the mean transit time according to Eq. (15).

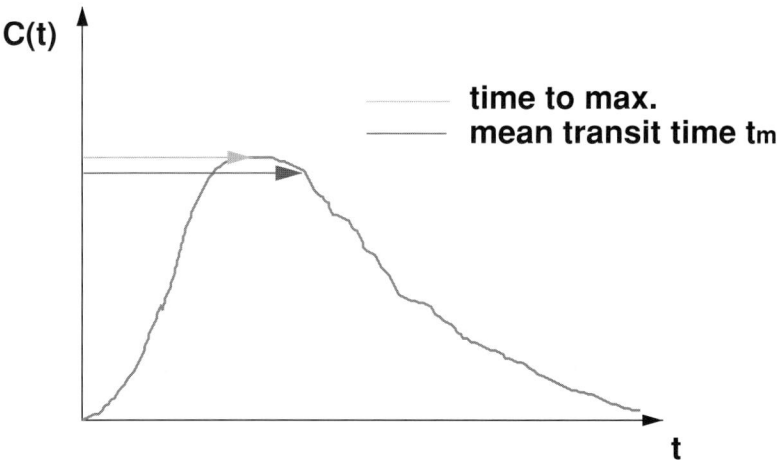

Figure 11. The mean trasit time in a skewed curve does not coincide with the time to maximum concentration, as would be the case in a symmetrical curve. The mean transit time is obtained by calculating the first moment of the concentration distribution function.

recirculation starts. However, this exponential decay is no longer a function of tissue perfusion alone but also of the shape of the bolus concentration curve injected; the wider the bolus, the slower is the exponential decrease in tissue concentration. The mathematical techniques necessary to separate the contributions to the widening of the tissue concentration curve by the tissue itself and the finite width of the bolus are the so-called deconvolution techniques mentioned earlier. This amounts to solving Eq. (4). Once input deconvolution has been performed, a semilogarithmic plot of the deconvolved data yields the value of tissue perfusion very much as in the height-over-area method described earlier. The fourth and final problem that has to be addressed when trying to extract perfusion data from CT or MRI bolus experiments is to relate the concentration of the marker substance injected to the measured signal intensities, since these two quantities are not directly proportional to each other. Signal intensity versus concentration curves have to be found for the CT and MRI contrast agents, while the number of counts measured per unit volume in a PET scan is directly proportional to the substance present.

$$t_m = \frac{rBV}{f} \tag{19}$$

Thus, if by measurement the mean transit time, t_m, and the regional blood volume are known, Eq. (19) yields the flow rate f. While this seems unproblematic, we have to apply a correction because in a "real life" experiment the intravenous bolus is not short compared with the mean tissue transit time but spread out, as discussed. It turns out (and this is a consequence of the fact that we are dealing with a mathematical convolution of the arterial input function with the exponential wash-out curve as given in Eq. 4) that the mean tissue transit time and the mean bolus time are additive. The correction can then be made by using the relation

$$t_{m_{obs}} = t_m + t_{bolus} \tag{20}$$

The most general approach to determine tissue flow using bolus techniques applies Eq. (4), which we recall to be

$$C_t(t) = C_t(0) \exp(-kt) + f \exp(-kt) * C_a(t)$$

The first term on the left in Eq. (4) is zero if no substance is present initially [$C_t(0) = 0$], which is the case when data taking over the tissue investigated begins as peripheral bolus injection is started. In the brain, the arterial input function $C_a(t)$ has to be measured either by arterial sampling, as is done in PET, or by measuring the signal intensity in a feeding artery, as in an imaging modality with higher resolution, such as CT or MRI

(36). In the heart, where the large intravascular blood pool is imaged together with the perfused tissue, all methods are performed without arterial sampling. The arterial as well as the tissue concentration curves will look something like the curve depicted in Fig. 10. As long as the temporal spread of the arterial input bolus function is small compared with the recirculation time (which is typically 10 to 20 seconds), that is, when recirculation effects occur only in the late part of the decaying limb of the tissue concentration curve, as depicted in Fig. 10, input deconvolution can be performed successfully. Under this condition, the tissue curve can be extrapolated in the "tail" region by fitting to it a decaying exponential curve (dashed line in Fig. 10) or a gamma variate function with a recirculation cutoff. Alternatively, Eq. (4) can be solved by using numerical integration techniques (4, 42). The interested reader is referred to the specialized literature for details of these techniques.

Tissue Perfusion Measurements: Conclusions

In this section we have seen that there are many ways how to extract perfusion information: the microsphere approach, the equilibrium method, wash-out methods, and dynamic substance bolus application experiments. The different approaches are variably suitable for in vivo experiments and clinical use as a result of limitations in the imaging techniques, the available tracer substances, and the ease of data analysis. The most widely used qualitative methods to assess tissue perfusion are clearly NM methods using single-photon tracers. Quantitative data can be obtained with xenon using NM as well as CT techniques, and the most readily quantifiable methods make use of PET imaging. The mathematics involved in the analysis of data obtained with bolus techniques are quite involved, which is particularly true when input deconvolution is necessary, but with increasing computing power, this no longer poses major limitations. Here, general results were obtained by making various realistic assumptions on how a perfusion experiment is carried out, and these assumptions were made mostly independent of the imaging method used.

The best tracer substances are the freely diffusible tracers with their relatively long tissue transit times, but strictly intravascular substances are also suited as perfusion markers because the extravasation kinetics of the substance into the interstitial space do not have to be modeled. If intravascular substances are used, care has to be taken that the arterial input bolus is as narrow as possible. From a marker substance point of view, the most suitable molecules for such studies are xenon (CT, NM) and water and carbon dioxide (PET), which are freely diffusible substances, and the iodine (CT) and gadolinium (MRI) compounds, which are suitable for brain perfusion studies because there they remain strictly intravascular as long as the blood-brain barrier is intact. From the imaging technology point of view, the NM/PET methods are currently the most simple to analyze. They are used mostly in clinical practice, although xenon-CT with its higher patient radiation dose is still used in some institutions. Methods using iodine and gadolinium compounds have been abandoned and are in experimental use, respectively. The clinical introduction of MRI contrast agents that stay strictly intravascular is currently pending.

We have noted that for dynamic perfusion measurements the quantitative determination of tissue perfusion also either requires a priori knowledge of regional blood volume or the regional blood volume has to be measured in a second experiment. The basics of how to determine blood volume experimentally are discussed in the next section. Further details on how to apply the techniques are given in the chapters on the specific imaging technologies.

BLOOD VOLUME MEASUREMENTS

Several methods have been devised to measure tissue blood volume, and as with perfusion, most efforts have been made to determine cerebral blood volume. Generally speaking, each organ is composed of several tissue components, one of which is the intravascular space occupied by the arterioles, capillaries, and venules. The fraction of the vascular space relative to other tissue in the volume under examination was termed *rBV* earlier, as an abbreviation for *regional blood volume*. It varies substantially from organ to organ and is highest for the kidney; large for liver, spleen, heart, lung, muscles, and the brain; but low in tissues such as fat. In the kidney, *rBV* is on the order of 0.10 to 0.15, while in the brain it is typically 0.03 to 0.05. It has to be noted that it is mainly capillaries and venules that compose the vascular volume, with the arterioles representing only a very small fraction of the total vascular space.

Obviously, an intravascular maker, such as radioactively labeled albumin, hemoglobin, or red cells, can serve as tracers, but blood volume also can be determined using CT or MRI in conjunction with intravascular contrast agents. Albumin and red cells can be labeled with technetium for NM investigations, while hemoglobin labeling is done with ^{11}C or ^{15}O carbon monoxide, which tightly binds to hemoglobin, thus gets stuck in the red blood cells, and remains intravascular in all organs. As noted, the CT and MRI contrast media currently in clinical use stay in the intravascular space only in the normal brain with its intact blood-brain barrier. In all other organs these contrast media will leak into the interstitium to a variable degree. However, there are currently several gadolinium-based compounds and ferrite particles under investigation that have a much longer biologic half-life of several hours compared with the Gd-chelates, which are rapidly eliminated by the kidneys and therefore have biologic half-lives of less than 1 hour. As with tissue perfusion measurements, there are several possibilities to determine blood volume, some based on equilibrium and others based on dynamic experiments. Obviously, the former require that a quasi-equilibrium or quasi-steady state is reached, while the latter can be performed with any tracer substance that stays intravascular during the measurements.

Equilibrium Determination of Blood Volume

Qualitative determinations of blood volume can be done using strictly intravascular compounds labeled with technetium. Most commonly used are Tc-labeled red blood cells, while Tc-labeled albumin has gone out of fashion. The clinical application is mainly in the heart, where the determination of ventricular ejection fraction is based on measurements of end-diastolic and end-systolic blood volume (3, 43). Another application is the diagnosis of liver hemangiomas, which usually have a large blood pool but little perfusion (18) and the pathology seen is a region with increased radioactivity. The large blood pool with relatively little perfusion also is at the base of the characteristic appearance of these lesions on CT and MRI examinations, where late filling in of the lesion with contrast material is observed (Fig. 12). Since the CT and MRI contrast media are quickly eliminated, hemangiomas with very small perfusive input may be missed. Qualitative blood volume determinations are also used occasionally in stroke patients to identify the regions where regional impairment of perfusion leads to an increase in regional blood volume. These standard NM techniques yield qualitative results, except for the ejection fraction determination in the heart, but the latter quantity is a ratio of volumes that does not require absolute quantitation.

The equilibrium approach to quantify blood volume lends itself to analyze data obtained with strictly intravascular tracers such as carbon monoxide. MRI also can potentially be used for this purpose (17) when using contrast agents with prolonged intravascular half-lives such as Gd-polylysine or ultrasmall ferrite particles. For these intravascular agents, the ratio between the concentration measured in the tissue region of interest and the concentration in arterial or venous blood must equal the *rBV* once a tissue distribution equilibrium has been reached after injection. This is obviously so because the tissue region consists of a mixture of blood vessels forming the intravascular space and extracellular and cellular tissue forming the extravascular space. As in perfusion measurements, this general principle is applicable to all intravascular compounds and imaging methods, but the experiments are most simply performed using PET because only in PET is there a simple quantitative relation between the radioactivity measured

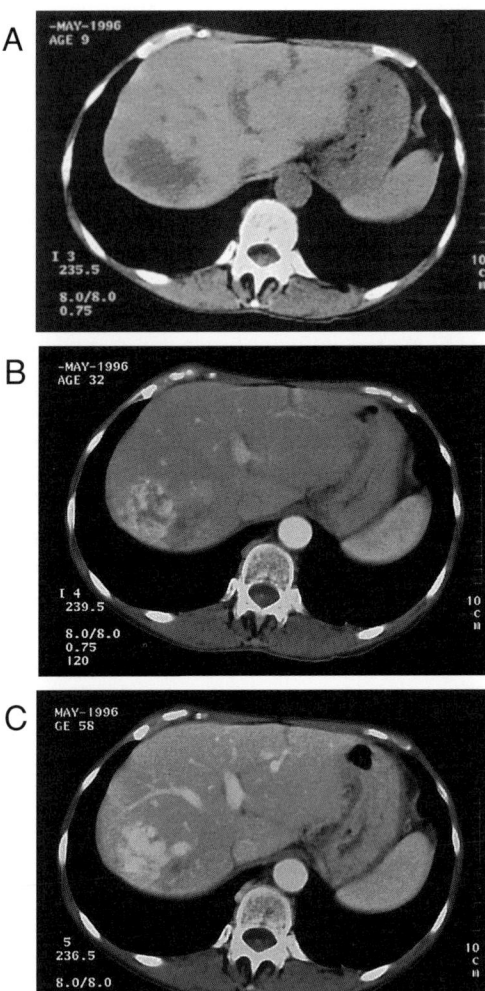

Figure 12. Liver hemangioma as imaged by contrast-enhanced dynamic CT. Note that the image prior to contrast media (CM) injection (**A**) shows a hypointense lesion. A few minutes after CM injection (**B**) the lesion enhances partly, demonstrating the slow inflow of CM. In delayed images almost the entire lesion shows enhancement (**C**). This is a typical example of a lesion with a large blood volume but relatively little perfusion, which results in the observed slow enhancement of the lesion.

in a given region of a scan and that measured in a blood sample. As in perfusion measurements, examinations using MRI need the additional knowledge of a signal-intensity change versus substance-concentration curve, which is strongly dependent on the tissue under consideration and the pulse sequence.

The quantitative description of blood volume determinations using an equilibrium approach is simple. If we call $C_t(t)$ the concentration of the substance in the tissue in grams per milliliter and $C_v(t)$ that in venous blood (which is equal to that of arterial blood but more easily accessible), the regional blood volume rBV is given by

$$rBV = \frac{C_t(t)}{\rho C_v(t)} \tag{21}$$

where ρ is a correction factor, typically on the order of 0.85, accounting for the fact that the hematocrit in capillaries is lower than in the large vessels. Hence not using this correction factor would result in an underestimation of rBV. Obviously, this correction has only to be made when the "tracer" is bound to red cells.

Dynamic Determinations of Blood Volume

Blood volume determinations also can be made by rapid dynamic measurements of the first pass of a tracer substance after a bolus injection. Again, the technique has been implemented quantitatively using PET, but it also turns out that this quantity is readily measured by dynamic tracer bolus studies using CT or MRI as imaging devices.

If a bolus is injected, the total amount of tracer substance delivered to the tissue is given by summing (integrating) the arterial concentration of the substance multiplied by the flow to the tissue over the time during which the bolus passes. Since it was assumed from the beginning that mass is conserved (i.e., what goes in, goes through, and comes out at the other side), the same is true for the tissue and venous concentrations integrated over time with the appropriate correction for the fact that in the tissue only a fraction corresponding to the regional blood volume *rBV* of the total volume consists of vascular space.

$$\int_0^\infty fC_a(t)\,dt \;=\; \int_0^\infty fC_v(t)\,dt \;=\; (1/rBV)\int_0^\infty fC_t(t)\,dt$$

$$\text{or}\qquad rBV = \frac{\displaystyle\int_0^\infty C_t(t)\,dt}{\displaystyle\int_0^\infty C_a(t)\,dt} = \frac{\displaystyle\int_0^\infty C_t(t)\,dt}{\displaystyle\int_0^\infty C_v(t)\,dt} \qquad (22)$$

The blood volume is thus obtained by measuring an arterial input curve to determine the denominator by using arterial sampling, as is commonly done in NM procedures, or alternatively, with higher-resolution modalities such as CT and MRI, larger arterial vessels present on the scan can be used for this purpose, and regions of interest can be drawn around these vessels directly or using some specific algorithms (36). Measurement of venous output curves is not practical. Measurements of signal-intensity versus time curves using intravascular markers are done readily using CT and MRI. Note that since tissues receive the same arterial input, Eq. (22) states that one can obtain relative tissue blood volumes by integrating images pixel-wise over the tissue-concentration versus time curve (2, 26, 46). In fact, this is the only information obtained unless the arterial input function is measured and an input deconvolution is carried out (see preceding section).

When a tomographic measurement of a tissue is performed, the quantity measured during the passage of a bolus of tracer substance is not the concentration of the substance in the tissue at some moment but rather the residual tracer remaining in each voxel in the tissue, provided that no larger vessel is present in it. Using the distribution function of tracer substance as defined in Eqs. (16) and (17), we note once more that it represents the tracer substance leaving the tissue at time t, while the fraction remaining in the tissue is the residue $R(t)$. $R(t)$ is one minus the total fraction of tracer substance that has left the tissue up to the time t:

$$R(t) = 1 - \int_0^t h(t')\,dt' = 1 - H(t') \qquad (23)$$

The rate of change of $R(t)$ must be the concentration in the draining veins, since everything which leaves the tissue must leave it by this path. The concentration in the draining veins is thus proportional to the time derivative of $R(t)$, that is, $-h(t)$, as readily derived from Eq. (23) (2, 44, 46). If a mass m_0 is delivered to the tissue voxel under consideration, the signal measured will be related to $m_0 R(t)$, provided that the zero signal value of that voxel has been subtracted. This zero value is obviously zero in NM tracer studies, since no radioactivity is present before the measurement begins, but has a finite value corresponding to the unenhanced voxel signal value if CT or MRI measurements are used.

Assuming that the relation between the voxel signal measured $S(t)$ and $m_0 R(t)$ is linear, that is,

$$S(t) \propto m_0 R(t)$$

the total residue signal measured over the entire experiment is

$$\int_0^\infty S(t)\,dt \propto \int_0^\infty m_0 R(t)\,dt = m_0 \int_0^\infty th(t)\,dt \tag{24}$$

where use has been made of partial integration and the fact that $\lim tR(t)|_{t\to\infty} = 0$. Comparing Eq. (24) with Eqs. (17), (18), and (19) used to prove the central volume theorem, we conclude that

$$\int_0^\infty S(t)\,dt \propto m_0 t_m = \frac{m_0 rBV}{f} = \frac{m_{inj} rBV}{F} \tag{25}$$

This relation signifies that the signal versus time curve derived from a tomographic measurement only yields the tissue volume to flow ratio if the amount of indicator reaching the voxel m_0 is known. While with a quantitative measurement from a PET system this is feasible using a calibration measurement, it is not possible with either CT or MRI. When performing dynamic contrast media measurements using these instruments, the total injected mass m_{inj} is known and the total flow F at the indicator injection site can be measured, which relate to each other like m_0 and f. It is concluded from this equation that measurement of the signal intensity only provides information proportional to the absolute tissue blood volume but no information on tissue flow. To determine tissue flow with bolus techniques, input deconvolution has to be performed.

PRINCIPLES OF REACTION KINETICS AND COMPARTMENT MODELING

Modern functional imaging is capable of depicting spatially localized biochemistry. While the paradigmatic imaging methods used to image biochemistry are NM and mainly PET, MRI using tissue-specific contrast agents and MRS with its substantial progress toward reasonably resolved chemical-shift images are quickly also moving into the field of ''biochemical'' imaging. Hence, MR specialists in the field of function studies also need familiarity with the methodology used to analyze imaging data on biochemical processes. The standard methodology required to extract quantitative information or even just understand what one measures is tissue compartment modeling. Substantial parts of compartment modeling will therefore be discussed in this section rather than in conjunction with NM methodology.

Biochemical processes are chemical reactions during which substances react to form new compounds or disintegrate. Not only does this hold when a molecule is synthestized, but the same quantitative formalisms also can be used to describe a very temporary binding of a molecule. Hence phosphorylation of glucose, binding to a membrane transporter molecule to be shuttled across a cell membrane, and nonspecific adsorption by hydro- or lipophilic binding of a molecule to a surface can all be described with the same quantitative formalisms. In a biologic system, all these reactions do not take place in a fluid where the substances can move around freely. Rather, biologic systems are compartmentalized into vascular, interstitial, and various cellular compartments. Typically, a substance being metabolized does not undergo a chemical reaction inside the vascular compartment. This compartment is used to transport the molecule to its destination, where it is transported into the cell. Only in the cells will the biochemical reactions involving this molecule occur. Take as an example the glucose molecule, which, once transported by an active transport mechanism into a cell, undergoes a series of reactions known as *glycolysis* and *oxidative phosphorylation* if used for energy generation. For each biochemical process to be described quantitatively, we have to conceptualize a series of model reactions and then solve the mathematical equations describing the reaction kinetics.

In this process, first the compartments are defined, in which the substance of interest is present (i.e., the intravascular compartment, the interstitial compartment, and any number of cellular compartments). This substance of interest will henceforth be termed the *ligand.* Then one identifies which compartments are relevant in order to minimize the parameters necessary to define the model (see Introduction, Chap 3). For example, when formulating a model for glucose metabolism, it is unnecessary to distinguish intravascular and interstitial spaces because glucose moves freely between these two spaces; for glucose, these two compartments are but one. Second, one has to identify what kind of biochemical process occurs within a compartment and quantitatively describe each particular reaction. This is accomplished by using the principles of chemical reaction kinetics, employing the simplest reaction types and the ones describing the vast majority of biochemical processes: the unimolecular and bimolecular reactions. The exchange of substances between compartments in these reactions is characterized by reaction rate constants that are generally used in the description of chemical processes. While the mathematical description of a single chemical reaction is simple (see below), the quantitative description of a combination of reactions as they occur in most biochemical processes is often very difficult. Solving the reaction kinetics equations of a complex biochemical process requires numerical integration of the equations for the most part using substantial computer power.

In this initial section we will formulate the principles of reaction kinetics, while the following sections lay down the principles of compartment modeling and examine various aspects relating to the reaction rate constants.

Fundamentals of Chemical Reaction Kinetics

The two most important chemical reactions are the unimolecular reaction and the bimolecular reaction. In a *unimolecular* reaction, a substance A is transformed into a substance B in whatever conceivable way. A simple example would be that the substance A present in the extracellular fluid crosses the cellular membrane to arrive in the intracellular fluid, where we call it B.

$$A \xrightarrow{k_{AB}} B \quad \text{and} \quad A \xleftarrow{k_{BA}} B$$

The temporal changes in the concentration of B are due to substance A being transformed into it and due to substance B being transformed back into substance A. It is intuitively clear that the generation of B out of A must be proportional to the concentration of substance A available to become transformed into B, and the same way it is clear that the removal of substance B must be proportional to the concentration of substance B available to become retransformed into A: The larger the amount of substance in form A, the more likely the substance will be transformed into substance B, and vice versa. The constants of proportionality in this process are called *unimolecular reaction rate constants*, which have been termed k_{AB} and k_{BA} in the preceding reaction schematics.

The reaction rate constants reflect the physicochemical nature of this transformation, and they are proportional to the probability that a single molecule A is transformed into B or B into A. For example, k_{AB} would be higher for a lipophilic molecule passing from the extracellular to the intracellular compartment than for a hydrophilic molecule. Notice, however, that this simple model reaction does not in general apply to transport across the cellular membrane. In the case of glucose, some amino acids, and many other substances, there are specific transporter mechanisms across the cell membrane. In such situations, binding of a molecule to the transporter on one side of the membrane and unbinding on the other side are required. While it is easy to imagine that if the transport capacity is very high and the molecules to be transported are present in low concentrations, the process actually looks like the one described above (there is no saturation of transporters or ''binding sites''), we also can imagine a situation where transport capacity is limited; then the interaction of the transporter molecule with the substance to be transported becomes relevant. In this setting, *bimolecular* rather than unimolecular reactions have to be considered. A more in-depth discussion of these issues will be presented below.

The quantitative description of a unimolecular reaction is as follows: Call C_A and C_B the respective concentrations in grams per milliliter (fluid or tissue) of the substances under consideration. Then the rates of change of C_A and C_B, dC_A/dt and dC_B/dt is given by

$$dC_A/dt = -k_{AB}C_A + k_{BA}C_B \qquad (26)$$

$$\text{and} \qquad dC_B/dt = +k_{AB}C_A - k_{BA}C_B \qquad (27)$$

The rates of change are proportional to the concentrations of the substances available to react and the rate constants k_{AB} and k_{BA}. Note that Eqs. (26) and (27) describe a set of coupled linear differential equations relating the concentrations of ligand in forms A and B. A and B could be different chemical entities or the same substance in different compartments.

In a *bimolecular* reaction, a substance A reacts with substance B to form a new compound that we call AB. In principle, many standard reactions belong to the category of bimolecular reaction. Examples are the reaction of antigens with antibody haptens, the binding of a neurotransmitter ligand to the receptor binding site, or the reaction of glucose with phosphate to form glucose-6-phosphate.

$$A + B \xrightarrow{k_v} AB \qquad \text{and} \qquad A + B \xleftarrow{k_r} AB$$

As in unimolecular reactions, the probability that a reaction occurs is proportional to the concentration of the reagents available. If many molecules of both types are around for the reaction, it is more likely to occur than when few are around. Hence the rate of appearance of a substance during a reaction must be proportional to the concentration of both reagents, and furthermore, in analogy to the unimolecular reaction rate constants, we have a bimolecular reaction rate constant k_v describing the probability that two molecules A and B will form AB and the constant k_r that describes the probability that a molecule AB will decay into its constituents A and B. Note that while the physical dimensions of the rate constants k_{AB}, k_{BA}, and k_r introduced earlier are all per minute, the dimension of k_v is liter per mole per minute. It is easy to show for both unimolecular and bimolecular reactions that if there is equilibrium, the equilibrium constant K_d is the ratio of k_{AB} to k_{BA} and k_v to k_r, respectively.

Let us briefly examine a special case that in order to simplify matters will be used over and over again when examining various compartment models. If the total number of available reaction sites B is called B_{max} and their availability is very high compared with substance A reacting with B, then the concentration of free sites B (i.e., the ones that are available for reaction) is very closely equal to the total number of B sites, that is, B_{max}, and thus virtually constant. Then the reaction really looks like an unimolecular reaction, and we can write

$$A_{\text{free}} \xrightarrow{k_w = k_v B_{max}} A_{\text{bound}}$$

where we have transformed the bimolecular reaction rate constant k_v into the unimolecular reaction rate constant k_w by multiplying it by B_{max}. Note that k_w also has the dimensions of $\min^{-1}$.

To quantitatively describe the bimolecular reaction, we call C_A and C_B the respective concentrations in grams per milliliter (fluid or tissue) of the substances under consideration and C_{AB} the concentration of the reaction product. Then the rates of change of substances AB, A, and B, dC_{AB}/dt, dC_A/dt, and dC_B/dt are given, respectively, by

$$dC_{AB}/dt = +k_vC_AC_B - k_rC_{AB} \qquad (28a)$$

$$dC_A/dt = -k_vC_AC_B + k_rC_{AB} \qquad (28b)$$

$$\text{and} \qquad dC_B/dt = -k_vC_AC_B + k_rC_{AB} \qquad (28c)$$

In these quantitative descriptions the rates of change are proportional to the concentration of the reagents, as postulated above.

Obviously, the conservation of mass also stipulates that

$$A_{max} = C_{AB} + C_A \quad \text{and} \quad B_{max} = C_{AB} + C_B \quad (29)$$

In the special case of $C_A \ll C_B$, that is, when the ligand to undergo reaction is available in much smaller concentrations than the receptor, and thus the concentration C_{AB} is very small even if k_1 is large, we see from combining Eqs. (28a) and (29) that $B_{max} \approx C_B$ and thus

$$dC_{AB}/dt = +k_v C_A B_{max} - k_r C_{AB} = +k_w C_A - k_r C_{AB} \quad (30)$$

$$\text{with} \quad k_w = k_v B_{max} \quad (31)$$

which is identical to Eq. (26); that is, the system behaves as if it were a unimolecular reaction.

If a reaction is in equilibrium, the rate of change of ligand becomes zero, that is, Eq. (28), or in the special situation with $C_A \ll C_B$, Eq. (30) must be zero. Then we have

$$C_{AB} = \frac{C_A C_B}{K_d} \quad \text{with} \quad K_d = k_r/k_v \quad (32)$$

which is called the *equilibrium binding constant* of the reaction.

Compartment Modeling: General Considerations

As stated, most physiologic and biochemical processes are very complex. The true model of such a process would contain a multitude of compartments, as is demonstrated schematically in Fig. 13. The models generally consist of vascular and tissue compartments. Ligand exchange between the compartments is described by the rate constants $K_1, k_2, \ldots, k_n$, and one uses the conservation of mass principle (see "Quantitative Description of Tissue Perfusion" above) as in the quantitative description of perfusion to arrive at the relations describing the temporal changes in ligand concentrations in the various compartments. Note that in the following section we will use the term *ligand* for

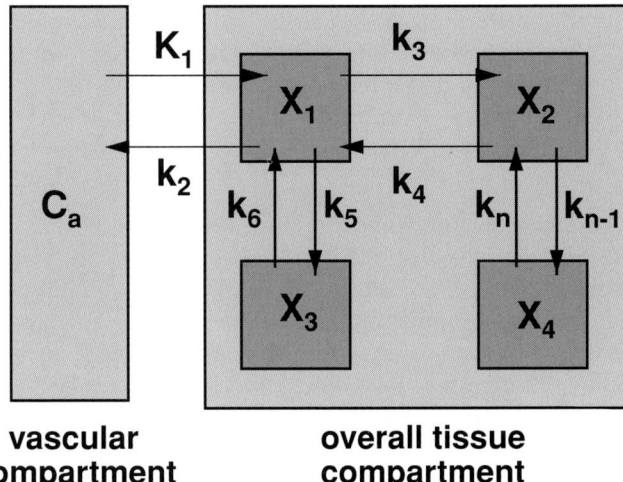

vascular compartment   **overall tissue compartment**

Figure 13. General compartmental model to describe ligand kinetics in a region of interest of a target organ. The model consists of n tissue compartments and the vascular compartment. The concentration in the vascular space is denoted C_a and the concentrations in the tissue compartments $X_1, \ldots, X_n$ with the reaction rate constants $K_1, k_2, \ldots, k_n$.

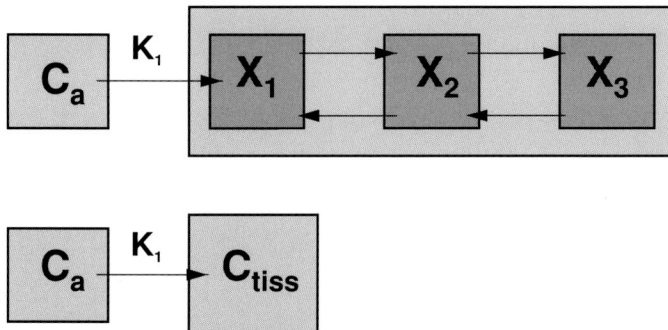

Figure 14. Tracer kinetics with strictly unidirectional transport from vascular space to tissue. The two biochemical systems described by the two different models shown cannot be distinguished from each other because the three compartments shown in the upper model cannot be separated from each other by imaging.

the molecule under study and *receptors* for the sites these molecules are reacting with. But the discussion is also valid in situations where the molecule undergoes metabolism. As an example, FDG takes the role of ligand and the phosphate molecule that reacts with FDG to form FDG-6P takes the role of receptor in the description of the phosphorylation reaction.

Imagine accounting for all the reactions occurring when a model with just four compartments has to be described quantitatively. In this case, eight reaction rate constants and the concentration of binding sites in each compartment would have to be determined, and we would clearly find ourselves in the "elephant" situation of Fig. 1: The model would have so many free parameters that it would be unlikely that enough data could ever be obtained so that inserting them into the model would yield accurate enough numbers to describe the biochemical system under study. The "trick" is obviously to try to find marker molecules for which a complicated model is not necessary or to find— as stated earlier—the simplest model describing the essential features of the behavior of the molecular system under examination. A simplified model requires determination of a smaller number of fit parameters, thereby greatly increasing the accuracy of the results of fitting model curves to the data.

When imaging, the spatial resolution of the imaging systems in use precludes the anatomic separation of individual kinetic compartments, since the partitions are typically of cellular or even subcellular size. As a result, we can only measure the average tissue concentration $C_{\text{tiss}}(t)$ and hence the sum of the signals coming from the relative concentrations of the ligand in each of the tissue compartments X_i:

$$C_{\text{tiss}}(t) = \sum_{i=1}^{n} X_i \tag{33}$$

Furthermore, the concentrations measured in a region of interest also contain some blood within the arterioles, venules, and capillaries in the area: the vascular compartment. Therefore, one observes the sum of the signal from the ligand in all tissue compartments $C_{\text{tiss}}(t)$ but has to add a contribution coming from the vascular compartment. The inability to separate different tissue compartments by imaging has a very important consequence: Several completely different reaction configurations can look identical when examined. If transport between the vascular and the tissue spaces is only unidirectional, it turns out that it is not possible to characterize the individual tissue compartments in a complicated model like the one in Fig. 14 at the top. The only information that can be obtained is that represented by the simple one-tissue compartment model depicted in Fig. 14 at the bottom: Any exchange of substance within the various tissue compartments of Fig. 14 (above) does not change the overall signal measured. This simple example already points to the importance of parameter k_2, which describes transport from the tissue space to the vascular space. On the other hand, if substance is released from the tissue compartment into the vascular compartment again—i.e., if k_2 is not zero—the rate of removal out of the region of interest affects the substance distribution among the various tissue compartments. In the discussion on receptor modeling, this issue will be examined in more detail.

Since the signal measured in a region of interest (ROI) is composed of tissue and vascular fractions, the concentration of ligand in such an ROI can be expressed as

$$C_{TAC}(t) = rBV \cdot C_a(t) + (1 - rBV) \cdot C_{\text{tiss}}(t)$$

$$= rBV \cdot C_a + (1 - rBV) \cdot \sum_{i=1}^{n} X_i \tag{34}$$

where $C_{TAC}(t)$ is the total ligand concentration in the region of interest (time-activity curve), rBV denotes the regional blood volume, and C_a and $C_{\text{tiss}}(t)$ are the concentrations of ligand in blood and tissue, respectively.

In NM including PET, no direct compartment separation is possible at all on the images, while with the higher-resolution modalities such as CT and MRI, at least larger vessels can be identified. Hence such images may contain information on the vascular compartment that can be measured separately, while in NM and PET information on the vascular compartment is obtained by arterial or venous sampling.

Equation (34) represents the central functional equation for modeling of an n-compartment biochemical reaction. Depending on the information desired, one approaches

---

Equation (34) represents a general equation for an n-compartment model. Since the tissue and vascular compartment concentrations are related to each other by the reaction rate Eqs. (26) through (28) and (30), Eq. (34) is a relation linking a set of differential equations. The ligand exchange between the compartments in the general model of Fig. 12 is described by a set of n differential equations. It can be shown by using general mathematical arguments (19) that these differential equations can be represented as follows:

$$dr_x/dt = Ar_x + r_b C_a(t) \tag{35}$$

where $C_a(t)$ is the arterial input function, $r_x = [x_1, \ldots, x_n]$ is the vector of ligand concentrations in the n tissue compartments, A is the matrix of transfer rates between compartments, and $r_b = [b_1, \ldots, b_n]$ is a vector of transfer rates from the input to the compartments. Note that Eq. (35) represents a system of linear differential equations, i.e., a set of unimolecular reactions or of bimolecular reactions that are linearized according to Eq. (30). This is advantageous because linear differential equations with constant coefficients can be solved analytically in most situations, while this is usually not the case for nonlinear (e.g., quadratic) differential equations.

The solution to the set of linear differential Eq. (35) is given by

$$r_x = e^{Mt} r_b * C_a(t) \tag{36}$$

where e^{Mt} is the matrix exponential and the asterisk denotes the convolution operation (9). Note the resemblance to Eq. (4), which also was arrived at by integrating the linear differential equation represented in Eq. (1).

In receptor binding when the receptor sites are nearly occupied, the situation becomes more complex. Then the differential equations may no longer be simplified using the approach leading to Eq. (30) but contain nonlinear terms, which appear when the full Eq. (28) (combined with Eq. 29) has to be used. In these situations the rate of change of bound substance depends nonlinearly (e.g., quadratically) on the concentration of the free substance. This situation will be discussed in more detail below.

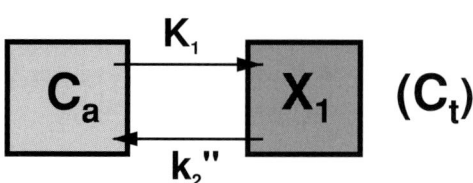

Figure 15. One-tissue compartment model. The vascular component C_a of the ligand is in exchange with the tissue ligand C_t, which denotes the total ligand, since in this model no distinction is made between free and specifically and nonspecifically bound ligand. The rate constants are K_1 and k_2'', where the " denotes that the ligand exiting the tissue compartments does not only come from the free tissue ligand.

solving this equation from either of two sides. The approach we have been taking so far is the experimental approach. In an experiment we can measure the time course of the concentrations C_{TAC} and C_a, and we would like to derive information on the kinetic constants K_1 to k_n, which are implicit in Eq. (34) because all the concentrations C and X in this equation are linked by unimolecular or bimolecular reaction kinetic relations, as discussed in "Equilibrium Determination of Blood Volume" above. The problem consists of finding the set of parameters K_1 to k_n for which the model-generated tissue concentration versus time curves for the concentrations C_{TAC} and C_a best approximate the measured ones. The method used to this end is mathematical curve fitting. As demonstrated in Fig. 1, curve fitting becomes more difficult and less conclusive the more parameters can freely change; hence the need to use substances that obey simple models if substantial information is to be derived from this curve-fitting process.

Note, however, that Eq. (34) also can be looked at from a different point of view. We can use Eq. (34) to make model predictions. One assumes values for K_1 to k_n and an arterial input function $C_a(t)$ and calculates the time course of $C_{\text{tiss}}(t)$. With the availability of powerful computers, this is achieved easily by numerical integration of the set of differential equations that Eq. (34) in fact constitutes. The advantage of this approach is that the complexity of the model is of no importance except that it can take shorter or longer to compute the results. In simple cases, the differential equations can be solved explicitly. This second approach lends itself perfectly to simulation studies. Such studies are extremely useful to examine the effects of varying the arterial input curve or the parameters K_1 to k_n on the time course of the tissue concentration.

Common Models Used in Receptor Imaging

Figures 15, 16, and 17 depict models commonly used in receptor imaging. They are composed of one, two, and three tissue compartments containing the concentrations X_1, X_2, and X_3 of ligand, respectively. Each model contains in addition the vascular compartment containing ligand at concentration C_a, which is obviously necessary because through it occurs delivery and removal of ligand to and from the region of interest. We

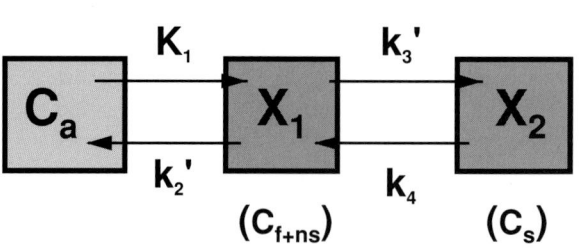

Figure 16. Two-tissue compartment model. The vascular component C_a of the ligand is in exchange with the ligand C_{f+ns}, which represents the sum of the free and nonspecifically bound ligand. In a further reaction, free and nonspecifically bound ligand is converted into specifically bound ligand C_s and back. The rate constants are K_1, k_2', k_3, and k_4, where the prime denotes that ligand exiting the tissue compartment does not only come from the free tissue ligand.

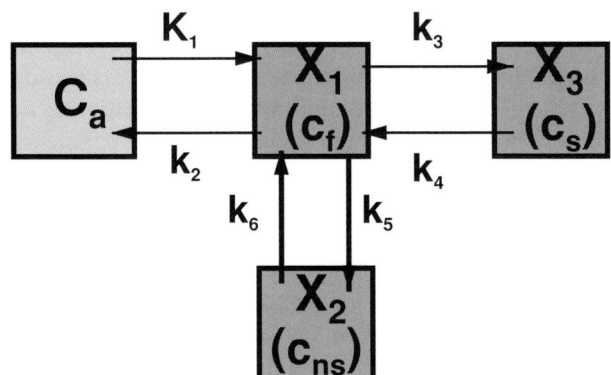

Figure 17. Three-tissue compartment model. The vascular component C_a of the ligand is in exchange with the free ligand C_f in tissue. The ligand can then further react to become nonspecifically bound ligand C_{ns} or into specifically bound ligand C_s and back. The rate constants are K_1, k_2, k_3, k_4, k_5, and k_6.

will denote the models A (one-tissue compartment model), B (two-tissue compartment model), and C (three-tissue compartment model). The notations with double primes are borrowed from Koeppe et al. (25) and signify that the compartment from which the ''double prime'' k values originate does not only represent free ligand. This is the case in the models depicted in Figs. 15 and 16, where the tissue subcompartments exchanging ligand with the vascular compartment are either not or only partly considered distinct entities.

One-Tissue Compartment Model

Let us first consider the one-tissue compartment model of Fig. 15, which we shall call model A and which is clearly the simplest of the three models depicted. Here ligand is brought to the tissue by the vascular compartment, is taken up into the tissue with the uptake constant K_1 and can leave the tissue again, and this is controlled by the rate constant k_2''. The rate of uptake also must be proportional to the concentration of ligand being supplied $C_a(t)$; hence the uptake is given by $K_1 C_a(t)$, while the rate at which ligand leaves the tissue is proportional to k_2'' and its concentration in the tissue X_1. The net rate of change of ligand in tissue is thus given by what comes in and what leaves it, that is,

$$dX_1/dt = -k_2''X_1 + K_1 C_a(t) \tag{37}$$

MATHEMATICAL ANALYSIS OF MODEL A

As already noted, the solution of linear differential equations like Eq. (37) can be given analytically if the arterial input function is given, and it involves the convolution operation denoted here with an asterisk:

$$X_1 = K_1 \exp(-k_2''t)*C_a(t) \tag{38}$$

This is equal to Eq. (4) if we assume that the ligand concentration in tissue was zero at the onset of the experiment. Let us examine the special case where $k_2'' = 0$. In this situation, ligand enters the tissue compartment but cannot leave it. Physiologically, it corresponds to the perfusion case where no substance leaves the tissue once it has entered it (i.e., the so-called microsphere case). Then the preceding solution simplifies to $X_1 = K_1*C_a(t)$, which when making use of the definition of the convolution operation yields

$$X_1 = K_1 \int_0^t C_a(s)\, ds \tag{39}$$

Comparing this expression with Eq. (5), the analogy to microsphere perfusion is again obvious, although there we were interested in the total substance accumulated at the end of the experiment; hence integration there was carried out up to infinity.

Note that this expression is identical to the one derived when analyzing tissue perfusion (Eqs. 1 and 2), since the problem analyzed there was identical: We equated the rate at which a perfusion marker entered and left the tissue to derive the mathematical expression there. Hence when analyzing the problem of tissue perfusion, we already made use of the most simple form of compartmental analysis; we investigated a model with a vascular and a tissue compartment. It turns out that the rate constant K_1 is very often closely related to tissue flow, but this will be evaluated in more detail in ''Model Reduction Illustrated in Receptor Imaging'' below. Since the mathematical equations describing ligand behavior in model A are the same as those describing perfusion, the solution is also the same. The same is true for the special cases. If we assume that $k_2'' = 0$, that is, the ligand sticks to the tissue and does not leave it, we find ourselves in the microsphere perfusion situation discussed in ''Mechanical and Biochemical Microspheres'' above. Note that if a ligand shows such behavior, rather than telling us something about the receptor system it is supposed to probe, it will merely act as a marker of perfusion. Further discussion of this point will come in ''Suitability of Ligands'' below.

Two-Tissue Compartment Model

The second model that we want to analyze is the two-tissue compartment model depicted in Fig. 16 and termed model B, which is simple to examine but more complicated to give the mathematical solutions. Conservation of ligand requires again that ligand can neither disappear nor appear from a compartment except by the reaction routes defined in Fig. 16. Let us start the analysis with compartment 2. Ligand appears there by being transformed by ''reaction'' out of compartment 1 in proportion to its concentration X_1 with the rate constant k_3', and it disappears in proportion to its concentration in compartment X_2 with a rate constant k_4:

$$dX_2/dt = k_3'X_1 - k_4X_2 \tag{40a}$$

The flux into and out of compartment 1 is more complicated because it is from and toward the vascular compartment as well as to and from compartment 2. The description of the flux of ligand from and into the vascular compartment was already obtained when deriving Eq. (37), but in addition, in model B there is flux from compartment 1 to compartment 2 according to $k_3'X_1$ and from compartment 2 to compartment 1 according to k_4X_2. Thus the net change of ligand in compartment 1 is given by

$$dX_1/dt = -(k_2' + k_3')X_1 + k_4X_2 + K_1C_a(t) \tag{40b}$$

Equation (40) is a set of two coupled linear differential equations whose solutions are relatively complicated and given below. Many systems can be quite adequately described with a two-tissue compartment model. Probably the most relevant example of a system

---

MATHEMATICAL ANALYSIS OF MODEL B

The solution of Eq. (40) is

$$C_{\text{tiss}}(t) = X_1 + X_2 = [K_1/(\alpha_1 - \alpha_2)][(k_3' + k_4 - \alpha_1)e^{-\alpha_1 t} \tag{41}$$
$$+ (\alpha_2 - k_3' - k_4)e^{-\alpha_2 t}]*C_a(t)$$

with $\quad \alpha_{1,2} = \left[k_2' + k_3' + k_4 \mp \sqrt{(k_2' + k_3' + k_4)^2 - (4k_2'k_4)}\right]\Big/2 \tag{42}$

In the special case where $k_4 = 0$, that is, when there is virtually no ligand released after it has bound to the receptors, the solution simplifies to

$$C_{\text{tiss}}(t) = X_1 + X_2 = [K_1/(k_2' + k_3')][(k_3' + k_2'e^{-(k_2'+k_3')t}]*C_a(t) \tag{43}$$

This is the case when modeling FDG metabolism for data acquired within the first hour after FDG injection (see Chap. 5).

that behaves according to model B is the phosphorylation of FDG to FDG-6P, a reaction that has been used extensively for in vivo quantitation of glucose metabolism. This example will be discussed in more detail in Chap. 5.

Four-Tissue Compartment Model

The third model, model C, is again simple to examine, but the mathematical solutions are very complicated. Conservation of ligand requires again that ligand can neither disappear nor appear from a compartment except by following the reaction routes as defined in Fig. 17. The rate equations for compartments 2 and 3 are in analogy with Eq. (40a):

$$dX_2/dt = k_5 X_1 - k_6 X_2 \qquad (44a)$$

$$dX_3/dt = k_3 X_1 - k_4 X_2 \qquad (44b)$$

The flux into and out of compartment 1 is even more complicated than in model B because there are three ways for ligand to enter and exit. Compared with model B, there is an additional exchange of ligand between compartment 1 and 3. Thus the net change of ligand in compartment 1 is given by

$$dX_1/dt = -(k_2'' + k_3 + k_5)X_1 + (k_4 + k_6)X_2 + K_1 C_a(t) \qquad (44c)$$

Equation (44) is a set of three coupled linear differential equations. General solutions exist but are so complicated that they are beyond the context of this book.

One-Tissue Compartment Model with Coupled Ligands: Oxygen Consumption

The fourth model, relevant when measuring the oxygen extraction fraction, is depicted in Fig. 18. This model accounts for two different substance fluxes rather than just one, as the models described above, namely, the flux of oxygen as well as water. This model has been used extensively for PET determinations of oxygen extraction fractions. The concept of oxygen extraction is discussed here because it also bears relevance to the BOLD effect observed in MRI studies (see Chap. 8), but the specific PET applications are discussed in Chap. 5.

The measurement of the oxygen consumption and the extraction fraction or ratio (OER) is of considerable interest to understand various disease states. In early cerebral ischemia, it is in fact the OER that first increases as a result of capillary dilatation. As a result, the blood and the brain cells are longer in contact, and the efficiency at which the oxygen is transferred from hemoglobin to the brain tissue is higher, representing a mechanism for the brain to protect itself against ischemia in addition to increasing the regional perfusion. While the OER is relatively low in brain in normal perfusion states, in the heart the OER is already high in the resting state, and much of the increased demand occurring during exercise is provided by increased flow. The model used to analyze OER is presented here for two reasons. First, it represents an interesting example for quantitative analysis of an important problem, and quantitative information on OER can be obtained with PET. Second, with the advent of MRI, issues of hemoglobin oxygenation have become relevant for the understanding of the BOLD effect (29). The PET

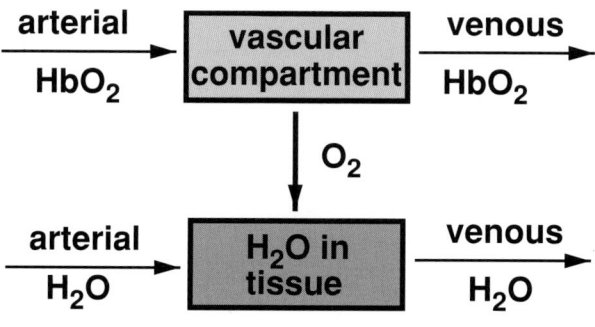

Figure 18. Compartment model for oxygen consumption in tissues. Oxygen enters the tissues through the vascular compartment and is completely converted into water on entry into tissues. Water, on the other hand, is freely diffusible, and therefore, it is described by the single-compartment model at the bottom of the figure.

methods devised to measure OER permit one to determine the oxygen removal from the bloodstream and thereby determine cerebral oxygen consumption. Once OER is known, we may obtain the oxygen consumption of the tissue under consideration, since it is simply the arterial concentration of oxygen multiplied by the tissue flow and the fraction OER. Similar to perfusion measurements using PET, an equilibrium approach and a dynamic approach have been devised, and both will be discussed here.

The events occurring during oxygen delivery to tissues can be conceptualized as in Fig. 18. When O_2 is inhaled, it is transported by the hemoglobin located in the red blood cells to the organ under consideration, enters the cells, and is transformed immediately and completely into water by oxidation so that it may be fairly assumed that the tissue contains virtually no oxygen. Thus k_2 is zero for oxygen. For O_2 we have therefore the simple situation of a one-tissue compartment model, as discussed in "One-Tissue Compartment Model" above. By looking at the vascular rather than the tissue compartment and using $k_2 = 0$, we derive in analogy to Eq. (37).

$$dC_a/dt = -K_1 C_a(t) \tag{45}$$

For H_2O the situation is as follows: It is produced by oxidation and is a freely diffusible substance, as already assumed when analyzing the problem of tissue perfusion. Hence it is in equilibrium with the venous bloodstream through which it leaves the cells and recirculates. When labeled O_2 is used (denoted here with an asterisk), the total O* concentration in the tissue compartment C_{O*t} is thus a sum of the H_2O* generated by the conversion of O_2* $[+K_1 C_a(t)]$ and of recirculating H_2O*. Conservation of substance applied to the H_2O* compartment requires that the difference of the flux of substance into and out of the tissue compartment equals the rate of change of the substance within the compartment. The flux into the compartment is the sum of the fraction of the oxygen converted into water by the metabolic conversion of O_2* into H_2O* in the tissue and the recirculating H_2O* (first term in Eq. 45). The flux leaving the tissue is equal to the tissue concentration C_{tH_2O*}, which again is presumed to be in equilibrium with the venous concentration divided by the tissue-blood partition coefficient for water P.

$$dC_{tH_2O*}/dt = \underbrace{f(C_{aH_2O*} + OER \cdot C_{aO*_2})}_{\text{Arterial influx}} - \underbrace{C_{tH_2O*}/P}_{\text{Venous outflux}} \tag{46}$$

where OER is the oxygen extraction ratio. Note that if the notation with K_1 is used, we have

$$K_1 = OER \cdot f \tag{47}$$

A quantitative analysis of this compartment model is provided in Chap. 5.

In MRI, the quantity of principal interest is the venous hemoglobin (HbO_2) concentration, since it can be safely assumed that the arterial hemoglobin concentration is equal for all perfused organs. In keeping with the preceding model, we note that the difference between arterial and venous hemoglobin is equal to the oxygen that has been removed in the tissue, and this is given by $C_{aO_2}OER$. In a steady-state situation, we have

$$C_{vO_2} = C_{aO_2}(1 - OER) \tag{48}$$

If the oxygen consumption of the tissue is constant and the flow is increased, the OER has to decrease, hence the increase in venous HbO_2, which by decreasing the amount of paramagnetic Hb leads to the signal enhancement observed on MRI images.

Like perfusion, the oxygen extraction fraction OER can be measured under steady-state conditions or using the bolus injection approach in PET and with ^{15}O-labeled oxygen. In both the steady-state and dynamic approaches, it may be deemed necessary to correct the final result for the oxygen activity bound intravascularly to hemoglobin. Such a correction requires a blood volume measurement in addition to the measurement of tissue flow and oxygen extraction. With the BOLD effect in MRI, a quantity is measured that ultimately is related to the concentration of deoxyhemoglobin in the tissue under study.

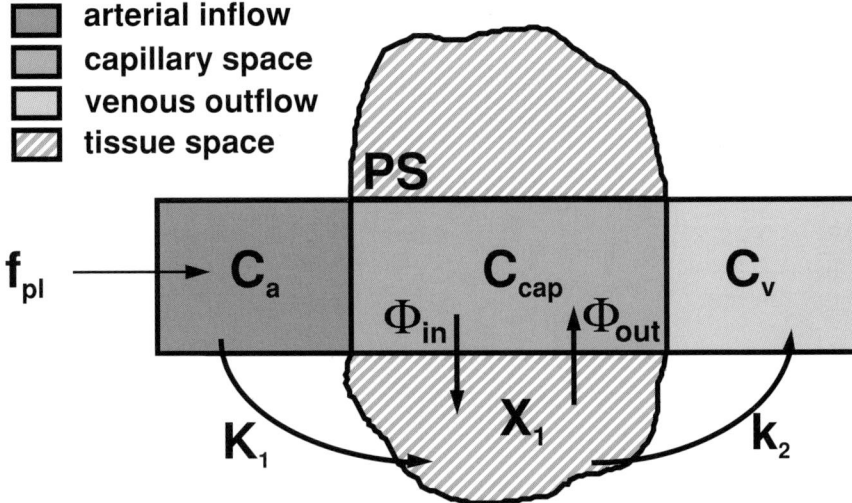

Figure 19. In reality, exchange of ligand occurs along the course of the capillary with an influx Φ_{in} and an outflux Φ_{out}. Ligand is present in the various vascular sections in concentrations denoted C_a, C_{cap}, and C_v and the arterial flow f_{pl}. How much of a barrier the capillary to tissue barrier is can be described by using the so-called permeability surface product *PS*. The rate constants K_1 and k_2 describe the exchange from the arterial to the venous rather than to the capillary compartment.

The Parameter K_1, Influx Rate Constant from Vascular into Tissue Compartment

In all the models discussed in "Common Models Used in Receptor Imaging" above, the parameter K_1 describes delivery of ligand from the vascular compartment to the tissue, and k_2, k_2', and k_2'' describe the rate of backdiffusion of ligand from the tissue to the vascular space and subsequent removal from the region of interest. The capital letter of K_1 underscores the different dimension of this parameter (ml/min/ml of tissue as opposed to min^{-1} for the other parameters k_i). K_1 relates the mass flux of ligand into tissue to the arterial concentration of ligand at the entrance to the target organ (C_a). However, the ligand exchange between the vascular compartment and tissue occurs in the capillary space rather than in the feeding arteries. A simplified model of this exchange is depicted in Fig. 19. If we assume passive diffusion as the transport mechanism, the permeability of the capillaries to the ligand as well as the total capillary surface area per tissue volume must be closely related to K_1. This so-called permeability surface product *PS* is one key factor determining the rate of ligand exchange between vascular space and tissue. The flow into the tissue through the arteries is denoted f_{pl}, the plasma flow.

The aim of the following section is to illuminate this relationship between K_1, *PS,* and f_{pl} to thereby understand more profoundly how ligand exchange between the capillary bed and the tissue occurs and to analyze how different exchange modes affect the binding of ligand to tissues. The fluxes of ligand into (Φ_{in}) and out of (Φ_{out}) tissue are defined by

$$\Phi_{in} = PSC_{cap} \tag{49}$$

$$\Phi_{out} = PSX_1 \tag{50}$$

In the models discussed above, the flux into the tissue was given in terms of K_1. Using the notation introduced previously, the flux into tissue is

$$\Phi_{in} = K_1C_a \tag{51}$$

It is of crucial importance which assumptions regarding the spatial profile of the capillary concentration C_{cap} are made as the capillary traverses from arterioles to venules. A simple assumption is that mixing in capillary space is instantaneous, leading to a homogeneous ligand concentration. A consequence of this assumption is an abrupt concentration change

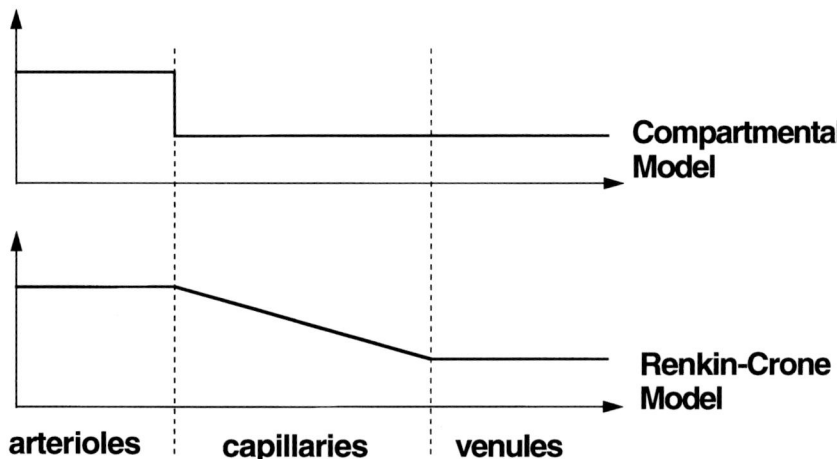

Figure 20. If equilibration of the ligand across the capillary membrane is instantaneous, there is an abrupt drop in ligand concentration at the entrance to the capillary. This is depicted in the top graph. If a more physiologic linear decrease of concentration along the course of the capillary is assumed, the concentration along the capillary looks like that depicted in the bottom graph. This model was proposed by Renkin and Crone.

at the entrance to capillary space (Fig. 20). Employing the conservation of mass principle then yields the differential equations for the concentrations in capillary and tissue space. An alternative assumption about the concentration of ligand in the capillaries is a linear decrease from arterial to venous concentration levels. This type of assumption is depicted in the bottom graph of Fig. 20.

A quantitative analysis of the situation where bolus injection is used yields the not very surprising result that K_1 is proportional to blood flow if the surface permeability is high, i.e., when the ligand is virtually extracted completely as it passes the capillary bed. On the other hand, if the surface permeability product PS is small compared with the capillary flow, the uptake of tracer becomes independent of perfusion. These results are derived under the assumption that capillary and venous concentrations are equal, which is the same assumption used to derive the perfusion equation in "Quantitative Description of Tissue Perfusion" above. If a more complex dependence of capillary concentration as a function of the course of the capillary is assumed (Fig. 20, bottom graph), the limit that K_1 is determined by plasma flow if the extraction of the substance is high and determined by the extraction if this is relatively low is still valid.

The quantitative analysis leading to these predictions is as follows: Using the definitions given earlier and remembering that rBV is the regional blood volume, the differential equation for the capillary concentration C_{cap} can be written as

$$rBV \cdot dC_{cap}/dt = -(f_{pl} + PS)C_{cap} + PSX_1 + f_{pl}C_a \qquad (52)$$

$$\text{and} \qquad (1 - rBV)dX_1/dt = PS(C_{cap} - X_1) \qquad (53)$$

The venous outflow does not appear here because it is assumed that C_{cap} and C_v are equal. These equations were again obtained simply by using conservation of mass and accounting for the fluxes into and from the capillary and the tissue compartments, as shown in Fig. 19. It should be noted that there is another simplification in Eq. (52). The left side describes the temporal change in the amount of tracer in capillary space. One should therefore correctly use the volume of capillary space, which is somewhat smaller than rBV, since the latter contains arterioles and venules in addition to capillaries. However, the consequences of this simplification are negligible, since the left sides of Eqs. (52) and (53) are neglected in the following derivation. In principle, Eqs. (52) and (53) could be solved explicitly.

For our purposes, another simpler approach shall be taken. The equations will be evaluated during the first pass of a bolus of ligand through the target organ.

During the first pass, transport of ligand is primarily unidirectional from the capillary to tissue ($X_1 \ll C_{cap}$). For simplification, we assume $X_1 = 0$. Since the regional blood volume in tissue is very small in most tissues, the temporal change in the mass of ligand in the capillary ($rBV \cdot dC_{cap}/dt$) can be expected to be small compared with the ligand fluxes. For practical purposes, $rBV \cdot dC_{cap}/dt$ can then be set to zero. With these assumptions, Eq. (52) becomes

$$0 = -(f_{pl} + PS)C_{cap} + f_{pl}C_a \tag{54}$$

and solving for C_{cap}, we obtain

$$C_{cap} = \frac{C_a f_{pl}}{f_{pl} + PS} \tag{55}$$

Inserting this expression into Eq. (49) and equating Eqs. (49) and (51) yields

$$K_1 = \frac{PSf_{pl}}{f_{pl} + PS} \tag{56}$$

This expression is interesting because it lends itself to a simple interpretation. K_1 is proportional to the probability per unit time that a molecule gets transported into the tissue from the vascular compartment. Apparently, this probability is a function of the probability that a molecule gets close to the tissue by plasma flow and the probability that it crosses from the vascular to the tissue compartments. If either flow or the permeability surface product are zero, then the transport probability becomes zero. If $PS \gg f_{pl}$, then $K_1 \approx f_{pl}$ and the process is dominated by flow of the ligand to the region, while if $PS \ll f_{pl}$, then $K_1 \approx PS$ and the kinetics of tissue compartment uptake are determined by the properties of the boundary between the vascular and tissue compartments and independent of tissue flow.

A useful expression is the *first-pass extraction fraction*. It is defined as the fraction of incoming ligand that is transported into tissue during the first pass of the bolus through the target organ:

$$E_{fp} = \frac{\Phi_{in}}{C_a f_{pl}} \tag{57}$$

Combining Eqs. (51) and (57) yields

$$K_1 = f_{pl}E_{fp} \tag{58}$$

which for the special case of $E_{fp} = OER$ was already intuitively derived in Eq. (47). Combining Eq. (58) with Eq. (56), we obtain

$$E_{fp} = \frac{PS}{PS + f_{pl}} \tag{59}$$

This signifies in analogy to the preceding that if the permeability surface product is high, i.e., the probability that the molecule gets into tissue across the compartmental boundary, E_{fp} becomes 1; hence K_1 is closely associated with blood flow. For freely diffusible tracers, the first-pass extraction fraction is high (>95%), and K_1 equals blood flow. For microspheres the same is true, but the model outlined in Fig. 19 is not valid because the microspheres do not cross into tissue space.

A more physiologic model for the concentration variation of a substance along the path of a capillary from the arteriolar to the venous side was developed by Renkin (37) and Crone (10). It allows for a concentration gradient between the arterial inlet and the venous outlet of the capillary (bottom graph in Fig. 20). With this model, Renkin and Crone derived the following expression for the first-pass extraction fraction:

$$E_{fp} = 1 - \exp(-PS/f_{pl}) \tag{60}$$

The first-pass extraction fraction is of major importance for perfusion tracers. Implications of a reduced E_{fp} are discussed in "Suitability of Ligands" above.

Model Reduction Illustrated in Receptor Imaging

Practical experience shows that in imaging experiments, the estimation of most parameters becomes unreliable or even impossible if the number of compartments exceeds two tissue compartments, i.e., if the model has more than three compartments (remember Fig. 1). For practical purposes, one therefore should try to find ligands whose fate can be described using such simple models, or—given a ligand—one has to reduce a per se

---

REDUCTION OF THE MATHEMATICAL MODEL

When there is rapid equilibration between the compartment with free and non-specifically bound ligand, model C can be reduced to model B. The following relationships exist between the rate constants of model C and model B.

$$k_2' + \quad = \frac{K_2}{1 + k_5/k_6} = \frac{K_1}{DV_f(1 + k_5/k_6)} = \frac{K_1}{DV_{f+ns}} \ (\text{min}^{-1}) \tag{60}$$

where $K_1/k_2 \ (=DV_f)$ is the distribution volume of the free ligand and DV_{f+ns} is the summed distribution volume of the free and nonspecifically bound ligand.

In general, the distribution volume is an often used and helpful entity in tracer kinetics. It is defined as the concentration in compartment A (C_A) relative to another compartment B (C_B) at equilibrium, e.g., $DV = C_A/C_B$. One often chooses the tracer concentration in plasma as C_B. At equilibrium, the net mass flux between any compartments is zero. Considering, for example, the compartments C_a and X_1 in model C, this means that the flux from blood to tissue ($=K_1C_a$) equals the flux of backdiffusion from the free tissue compartment to blood ($=k_2X_1$), for example,

$$K_1C_a = k_2X_1 \tag{61a}$$

The distribution volume DV_f of compartment X_1 relative to blood is X_1/C_a, which according to Eq. (61a) is K_1/k_2:

$$DV_f(1 + k_5/k_6) = DV_{f+ns} \tag{61b}$$

Furthermore, k_3' is given by

$$k_3' = \frac{k_3}{1 + k_5/k_6} = \frac{k_{on}B_{max}}{1 + k_5/k_6} \ (\text{min}^{-1}) \tag{62}$$

where k_v, defined in "Fundamentals of Chemical Reaction Kinetics" above, is called k_{on} in receptor kinetics, and k_3 takes the role of k_w.

A useful measure for receptor density is the distribution volume of specifically bound ligand relative to ligand concentration in blood (DV_s). In terms of the rate constants, DV_s can be expressed as follows

$$DV_s = \frac{K_1k_3'}{k_2'k_4} \ (\text{ml/g}) \tag{63}$$

If there is rapid equilibration between the two tissue compartments of model **B,** a further reduction to model **A** is possible.

$$k_2'' = \frac{k_2'}{1 + k_3'/k_4}$$

$$= \frac{k_2(1 + k_3'/k_4)}{1 + k_5/k_6} = \frac{k_2}{1 + k_3/k_4 + k_5/k_6} \ (\text{min}^{-1}) \tag{64}$$

$$\text{and} \quad DV'' = \frac{K_1}{k_2''} = DV_s + DV_{ns} + DV_f$$

is the total distribution volume of ligand in tissue.

complicated biologic model describing the ligands' fate to one or two tissue compartments. This has implications for the interpretation of the parameters, as shall now be demonstrated.

When describing ligand binding to receptor sites, one has to consider that depending on the amount of ligand injected, a considerable fraction of receptor sites may become occupied during the experiment. This leads to nonlinear kinetics, as will be discussed below. The case with a negligible amount of ligand relative to the available free receptor sites shall be considered first (see "Model Reduction Illustrated in Receptor Imaging" and "Receptor Kinetics with Minimal Receptor Occupation" above). It is obvious, for example, that when there is rapid equilibration between the compartments containing free and nonspecifically bound ligand, model C in Fig. 17 reduces to model B in Fig. 16.

Receptor Kinetics with Minimal Receptor Occupation

In receptor kinetics, the situation with minimal receptor occupation must be distinguished from the case with major receptor occupation. In the latter case, the number of available receptor sites decreases during the course of the experiment, leading to progressively slower binding of ligand to receptors, as will be discussed later in "Receptor Kinetics with Major Receptor Occupation." Compartmental modeling of receptor-ligand binding usually starts with model **C** shown in Fig. 17. The four compartments correspond to extractable ligand in arterial blood (C_a), free ligand in tissue (C_f), and ligand bound nonspecifically (C_{ns}) and specifically (C_s). The six rate constants describe the exchange of ligand between the different compartments. The physiologic meaning of the parameter K_1 was discussed earlier.

In receptor imaging, the major interest in compartment modeling is usually to obtain information on the receptors involved, notably their concentration and the affinity of the ligand to the receptor site. This information is contained in parameters k_3 and k_4, which are related to the receptor characteristics; e.g., k_3 denotes the product of k_{on} and B_{max} ($k_3 = k_{on}B_{max}$) (Eqs. 31 and 62), and k_4 represents the dissociation rate of ligand from receptor k_{off}. In practice, it is usually not possible to employ the complex model **C** required to estimate k_3 because too many parameters have to be determined, leading to inaccuracy. An alternative is to use the simplified two-tissue compartment model **B** and take k_3' and related parameters as a measure for receptor density. A summary of useful receptor measures and their relation to B_{max} is given in Table 2.

One of the simpler measures for receptor density is the distribution volume of total ligand binding determined with the one-tissue compartment model **A** (DV''). Advantages of this measure are the reliability and simplicity with which it can be calculated. The measure can even be estimated on a pixel-by-pixel basis, allowing the calculation of parametric maps (25). A disadvantage is that a clear separation of specific and nonspecific

Table 2. *Useful quantities describing receptor characteristics and their relation to the receptor density B_{max}*

Model	Parameter	Relation to B_{max}
B	k_3'	$k_3' = \dfrac{k_{on}B_{max}}{1 + \dfrac{k_5}{k_6}}$
B	$\dfrac{K_1}{k_2'} k_3'$	$\dfrac{K_1}{k_2'} k_3' = \alpha k_{on}B_{max}$
B	DV_s	$DV_s = \dfrac{K_1}{k_2'} \dfrac{k_3'}{k_4} = \dfrac{\alpha}{K_d} B_{max}$
C	DV''	

binding is not possible. The method is therefore most suitable for tracers with low non-specific binding.

Receptor Kinetics with Major Receptor Occupation

The concepts discussed above no longer apply when receptor binding occurs in the presence of major receptor occupation (see "Fundamentals of Chemical Reaction Kinetics" above). In fact, the probability that binding occurs is proportional to the available receptor sites, and this number becomes very small once most sites are already occupied. The important point to note is that k_3, the rate constant reflecting binding to specific receptor sites, is no longer a constant. As more and more receptors become occupied, the apparent k_3 gets progressively smaller because k_3 not only reflects binding but is the product of a rate constant and the available receptor sites. In this setting, then, the basic tracer kinetic principle, namely, that the process of interest is not disturbed by the tracer, is no longer fulfilled. However, kinetic experiments with receptor saturation are necessary if one wants to estimate B_{max} and k_{on} separately. A standard procedure to this aim consists of two separate experiments, one with major and one with negligible receptor occupation. From these two experiments, B_{max} and k_{on} are then indeed obtained separately using the formalism outlined in the following box. This approach was applied successfully to measure B_{max} of various receptor types, such as dopaminergic (15), muscarinic (11), and benzodiazepine (12) receptors.

QUANTITATIVE ANALYSIS OF RECEPTOR KINETICS WITH MAJOR RECEPTOR OCCUPATION

In the presence of high ligand concentrations, most receptor sites can become occupied by ligand. Then the approximate form of the biomolecular reaction equation given by Eq. 3 is no longer applicable. Rather, we cannot neglect C_{AB} and therefore have to retain the full reaction equation (Eq. 28). Calling the bound ligand concentration C_s rather than C_{AB} and the free concentration C_f rather than C_A, Eq. (28) becomes

$$dC_s/dt = k_{on}(B_{max} - C_s)C_f - k_{off}C_s \qquad (65)$$

Comparing Eq. (65) with the standard equation in the four-compartment model (model **C**) for the rate of change of bound ligand (Eq. 40a), we note that

$$k_3 = k_{on}(B_{max} - C_s) \qquad (66)$$

which amounts to incorporating the nonlinearity introduced into the problem by receptor saturation conditions into the reaction rate constant k_3. C_s is time-dependent; hence k_3 also becomes time-dependent, and as a result, the differential equations describing the ligand exchange in the compartment model considered become nonlinear. In terms of model **B**, k_3' is obtained by comparing Eq. (66) with Eq. (62) and remembering that for small receptor occupancy $k_3 = k_{on}B_{max}$:

$$k_3' = \frac{k_{on}(B_{max} - C_s)}{1 + k_5/k_6} \qquad (67)$$

Basically, experiments with negligible receptor binding allow one to determine k_3, i.e., the product of k_{on} and B_{max}. If one wants to measure B_{max} and k_{on} separately, two experiments are needed. The first is one with minimal receptor occupation and yields $k_{on}B_{max}$. The second is one with major receptor occupation. Parameter k_3 is then given by Eq. (66), or written slightly differently,

$$k_3 = k_{on}B_{max} - k_{on}C_s \qquad (68)$$

Since $k_{on}B_{max}$ is known from the experiment with minimal receptor occupation, k_{on} can now be determined in the experiment with major receptor occupation. Once

k_{on} and $k_{on}B_{max}$ are known, it is easy to calculate B_{max}. It is obvious that the described method has limitations. For instance, human experiments with major receptor occupation can only be performed if the side effects of receptor occupation are negligible. This is, for instance, the case with benzodiazepine receptors, whereas major occupation of cholinergic receptors may be intolerable.

Suitability of Ligands

The success of quantification depends to a great deal on the kinetic properties of the ligand used. It is obvious that a tracer must have a high extraction fraction to serve as a good flow tracer or "chemical microsphere" (see "Mechanical and Biochemical Microspheres" above). In fact, the first-pass extraction fraction (EF_{fp}) should be close to 100%. This requirement is ideally met by microspheres. Of the clinically available tracers, only the PET agents [^{15}O]H$_2$O and [^{13}N]NH$_3$ show a first-pass extraction fraction greater than 90%. The first can be used to quantify perfusion in almost any organ; the latter is suitable to assess myocardial perfusion. If the EF_{fp} is lower, exact quantitation of perfusion is impaired. This is easily seen by considering Eq. (58). The parameter related to perfusion is K_1, which is the product of perfusion and first-pass extraction fraction. The latter is itself dependent on blood flow, as described by Eqs. (59) and (60). The degree of this dependence grows with decreasing extraction fraction. This is illustrated in Fig. 21.

The requirements for a suitable receptor ligand are more subtle. There are two main aspects that have to be considered. First, one would like to produce images of the regional distribution of the receptor in question. This requires that most of the ligand binds specifically to the receptor under examination and that at the same time nonspecific binding is low. This second condition is met if the affinity of the ligand for the receptor is sufficiently high. A common measure for affinity is the equilibrium binding constant K_d, which was defined in Eq. (32) as

$$K_d = k_{off}/k_{on}$$

with k_{on} being the bimolecular association rate and k_{off} the dissociation rate describing

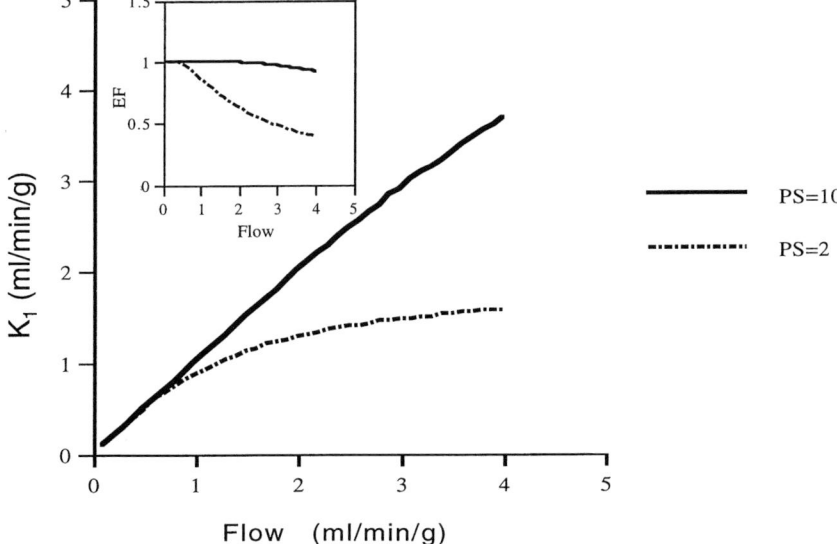

Figure 21. Plot of K_1 as a function of flow. We note that for low-flow states, K_1 is directly proportional to the flow. However, at higher flows, K_1 no longer increases linearly with flow. Depending on the magnitude of the surface permeability product, this breakdown of linearity occurs at lower or higher flow rates. In the insert, the same plot is given for the extraction fraction rather than K_1. The deviation from unity is noted at higher flow rates.

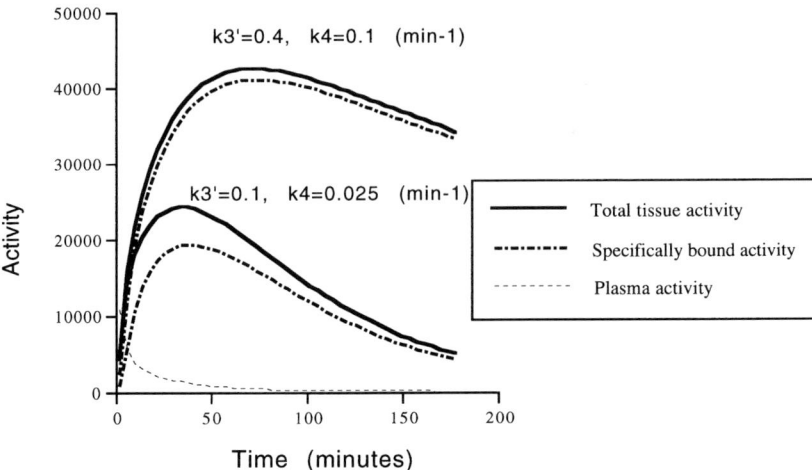

Figure 22. Total tissue activity and specifically bound ligand for two ligands with the same K_d but different values for k_{on} and k_{off}. The curves were generated with model **B** and values $K_1 = 0.4$ ml/min/g, $k_2' = 0.1$ min^{-1}, and k_3' and k_4 as indicated.

the biochemical reaction between ligand and receptor. From the definition it follows that K_d and affinity are inversely related: The lower K_d, the more likely it is that the ligand will be found in the bound state, and the higher K_d, the more likely it is to find the ligand in the unbound state. Increased affinity therefore can be achieved by increasing k_{on} or lowering k_{off}. However, the two cases are not equivalent when looking at them from a kinetic viewpoint. This is illustrated in Fig. 22, which depicts the tissue time activity curves for ligands with the same K_d but different values for k_{on} and k_{off}. A serious problem may arise if k_{off} is very small, as shall be illustrated for the case $k_{off} = 0$.

The time course of tissue activity is then described by Eq. (41). As long as the back-diffusion rate k_2' is sufficiently large relative to k_3' ($= k_{on}B_{max}$), ligand uptake is determined by all parameters K_1 to k_3'. If, however, $k_2' << k_3'$, practically all ligand transported into tissue space will bind to the receptors. Consequently, ligand uptake in this case will only reflect blood flow, or expressed differently, ligand uptake is flow-limited. Mathematically, this is easily seen in Eq. (41). If $k_2' << k_3'$, the denominator is dominated by k_3' and the expression is reduced to $C_{tiss} = K_1 * C_a(t)$. This is the equation of a flow tracer in which all information on k_3', the receptor-related parameter, is lost. The conclusion is that high affinity is not a sufficient criterion for a suitable receptor ligand. The relation between k_3' and k_2' is of great importance, especially for small dissociation rates k_{off}.

Parameter Estimation in Kinetic Modeling

Kinetic models, as discussed in the preceding sections, provide a mathematical description of tracer exchange between the different compartments considered in the target organ. They are fully specified by the rate constants. Hence the aim of tracer kinetic modeling is to determine the rate values of a specific system under investigation.

In an actual study, experimental data are acquired with one or more recording devices. An essential aspect of these data is the *input curve,* which is the temporal concentration $C_a(t)$ of tracer in plasma. Given $C_a(t)$, the kinetic model predicts the time course of tracer concentrations in the other compartments. In most situations, the recording device cannot distinguish between contributions from the different compartments. Rather, the total tracer concentration within a resolution element is recorded at one or more time points according to the sampling protocol. The task then is to find those rate constants of the prescribed kinetic model which provide the best match between the predicted and the observed data. In this sense, the ''constants'' are parameters that have to be adjusted, and the task is a parameter-estimation problem.

In what follows we will discuss the different issues of parameter estimation in kinetic modeling. Although the discussion is general, the two-tissue compartment model as applied to PET data is chosen as a paradigmatic example. First, the differential equations of the compartment model are specified. Then an operational equation is derived that must be matched against the acquired data with a fitting algorithm. The resulting parameters may not be accepted without some measure of error. Therefore, the section continues with a discussion of identifiability problems in kinetic modeling. It concludes with the outline of a software environment for interactive kinetic modeling of NM-type data.

This section is introductory in nature. For a more thorough review of parameter-estimation problems, the reader is referred to Carson's excellent summary (8), and detailed algorithmic information is available in Press et al. (34).

Model Specification

The two-tissue compartment model shown in Fig. 16 is specified by the system of linear differential equations given in Eq. (40), which are recalled here to be

$$dX_1/dt = K_1 C_a(t) - (k_2' + k_3')X_1 + k_4 X_2$$
$$dX_2/dt = k_3'X_1 - k_4 X_2 \tag{69}$$

Assuming that no tracer is present in tissue compartments X_1 and X_2 at the beginning of the experiment, the initial conditions are $X_1(0) = 0 = X_2(0)$. After administration, tracer is carried to the vascular compartment, from which it can exchange with the tissue compartment X_1. Actually, it is only the free ligand in plasma, the input curve $C_a(t)$, that can exchange with compartment X_1. For a kinetic analysis, the time course of $C_a(t)$ must be monitored. Then the evolution of the tracer concentration in the different regions can be calculated by integrating the system [Eqs (69)] for a specific set of parameters K_1 to k_4.

It is important to note that in the present formulation, tracer leaving the tissue compartment does not add back to the input curve. Thus the input curve is not affected by the actual model configuration. If the tracer does not bind intravascularly, the input curve is in constant relation to the tracer concentration in whole blood. In this case it is sufficient to measure the total tracer concentration in blood $C_B(t)$ and to determine the relationship to $C_a(t)$ for one blood sample. Otherwise, the free fraction in plasma must be determined experimentally from the time of injection to the end of the acquisition.

Operational Equations

An operational equation is an explicit mathematical solution to the model to which the measured data can be compared in order to extract the parameters of interest. How the operational equation is set up depends on the actual acquisition device and protocol. In the example considered here, we assume a dynamic NM-type study. This means that after tracer administration, data are collected and averaged in a sequence of succeeding time intervals, so-called frames. As a result, the average concentration of total tracer per resolution element is sampled at the frame midpoints, providing the *time-activity curve* (TAC; see Fig. 23). The TAC therefore includes contributions from both tissue compartments X_1 and X_2 but also from blood in the vascular bed, and the operational equation can be specified as

$$C_{TAC}(t_i) = \frac{1}{(tE_i - tB_i)} \left\{ rBV \int_{tB_i}^{tE_i} C_B(t) \, dt + (1 - rBV) \int_{tB_i}^{tE_i} [X_1(t) + X_2(t)] \, dt \right\} \tag{70}$$

where tB_i and tE_i denote beginning and end of frame i, rBV is the regional blood volume, and C_B is tracer concentration in total blood. In this operational equation, the values $C_{TAC}(t_i)$ directly model the measured TAC samples. During the estimation task, Eq. (70) is evaluated for a specific kinetic model (i.e., for fixed parameters K_1 to k_4), and these predicted values are compared with the measured values.

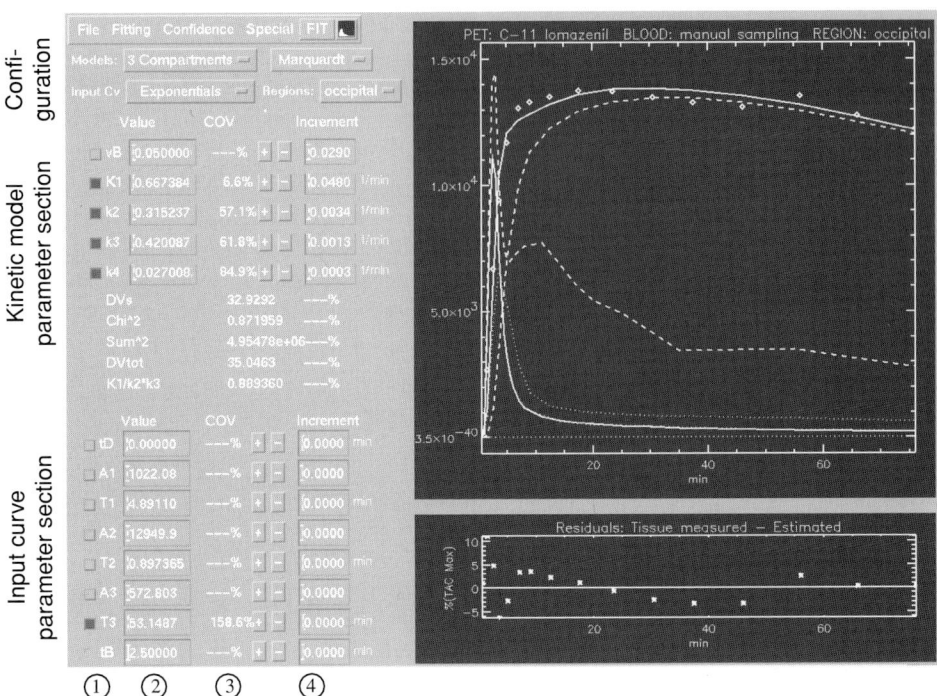

Figure 23. Example of an interactive kinetic modeling package (7). In the configuration section a kinetic model and an input-curve model can be selected from a list. Their parameters are displayed below. ① Buttons allow one to specify which parameters are fitted and which are fixed. ② The resulting fixed parameter values. ③ Standard error estimated from the covariance matrix or from a Monte Carlo study. ④ Interactive incrementation/decrementation of parameter values followed by a model curve update. This feature is used to study the sensitivity of the model to the different parameters and to manually find an initial guess. ⑤ Selection of the fitting algorithm. ⑥ Selection among several regional TACs. See text for the notations.

The evaluation of the operational equation for the example model configuration requires the time course of X_1 and X_2. It can be obtained in two ways. The first is based on solving the system (69) explicitly; the second applies numerical integration techniques. The analytical solution in the present two-tissue compartment example is well known and has been given in Eq. (41). In general, linear kinetic models can be solved using the Laplace tranformation (5) and result in a convolution of the input curves with a sum of exponentials (8). However, the complexity of this approach increases rapidly with the number of compartments. Therefore, it is more convenient to employ direct numerical integration, although a software system for computing the analytical solution also has been devised (9). Numerical integration has the further advantage that nonlinear models applying to receptor systems near saturation also can be handled.

Other examples for operational equations can be found in Chap. 5 for calculating tissue perfusion with $H_2{}^{15}O$ water bolus measurements and PET and pp. 109–111 describing the graphic (Patlak) analysis. They require further processing of the acquired data.

Fitting

Once the operational equation has been specified, the optimal parameters for adjusting the model to the measured data must be found. In the preceding example, *rBV* is a parameter that explicitly appears in the operational equation. However, rather than being estimated, *rBV* is often set to a predefined value, e.g., to 5% for brain studies. The parameters K_1 to k_4 enter indirectly through the calculation of X_1 and X_2.

A measure must be defined for quantifying the match between model and data, also called a *cost function.* Most commonly, the least squares function is employed, in the example defined by

$$X^2(K_1, k_2', k_3', k_4) = \sum_{\forall\text{frames } i} w_i [C_{\text{TAC}}(t_i) - \hat{C}_{\text{TAC}}(t_i, K_1, k_2', k_3', k_4)]^2 \qquad (71)$$

This means that the residuals are formed between the measured values and the predicted values (indicated by ^) at the frame midpoints (see Fig. 23). The residuals are squared, weighted by w_i, and summed to form the cost function, which must be minimized. It can be shown that the ideal weights are proportional to the variance of the measurement error e_i for each sample i:

$$w_i = \frac{1}{\text{var}(e_i)} \qquad (72)$$

In the case of pure radioactivity counting, for instance, the weights would be inverse to the number y_i of detected counts, $w_i = y_i^{-1}$ (Poisson statistics). This noise model, however, does not apply to reconstruced emission tomograpy, as discussed in Chap. 5. In most cases, the proper specification of weights is very difficult, so unweighted ($w_i \equiv 1$) rather than weighted least squares estimation is commonly applied.

The parameter-estimation problem is now reduced to finding that set of model parameters that results in minimal X^2. Except for some special model configurations (no clearance), this generally is a nonlinear problem. Therefore, no closed-form solution exists, and the optimal parameter set must be found by iterative methods. The principle is to start from an initial guess, evaluate X^2, and try to search for new parameter combinations that successively reduce X^2. There are many algorithms implementing different search strategies. They are not discussed here, since an excellent introduction to this topic as well as implementation code is easily available (34), but some common problems must be emphasized: The multidimensional cost function may have several local minima into which the search may be trapped. Therefore, it is desirable to start from a reasonable guess already in the neighborhood of the global optimum. For complex models such a guess may be obtained by bootstrapping parameter estimates (8). A reduced model is first fitted. The resulting rate constants are translated into a more complex model and serve as starting values for adjusting that model. This process continues until the target model is reached. The stability of the estimation algorithms can be improved further by restricting the search within physiologically meaningful parameter ranges. Negative rate constants, for instance, obviously can be excluded.

Analysis of the Estimation Results

Estimation results may not be accepted without further analysis. Crucial points are the adequacy of the model for the measured data and the identifiability of the model parameters. An adequate model for a specific study includes as few compartments as possible. This situation is accompanied by residuals randomly distributed about the zero line. If the model is further reduced, the residuals will become systematically biased, as illustrated in Fig. 24. On the other hand, if the model includes too many compartments, the parameters get poorly identified. This means that several parameter combinations produce almost identical predicted model curves; hence a unique solution cannot be identified. The same situation, however, also may arise due to unfavorable kinetics, although the model is adequate. In particular, slowly exchanging compartments tend to obscure subsequent fast exchanges. As a guideline, compartments can best be resolved if their exchange rates are neither too different nor too similar (16).

Assessment of parameter identifiability is an intricate problem. Two methods are outlined briefly that try to calculate the standard error of the parameter estimates. The first approach is based on the formal covariance matrix of least squares fitting. If the measurement errors are normally distributed and the problem is linear, then the diagonal elements of the covariance equal the variance (squared standard error) of the parameter estimates (34). It is therefore desirable that a fitting method calculates not only the

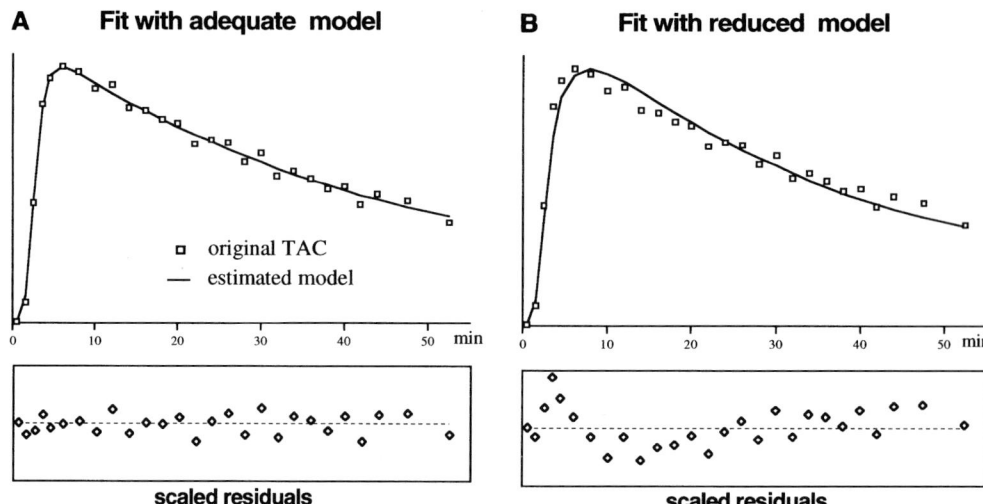

A   Fit with adequate model

B   Fit with reduced model

□ original TAC
— estimated model

scaled residuals

scaled residuals

Figure 24. Examination of the residuals after fitting a kinetic model to a TAC. The TAC was synthetically generated from an input curve and a three-compartment model by adding Gaussian noise of constant variance to the ideal values. (**A**) This synthetic TAC was fitted with the adequate three-compartment model. The residuals are randomly distributed around the zero line. (**B**) The same TAC was fitted with a two-compartment model. The significantly biased residuals indicate inadequacy of the model.

parameter estimates but also the covariance matrix. The Levenberg-Marquardt algorithm is particularly convenient because this information is a by-product of fitting. However, the assumptions for interpreting the covariances as standard errors are normally not fullfilled in tracer kinetic modeling. Hence it should correctly be termed as "formal" covariance and the values used with caution.

The second approach employs Monte Carlo simulations as follows (34): From the fitted parameters a synthetic TAC is generated that is assumed to represent the true process. Then many TACs are created that might be measured if one performed many experiments. To this end, measurement noise is added to the synthetic TAC. Each of these "experimental" TACs is then fitted, and the resulting parameter estimates are recorded. After enough runs, the distribution of the estimates for each parameter is analyzed. Provided that the noise model employed is realistic, the resulting confidence limits represent valuable measures of parameter uncertainty.

Software Environment

Tracer kinetic modeling can be subdivided into two data-processing categories. Interactive data processing is required in the early stage of model development and verification. Thus *TAC*s from different tissues of interest are analyzed using various model configurations. This task should be supported by a flexible interactive software environment including the following features:

- Ease of switching between kinetic models. Transfer of model parameters from one model to another supports parameter bootstrapping.
- Support for restricting the parameter search to physiologic ranges.
- Implementation of different search strategies. If results are in a suspected local minimum, another algorithm will pursue a different search path and may end up with a better solution.
- Smoothing of the noisy input curve. Acquisition noise is usually quite significant in the input curve. It can be reduced by fitting analytical functions to the measured data points or by treating the input curve as a separate kinetic model.
- Assessment of parameter identifiability by covariance calculation and Monte Carlo simulations.

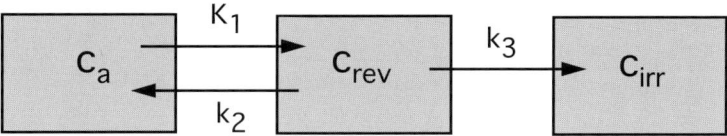

Figure 25. Compartment model typically used in Patlak analysis. Arterial tracer C_a exchanges with a reversible compartment C_{rev} and gets trapped in an irreversible compartment C_{irr}.

- Export of results into statistical analysis tools. The most important application is to decide on which model is adequate and provides sufficient parameter identifiability for a study protocol. To this end, a series of studies is fitted with different models, and the parameters, their standard errors, and X^2 are exported and analyzed by statistical methods such as F statistics.
- Generation of synthetic studies. For a specific model configuration and acquisition protocol, the predicted TAC can be calculated and parameter identifiability analyzed. This helps in setting up an optimal study protocol.

An application that includes the preceding requirements was implemented in the authors' laboratory. It is illustrated in Fig. 23 (7).

After careful evaluation of adequacy and parameter identifiability, a model may be applicable without user interaction. A highly desirable application is the calculation of parametric images. In this case the functional equation is fitted for each image pixel, and the estimated parameters are presented as images. Two examples for calculating perfusion maps are given in Chap. 6. It is clear that only simple models qualify for pixel-wise modeling due to signal-to-noise constraints.

Graphic Analysis of Dynamic Data: Patlak Plot

The graphic method loosely known as a *Patlak plot* is a special form of setting up the operational equation. It has been developed by Patlak et al. (30, 31), and can be applied if at least one compartment in the system under investigation displays irreversible kinetics, meaning that the tracer is trapped in this compartment. The mathematics for a general system consisting of an arbitrarily high number of reversible and irreversible compartments is given in Patlak, Blasberg, and Fenstermacher (30). In general, it turns out that the long-term behavior can be described by considering one reversible and one irreversible component.

One important result is that there exists a time point t^* after which the ratio total tracer concentration in the reversible compartments versus tracer concentration in plasma (C_{rev}/C_a) is stable. This is true for any shape of the time course of the arterial tracer concentration. The consequences of this result shall be illustrated for the case of a step input function, demonstrated in Fig. 26. A stable ratio in this case implicates that the amount of tracer in the reversible compartments C_{rev} is constant. The rate of tracer accumulation in the total system (dC_{tiss}/dt) equals therefore the rate at which the tracer enters the irreversible compartments. Furthermore, this rate is proportional to the arterial tracer concentration C_a. Mathematically, this is expressed by the following expression:

$$\frac{d}{dt}C_{tiss} = \frac{d}{dt}C_{irr} = K_iC_a \qquad (73)$$

The influx constant K_i is easily expressed in terms of the rate constants K_1 to k_n of the compartment model, as shall be demonstrated for the case of the two-tissue compartment model shown in Fig. 25. This model and Patlak analysis are often employed to analyze FDG kinetics with PET. Once the concentration in compartment C_{rev} has reached a stable value, the total of all ligand exchanging with compartment C_{rev} equals zero.

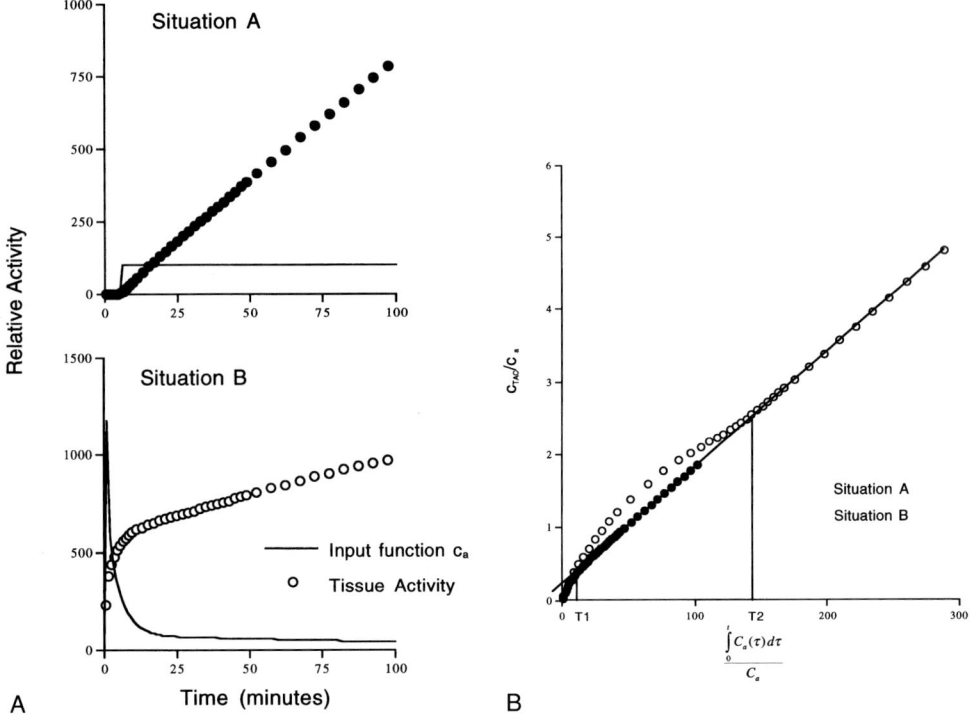

Figure 26. The left panel demonstrates tissue time-activity curves generated with the model depicted in **A** and two different input functions. In situation **A** the input function is a step function; in situation **B** an initial steep increase is followed by a multiexponential decline. The k values used were the following: $K_1 = 0.1$ ml/min/g, $k_2 = 0.013$ min^{-1}, $k_3 = 0.06$ min^{-1}, and $rBV = 0$. The Patlak plots for the two situations are displayed on the right. T_1 and T_2 represent the time points at which the plots converge toward a straight line.

$$K_1 C_a - C_{\text{rev}}(k_2 + k_3) = 0 \tag{74}$$

From this expression, C_{rev} following time point t^* is calculated as

$$C_{\text{rev}}(t > t^*) = \frac{K_1}{k_2 + k_3} C_a \tag{75}$$

The flux of tracer into the irreversible compartment C_{irr} is given by $k_3 C_{\text{rev}}$ and equals the flux of tracer from plasma to C_{rev}:

$$F = k_3 C_{\text{rev}} = K_i C_a \tag{76}$$

Reordering terms yields the following expression for influx constant K_i:

$$K_i = \frac{C_{\text{rev}}}{C_a} k_3 \tag{77}$$

or considering Eq. (8),

$$K_i = \frac{K_1}{k_2 + k_3} k_3 \tag{78}$$

The time course of the ligand concentration in C_{irr} is simply the integration of the flux over time:

$$C_{\text{irr}} = K_i \int_0^t C_a(\tau)\, d\tau \tag{79}$$

The total tracer concentration in tissue is now obtained by adding the amount of tracer in the reversible compartment C_{rev}. Since a region of interest often also contains vascular space besides tissue, the total tracer concentration C_{TAC} in such a region is given by

$$C_{TAC} = C_{irr} + C_{rev} + rBV \cdot C_a \qquad (80)$$

For each model, C_{rev} following t^* can be expressed in terms of C_a as in Eq. (75):

$$C_{rev} = V_0 C_a \qquad (81)$$

where V_0 is the steady-state space (distribution) volume of the reversible compartment. The total concentration in a region of interest following t^* is therefore given by

$$C_{TAC}(t > t^*) = K_i \int_0^t C_a(\tau)\, d\tau + (V_0 + rBV)C_a \qquad (82)$$

The final form of the operational equation is now obtained by dividing both sides of Eq. (82) by C_a:

$$\frac{C_{TAC}}{C_a}(t > t^*) = K_i \frac{\int_0^t C_a(\tau)\, d\tau}{C_a} + (V_0 + rBV) \qquad (83)$$

This formula means that plotting C_{TAC}/C_a versus $[\int_0^t C_a(\tau)\, d\tau]/C_a$ (Patlak plot) results in a straight line with slope K_i and y intercept $V_0 + rBV$ after t^*. The preceding derivation has been given for the simplest configuration of constant arterial concentration and a two-tissue compartment model. However, the result as presented above holds for any shape of the input curve and model configuration (see Fig. 26). Therefore, the Patlak plot can be applied to examine whether there exists an irreversible component in the model. If it does, it is represented by a linear segment in the Patlak plot. Its influx constant K_i can then be obtained as the slope of the regression line fitted to that segment. Apart from its simplicity, this graphic approach has the further advantage that the vascular volume rBV must not be predetermined. Rather, information related to rBV can be derived from the y intercept of the regression line. For a short communication on applications of the Patlak plot in PET, SPECT, and CT, the reader is referred to Peters (32).

Reaction Kinetics and Compartment Modeling: Conclusions

The basics of reaction kinetics are simple. The probability that a reaction occurs is proportional to the concentration of the reagents and a rate constant characteristic of the reaction. As long as one of the reagents (which we called *receptor,* but it also could be called *substrate*) is present in excess, the system behavior can be quantitatively understood without being forced to perform computer simulations. When examining a multicompartment system, this analysis gets cumbersome very quickly because too many free parameters have to be determined using the relatively sparse experimental data that can be obtained from an imaging experiment. In fact, the data obtained are at best the tissue concentration of a substance as a function of time and the arterial input function of the substance as a function of time. These curves can then be fitted to estimate the parameters characterizing the system under study. In this situation, the mathematical formalism needed to analyze biochemical systems is the theory of linear coupled differential equations. In receptor studies in the widest sense, the most relevant parameters are the density of the receptors and the affinity constants with which the ligand binds to the receptor. Note, however, that whenever an experiment is done with a labeled substance, this substance has to first get to the tissue under consideration, and flow into tissue therefore has always to be considered when analyzing a compartment model. The easier a substance is taken up by tissue, the more the uptake becomes flow-determined. Furthermore, compartment analysis shows that it is important when examining a ligand-receptor system that the backdiffusion of the substance into the bloodstream is not negligible. If this is the case, a potentially good receptor marker often ends up just being a good perfusion marker.

While much of the discussion in the preceding sections is predominantly relevant to tracer studies, the concepts will potentially start to have some impact on MRI experiments as well. Specific methodologies will be discussed in more detail in the corresponding chapters.

REFERENCES

1. Albert MS, Schepkin VD, Budinger TF. Measurement of 129Xe T1 in blood to explore the feasibility of hyperpolarized 129Xe MRI. *J Comput Assist Tomogr,* 19(6), 975–978 (1995).
2. Axel L. Cerebral blood flow determination by rapid-sequence computed tomography: Theoretical analysis. *Radiology,* 137(3), 679–686 (1980).
3. Benedetto AR, Nusynowitz ML. Correlation of right and left ventricular ejection fraction and volume measurements. *J Nucl Med,* 29(6), 1114–1117 (1988).
4. Berninger WH, Axel L, Norman D et al. Functional imaging of the brain using computed tomography [Erratum: *Radiology,* 171(3), 878 (1989)]. *Radiology,* 138(3), 711–716 (1981).
5. Braun M. *Differential equations and their applications* (3rd ed.). New York: Springer (1983).
6. Bronstein IN, Semendjajew KA, Musiol G, Muehlig H. *Taschenbuch der Mathematik.* Frankfurt am Main: Harri Deutsch (1993).
7. Burger C. *KMZ: An interactive kinetic modeling environment.* Zurich, Switzerland: University Hospital Zurich (1996).
8. Carson RE (Ed.). Parameter estimation in positron emission tomography and autoradiography. In: M Phelps, J Mazziotta, H Schelbert (Eds.). *Positron emission tomography and autoradiography: Principles and applications for the brain and the heart.* New York: Raven Press 347–390 (1986).
9. Coxson PG, Salmeron EM, Huesman RH. A strategy for using closed form solutions for compartmental models of dynamic PET data. In: *IEEE Conference Record Nuclear Science Symposium & Medical Imaging Conference* 1577–1578 (1990).
10. Crone C. Permeability of capillaries in various organs as determined by the use of the indicator diffusion method. *Acta Physiol Scand,* 58(4), 292–305 (1964).
11. Delforge J, Le Guludec D, Syrota A et al. Quantification of myocardial muscarinic receptors with PET in humans. *J Nucl Med,* 34(6), 981–991 (1993).
12. Delforge J, Pappata S, Millet P et al. Quantification of benzodiazepine receptors in human brain using PET, [11C]flumazenil, and a single-experiment protocol. *J Cereb Blood Flow Metab,* 15(2), 284–300 (1995).
13. Drayer BP, Wolfson SK, Reinmuth OM et al. Xenon enhanced CT for analysis of cerebral integrity, perfusion, and blood flow. *Stroke,* 9(2), 123–130 (1978).
14. Eichenberger AC, Schuiki E, Kochli VD et al. Ischemic heart disease: Assessment with gadolinium-enhanced ultrafast MR imaging and dipyridamole stress [Comments]. *J Magn Reson Imaging,* 4(3), 425–431 (1994).
15. Farde L, Eriksson L, Blomquist G, Halldin C. Kinetic analysis of central [11C]raclopride binding to D2-dopamine receptors studied by PET: A comparison to the equilibrium analysis. *J Cereb Blood Flow Metab,* 9(5), 696–708 (1989).
16. Gjedde A. Compartmental analysis. In: HN Wagner, Z Szabo, JW Buchanan (Eds.). *Principles of nuclear medicine.* Philadelphia: Saunders, 451–461 (1995).
17. Gore JC, Majumdar S. Measurement of tissue blood flow using intravascular relaxation agents and magnetic resonance imaging. *Magn Reson Med,* 14(2), 242–248 (1990).
18. Groshar D, Ben Haim S, Gips S et al. Spectrum of scintigraphic appearance of liver hemangiomas. *Clin Nucl Med,* 17(4), 294–299 (1992).
19. Hearon JZ. Theorems on linear systems. *Ann N Y Acad Sci,* 108, 36–68 (1963).
20. Herscovitch P, Markham J, Raichle ME. Brain blood flow measured with intravenous $H_2^{15}O$: I. Theory and error analysis. *J Nucl Med,* 24(9), 782–789 (1983).
21. Heyman MA, Payne BD, Hoffman JE, Rudolph AM. Blood-flow measurements with radionuclide-labeled particles. *Prog Cardiovasc Dis,* 20, 55–79 (1977).
22. Kalender WA, Polacin A, Eidloth H et al. Brain perfusion studies by Xenon-enhanced CT using washin/washout study protocols. *J Comput Assist Tomogr,* 15(5), 816–822 (1991).
23. Kanno I, Lammertsma AA, Heather JD et al. Measurement of cerebral blood flow using bolus inhalation of $C^{15}O_2$ and positron emission tomography: Description of the method and its comparison with the $C^{15}O_2$ continuous inhalation method. *J Cereb Blood Flow Metab,* 4(2), 224–234 (1984).
24. Kety SS. The theory and applications of the exchange of inert gas at the lungs and tissues. *Pharmacol Rev,* 3, 1–41 (1951).
25. Koeppe RA, Holthoff VA, Frey KA et al. Compartmental analysis of [11C]flumazenil kinetics for the estimation of ligand transport rate and receptor distribution using positron emission tomography. *J Cereb Blood Flow Metab,* 11(5), 735–744 (1991).
26. Lassen NA. Cerebral transit of an intravascular tracer may allow measurement of regional blood volume but not regional blood flow [Letter]. *J Cereb Blood Flow Metab,* 4(4), 633–634 (1984).
27. Lauritzen M, Henriksen L, Lassen NA. Regional cerebral blood flow during rest and skilled hand movements by Xenon-133 inhalation and emission computerized tomography. *J Cereb Blood Flow Metab,* 1(4), 385–387 (1981).

28. Meier P, Zierler KL. On the theory of the indicator-dilution method for measurement of blood flow and volume. *J Appl Physiol,* 6, 731–744 (1954).
29. Ogawa S, Tank DW, Menon R et al. Intrinsic signal changes accompanying sensory stimulation: Functional brain mapping with magnetic resonance imaging. *Proc Natl Acad Sci U S A,* 89(13), 5951–5955 (1992).
30. Patlak CS, Blasberg RG, Fenstermacher JD. Graphical evaluation of blood-to-brain transfer constants from multiple-time uptake data. *J Cereb Blood Flow Metab,* 3(1), 1–7 (1983).
31. Patlak CS, Goldstein DA, Hoffman JF. The flow of solute and solvent across a two-membrane system. *J Theor Biol,* 5, 426–442 (1963).
32. Peters AM. Graphical analysis of dynamic data: The Patlak-Rutland plot. *Nucl Med Commun,* 15, 669–672 (1994).
33. Phelps ME, Huang SC, Hoffman EJ et al. Cerebral extraction of N-13 ammonia: Its dependence on cerebral blood flow and capillary permeability—surface area product. *Stroke,* 12(5), 607–619 (1981).
34. Press WH, Teukolski SA, Vetterling WT, Flannery BP. *Numerical recipes in C.* Cambridge: Cambridge University Press (1992).
35. Raichle ME, Martin WR, Herscovitch P et al. Brain blood flow measured with intravenous $H_2{}^{15}O$: II. Implementation and validation. *J Nucl Med,* 24(9), 790–798 (1983).
36. Rempp KA, Brix G, Wenz F et al. Quantification of regional cerebral blood flow and volume with dynamic susceptibility contrast-enhanced MR imaging. *Radiology,* 193(3), 637–641 (1994).
37. Renkin EM. Transport of potassium-42 from blood to tissue in isolated mammalian skeletal muscles. *Am J Physiol,* 197, 1205–1210 (1959).
38. Rosen BR, Belliveau JW, Vevea JM, Brady TJ. Perfusion imaging with NMR contrast agents. *Magn Reson Med,* 14(2), 249–265 (1990).
39. Shah A, Schelbert HR, Schwaiger M et al. Measurement of regional myocardial blood flow with N-13 ammonia and positron-emission tomography in intact dogs. *J Am Coll Cardiol,* 5(1), 92–100 (1985).
40. Shirahata N, Henriksen L, Vorstrup S et al. Regional cerebral blood flow assessed by 133Xe inhalation and emission tomography: Normal values. *J Comput Assist Tomogr,* 9(5), 861–866 (1985).
41. Sorensen MB, Bille Brahe NE, Engell HC. Cardiac output measurement by thermal dilution: Reproducibility and comparison with the dye-dilution technique. *Ann Surg,* 183(1), 67–72 (1976).
42. Starmer CF, Clark DO. Computer computations of cardiac output using the gamma function. *J Appl Physiol,* 28(2), 219–220 (1970).
43. Verani MS, Gaeta J, LeBlanc AD et al. Validation of left ventricular volume measurements by radionuclide angiography [Erratum: *J Nucl Med,* 28(3), 401–402 (1987)]. *J Nucl Med,* 26(12), 1394–1401 (1985).
44. Weisskoff RM, Chesler D, Boxerman JL, Rosen BR. Pitfalls in MR measurement of tissue blood flow with intravascular tracers: Which mean transit time? *Magn Reson Med,* 29(4), 553–558 (1993).
45. Wilke N, Jerosch Herold M, Stillman AE et al. Concepts of myocardial perfusion imaging in magnetic resonance imaging. *Magn Reson Q,* 10(4), 249–286 (1994).
46. Zierler KL. Equations for measuring blood flow by external monitoring of radioisotopes. *Circ Res,* 16, 309–321 (1965).

Functional Imaging, edited by
Gustav von Schulthess and Jürgen Hennig.
Lippincott–Raven Publishers, Philadelphia, © 1998.

4

Digital Image Processing for Functional Analysis

Guido Gerig, Gábor Székely,
and Cyrill Burger

Digital image processing can be defined as a postprocessing of digital image data in order to do image restoration or to extract implicit information that is not directly accessible by visual inspection. With digital imaging modalities, computerized processing is already a part of the acquisition devices, since measured data only become images after computerized processing of the sensor signal. However, it is reasonable to make a distinction between processes that create digital image data that are directly observable on film or on the screen and computer-assisted methods to further analyze the content of the data. Such a distinction also can be justified from the doctors' point of view. In this book basic aspects of image formation have been discussed in Chap. 1, while the methods used to obtain the basic image data are discussed in the methodologic chapters (Chaps. 5 to 11). Fullerton et al. (10), for example, remind us that ''medical imaging is, has been and always will be a two step process.'' In a first step, a camera or scanner device creates a recorded image, whereas in a second step the recorded image is observed by the doctor to form a perceived image. A computer-assisted analysis of the recorded images converts data into new perceivable images and quantitative measurements that support the clinician's task.

DIGITAL IMAGE DATA

This section systematically characterizes digital image data and introduces a terminology that forms the basis for the presentation of computerized image analysis procedures.

G Gerig and G Székely: Communications Technology Laboratory, ETH Zentrum, Zurich, Switzerland.

C Burger: Department of Medical Radiology, University Hospital, Zurich, Switzerland.

Quantization of Brightness Values. In digital systems, the measurements observed as brightness values are stored as discrete numbers. The range between minimum and maximum brightness is quantized into a set of intervals, depending on the depth of a number expressed as the number of bits. Common choices for medical image data are 8-bit (256 intervals), 12-bit (4096 intervals), or 16-bit numbers (65,536 intervals).

Sampling. Digital image data form a regular raster grid composed of picture elements (pixels). Each pixel covers a small region of the original scene that is given by the sampling widths of the spatial axes (Δy, Δy). The number of pixels of a two-dimensional (2D) image is easily calculated by multiplying the number of discretization steps in x and y. In a three-dimensional (3D) image, volume elements are called *voxels* with spatial extension (Δy, Δy, Δz).

Spatial Dimension. Original scenes observed by the human visual system are scenes projected onto the 2D retina. Since due to hidden surfaces the whole 3D information is not available in these projections, one usually speaks from $2\frac{1}{2}$D scenes. Radiologic images, on the other hand, are most often recorded as 2D images from projections or from a scanning process. Stacks of 2D images with constant slice distance form full 3D volumes. The 2D images are stored as a regular grid of picture elements (pixels) and are printed to a film or viewed on a computer screen. Stacks of 2D images covering a slab or a volumetric section of the patient are represented either as a series of slices or as a 3D volumetric data structure after postprocessing.

Spectral Dimension. Medical images usually viewed on a black and white film or a screen carry a single piece of physical information per pixel. In computed tomography (CT), for example, the brightness information is proportional to the absorption, which is measured in Hounsfield units. In magnetic resonance imaging (MRI), the brightness of a pixel may represent the proton density, T1 or T2 relaxation times, or mixtures thereof. These types of single-valued images will be called *scalar images*.

Sensors and scanners often measure not only one scalar value at each pixel but also multiple values. The best known example is a digitized color photograph with the components red, green, and blue forming a vectorial value per pixel. MRI is an extremely versatile imaging technique and can provide multiple parameters per pixel. In spin-echo acquisitions, multiple echoes representing different tissue characteristics can be measured and stored as vectorial information at each pixel. Although these multiple images are usually represented as separate images on film, one should consider that the vector measurement at each pixel represents different tissue properties. If the images are acquired in one acquisition, the image channels are perfectly registered and can be overlayed pixel by pixel.

Temporal Dimension. Another parameter of increasing importance relates to time sequence or serial data. High-speed image acquisitions can acquire multiple images during a short time interval and therefore measure dynamic changes and yield functional information. As a different application, monitoring a patient requires a screening in certain

---

FORMAL SPECIFICATION OF DIGITAL IMAGE DATA

Digital raster image:	$\vec{I}[\vec{x};\, t]$
Spatial dimensionality:	$\vec{I}[\vec{x}]$
	$\vec{x} = \{x_1, x_2, \ldots, x_k\} \in \mathcal{R}^k$
	k: spatial dimension
	$\vec{x}$: spatial location
Spectral dimension:	$\vec{I}[\vec{x}]$
	Single scalar measurement: $I[\vec{x}]$
	Multiple measurements: $\vec{I}[\vec{x}] = (i_1[\vec{x}],$
	$i_2[\vec{x}], \ldots, i_c[\vec{x}])$
	c: number of spectral channels
Temporal dimension:	$\vec{I}[x;\, t]$
	t: time variable, $t \in \mathcal{R}$

CALCULATION OF THE SIZE OF DATA SETS

Number of image
  elements:
$$np_{\text{tot}} = np_1 * np_2 * \ldots *np_k$$
  k: spatial dimensionality
  Δx_i: sampling width
  $x_{(i,\min)}, \ldots, x_{(i,\max)}$: sampling range
  $np_i = x_{(i,\max)} - x_{(i,\min)}/\Delta x$: number of samples in x_i

Spectral dimension: $nc * np_{\text{tot}}$
  nc: number of spectral channels

Temporal
  dimension: $nt * np_{\text{tot}}$
  nt: number of time steps

Quantization of
  brightness: $nb * np_{\text{tot}}$
  nb: number of bytes per pixel or voxel, 1 byte $= 8$ bits
  $2^{n\text{bits}}$: quantization resolution (e.g., 8 bits $= 256$ steps)

Total amount of
  data: $\text{Size} = np_{\text{tot}} * nc * nt * nb$
  Size measured in bytes or megabytes (Mbytes)

Examples:
  (a) Temporal series of twenty scalar 2D MRI images,
      2 bytes per pixel: $np_1 * np_2 = 256^2$ pixels, $nt = 20$,
      $nc = 1$, $nb = 2$
      $\text{Size} = np_{\text{tot}} * nc * nt * nb = 256^2 * 1 * 20 * 2 =$
      2,621,440 bytes ($= 2$ Mbytes)
  (b) 3D MRI volume data set, spin-echo double echo (nc
      $= 2$), 128 slices with 256^2 pixels, 2 bytes per
      pixel: $np_{\text{tot}} * nc * nt * nb = 256^2 * 128 * 2 * 1 * 2$
      $= 33,554,432$ bytes ($= 32$ Mbytes)

---

time intervals. The series of images, if perfectly registered pixel by pixel (image registration will be explained later), represents a stack of 2D images or a 3D image volume with the coordinate axes $[x, y]$ and t.

Today's scanners can produce huge amounts of data in short time intervals. Several measurements of 3D volume data taken at different times even represent 4D data sets. Details and formulas concerning the calculation of the size of a medical data set are illustrated in the accompanying boxes.

OBJECTIVES FOR DATA POSTPROCESSING

Computer-assisted methods can support image interpretation and description by *supporting the cognitive abilities* of physicians with advanced visualization of multidimensional and multimodality data. Another important domain will be the *access to quantitative information* by providing multidimensional measurement and manipulation tools, supporting morphometric applications.

Representation of Anatomic and Functional Structures

Digital imaging devices are capable of forming multidimensional images with several spectral channels measuring a variety of different morphologic and functional properties of the human body. The higher dimensionality and the complex interrelationship between the structures being imaged and the resulting intensities require a complex reasoning process to perceive and understand the image contents. The difficult task of interpreting measurements in three spatial dimensions plus possibly time and the integration of information from multimodalities clearly demonstrate the need for new computerized exploration methods.

MR angiography (MRA) may serve as a typical example to express the dilemma between a 3D acquisition and the visual analysis of slice series. Images are acquired as true 3D data, but because of the difficulty to mentally combine vessel cross sections to vascular systems, data have to be analyzed as projections (MIP: maximum-intensity projection) or rendered surfaces to make the information accessible to recognition.

Shape, Measurements, Morphometry

The image-based diagnostic process can be described as an interpretation task. Shapes, forms, and interrelationships among them are recorded and identified, but their etiology and implications have to be understood as well. To extract the ''message'' from an image, i.e., to detect changes from normality or plan interventions relative to the anatomic structure, a complex reasoning process integrating information from a huge knowledge base becomes necessary. Computer analysis will help not only in analyzing the image data but also in integrating them as a knowledge source into the therapeutic process, potentially supporting the development of minimally invasive techniques with higher accuracy.

Digital image data carry quantitative information. They represent the basis for quantitative measurements because they measure the extent of anatomic objects and capture pathologic changes. Based on images depicting individual anatomic variations and pathologic morphologies, physicians make a diagnosis or plan surgery either as an imaginative process or by measuring absolute distances, angles, and areas. In radiation therapy, the directions and intensity distribution of the beams are optimized to treat the target object under consideration and to minimize the radiation burden to neighboring tissues sensitive to exposure to ionizing radiation. Measurements and planning in multiple spatial dimensions and possibly time are beyond the cognitive abilities and require new computer-assisted tools.

Computer-Assisted Medical Image Analysis

Early work on computerized analysis was directed at developing tools for rapid 3D visualization. Technical development has since progressed very fast so that visualization tools are now offered by all medical equipment manufacturers. Given modern powerful hardware, research and development efforts now focus on analysis rather than display. In terms of clinical potential and achievement, many useful results have been presented that do not propose a general approach but a domain-dependent judicious combination and integration of methods.

Computerized image analysis tools represent an aid for processing radiologic data. They have to support, amplify, and expand perceptual and cognitive abilities of physicians and permit quantitative measurements. The key issues are expressed by the following points:

- Optimally supporting tedious manual tasks (automated processing) as the definition of regions of interest
- Helping intuition and communication (visualization and manipulation)
- Providing segmentation, description, and analysis of anatomic and functional structures (model-based interpretation)
- Deriving qualitative description and quantitative parameters (morphometry and shape description)
- Combining information from multiple acquisition devices (multisensor fusion)
- Guiding therapeutic procedures based on image information (image-guided therapy)

Image analysis goes far beyond simply representing image slices on a computer monitor. The computerized processing of images converts image data into a description that *explicitly enhances, represents, and describes features important for understanding and measurements.* Computerized systems support the task of medical image analysis by segmenting medical image data into meaningful regions and objects, by recovering organs and providing a description encoding shape and quantitative measurements, by characterizing invariant landmarks, by multimodality analysis, and by applying the latest visualization techniques to support cognitive abilities of human interpreters (23). Especially, we should follow the paradigm of letting the computer solve problems where humans have no access to or cannot compete. Computers are very strong in number "crunching," in analyzing multidimensional scenes, and in generating $2\frac{1}{2}$-dimensional (surface shaded) displays from 3D data, respectively.

VISUALIZATION METHODS

Visual data are probably the most important source of information about the world around us. The human visual system is extremely powerful in interpreting the image signal information produced by the eyes as sensors of the human visual system. In the process of evolution, the further processing of this information has been adapted to some characteristics of these images to ensure optimal processing of the visual information received from our environment:

- The image signal formed on the retina of the eye is inherently two-dimensional (2D).
- The left and right retinas produce a pair of stereo images, i.e., a pair of 2D views of a 3D scene from slightly different points of views.
- The basic task of the human visual system is the reconstruction of 3D scenes from the primary information. In a pure mathematical sense, this problem cannot be solved uniquely. In order to still perform the task, the visual processing of the brain uses several additional sources of information in the images (so-called image cues) which, together with a priori expectations (knowledge) about the surrounding world, usually allow a correct interpretation of the images sensed. The most important visual cues are object color and texture, object shading (change of the apparent object brightness due to surface curvature or shadows), and object motion, allowing the extraction of additional information from the dynamics of an animated scene.

Imaging data are usually presented on 2D devices such as the traditional light boxes or on computer screens. As long as the acquired images are two-dimensional (as traditional x-ray images), the presentation of the complete information can be solved easily just by displaying them on the selected device. Postprocessing techniques may only be necessary for the enhancement of some visually less obvious image features.

Modern image-acquisition techniques can produce much more complex image data that are not directly accessible by the human visual system trained for the interpretation of visual scenes. Recognition of 3D structures from cross-sectional views or understanding blood flow from single components of flow vectors is not a spontaneous cognitive task. Even after extensive training, one can hardly expect to be able to extract the complete information hidden in such complex image data.

The role of specialized visualization algorithms is a conversion of the sensed raw data into images that can be interpreted directly based on the capabilities of the human visual system. These techniques should allow an easier and more complete comprehension of the information contained in the raw data.

The use of advanced visualization methods can deliver unprecedented diagnostic and surgical information providing a major contribution to better and more efficient patient care. One has to realize, however, that these "pretty images" are most often generated under certain assumptions and can be highly dependent on several hidden parameters. The influence of these parameters on the resulting images is often far from obvious, and a bad selection can lead to erroneous interpretation.

In this section we first give an overview of some simple preprocessing techniques that are broadly used for image enhancement. Then the most important methods for visualization of volumetric data will be presented The last part of the section gives a short summary of special visual cues for more realistic perception of image data. The image examples have been created using the ANALYZE package developed by the Biomedical Image Resource of the Mayo Foundation (22).

Image Enhancement

The digital representation (see ''Digital Image Data'' above) of the brightness values of images cannot always be used directly for their presentation on a computer screen. There are two major reasons why a conversion of the original output of a digital imaging device to an image representation on a computer screen is necessary:

1. The representation of gray-scale values in images on a computer screen is most often limited to 1 byte (8 bits). Raw data of today's imaging devices have a higher dynamic range (usually 12 bits, sometimes even 16 bits). This makes a conversion from a 12-bit to an 8-bit representation mandatory.
2. The brightness of the measured pixels in the raw data is determined by the physics of the imaging process. Usually, they are not optimally adapted to human visual perception and need some adjustment in order to optimally support image interpretation by a clinician.

The above-mentioned adjustments are always performed by applying an appropriate function transforming the measured brightness value at every pixel in an image $I[x, y]$ into a brightness value that will be presented on the screen. Figure 1 demonstrates some possible transfer functions that map the Hounsfield values measured by a CT unit coded in 12 bits (capable of coding 4096 distinct values) into an 8-bit quantized display brightness (values between 0 and 255).

The function shown in Fig. 1A may seem to be an optimal choice because it handles the whole 12-bit range equally. This, however, is far from optimal for CT images, since the usual range of Hounsfield units (-1000 to 1000) covers only part of this range. This demonstrates that a transfer function cannot be selected independently of the type of images to be presented. It is always necessary to adapt them to the imaging modality. In some cases even adjustment to the individual images may be justified.

The individual images can be characterized by the statistics of the measured values at the single pixels. A simple way to describe these statistics is to count the occurrence of the different brightness values over the whole image and present it as a bar chart. This representation of the image values is called a *histogram* and provides a general overview of the intensity distribution throughout the image. Figure 2A shows a CT slice through a lumbar vertebra together with the calculated histogram of the image.

The mapping function for the individual images is most often selected manually. The user then selects a range of measured values regarded to be interesting (the window) that

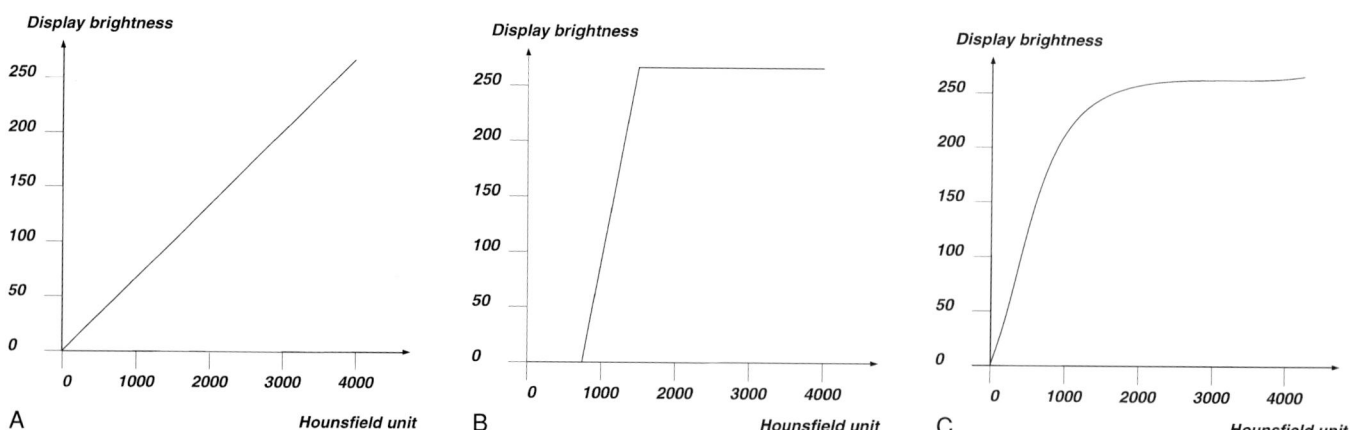

Figure 1. Different transfer functions mapping Hounsfield units as measured by CT imaging (*horizontal*) into brightness presented on a display screen (*vertical*).

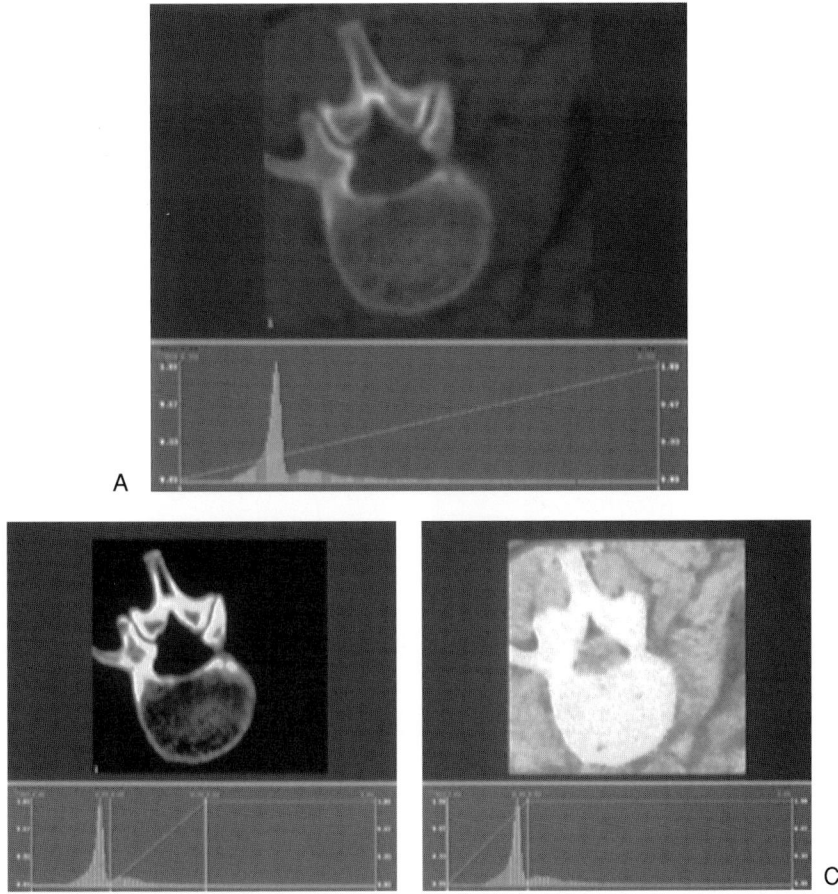

Figure 2. Manual adjustment of the brightness transfer function (windowing). See Color Plate 2.

is mapped linearly to the whole brightness range of the display. Intensities below the lower limit of the window will all be shown as black, while intensities above the higher window limit will show up as white on the screen. Figure 1B shows such a windowing function for the window range between 750 and 1250 Hounsfield units. The effects of such manual adjustments on the image are shown in Figure 2 (see Color Plate 2). The mapping function is overlayed with the calculated histogram, showing that example Fig. 2B concentrates on high densities (bone window), while 2C emphasizes the low-density range (soft-tissue window with the bone structures "washed out" in the image).

Image intensity adjustment also can be performed automatically by creating mapping functions that optimize the resulting distribution of display brightness values, i.e., the histogram of the image presented on the screen. Figure 3 illustrates two attempts at image enhancement by such histogram manipulation techniques. The intensities of the original image (mapped linearly in the whole intensity range in Fig. 3A) were mapped to display brightness values while optimally preserving the original intensity distribution (histogram) (Fig. 3B). Figure 3C shows the effect of trying to achieve a homogeneous intensity distribution throughout the whole brightness range (histogram equalization). While this technique guarantees optimal contrast in the whole image, it cannot differentiate between anatomic structure (where contrast should be enhanced) and noise (where contrast should be suppressed) and often leads to questionable results.

It should be noted that any adjustment of intensity mapping on individual images is potentially dangerous and should be applied very carefully. Clinicians are usually accustomed to specific intensity and contrast properties for a given imaging modality. Individual changes across images can be very disturbing and even misleading.

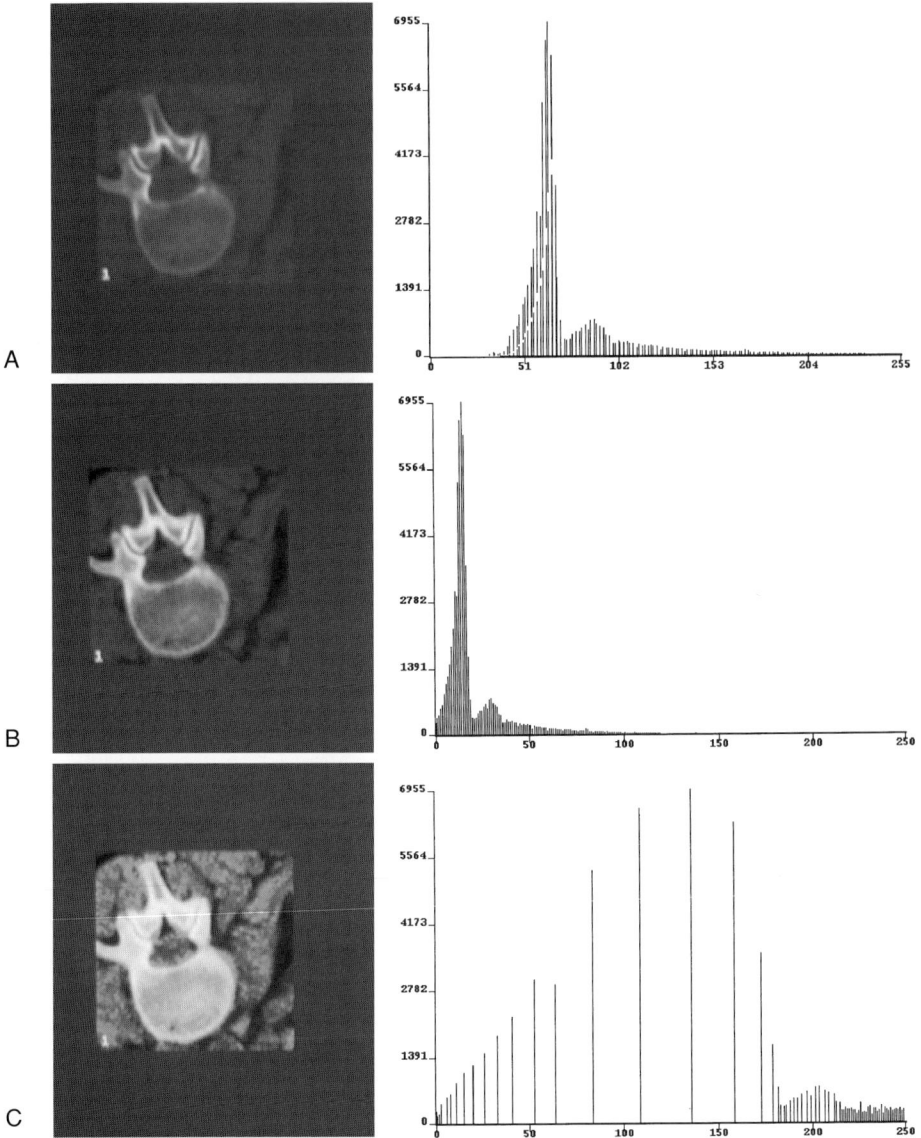

Figure 3. Automatic intensity mapping based on histogram manipulation.

Visualization of Volumetric Data

Volumetric data traditionally are presented as series of image slices on film. While this can be partially justified for highly anisotropic image data (where the distance between slices is much larger than the pixel size), the mental recognition of 3D structures from this series is very demanding and needs extensive training even for well-defined slicing directions and simple object structures. Modern imaging devices can produce nearly or completely isotropic data where such a distinction between spatial directions is no longer technically justified although still can be useful for image interpretation.

The simplest techniques for visual inspection of volumetric data allow one to roam through the original volume from any direction. This allows the investigation of the data in any orthogonal direction (coronal, axial, or sagittal) independently of the slicing direction during acquisition. At the same time, any oblique slicing direction can be selected if it is better adapted to the local anatomy under investigation. Figure 4 shows the result of such an oblique slicing. The position of the selected slice is shown in 3D space for better comprehension.

A better understanding of the 3D structure of anatomic objects can be gained by showing simultaneously more than one orthogonal slice through the data volume together

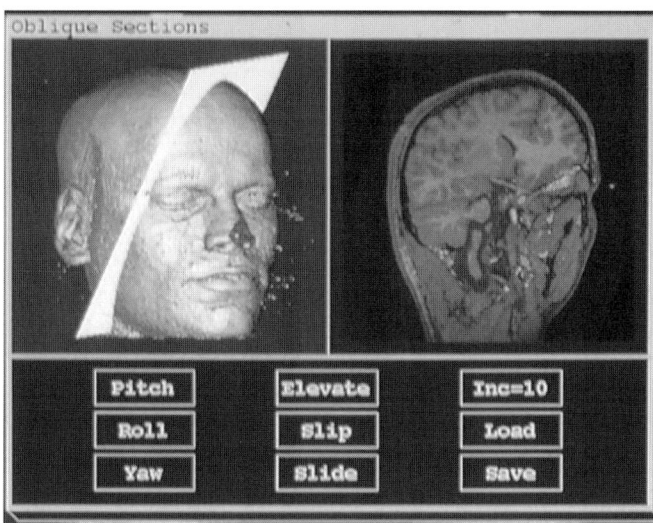

Figure 4. Oblique slice through an MRI image volume.

with their spatial relationship. A simple way to reach pseudo-3D effects is to present a clipped data volume as a projected cube where the original image data are painted on the clipping surfaces, as shown in Fig. 5A. A more advanced tool allows the arbitrary positioning of a 3D point (the so-called cursor) in the data volume and to display simultaneously the three orthogonal anatomic planes (coronal, axial, and sagittal) cutting the volume at the selected point. The cursor position can be adjusted in any two orthogonal directions simultaneously by pointing to the desired position on the third image plane. This multiplanar reconstruction method is illustrated in Fig. 5B.

More sophisticated volume visualization can be obtained by data-projection techniques. These methods simulate the effect of traversing the data volume with a bundle of rays in a parallel or perspective projection. The interaction between the rays and the intersected single voxels is estimated and integrated along the traversal paths. The simplest possibility is the simulation of x-ray traversal through the volume, where the local absorption of the x-ray energy is summed up for all voxels that are hit by the ray during traversal.

Figure 6 shows the result of a simulated x-ray projection by ray tracing on a pelvic

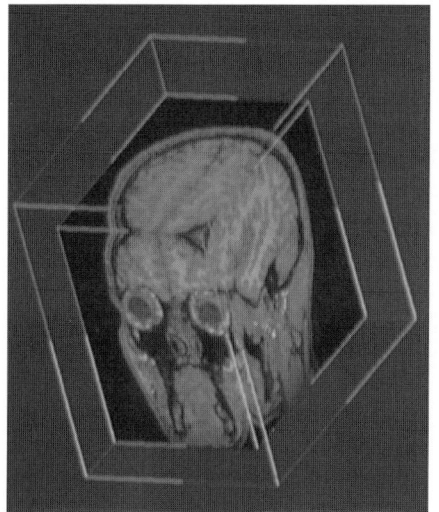
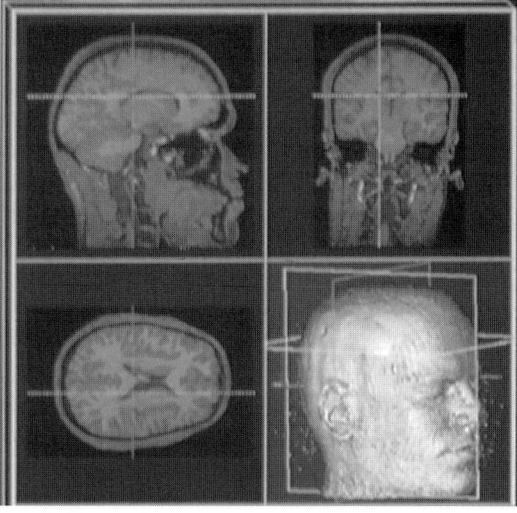

A   B

Figure 5. Simultaneous presentation of orthogonal slices through a data volume as a clipped data cube (**A**) and a multiplanar reconstruction (**B**).

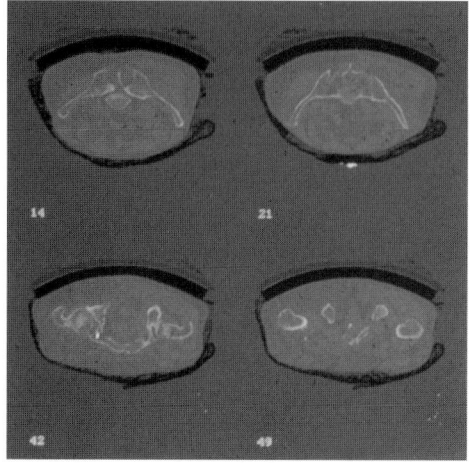 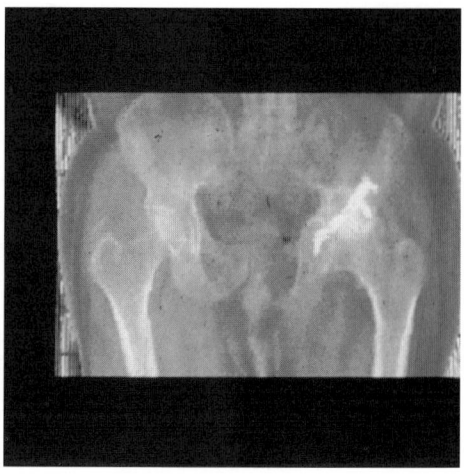

A   B

Figure 6. Radiographic projection (**B**) of a pelvic CT data set (some original slices shown in **A**).

The figure below illustrates the principle of ray tracing that provides the basis for more sophisticated volume-rendering procedures. The display screen is represented by the image plane with the pixel coordinates (u, v). From every pixel of the screen a ray $(\mathcal{R}_j)$ is sent into the data volume parallel to the actual viewing direction, i.e., orthogonal to the viewing plane. Some examples of such projection rays are shown as dashed arrows. For each ray, image data voxels $(\mathcal{V}_i)$ hit by the ray are selected and their intensity values $(I[x_i, y_i, z_i])$ are summed up to provide the actual brightness value on the scene at the given position $(D[u_j, v_j])$:

$$D[u_j, v_j] = \sum_{\mathcal{V}_i \cap \mathcal{R}_j \neq 0} I[x_i, y_i, z_i]$$

In the figure, voxels that are hit by the selected ray (solid arrow) (i.e., those satisfying the condition $\mathcal{V}_i \cap \mathcal{R}_j \neq \emptyset$) are denoted by solid lines. Voxels that are avoided by this ray are shown as dotted cubes.

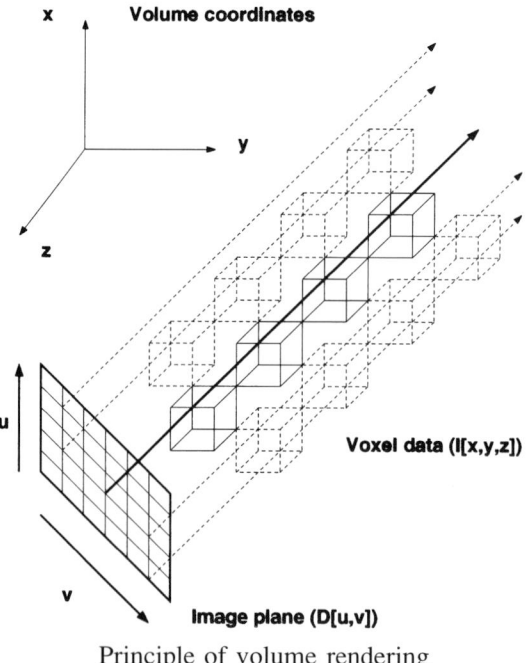

Principle of volume rendering

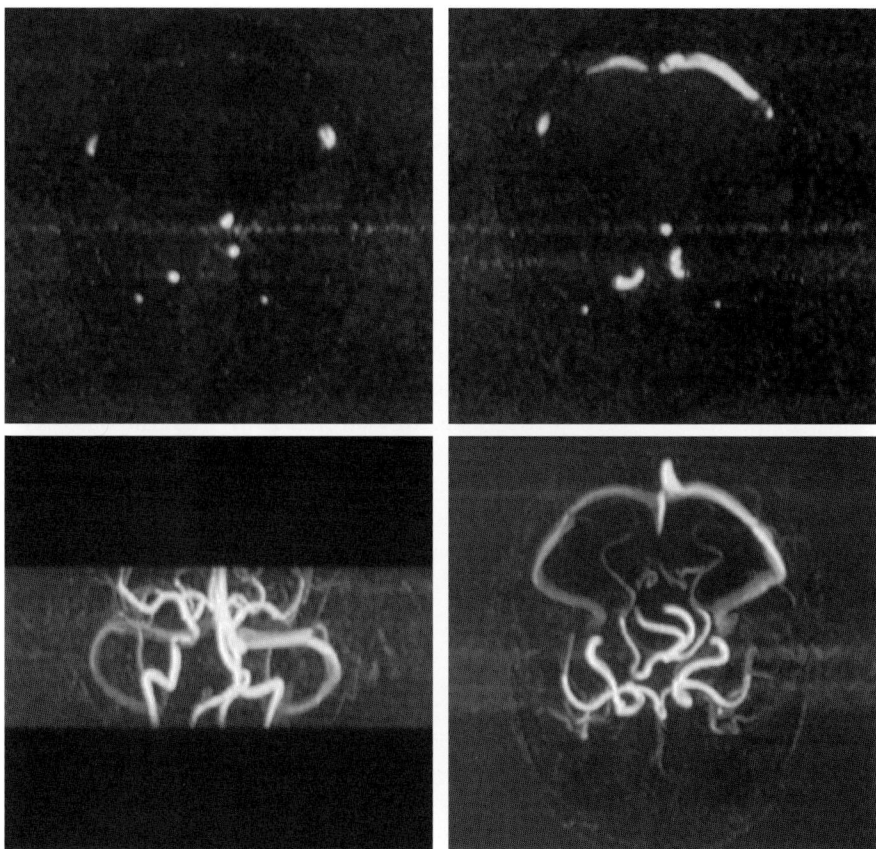

Figure 7. Two slices from an MR angiography data set (*upper row*) and its maximum-intensity projections (*lower row*).

CT data set. On the left image some selected slices from the original data set are presented. On the right the simulated frontal x-ray image is shown.

The ray-tracing principle allows more sophisticated combinations of information extracted during the ray traversal. The visualization of volumetric angiographic data as acquired in MR angiography, for example, cannot be solved satisfactorily by the visualization techniques discussed above. The mental reconstruction of fine linear 3D vessel structures from a sequence of image slices (a few examples are shown on the top row of Fig. 7) poses a serious challenge even for the experienced physician. Due to limited contrast at fine vessel structures, a lot of important details are lost while summing up intensities during radiographic projection. The maximum-intensity projection (MIP) method provides a simple and efficient visualization technique to overcome these difficulties. This technique is a specialized ray-tracing procedure that is searching for a maximal intensity value along the traversed ray and uses this as intensity value in the projected image. In this way one can avoid summing up a large amount of background intensity and completely preserve the contrast between rays hitting a vessel and those traversing through background. The lower row on Fig. 7 shows two MIP images generated from the MR angiography data set clearly demonstrating how fine details are preserved by this projection technique.

All the presented ray-tracing methods for the visualization of volumetric data up to this point result in a general loss of depth information as a consequence of the projection procedure. If some 3D organs have been isolated and identified using segmentation techniques discussed later in the chapter, ray tracing also can provide means for their nearly photorealistic shading resulting in a detailed 3D impression of the anatomic scene under investigation.

These surface-rendering techniques are based on calculating the visibility of different parts of the organ surfaces and removing surface patches hidden behind other object parts in the foreground. Additionally, the modeling of light-reflection properties of the visible surfaces of segmented organs provides the basis for their realistic rendering. The components of the light-reflection model are usually the following:

- The amount of reflected *ambient light* is independent of specific light sources and depends only on the reflection coefficient of the visible surfaces.
- The amount of light resulting from *diffuse reflection* depends on the angle between the surface and the direction of illuminating light. The intensity of the reflected light is identical in all directions.
- In case of *specular reflection* (characteristic for metallic surfaces), the amount of reflected light is not distributed homogeneously, providing strong reflection around the mirror direction.
- Absorption of light through the surrounding medium can be accounted for by reducing reflected light intensity for object surfaces that are far away from the observer. This *depth-shading technique* can be used for supporting better depth perception.
- Ray-tracing techniques also can be used for shadow calculations. In many cases, however, it is assumed that the light source is exactly behind the observer, in which case no shadows can be cast on visible surfaces.

The calculation of the reflected light by a given surface can be summarized as follows:

- Ambient light is a result of multiple reflections on surfaces and is modeled as a constant term $c_a I_a$ independent of light incidence and reflection directions, where I_a is the amount of ambient light present in the scene and c_a is the reflectivity of the surface.
- Diffuse reflection is calculated by Lambert's law as $I_d = c_d I_l \cos(\theta)$, where I_l is the intensity of the light source, c_d is the diffuse reflectivity of the surface, and θ is the angle between the surface normal and the incidence direction of the light (see illustration a). The amount of reflected light is the same in all spatial directions.
- Perfect mirror reflection on specular surfaces is only visible if viewed from the mirror direction. Specular reflection on real surfaces is not perfect and will be visible in a finite cone of view around the mirror direction. This reflection is usually modeled as $c_s I_l \cos^n(\phi)$, where ϕ is the angle between the viewing direction and the perfect mirror direction of the surface (see illustration b).
- The reduction of reflected light due to growing surface distance is usually modeled by $I_r/(d + d_0)$, where d is the distance between the observer and the object surface and d_0 is an appropriately selected constant.

In summary, apparent surface brightness can be calculated as

$$I = c_a I_a + \frac{I_l}{d + d_0} [c_d \cos(\theta) + c_s \cos^n(\phi)]$$

a: diffuse reflection   **b: specular reflection**

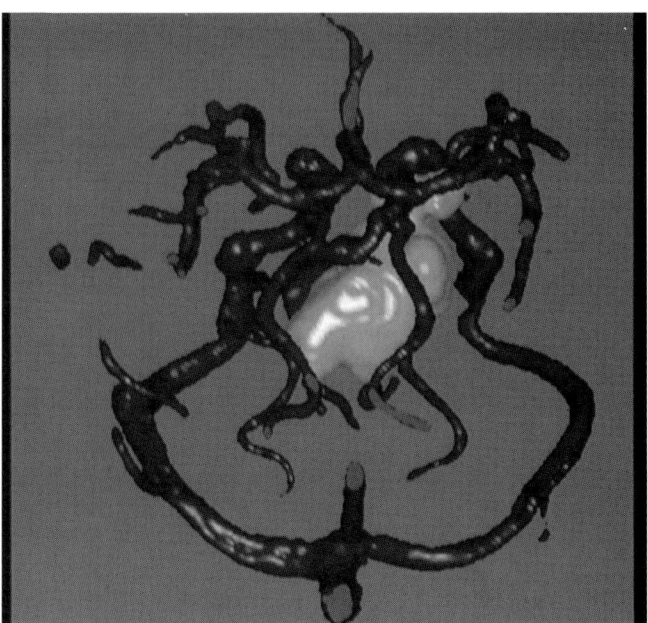

Figure 8. Surface rendering of a tumor with the surrounding vascularity obtained from a Gd-enhanced MRA acquisition. See Color Plate 3.

Figure 8 (see also Color Plate 3) illustrates the result of the surface-rendering technique. The image shows the shaded 3D surface of a tumor with the surrounding vascularity. The tumor and the vessels were first segmented out of a Gd-enhanced MR angiogram and then rendered as arbitrarily colored specular surfaces.

The basic difficulty of applying surface rendering is the necessity of preliminary segmentation. *Volume-rendering techniques* combine the possibilities of volumetric ray tracing with the photorealistic presentation capability of surface rendering. The technique relies on calculating light intensity along rays influenced by the following properties of image voxels:

- Transmission of light arriving from the voxels behind the one under consideration. The transparency of the voxel is usually related to the actual data value allowing its adaptation to different tissue types.
- The reflectance of external light is calculated by the same illumination models as in the case of surface rendering. The local surface direction and the surface reflectivity are calculated from the strength and direction of an edge centered at the voxel under investigation (see "Contour-Based Computer-Assisted Segmentation" following).

Volume rendering allows highly realistic visualization of complex anatomic scenes directly from the acquired data. However, one should be aware of the limitation that the objects identified by the observer on the generated images are only virtual and—in contrast to surface-rendered scenes—cannot be manipulated directly in subsequent simulation processes.

Advanced Visualization Cues

While elaborate surface- and volume-rendering methods allow excellent 3D visualization of anatomic scenes in many cases, impressively realistic depth perception can be achieved by the application of one (or both) of the following visual cues in many cases even without computationally expensive surface-shading techniques:

- Object motion, especially rotation around an axis parallel to the viewing plane, can provide very good depth perception. The visual system can very effectively extract this information even from simple projection sequences as radiographic or maximum-intensity projections. The generation of animated image sequences (movies) is already in everyday use, while modern (and at the moment still very expensive) graphic hardware can perform the generation of single images in real time, allowing interactive exploration of the anatomic scene.

- Specialized display screens allow one to present different images parallel to the left and right eyes of the observer by using separate screens for the two eyes (head-mounted display devices) or interlacing the two images on a single screen with different light polarization. The images can then be viewed through polarized glasses, allowing their separation for the left and right eyes. The eye disparity, which is the basis of stereoscopic perception, can be simulated by generating images for the two eyes from a slightly different point of view. Very realistic immersion into the 3D scene can be achieved through the presentation of these images through a stereoscopic display device.

Visualization Techniques for Image Fusion and Multivalued Data

All the techniques presented up to this point are aimed at the generation of optimally perceivable images from 2D and 3D data sets containing a single data value at every measurement position (pixel/voxel). In many cases, however, simultaneous presentation of several measurement values at the single positions is required. Visualization tasks demanding such techniques can be categorized into the following classes:

- Presentation of independently acquired images providing complementary information as, for example, overlay of anatomic and functional image data. Before presentation, such images have to be spatially perfectly aligned, requiring special registration techniques discussed in detail in ''Image Fusion'' below.
- Supporting manual registration of images by efficient visual control.
- Visualization of data sets containing several measured values at single measurement points as multiecho MRI acquisitions or flow vector measurements by phase-contrast MR angiography.

Presentation of dense vectorial data as flow usually requires the combined use of complex visualization and simulation techniques and is beyond the scope of this chapter.

The simplest way is to present different measurement values next to each other on the same screen. The connection between the images can be established by coupling every interactive image manipulation such as rotation and projection that are then performed in parallel and in identical fashion on all data sets. Especially efficient is the rigid coupling of the cursors on the different images, guaranteeing that any change in position on one image leads to an immediate update on the other images. An important advantage of this method, which can be very efficiently used for checking image registration, is that the number of data values to be presented is in principle unlimited.

In many cases it is important to combine all available information on a single image. Combination of different data channels in a single image always requires the characteristic use of color, which then can be used by the eye to discriminate and identify the source of information. Usually the selection of color is arbitrary and serves only the purpose of optimal information presentation through the color perception of the human visual system without claiming any physical meaning for the color selection. The most common methods for this presentation of fused images are the following:

- *Overlay methods* generate two separate images using different colorization. Areas of importance on the image to be overlayed are identified, and the color of the corresponding pixels on the background image is overwritten by them. Overlaying functional information onto anatomic images as presented, for example, on Fig. 30 is a typical example for the application of this technique. The anatomic images are colored by gray-scale values, while the overlayed functional images are colored according to the strength of the detected activation. Color coding of activation strength is arbitrary; in

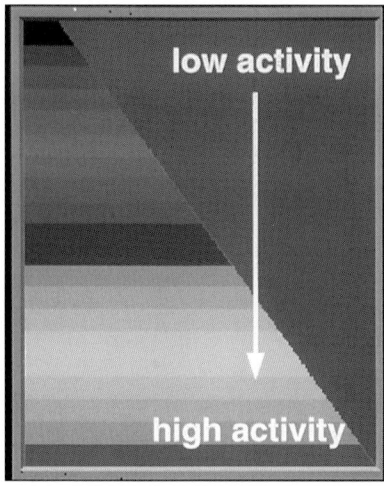

Figure 9. Mapping of functional activation strength to color. See Color Plate 4.

the presented example it grows from blue through green to red, as shown in Fig. 9 (see also Color Plate 4). Later sections provide some examples for the optimal presentation of fused images using color overlay technique.

• Two independently colored images can be composed into a single image by calculating the weighted average of their colors at every pixel position (blending). The weighting factors in the blend can be used to stress the content of one image over the other. Interactive adjustment of the blending coefficients can provide additional support for relating the images under investigation.

• The principle of representing colors by mixing of an appropriate set of primary colors also can be used for the visualization of fused data. Every color presented on the display screen is mixed together from the red, green, and blue principal color components representing three separate and independent data channels. Accordingly, up to three individual scalar images can be combined to a single color image using the principal colors to represent them. Figure 10 illustrates this principle on the registration of dye-painted retinal images. Color Plates 5A and B show the two images to be registered rendered in red and green. They are shifted for registration and combined for a single color image as shown on Figs. 10C (aligned) and 10D (misregistered). Areas of perfect agreement show up as yellow regions, while misregistration can be well identified as red or green boundaries.

SEGMENTATION TOOLS

The requirements for computer-assisted medical image analysis are

• Limited user interaction (high degree of automation)
• Efficient procedures running on standard computer hardware
• Robustness (insensitivity to noise, to imaging artifacts, and to variations among patients)

The following subsections describe computerized image-processing tools that are established in the field of medical image analysis. Segmentation techniques may be divided into two areas: (a) region-based segmentation from homogeneity criteria and (b) structure segmentation by discontinuity detection and contour grouping. This basic distinction is also reflected in the structure of the following subsections.

Interactive Segmentation

The human visual and cognitive system is by far superior to any computerized analysis procedure for the evaluation of structures in 2D image data. A pure manual outlining

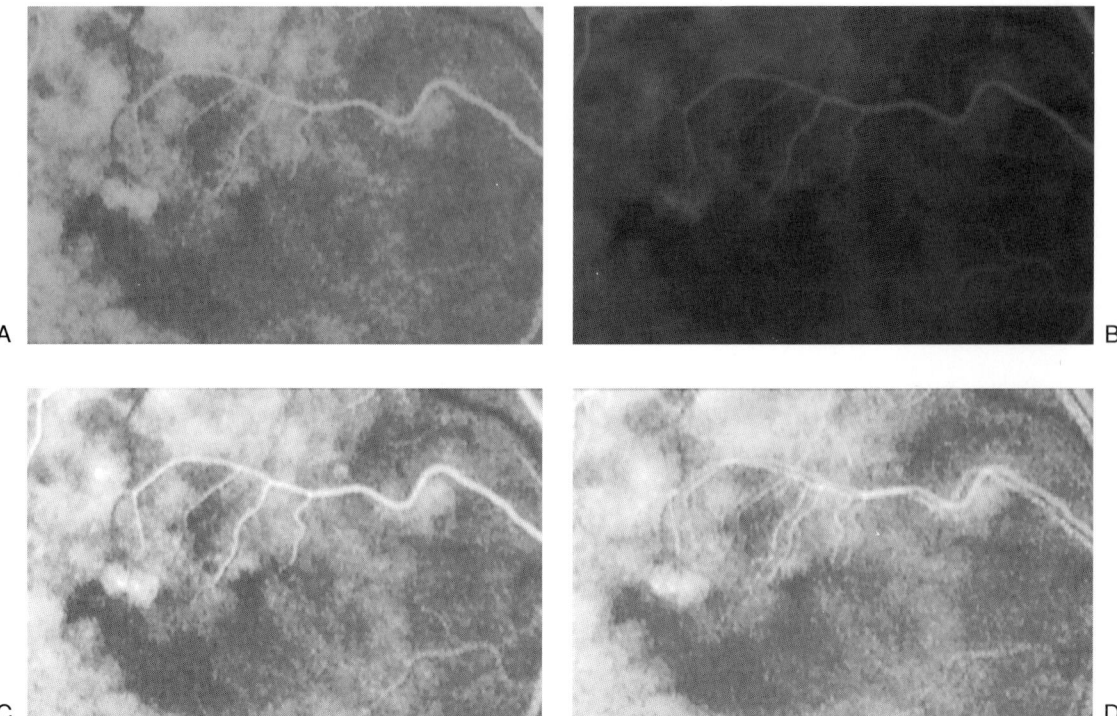

Figure 10. Combination of misaligned retinal images for visual registration. Images **A** and **B** show the images to be aligned in red and green. They are combined as color channels to a single color image as demonstrated in images **C** (aligned) and **D** (misregistered). See Color Plate 5.

of structures on a computer screen is therefore still regarded as the "gold standard" against which all the automated procedures have to compete. Interactive editing devices are part of most software systems and allow, in addition to fully interactive object definition, one to control automated procedures and to correct for segmentation errors. Interestingly, large studies (16) indicated that manual segmentation by clinicians—used for blind tests of segmentation algorithms—is not always guided primarily by the image-intensity function but from mental models where there is no contrast. A simulation of this behavior is approached by developing model-based segmentation techniques.

As a disadvantage, purely interactive segmentation is extremely tedious and time-consuming, lacks reproducibility, and largely depends on subjective criteria of the observers. Results can be significantly influenced by the intensity transfer function of the computer screen (brightness, contrast, and windowing) and by the mechanics of the user interface. Further, appropriate user interfaces for the interactive segmentation of 3D data, of time series, and of multimodal data are not yet available.

Region-Based Computer-Assisted Segmentation

In general, manual segmentation of high-resolution images from different imaging devices by far exceeds practical time limits and must be supported by automated procedures. A subgroup of medical image data is being composed of relatively homogeneous areas representing different tissue classes. This simplified world model leads to the development of segmentation techniques based on one- and multidimensional global thresholding, called *statistical classification.* Statistical pattern recognition, although a standard method with an elaborate mathematical basis and in widespread use in image-analysis applications (mainly in remote sensing), plays a significant role in the analysis of multidimensional medical data. In statistical pattern recognition, a priori knowledge about the physical measurements of voxels (MRI or CT voxel values) can be

A: Segmentation by thresholding   B: Segmentation by region growing

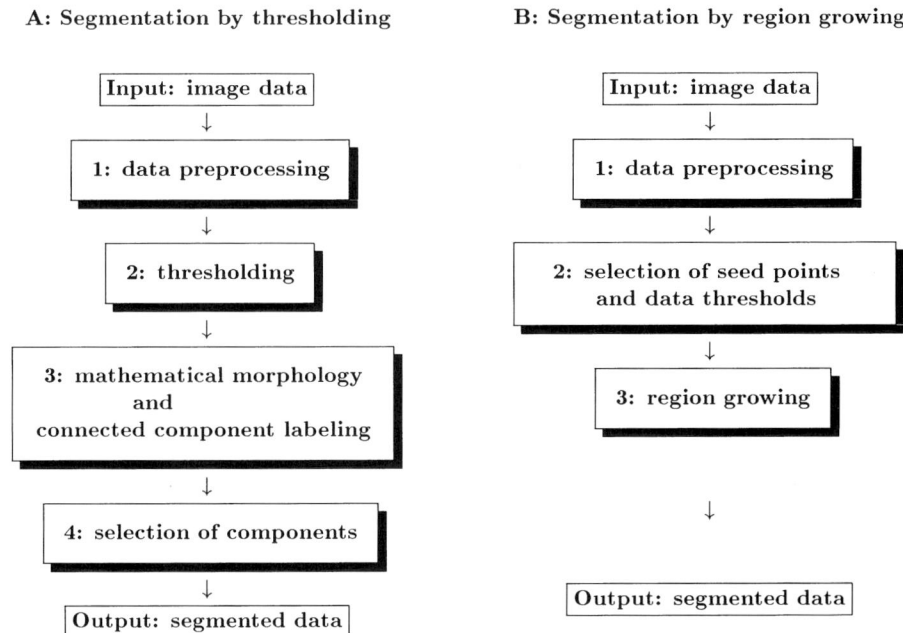

Figure 11. Most commonly used multistage segmentation schemes.

included in the task of image segmentation by choosing a supervised approach with training or an unsupervised clustering with initial estimates. The automatic selection of thresholds based on maximum a posteriori classification is often replaced by a purely interactive technique where a user manually selects thresholds.

Multistage System

Segmentation of medical image data into anatomically and functionally distinct regions requires a *multistage processing scheme.* Most of the successfully presented segmentations follow one of the two basic processing schemes presented in Fig. 11. The processing chains require only minimal user interaction and are known to produce better reproducible results than purely manual object definition. The processing stages can be regarded as a protocol, similar to acquisition protocols with predefined parameters in radiology. The choice of methods may be considered heuristic and tailored to a very special application. It illustrates, however, the strategy of exploiting the original measurements by extracting their information content with optimally suited procedures.

Preprocessing

Preprocessing largely depends on the individual application. Common preprocessing methods are corrections for geometric and radiometric distortion, resampling of digital data, or suppression of noise. Noise suppression has always been a basic issue in image processing. Linear smoothing as a preparatory step is often of little value because contours and fine details are blurred. A number of discontinuity-preserving nonlinear smoothing methods have been proposed, the most effective of which appears to be an iterative system based on the multidimensional anisotropic diffusion equation (11). It shows considerable noise suppression while retaining relevant structural features.

Thresholding

A special case of methods based on statistical classification is *windowing* or *thresholding* of one-channel image data, which is a well-known technique in the bone to soft-

Cut through a healthy vertebra (slice 19)

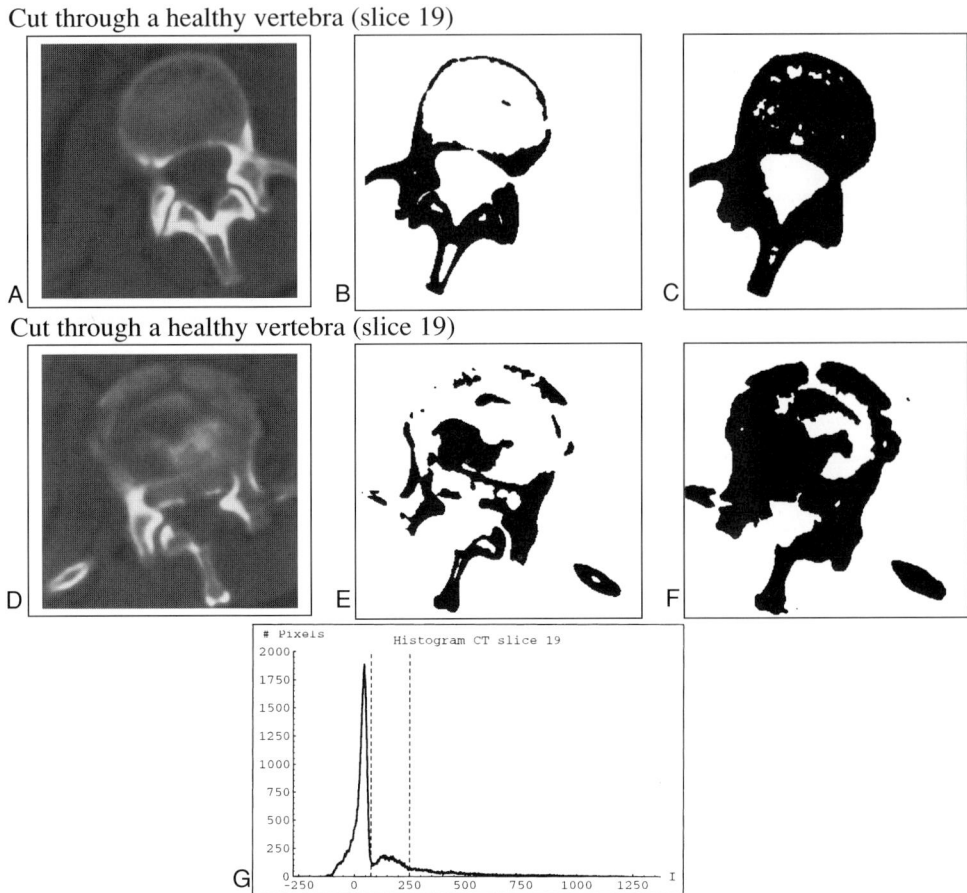

Cut through a healthy vertebra (slice 19)

Figure 12. Classification of bone and soft tissue in a CT data set presenting a compression fracture of a vertebra. Images **A** and **D** present the original CT slices and binary segmentations using thresholds of 75 HU (**B, E**) and 250 HU (**C, F**), respectively. Plot **G** presents the histogram of the original CT image. The two thresholds at 75 and 250 HU are marked with vertical dashed lines.

tissue discrimination in 3D CT image analysis. The image data have to fulfill two basic criteria: They must be radiometrically homogeneous over their full spatial extent, and different tissue categories must have characteristic brightness signatures. Thresholding is a pixel-by-pixel classification technique, assessing only the brightness value $I(x, y)$ at each pixel. Categories of individual data elements are assigned without any regard to those of their neighbors. The procedure is extremely fast and can be interactively controlled on the screen. Human observers immediately reconstruct structural properties from the classified images that are, however, not represented in the data at this stage of processing (see later discussion of connected component labeling). Figure 12 illustrates a classification of bone structures of CT data based on simple thresholding. The choice of the threshold is critical to the diagnosis of bone fragments in the spinal canal. The horizontal axis of the histogram reflects the quantization of the brightness in Hounsfield units that is usually stored as a 12-bit number.

Mathematical Morphometry

The main operations in *mathematical morphometry* are the nonlinear filtering operations: erosion, dilation, opening, and closing. *Erosion* decreases the size of objects by placing a kernel at each pixel position and by deleting object pixels at positions where the kernel mask is not completely included in the object. A circular (2D) or spherical

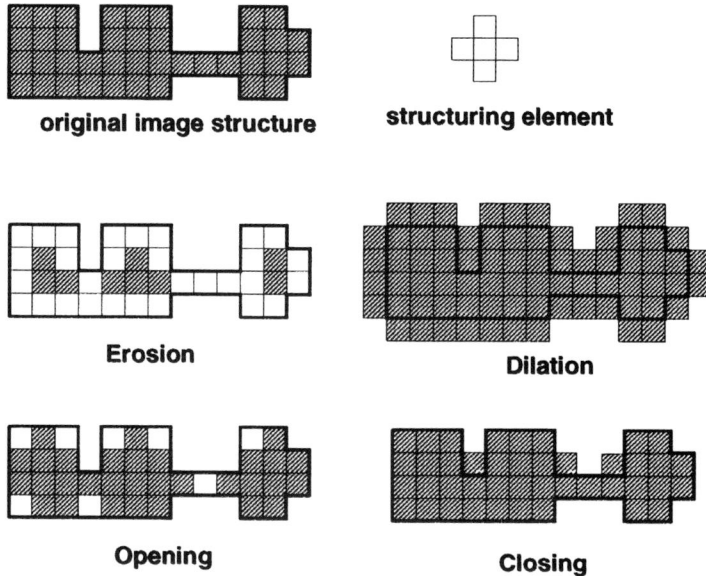

Figure 13. Mathematical morphology. The shaded areas represent the test object (*dark line*) after erosion (*middle left*), dilation (*middle right*), opening (*bottom left*), and closing (*bottom right*). The crosslike structuring element is shown upper right.

(3D) kernel with radius *r* "peels" off a skin of thickness *r*. Objects or object parts smaller than the kernel width are removed. *Dilation,* on the other hand, reverses the erosion process by growing the object or, as a duality, eroding the background rather than the object. The combination of an erosion process followed by dilation removes objects or object parts smaller than the kernel size while preserving the general shape of large structures, known as *opening.*

The effect of *opening* and *closing* can be explained in a much simpler way without using the mechanisms of erosion and dilation (Fig. 13). Two instructions suffice, namely (a) find each place where the structuring element *B* is entirely contained by the structure *X,* and (b) mark all the points in *X* that are covered by *B.* The set of marked points in *X* represents the opened structure or closed structure (bottom illustration in Fig. 13). A typical segmentation procedure that applies erosion, connected component labeling, and dilation is presented in Fig. 15. Most often the methods of mathematical morphology are applied as a correction of the binary segmentation to remove unwanted thin connections between different anatomic objects.

Connectivity

Connectivity defines a set of connected elements and depends on the definition of the topology. In a pixel grid we usually assume that we have quadratic or rectangular pixels. The pixels are connected to neighboring elements by common edges and common corners, as illustrated in Fig. 14.

A connected-component labeling procedure assigns unique labels to regions that are connected using either 4- or 8-connectivity. The regions are the result of a preceding binary segmentation, e.g., of a windowing or thresholding operation on the original image.

Region Growing

Region growing is a region-based segmentation technique that lets regions develop around previously defined seed points (1). Similar adjacent atomic regions are merged sequentially until the resulting regions exceed a predefined homogeneity criterion or, as

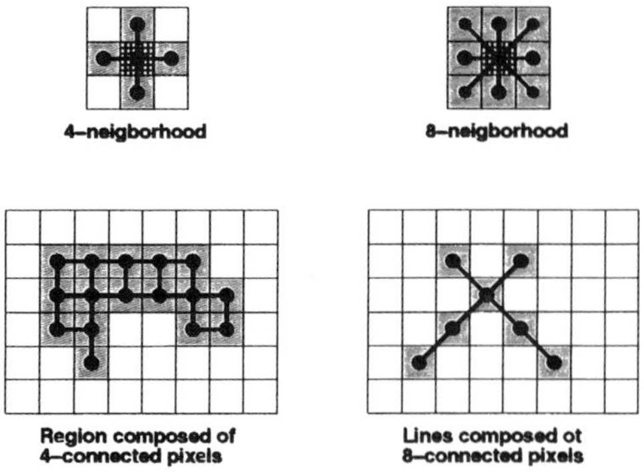

Figure 14. Topology of the pixel grid. Using 4-connectivity, a pixel is connected by edges to its four immediate neighbors (*top left*). Eight-connectivity defines the complete neighborhood (*top right*) with eight surrounding pixels. A region can be composed of a set of 4-connected pixels, whereas 8-connectivity is preferred for the representation of thin digital lines.

a dual constraint, adjacent regions become sufficiently different. In practice, many region-growing procedures let a user define lower and upper brightness thresholds and a seed pixel. An iterative procedure grows a region around the seed point by adding pixels that are connected (either 4- or 8-connected; see previous discussion on connectivity) and if they meet the similarity criterion (e.g., have a brightness value within the predefined thresholds). In this simplest form, region growing can be considered to be very similar to the multistage processing based on thresholding and connected component labeling.

The region-growing concept can be extended to include other homogeneity constraints, e.g., evaluating the standard deviation of the brightness values or the inclusion of boundary pixels (19). In its most general form, region growing can start at each pixel and can perform an image partition based on an iterative split-and-merge technique.

Application: Region-Based Segmentation of Brain Structure. A multistage segmentation procedure (Fig. 11, type A) has been applied to segment the intracranial cavity from MRI image data. The procedure is illustrated by 2D axial slices but actually was carried

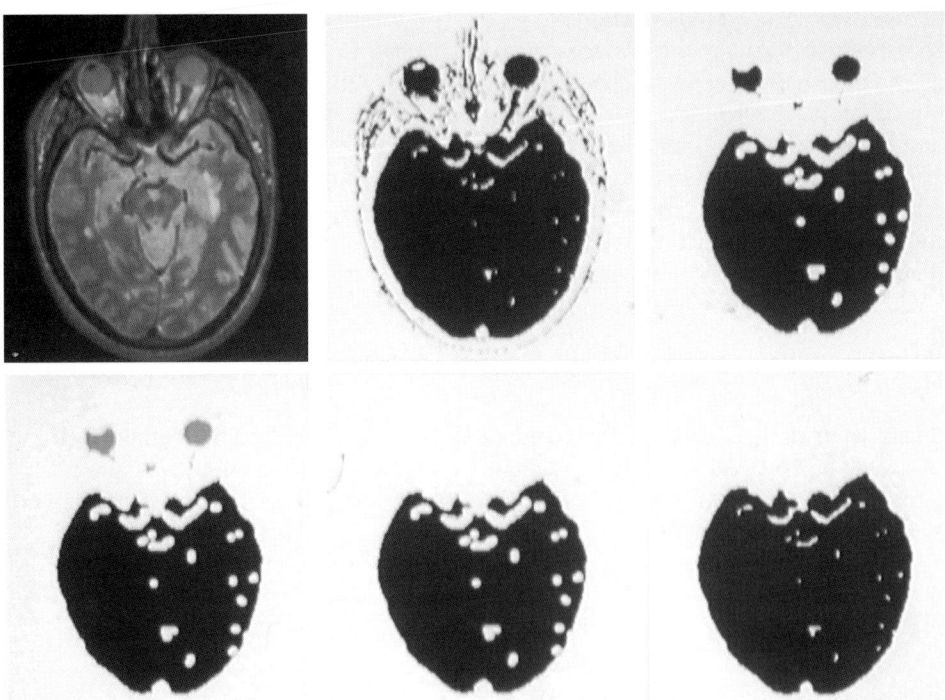

Figure 15. Application of mathematical morphology to brain segmentation. (*Upper row*) Original MRI image, thresholding and dilation. (*Bottom row*) Connected component labeling for assigning different labels to disconnected components, selection of largest component, and erosion to recover the original size of the brain structure. (*Medical image data courtesy of Dr. Ron Kikinis, Brigham and Women's Hospital, Boston.*)

out in 3D on volumetric data. After isolating the intracranial cavity, soft tissues and fluid can be segmented by applying further segmentation based on intensity thresholding.

Contour-Based Computer-Assisted Segmentation

A region-based segmentation assumes that objects to be segmented are represented as regions with constant brightness. This simple assumption is often violated because most anatomic objects possess a complex interior structure. A dual approach to region segmentation is structure segmentation based on discontinuity detection and grouping. Edge detection, which is most often a smoothing and differentiation of the image signal (3), marks discontinuities in image structure, i.e., boundaries between regions of different brightness. The first two images in Fig. 16 (see also Color Plate 6) illustrate an original image and the result of edge detection. In contrast to the previously discussed thresholding methods, edge detection is a technique that includes a small local neighborhood of each pixel into the analysis. The image is *filtered* with a neighborhood mask that assigns

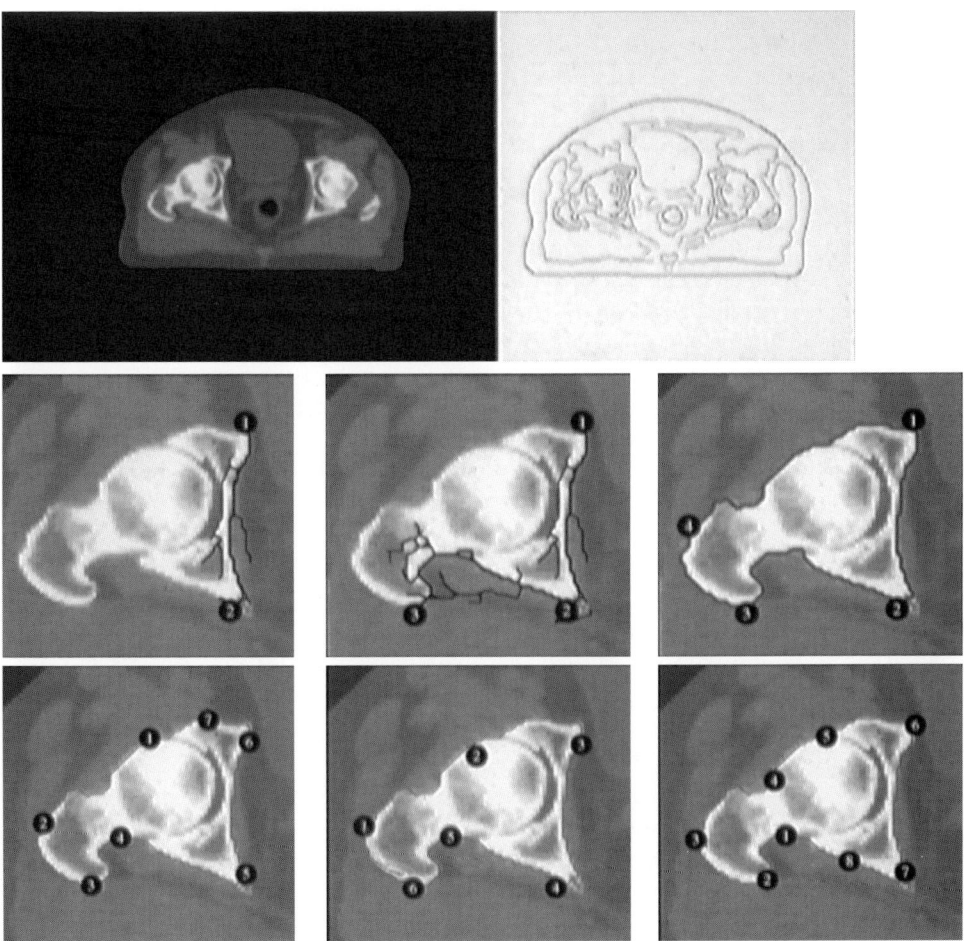

Figure 16. Examples of constrained interactive search. (*Top row*) The original CT image of the pelvis is transformed into a contour image using standard edge detection. (*Middle row*) A precomputed graph of contour fragments and possible links guides the interactive segmentation. A user selects a start point (left image, point 1) and additional control points (points 2–4). The procedure calculates an optimal closed path (right image) based on the precomputed contour fragments and shape criteria. The thin lines indicate structures evaluated as potential paths during the search. The three results shown in the bottom row are obtained by different users and nicely demonstrate the robustness and reproducibility of the procedure, which is not sensitive to the location and number of control points. See Color Plate 6.

a weighted sum of neighboring pixels to each new center pixel (see the following box). Images can be filtered by a linear filtering process or by nonlinear filters, where a filter is adapted to the local structure. Edge detection by smoothing and local differentiation is a linear operation that allows one to adopt highly efficient implementation schemes.

FILTERING OF DIGITAL IMAGE DATA

$$\hat{I}(x, y) = \sum_{k=-m}^{m} \sum_{l=-m}^{m} I(x, y) * \text{mask}(x-k, y-l)$$

where   mask(k, l): weights of neighborhood mask centered at (x, y)
        m, l: half extension of symmetrical mask in pixel space

Example: Detection of vertical and horizontal discontinuities using a 3 × 3 mask:

1/6	1	0	−1
	1	0	−1
	1	0	−1

1/6	1	1	1
	0	0	0
	−1	−1	−1

It is obvious from the edge image shown in Fig. 16 that edge detection itself is not sufficient. The multiple objects are represented by a set of contour fragments that have to be grouped to closed contours. A new grouping procedure developed by Vehkomäki (26) illustrates the concept of a computer-assisted structure segmentation method with only minimal user interaction. Local contour fragments and a graph of connected regions are precalculated but hidden to the user. A user selects a starting point near the desired object contour and a few control points to guide the procedure (see Fig. 16). The resulting closed contour follows the edge fragments and is therefore not sensitive to the exact choice of the control points (Fig. 16, bottom row). The procedure has the advantage of minimizing the interaction to a few simple mouse clicks, to be fully controlled by the observer, while still producing robust and reproducible segmentation results.

IMAGE FUSION

There is a growing need in medical practice and science to compare different images representing the same tissue structures. Picture archiving and communication systems (PACS) provide long-term storage of the digital images acquired in patient studies. If a patient returns for a new diagnosis or treatment, the images showing his or her former condition can be recalled, interpreted to guide the acquisition, and presented together with the newly acquired images.

More and more modalities are able to acquire images that represent functional properties. Often they show too little anatomic information to be interpreted without referring to morphologic images of the same tissue. Striking examples where the depicted tissue function does not change parallel to organ boundaries are the tissue pH or the temperature as accessible in MRI or the oxygen extraction fraction in positron-emission tomography (PET).

Some of the functional techniques involve the acquisition of an entire time sequence of measurements. Typical examples are neural activation experiments in PET or MRI. Here, the brain perfusion as a measure of brain activation is monitored for different conditions. The time course of the response to the stimuli is then analyzed within each image pixel using methods analyzed in "Analysis of Time Series of Image Data" below, resulting in a functional pixel value. It is clear that dislocation of the head during the successive experiments mixes the contents among pixels and thus compromises the anal-

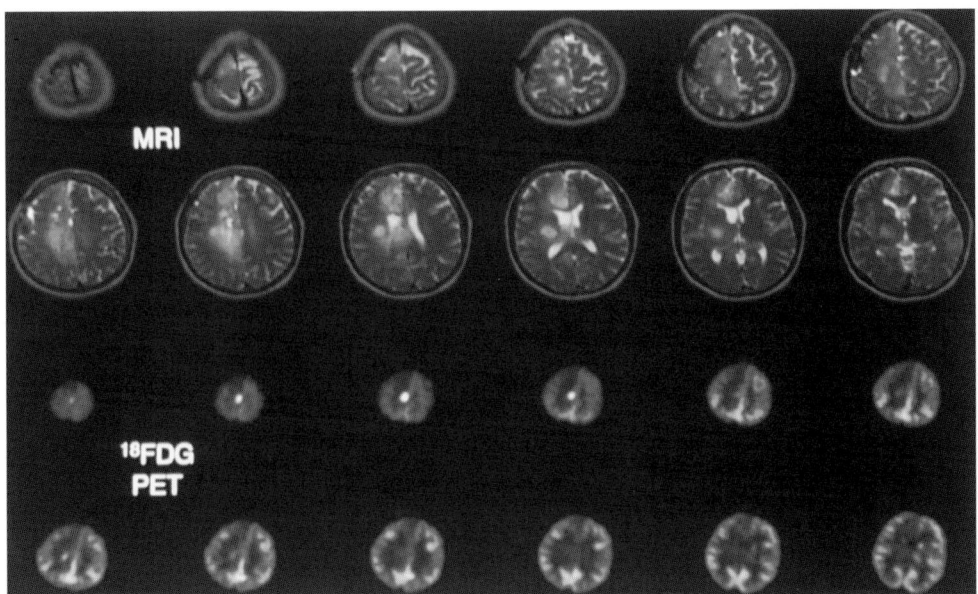

Figure 17. Typical situation in correlative imaging. The tissue structures in PET appear oriented and reduced relative to those in MRI due to different patient positioning and field of view. Accurate anatomic localization of the lesion visible in PET is therefore difficult. See Color Plate 7.

ysis. To avoid artefacts, a motion correction is therefore required that realigns all the data sets such that an image pixel represents the same tissue in each of the data sets.

Another domain with the need to integrate the information of different imaging modalities is radiation therapy (13). In radiotherapy, CT images are required because they provide the attenuation coefficients that are the input for the radiation plan calculation. However, the CT tissue contrast is often not optimal for delineating small tumors, particularly those which can be much better located on appropriately weighted MRI images. Obviously, then, it is desirable to have both a CT and an MRI data set, but again, they must show the organs in exactly aligned locations and orientations.

All the situations presented share the common task of image correlation. Given are two (or more) 3D image sets from an overlapping tissue volume of a patient. The information content in both data sets must be optimally combined in view of a clinical question. Let us illustrate the involved tasks with a typical example, the correlation of an FDG brain PET with a corresponding T1-weighted MRI (Fig. 17) (see also Color Plate 7). While PET shows the glucose turnover with a resolution of 5 mm, MRI yields much better resolved anatomic images. Since the patient had been differently positioned in the two scanners, the head was differently oriented within the field of view (Fig. 18) (see also Color Plate 8), resulting in PET images that appear rotated and reduced relative to the MRI images. When reading these images in a traditional way by just showing the slices in a viewbox, it is therefore difficult to precisely localize the lesion visible in PET. Image fusion supports this comparison in two steps. First "registration" brings the tissue structures in the two data sets into spatial alignment; that is, it undoes the acquisition-related geometric differences. As a result, it comes up with two directly comparable ("registered" or "matched" or "aligned") image stacks. The congruent slices could now be presented in the traditional side-by-side fashion, but this would still burden the observer with the task of information integration. Thus the second task, confusingly often itself called *image fusion,* is to support this process by visualization tools. For the example mentioned, a simple solution would be to transfer the lesion itself or its outlines from PET into the MRI images. This allows one to better assess its extent and severity and can help in surgical planning.

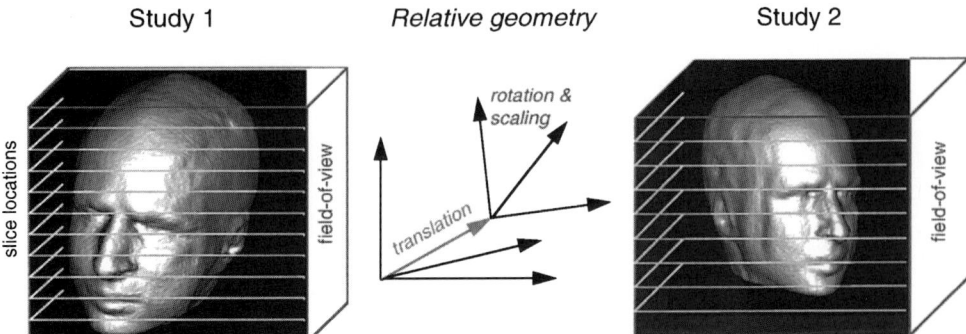

Figure 18. The problem posed in rigid image registration. The same head is imaged in two different acquisitions. Its position and orientation within the field of view differ. Therefore, the brain structures in the two image sets share the following relations: The center of the head is dislocated by δ_x, δ_y, δ_z; it is rotated about the angles ϕ, θ, ψ; and the lengths of the pixel edges differ by scale factors s_x, s_y, s_z. While the scale factors are normally known from the acquisition setup, the other six parameters making up the differences in the acquisition geometry must be estimated by an image registration procedure. Then one data set can be transformed into the coordinate space of the other data set and resliced along those slice positions. As a result, the tissue structures in both image sets are aligned. See Color Plate 8.

Registration for Geometric Realignment

Image registration is always required for data sets acquired in different studies because a patient will always be differently positioned, unless very cumbersome and invasive procedures are applied as required for stereotactic applications. Similar (although smaller) dislocations are likely to happen between consecutive acquisitions of one study due to involuntary movements of the patient. In order to set the stage for the ensuing discussion of different registration techniques, let us start with a quick summary of the conceptual models and rating criteria involved.

Overview of Registration and Rating Criteria

A registration procedure that allows one to match two data sets consists of the following steps:

- *Decide on the role of the data sets.* While registration means that both data sets end up aligned in a common coordinate space, it does not mean that both should actually be transformed. Transformations such as rotations involve interpolations that may degrade image quality, especially if the spatial resolution is not isotropic. Therefore, only one data set (the *model*) is transformed, while the other one (the *reference*) is kept fixed.
- *Decide on the type of information to register with.* Registration procedures often do not operate on the full images but rather use a set of derived information features common to the objects represented in the two data sets. Examples are anatomic landmarks or the surface of an organ. However, the pixel values themselves are sometimes also directly used.
- *Define the allowed transformation between the model and the reference.* There are two classes of transformations, namely, *rigid* and *elastic transformations*. Rigid transformations assume that the object's geometry is identical in both acquisitions and that the acquisition is distortion-free. In this case, the transformation sought consists of a 3D displacement (three parameters) and a 3D rotation (another two parameters). Differences in the size of the pixel edges are accounted for by three scaling factors. A rigid transformation is therefore determined by eight parameters, yet the scaling factors are known from the acquisition setups in many cases.

- *Define the "goodness-of-match" criterion.* For an automatic registration method, the goodness of the alignment after a candidate transform must be measurable. Only then can the transform parameters be found that provide the best match between the reference features and the transformed model features.
- *Collect the information features selected for registration if features other than the pixel intensities are used.* In this preprocessing step user interaction may be required, for instance, to point out corresponding anatomic landmarks or to guide segmentation procedures.
- *Perform the optimization.* Apart from the purely interactive registration, the technique usable for optimization depends on the selected information features, the transformation, and the matching criterion. Often iterative schemes are employed whereby the transformation parameters are systematically varied, driven by the matching criterion. The iteration is stopped when no better match within a certain accuracy can be found. One problem with these algorithms is that they can get stuck locally and miss the global optimum. For some formulations of the matching problem, closed-form solutions exist.

This outline suggests that a registration method can be characterized by six entities that describe its way of operation. With respect to a clinical application, however, there are some further relevant criteria of a registration method:

- *Prior requirements and retrospective registration.* The question is, to what extent does the registration method depend on special setups of the acquisitions? Examples are patient fixation techniques or the placement of external landmarks visible in the images. Further requirements might be related to image contrast and resolution or to the extent of organ coverage. If there are no such requirements, image data sets from previous studies or acquired at remote institutions can be matched anytime with newly generated images. It is clear that this ability of retrospective registration is very helpful in a clinical environment.
- *Reproducibility and automation.* Fully automatic registration techniques are highly desirable. Besides comfort, they also offer operator independence and hence exact reproducibility. On the other hand, it has to be ensured that the automatically found registrations are reasonable. In general, therefore, the input data for fully automatic methods cannot be acquired arbitrarily but must obey strict quality criteria.
- *Similarity of the modalities to be registered.* Image registration is easiest for images acquired with one protocol on a similar scanner because the same information is shown with like resolution. If these conditions are not fulfilled, registration becomes more difficult. Differences in resolution may not be a severe obstacle within certain limits. More difficult is the case frequently met when comparing functional and anatomic images where the tissue parameters shown have distinct distributions.
- *Preprocessing steps.* The importance of the preprocessing steps analyzed previously must be emphasized. Except for the image acquisition, here is the point where work must be done during a registration. The quality of preprocessing decides on the success of the registration. If, for instance, the segmentation of an organ yields a poor organ surface, little can be expected from a registration process trying to match such surfaces between model and reference.

In the rest of this section some widely used registration techniques are discussed (Table 1). We begin with rigid registrations and end with an elastic transformation that is frequently applied to transform functional patient data into the normalized coordinate space of the stereotactic Talairach atlas (24). For a more thorough review, the reader is referred to a recent review by A. C. Evans (4).

Interactive Registration

Interactive registration fully relies on the pattern-matching capabilities of a trained human professional, which is hard to surpass. Such a registration tool supports the cli-

Table 1. *Characteristics of rigid registration techniques*

	Interactive	Internal landmarks	Surface matching	AIR
Information	Visual features	Anatomic points	Organ surface	Pixel value
Transformation	Rigid	Rigid	Rigid	Rigid
Criterion	Subjective match	Distances between point pairs	Distances between surfaces	Variance of image
Preprocessing	None	Interactively define points	Surface segmentation	No
Optimization	None	Iterative	Iterative	Iterative
Retrospective	Yes	Yes	Yes	Yes
Reproducibility	Low	Low	High	High
Multimodality	Yes	Yes	Yes	After segmentation
Reported accuracy	0.6–2.2 mm	2–3 mm	0.7–2.5 mm	1.7 mm

nician in two ways. One is that it allows one to specify trial transformation parameters and calculates the transformed model data set. The other one is that it offers some presentation of the reference and the transformed model, which helps to judge the goodness of the match. An example is illustrated in Fig. 19 (see also Color Plate 9) using a tool developed by Pietrzyk et al. (21). A rigid transformation is assumed. The translation and rotation parameters can be specified using buttons of the user interface, while the scaling factors are taken from the acquisition setup. Three orthogonal slices of both data sets are shown in parallel. Once the match is completed, they will show corresponding slices. Assessment of the match is facilitated by exchanged contours that can be generated most easily using threshold values. The user incrementally modifies the transformation until the PET contours exactly follow the MRI structures, and vice versa.

The only prerequisite for interactive registration is a trained user understanding the anatomy and the characteristics of the two modalities and sufficient common features in the two studies. Retrospective and multimodality registration is thus possible. According to the procedure, there is some subjectivity in the resulting match. However, systematic studies of intra- and interobserver variability (21) have shown that its influence is not significant if a standard processing protocol is followed. The authors concluded that the

MRI: "Reference"

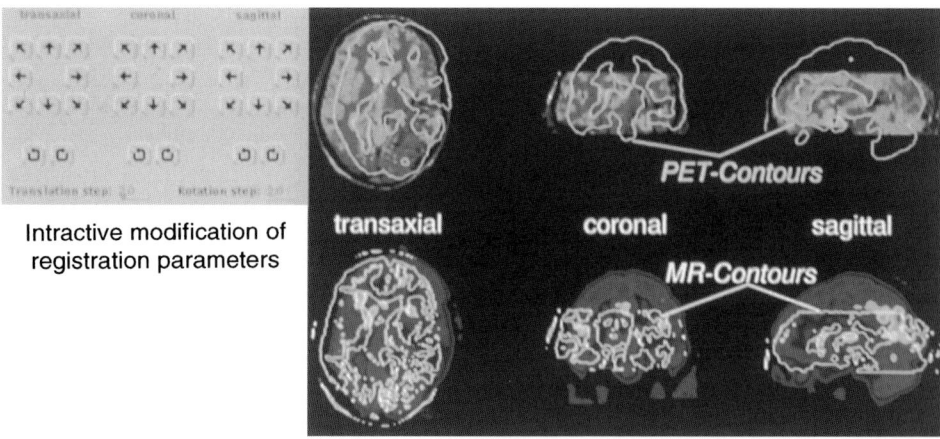

Intractive modification of registration parameters

¹⁸FDG PET: Resliced "model"

Figure 19. Purely manual image registration by an experienced user. Button presses update the transformation parameters and trigger reslicing of the model study. The exchanged contours allow one to evaluate the match visually. The user shifts and rotates the model volume until he or she is satisfied with the alignment. See Color Plate 9.

reproducibility and accuracy are comparable or better than those of published automatic registrations or fixation systems such as head holders or face masks in a large variety of registration situations.

Landmark-Based Registration

The information features used in landmark-based registration are homologous point pairs. Such a point pair identifies the same spatial location in both data sets. In order to calculate the registration parameters, a whole set of point pairs is needed. Thus the two image sets are reduced to two spatial arrangements of points, the reference and model points, which must be brought into optimal agreement. We assume here that the transformation performing this alignment is rigid, but this is not mandatory, and approaches with elastic transformations also have been described. The criterion for the match is some norm based on the distance between the model points and the corresponding reference points after transformation. Usually the sum of the squared distances is minimized by an iterative algorithm.

In general, the point pairs are obtained in an interactive preprocessing step. A trained user repetitively explores the two image sets and in each repetition tries to locate a point in both of them. This assignment happens in three dimensions and is therefore quite difficult to perform. Consequently, the point locations are specified with a measurement error s that has an impact on the registration accuracy. It is clear that the number N of point pairs used also affects the accuracy, since measurement errors tend to cancel themselves out on average. These issues have been investigated by Evans et al. (4, 5). They found that the registration accuracy is proportional to $s/\sqrt{N}$ and proposed to use about 10 to 20 point pairs. Since the quoted measurement error is in the range of 5 to 15 mm, a registration accuracy of 2 to 3 mm thus can be expected.

The interactive definition of the point pairs is crucial for this registration method. The user must therefore be supported by powerful visualization tools to efficiently browse through the image volume. With dedicated systems, 10 to 20 point pairs can be specified in about 15 to 20 minutes. Retrospective and multimodality registration is thus possible provided that enough anatomic landmarks can be located in the two studies. If one of the studies has poor anatomic information, one can resort to preplanned acquisitions with external landmarks. These are devices that are attached to the patient during both studies and which contain material visible in the acquired images. They show up as fiducial structures in the images and can be used to define landmarks additional to the anatomic ones.

Surface Matching

The information feature used in this popular registration method is the 3D surface of an object visible in both image sets. A rigid matching transform is assumed and estimated together with the scaling factors (20). The criterion to measure the goodness of match can be illustrated by the "hat over head" metaphor in Fig. 20: The surface from the modality with higher resolution usually takes the role of the "head." The other, the "hat," is considered to consist of points. For each of the "hat" points the residual is defined as the distance between the point and the "head" surface along the direction of the "head" centroid. The sum of all squared residuals yields the criterion that is minimized to find the optimal match. During an iterative optimization procedure, the transformation parameters are varied until the residual criterion of the transformed "hat" points is minimal.

As with most other techniques, this registration is mostly applied in the head, using the outer skull or the brain surface. The required contour lines are relatively easy to segment in most modalities without the interaction of a trained user. In PET, the transmission images are more adequate for segmentation than the emission images. Retrospective and multimodality registration is possible provided that a common object can be located in the two studies. It should be pointed out that the technique does not require

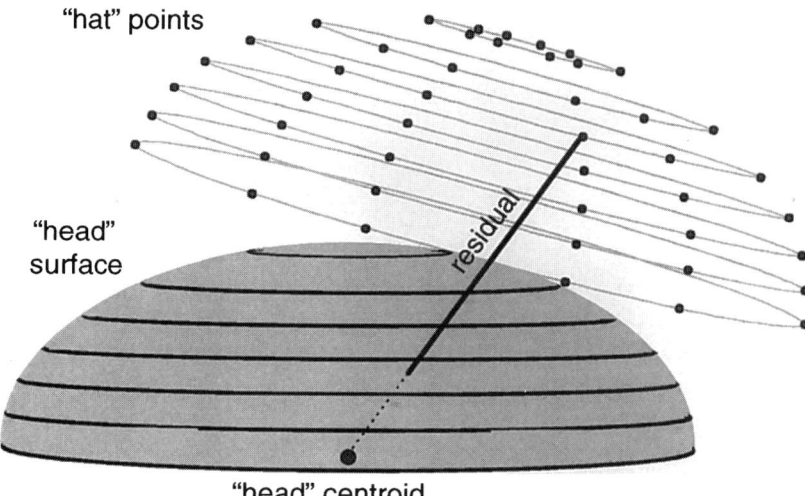

"hat" points

"head"
surface

residual

"head" centroid

Figure 20. Illustration of registration by matching the surface of an organ visible in both studies. The lower-resolution surface is represented by the "hat" points. The "hat" matches the "head" when the sum of the squared residuals is minimal.

the object to be covered to the same extent in both studies. A common part of the surface may be sufficient if there is not too much symmetry that prevents the calculation of a unique solution. The registration accuracy is limited by the lower-resolution pixels' size and slice thickness. In phantom studies, Pelizzari et al. (20) found errors in the range of 0.7 to 2.5 mm for various cross-modality registrations (MRI, CT, PET).

Automatic Image Registration (AIR)

This widely used registration method was introduced by Woods et al. (27) and aimed at PET studies of the brain. As the name suggests, it was developed for fully automatic registration. AIR directly uses the values of all pixels in the image volumes as the information feature. It is based on the assumption that both data sets show the objects very similarly and that they are related by a rigid transformation. To be more specific, the idealized assumption is that the pixel value in each model point equals the value in the corresponding reference pixel multiplied by a global factor F. In practice, the two data sets will differ by noise, sampling effects, and probably physiologic differences. Therefore, the assumption is relaxed to the criterion that the match is optimal if the variance of the ratio transformed model/reference (which has the value F in the ideal case) is minimal. An iterative optimization algorithm is applied that updates one parameter at a time to approach a better match until the further improvements as expected by the derivatives fall below a preset threshold. In the practical implementation, areas outside the head pose a practical difficulty when forming the ratio. Therefore, the ratio is only considered within a masked area obtained by applying an empirical threshold value to the reference data set.

The registration, as described before, is fully automatic. The only input value is the mask threshold, which can be determined empirically once for a certain study type. Retrospective registration is possible with AIR, but cross-modality registration is not directly supported. However, there exists an extension of the technique that makes it suitable for MRI-PET alignment (28). Besides modifications of the criterion that incorporates grouping of pixels with similar behavior in MRI, manual preprocessing of the MRI data is involved to mask out structures not visible in PET. The accuracy as determined in phantom experiments simulating $H_2{}^{15}O$-PET studies is reported as 0.7 mm in Woods, Cherry, and Mazziotta (27). There it is also shown that prior smoothing of the images improves the registration for high noise levels.

Elastic Registration with Talairach Atlas

The basis for this stereotactic normalization is the work of Talairach and Tournoux (24). They set up a proportional system that adapts itself to the proportions of each individual brain. This means that each pixel in a brain image can be mapped into a coordinate of the stereotactic "average" brain, the *brain atlas*. In order to estimate the mapping transform, it is important to localize the line passing through the anterior and posterior commissures (AC–PC line). In PET this has been accomplished by an additional lateral skull radiograph in the first approach (6), but automatic methods have since been developed (9, 18) that estimate the AC–PC line directly from the PET images. After this line has been found and realigned with that of the atlas by rotations and translations, the stereotactic transformation only consists of linear scaling along the three dimensions. While a certain degree of anatomic alignment is ensured by this transform, some regional variations among subjects still remain. When averaging such normalized images of different subjects, the mismatches might cause artefacts. As a remedy, an additional step has been introduced. It minimizes the shape differences of structures in the atlas images (the reference) and in the normalized patient images by applying a nonlinear "plastic" (7) or "warping" transformation (17). The implementations of stereotactic normalization differ in the information feature they use for estimating the plastic deformation. While Friston et al. (7) use the pixel values themselves, landmarks are employed by Minoshima et al. (17). Consequently, they also apply different matching criteria. Stereotactic normalization is most commonly applied within a modality, whereby the atlas images serving as a reference and the actual images to normalize share similar features. In this case the differences are primarily due to the brain shapes and only to a lesser extent caused by variations in pixel intensity. The methods referred to above are fully automatic and can operate retrospectively.

A typical domain of stereotactic normalization is in stimulation experiments. There the provoked signal changes are often too small to be reliably assessed by few acquisitions. Study data from several subjects must therefore be pooled for a single analysis in modalities such as PET where experiments cannot arbitrarily often be repeated. Hence all the images are first normalized and then subjected to statistical analysis. The results can then be reported directly in stereotactic coordinates.

Fusion Techniques for Correlative Image Interpretation

Once the parameters of the geometric transform between two data sets have been estimated by a registration procedure, either of them can be transformed into the coordinate space of the other. There are 2D and 3D methods for the subsequent task of image interpretation. Currently, the 2D approaches are much more widespread. They reslice the transformed model according to the slices of the reference study. The organ structures in the obtained images are now aligned with those in the reference study. Corresponding slices therefore can be arranged side by side and visually correlated without the need to take geometric distortions into account. Several visualization tools can be employed to improve the objectivity of this comparison (12, 21). The previously discussed "linked cursor" simultaneously marks the same anatomic location in both data sets and allows transfer of regions of interest from one study into the other. Although simple, the linked cursor supports rapid and accurate examination of the data. It has proven helpful to parallelly view images wherein the information from both studies is explicitly integrated. Different types of encoding are in use. Figure 21 (see also Color Plate 10) illustrates a straightforward approach where the composed image consists of pixels that are alternately taken from either study. The pixel colors are retained and change with the color table of the original studies. Another approach is to encode the two available pieces of information into different properites of a pixel, such as brightness for the anatomy and chromatinicity for the function. The resulting images show a transparency effect that is visually pleasing but difficult to interpret. Techniques to generate 3D fused displays are reviewed in Evans (4). They generally require further preprocessing steps whereby in-

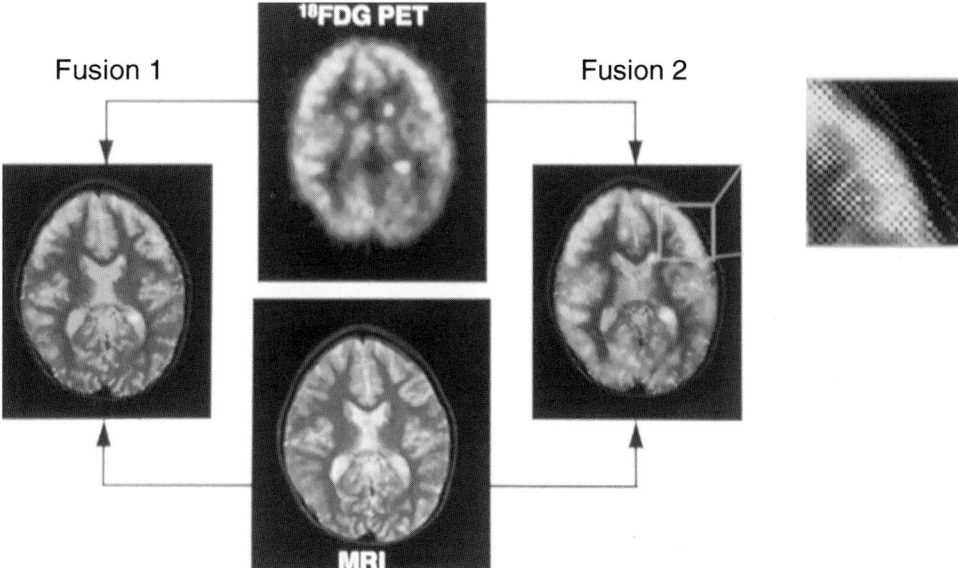

Figure 21. Fused image presentation using alternating pixels. In this example a fused image contains MRI information in gray and PET information in color. The color tables can be modified separately during interactive evaluation. Two of the resulting fused images are shown to the left and the right of the original images. See Color Plate 10.

formation might be discarded or artefacts might be introduced. Furthermore, they are computationally demanding such that interactive examination of the data set is more difficult to attain than with 2D methods.

ANALYSIS OF TIME SERIES OF IMAGE DATA

The acquisition of image sequences covering the same anatomic region of a patient allows the recording and subsequent analysis of time-related changes caused by different things, such as, for example,

- Morphologic changes due to developing pathology, surgical interventions, aging, prosthesis movement
- Image-intensity changes due to injection of contrast agents (as bolus injection for PET or traditional angiography)
- Image-intensity changes caused by physiologic reaction induced by some controlled activity (as in the case of functional MRI acquisitions)

Computerized analysis of image variation resulting from morphologic changes is very difficult and subject of current research. In this section we will concentrate on the analysis of time series restricted only to contrast variations without morphologic distortions of the underlying anatomic scene. Such time series form the basis for pixel-wise modeling as discussed in Chap. 3.

Differential Images

The simplest way to enhance and identify changes between subsequent images is to subtract them. Exactly identical structures will completely disappear from the resulting differential image, providing high contrast in areas of intensity change.

The resulting image enhancement is demonstrated on a digital subtraction angiography (DSA) sequence. The upper row of Fig. 22 shows a part of an acquired image sequence during a contrast agent bolus injection. The lower row shows the images resulting after the subtraction of the first image followed by an appropriate adjustment of the intensity window.

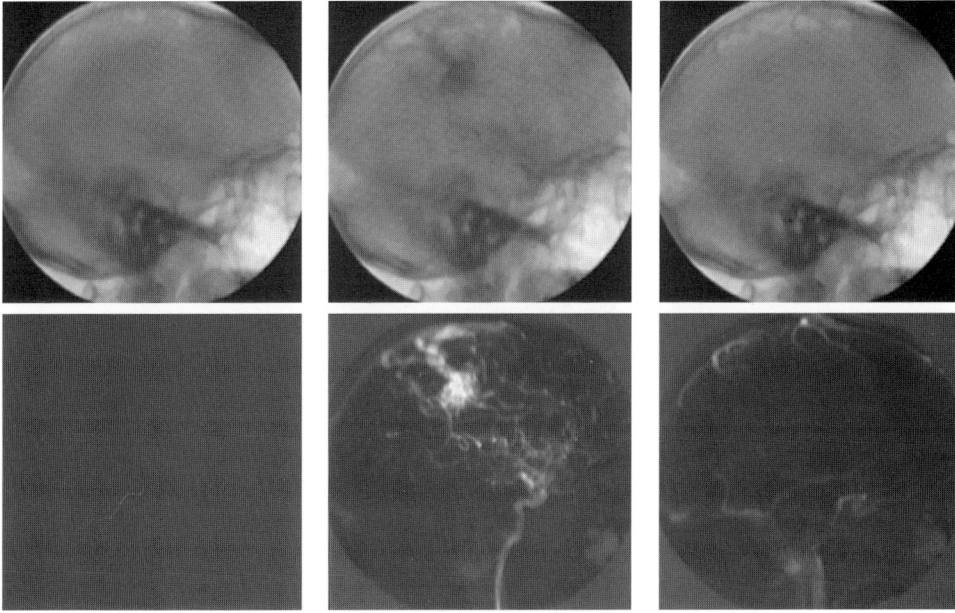

Figure 22. Differential images generated from a digital subtraction angiography (DSA) sequence. The upper row shows the original images; the lower, the result of the subtraction of the image on the left.

As this example demonstrates, image subtraction provides in many cases a simple and efficient way for identification of contrast changes in image sequences. However, one has to realize that two basic requirements have to be satisfied in order to get sufficient data quality for differential analysis:

• The images to be subtracted should reflect exactly the same anatomy. This means not only that no morphologic changes are allowed but also requires that the analyzed images are perfectly registered.
• The signal-to-noise ratio in the analyzed image sequence should be high.

Techniques described in the ''Image Fusion'' section possibly can be used to correct for image misregistration if the first condition is not fulfilled. Low signal-to-noise ratio, however, causes a major difficulty. Subtraction efficiently amplifies the noise present in the single images, which can lead to complete dominance of noise over the already weak signal. Figure 23 (see also Color Plate 11) shows the result of the subtraction of two functional MRI images of the brain. Figure 23A shows an acquisition without activation; this is the same slice acquired during visual stimulation. The signal change due to activation is completely lost in the very noisy difference image shown in Fig. 23C (color coded in Color Plate 11).

Improvement of the signal-to-noise ratio can be achieved by image-accumulation techniques. Periodic repetition of MRI acquisitions in the resting and activated states allows one to sum up several images of the same activation state leading to selective reduction of noise. The upper row of Fig. 24 (see also Color Plate 12) shows a few images from a complete functional MRI sequence obtained during visual stimulation by a flickering light. The sequence consists of eight periods. Each period contains four images acquired without (Figs. 24A and 24C) and four with stimulation (Figs. 24B and 24D). The result of the evaluation is shown by the lower row, where Fig. 24E shows the average of the resting and Fig. 24F shows the average of activated images. The result of subtraction is shown in Figs. 24G (in gray-scale) and 24H (to be compared with Fig. 23C. (See also Color Plates 11 and 12.)

Similarity of Time Sequences: Correlation

In many cases the measured signal is too weak to be enhanced by noise reduction through data accumulation. Figure 25 (see Color Plate 13) illustrates the result of the

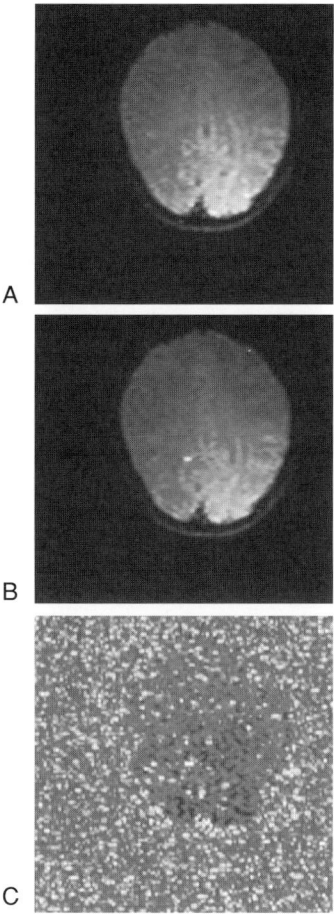

Figure 23. The result of direct subtraction of functional MRI images. Images **A** and **B** show the acquired images without and with visual stimulation. The result of the subtraction is shown on image **C** (growing from blue—negative—to red—positive—values). See Color Plate 11.

same procedure as shown in Fig. 24 on a different data set with less pronounced signal enhancement due to visual activation. In this case, more sensitive procedures are required for reliable extraction of activated regions from the acquired image sequences.

Periodic activation studies, as already used for the generation of accumulated images, provide a promising possibility for more advanced data evaluation for the study of the time behavior of single pixels of a 2D image slice. The acquired data can be regarded as a 3D data array with two spatial dimensions and one time dimension. This data cube can then be reformatted along the time axis, resulting in a 2D array of time-evolving functions, as illustrated in Fig. 26.

Figure 27 shows such reformatted functions obtained from the experiment in Fig. 24 extracted on a pixel position showing the activation clearly (A) and another (B) without response to the stimulus (C). The basic idea of correlation-based analysis is to search for pixels showing similar time behavior.

Searching for similar behavior of time sequences requires the definition of a measure allowing the quantification of similarity between 1D time functions. Calculation based on deviation of signal intensities at the same time position is a natural way to express distance between functions that has to be as small as possible. Figure 28 illustrates, however, how inappropriate this measure is to express similarity in the time behavior of signals. The upper sinusoidal activation signal (a) behaves identical to the lower one

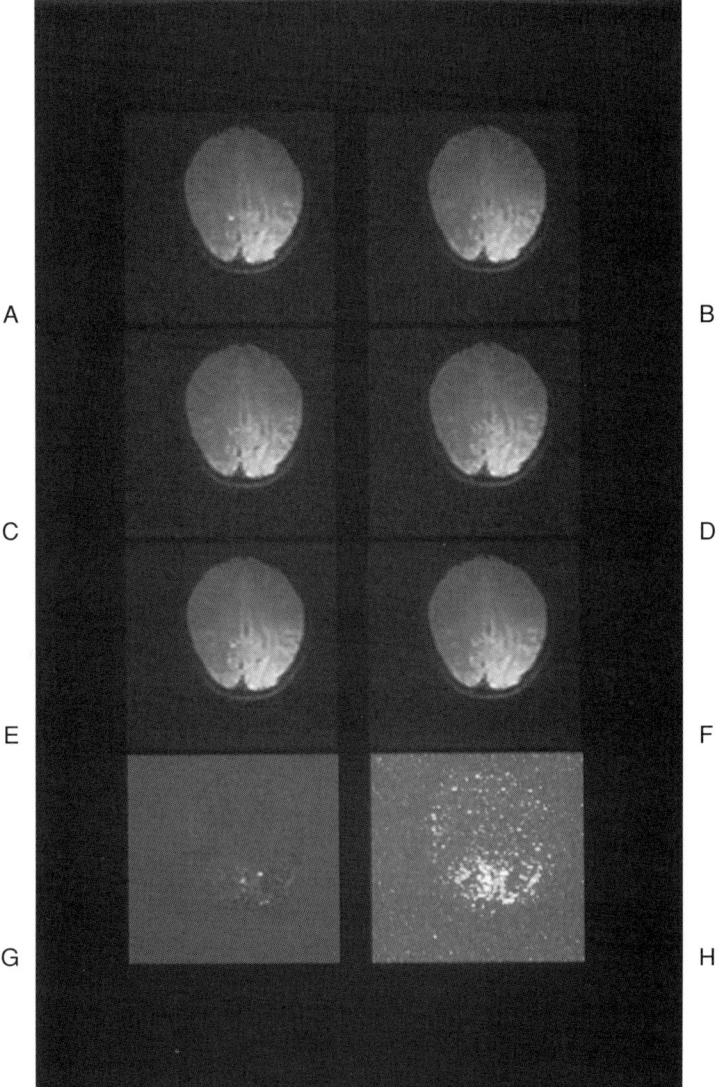

Figure 24. Example of a functional MRI acquisition (**(A–F)**) and the result of its evaluation by subtraction of accumulated images (**G–H**). See Color Plate 12.

passing through the origin (b). At the same time its distance to the straight line (showing no activation at all) (c) is much less. The example demonstrates clearly that we are looking for a measure reflecting parallel changes in signals instead of emphasizing their deviation.

Correlation between time series is one widely used possibility to express such coupled changes in the signals under investigation. The correlation coefficient is in principle calculated as the normed sum of the multiplied signal values (for a formal definition, see the following box). It varies between -1 and 1, where the value 1 expresses perfectly parallel, -1 perfectly antiparallel behavior of signals. Value 0 indicates that no similarity between signal behavior can be found. The correlation coefficient between the (a) and (b) signals is 1, while between (a) and (c) it is 0, showing exactly the desired behavior. One should, however, be warned that our understanding of signal similarity is too complex to be expressed completely by the correlation coefficient. One example is its extreme sensitivity to phase shifts. The calculated correlation coefficient between the signals (b) and its shifted version (d) in Fig. 28 is also 0 clearly demonstrating the limitations to be expected when using correlation in activation analysis.

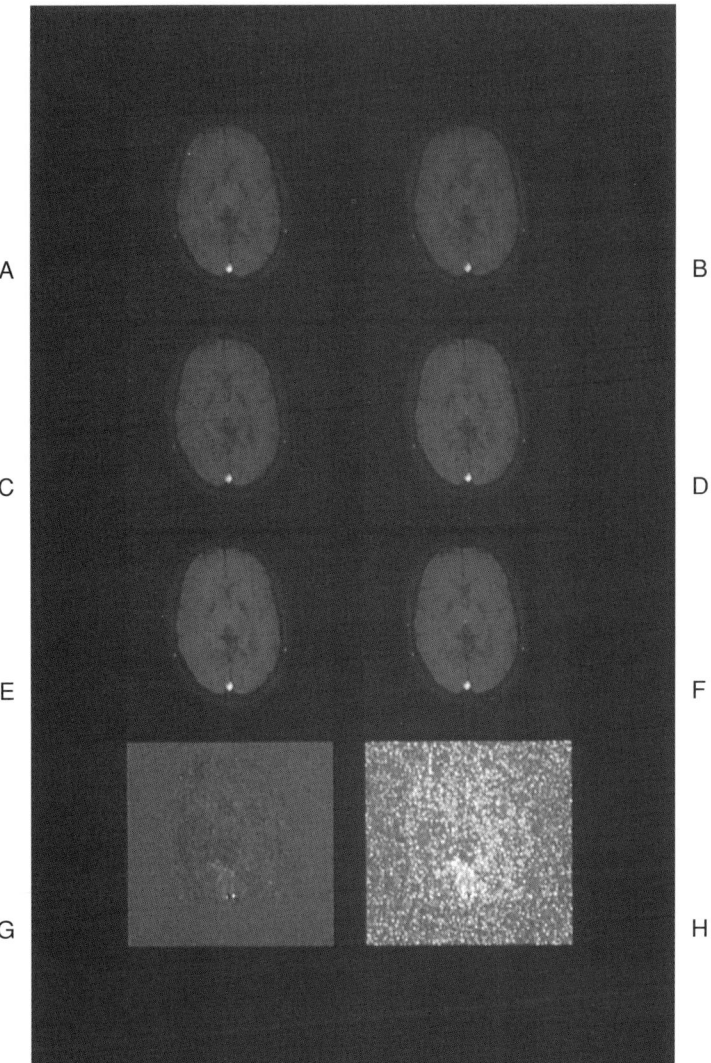

Figure 25. Example of another functional MRI acquisition (**A–F**) and the result of its evaluation by subtraction of accumulated images (**G–H**). For this sequence, data accumulation does not provide a satisfactory solution for the detection of activated brain regions. See Color Plate 13.

COMPARISON OF DISCRETE TIME SERIES (CORRELATION AND DEVIATION)

Let $\{f[t_i] \mid i = 1, \ldots n\} = f[t_1], f[t_2], \ldots, f[t_n]$

and $\{g[t_i] \mid i = 1, \ldots n\} = g[t_1], g[t_2], \ldots, g[t_n]$

be two discrete time series. If

$$\hat{f} = \frac{\sum_{i=1}^{n} f[t_i]}{n} \quad \text{and} \quad \hat{g} = \frac{\sum_{i=1}^{n} g[t_i]}{n}$$

denote the average of the signal values, the correlation coefficient is defined as

$$C_{[f,g]} = \frac{\sum_{i=1}^{n} (f[t_i] - \hat{f})(g[t_i] - \hat{g})}{\sqrt{\left[\sum_{i=1}^{n} (f[t_i] - \hat{f})^2\right]\left[\sum_{i=1}^{n} (g[t_i] - \hat{g})^2\right]}}$$

signal intensity

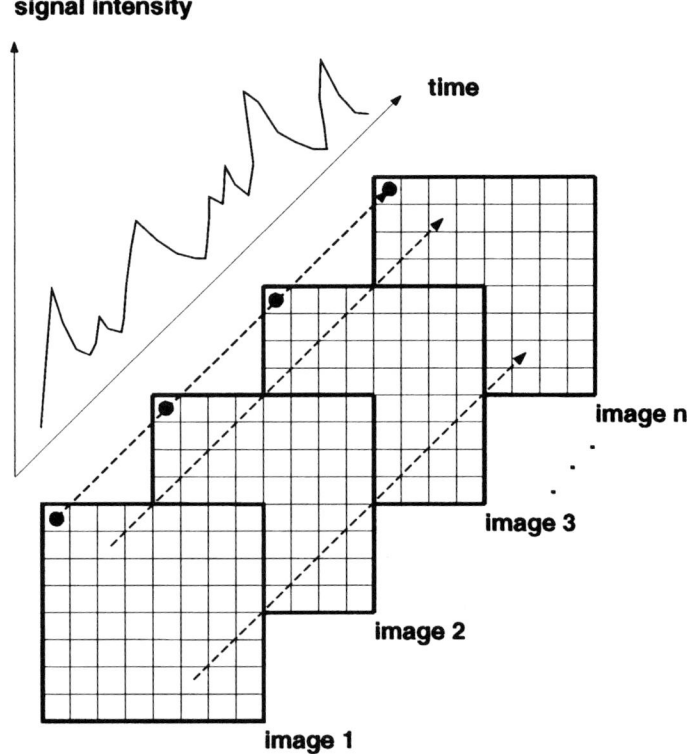

Figure 26. Reformatting a functional MRI acquisition into a matrix of 1D time functions.

The sequences $(f[t_1], f[t_2], \ldots, f[t_n])$ and $(g[t_1], g[t_2], \ldots, g[t_n])$ can be seen as vectors in an n-dimensional euclidean vector space using the measured function values as coordinates. The two similarity measures between them discussed above can be well visualized in terms of linear vector spaces, as illustrated in the following figure for two dimensions ($n = 2$). The similarity based on the deviation of the measurement values is

$$D_{[f,g]} = \sqrt{\sum_{i=1}^{n} (F[t_i] - G[t_i])^2}$$

nothing else than the length of the difference between the zero-mean vectors $\vec{F}$ and $\vec{G}$, while the correlation coefficient as defined above is the angle between them.

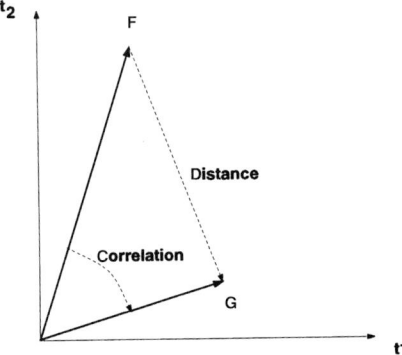

Similarity measures between the vectors $\vec{f}$ and $\vec{g}$.

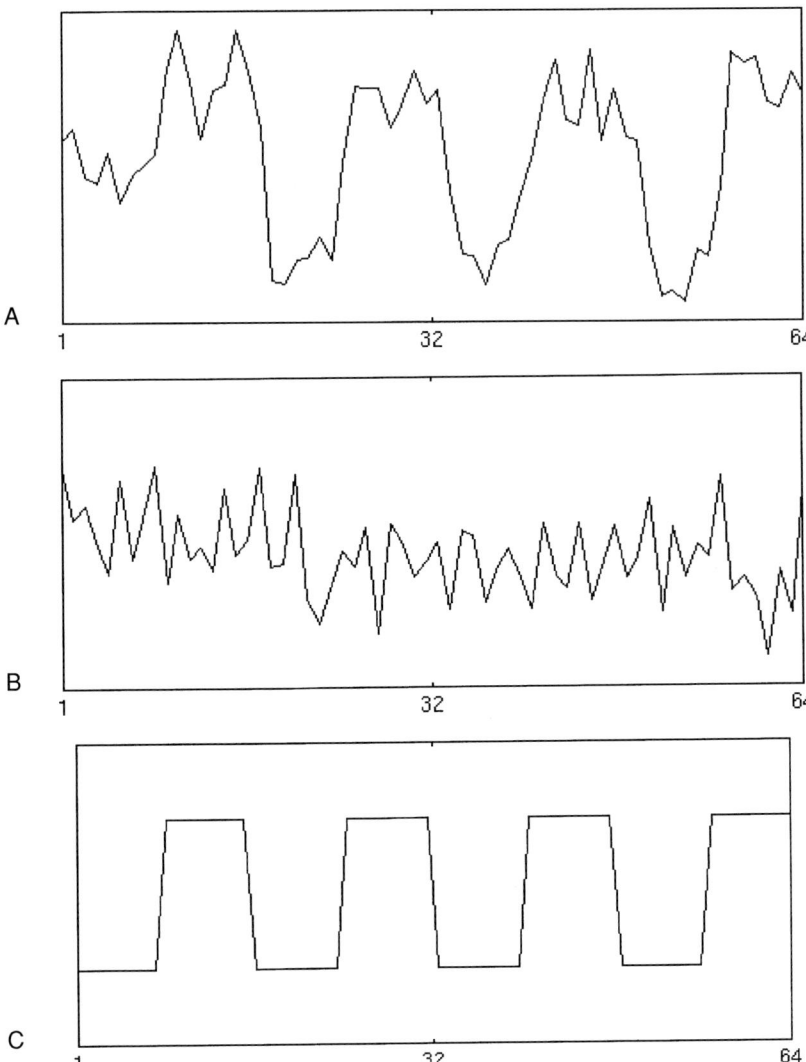

Figure 27. Time response to a visual stimulus shown in **C.** Figures **A** and **B** display the response of pixels with and without activation, respectively.

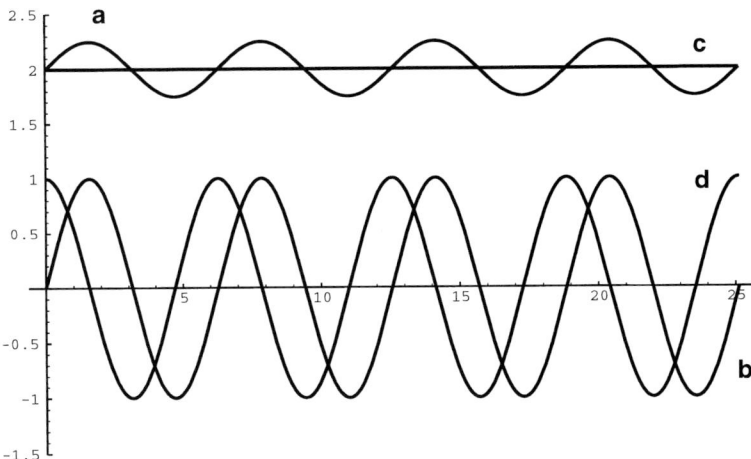

Figure 28. Similarity between different synthetic time series.

Correlation-Based Activation Analysis

Application of correlation-based techniques for the identification of active regions in functional image sequences requires a *reference signal* that will be used for the comparison with the measured time function at each pixel position. The proposed methods for correlation analysis differ in the way this reference signal is selected. The major alternatives investigated in the literature are the following:

- The simplest way to define the reference signal is use of the time function of the stimulation in the experiment. For periodic alternation of stimulated and rest phases, this function usually looks like the one presented in Fig. 27C.
- Bandettini et al. (2) proposed to select one pixel from the measured data and use this as a reference. In this case, areas in the functional image will be identified that show similar behavior to this manually selected pixel. This method can be used for the refinement of unsatisfactory activation maps resulting from the subtraction of accumulated images. Pixels clearly showing activation in this preliminary evaluation can then be selected as reference for correlation-based analysis. The method can be made more robust by selecting several pixels (image areas) showing activation, calculating the average of the selected time functions, and using it as a reference. The advantage of this method is that no a priori assumptions about the physiologic response to the stimulus have to be taken. At the same time, the somewhat arbitrary selection of reference data may lead to unstable results.
- The use of the stimulus function as reference signal relies on the implicit assumption that the physiologic response to this stimulus is immediate without any distortion. It is clear that this cannot be true under any realistic measurement circumstances. Consequently, Friston et al. (8) proposed using some a priori knowledge about the hemodynamic response to the neuronal activation in functional MRI sequences. The stimulus function can then be modulated by this physiological response function and used as reference for activation analysis.

Advanced Signal Analysis for Detection of Activation

During the past few years, a lot of different signal analysis techniques have been proposed and investigated in the literature to achieve optimal performance in the calculation of activation maps. While a detailed overview of these methods is beyond the scope of this chapter, the following list provides a selection of some techniques that have been applied with some success to functional data:

- The correlation-based analysis used the underlying assumption that the activated pixels show a rise and fall of intensity parallel to the activation. This requirement can be weakened by only requiring that the response signal shows the same frequency behavior as the stimulus function. In this way the notorious sensitivity of the correlation coefficient to phase changes (which, in general, should be expected because of the hemodynamic response developed in relation to the activation stimulus) can be overcome. Methods using this assumption perform signal analysis in the frequency space (the Fourier transform of the time sequences) and search for signals containing high energy in a band around the stimulation frequency or investigating the autocorrelation function of the response (the correlation of the signal with its phase-shifted copies).

• If the similarity of time series can be reasonably measured by the sum of their deviation at every point (i.e., their distance), principal component analysis provides a statistical method for the identification of clusters of similarly behaving pixels in the image. The basic idea of the method is to regard every time series as a vector in the n-dimensional Euclidean space and search for directions of maximal spatial variation. If similarly behaving pixels form tight, well-separated clusters, the identified directions of large variations, the *principal components* should correspond to the influence of activation over the random noise. A clear advantage of this method is that it is completely automatic and provides results *without any a priori assumptions* about the activation process. This fact, however, also restricts the specificity of the procedure. Together with the questionable basic assumption (relying on distance instead of correlation), it poses serious limitations for the applicability of this method.

Figure 29 (see also Color Plate 14) provides a comparison of results by some of the methods analyzed above on the two different data sets shown in Fig. 24 (see also Color Plate 12) and Fig. 25 (see also Color Plate 13). Evaluation results are shown for subtraction of accumulated images (Fig. 29A, E), for correlation analysis using reference

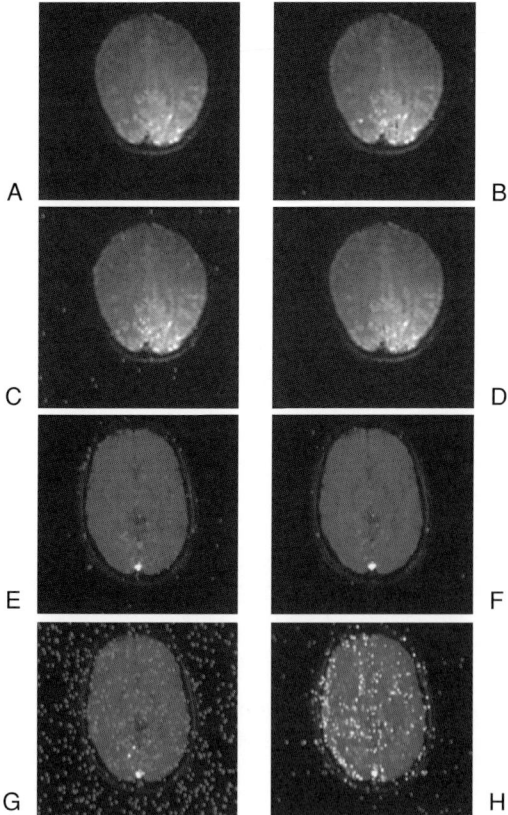

Figure 29. Evaluation results on the two previously presented functional MRI data sets. The activation map generated by subtraction (**A, E**), correlation analysis (**B, F**), bandpass filtering (**C, G**), and principal component analysis (**D, H**) were thresholded and overlayed as a color-coded activation map onto the acquired images. See Color Plate 14.

pixels (Fig. 29B, F), for bandpass filtering around the stimulation frequency (Fig. 29C, G), and for principal component analysis (Fig. 29D, H). The thresholded activation maps are overlayed in color (activation growing from blue to red) onto the gray-valued anatomic images in Color Plate 14.

Postprocessing of Activation Maps

The methods of time series analysis provide results in form of activation maps. Instead of the original intensity values, every pixel represents the strength of the activation estimated by the applied procedure.

Activated regions are generally identified from those maps by using some manually selected threshold value. Due to the usually low signal-to-noise ratio, the selection of this threshold is not obvious, and inappropriate selection could lead to a questionable result.

One has to realize that up to this point all pixels of the acquired data volume were handled totally independently, and no information has been used about their relative spatial position. It is usually assumed, however, that activation is not independent between neighboring pixels but highly correlated between pixels not too far away. This spatial coherence of the response to the stimulus can be used to reduce the effects of noise on the resulting activated regions. Two different procedures are used for this purpose:

* Smoothing of the activation map before thresholding by some selected filter. Gaussian filtering is applied in most of the cases.
* Thresholding can be performed in two stages to allow the selection of relatively low threshold values without generating small isolated regions resulting purely from weaker noise pixels (hystheresis thresholding). The image is thresholded with two different values. Pixels above the higher threshold value (category 1) are regarded as the surely activated ones and will be kept, while pixels below the lower threshold (category 2) are categorized as noise and will be left out. Pixels having activity values between the higher and lower thresholds (category 3) are possible candidates for detecting activations but will only be taken into account if they are connected to a pixel belonging to category 1. In this way, questionable pixels in category 3 can be left out if they are isolated without making connected activation regions smaller.

Figure 30 (see also Color Plate 15) illustrates the effect of applying postprocessing techniques as simple thresholding (Fig. 30A, D, thresholding after Gaussian smoothing (Fig. 30B, E), or hystheresis thresholding (Fig. 30C, F) to an activation map resulting from subtraction of accumulated images.

VALIDATION

From the description of the segmentation scheme so far, we could only conclude that it is possible to segment anatomic and functional objects. The fact that the segmentation methodology works routinely may lead to the incorrect conclusion that the segmentation is *reliable and accurate.* The characterization of the performance of the algorithms in terms of reliability and accuracy, however, needs the development of objective and quantitative methods evaluating these criteria after designing a statistical error-analysis technique.

Several articles (14, 15, 25) carefully discussed the validation of volumetric results as well as the reliability of segmentation schemes operated by different observers. These results are very important to demonstrate the potential benefit of computer-assisted postprocessing of medical image data to the medical community.

As illustrated by Kohn et al. (15), segmentation methods that give adequate qualitative results may not give satisfactory quantitative information. This statement was accompanied by an illustrative example demonstrating that a large variation of the threshold to

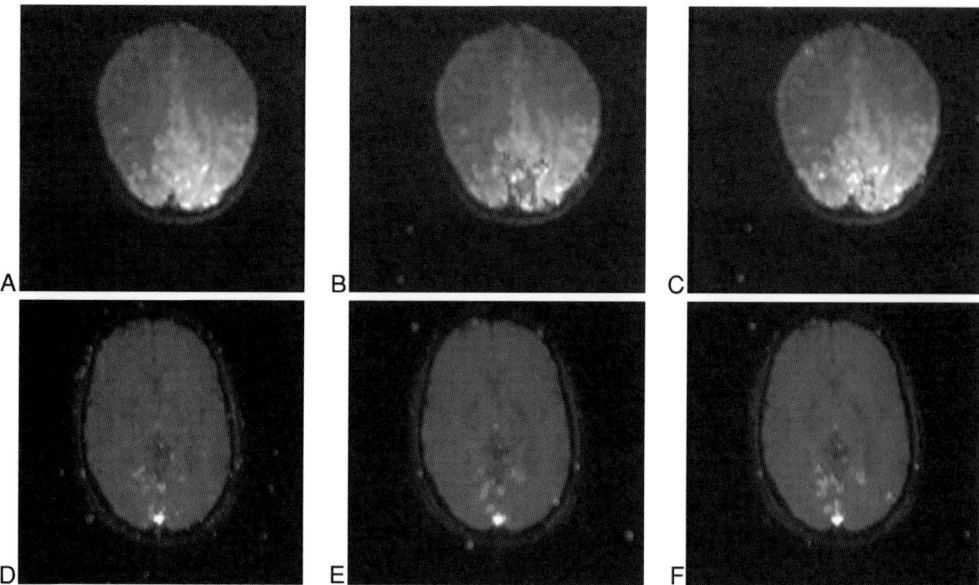

Figure 30. Effects of postprocessing on the two previously presented functional MRI data sets. The overlayed activation map is shown for simple thresholding, thresholding of the Gaussian blurted activation map, and hystheresis thresholding (*left* to *right*). See Color Plate 15.

segment brain tissue from cerebrospinal fluid (leading to a decrease of the volume by 25%) resulted in a barely perceptible difference in the appearance of the brain surface.

The scientific method of evaluating the performance includes the formulation and the objective evaluation of a hypothesis. The hypothesis is strongly related to the goal of the analysis, e.g., quantifying the deviation between the result of a segmentation algorithm and the real pathology or identifying significant changes when comparing data sets.

Two main aspects of the evaluation and validation of image analysis algorithms have to be analyzed, reproducibility and accuracy.

- *Reproducibility* characterizes deviations of results in repeated experiments and/or evaluations. The reproducibility of the segmentation process of the ''objects'' from the MRI data, including intra- and interoperator variability, has to be tested to analyze variations of the data-acquisition process and of the user interaction. The random and the systematic errors have to be propagated through the sequence of algorithms to find the standard deviation (SD) of the output. The analysis of the experimental results will be a quantitative statistical measure of confidence in the values obtained.
- *Accuracy* measures deviations of results of the image-acquisition and evaluation process from the reality, e.g., the investigated anatomy or pathology of the patient (the ''ground truth''). The output of the algorithm with its error bounds must be calculated and compared with this ground truth. If one formulates the hypothesis that the segmentation approach performs well in extracting an organ, a reference describing the ''truth'' has to be available. This hypothesis is evaluated objectively on the basis of the experimental results. The statistical confidence interval decides as to the acceptance of the hypothesis and determines whether the segmentation result is consistent with ground truth.

Whereas for numerical data, error-analysis and hypothesis-testing procedures are standard tools, the transfer of the statistical concept to image-analysis procedures is not straightforward and poses many difficult questions such as

- How can one describe the result of a segmentation experiment if *the result is not a numerical quantitative value but a complex image structure* (e.g., a boundary map)?
- How close are different experiments, or how are variations among them defined?

• How does one introduce costs or penalties of a wrong decision (or a decision that is partially wrong across a segmented object)?

In image segmentation, results are often evaluated subjectively because of a lack of ground truth. The estimation of a possible ground truth is often left to the imaginative vision of the reader of an article. The comparison of expectation and observation, however, is impossible without knowing what the correct result should be requiring carefully designed validation studies.

REFERENCES

1. Ballard DH, Brown CM. *Computer vision.* Englewood Cliffs, NJ: Prentice-Hall (1982).
2. Bandettini PA, Jesmanowicz A, Wong EC, Hyde JS. Processing strategies for time-course data sets in functional MRI of the human brain. *Magn Reson Med,* 30, 161–173 (1992).
3. Canny JF. A computational approach to edge detection. *IEEE Trans Pattern Anal Machine Intelligence,* 8(6), 679–698 (1986).
4. Evans AC. Correlative imaging. In: HN Wagner, Z Szabo, JW Buchanan (Eds.). *Principles of nuclear medicine.* Philadelphia: Saunders (1995).
5. Evans AC, Marrett S, Torrescorzo J et al. MRI-PET correlation in three dimensions using a volume-of-interest (VOI) atlas. *J Cereb Blood Flow Metab,* 11(2), 78 (1991).
6. Fox JS, Perlmutter PT, Raichle ME. A stereotactic method of anatomical localization for positron emission tomography. *J Comput Assist Tomogr,* 9(1), 141–153 (1985).
7. Friston KJ, Frith CD, Liddle PF, Frackowiak RS. Plastic transformation of PET images. *J Comput Assist Tomogr,* 15(4), 634–639 (1991).
8. Friston KJ, Jezzard P, Turner R. Analysis of functional MRI time-series. *Hum Brain Mapping,* 1, 153–171 (1994).
9. Friston KJ, Passingham RE, Nutt JG et al. Localisation in PET images: Direct fitting of the intercommissural (AC-PC) line. *J Cereb Blood Flow Metab,* 9(5), 690–695 (1989).
10. Fullerton GD, Lancaster JL. Radiology in the year 2000: Achievement, progress and potential. *Radiology,* 173(P), 47–48 (1989).
11. Gerig G, Kübler O, Kikinis R, Jolesz FA. Nonlinear anisotropic filtering of MRI data. *IEEE Trans Med Imaging,* 11(2), 221–232 (1992).
12. Hawkes JD, Hill D, Lehmann ED et al. Preliminary work on the interpretation of SPECT images with the aid of registered MR images and an MR derived 3D neuro-anatomical atlas. In: *NATO ASI* New York: Springer Verlag (1993).
13. Kessler ML, Pitluck S, Petti P, Castro JR. Integration of multimodality imaging data for radiotherapy treatment planning. *Int J Radiat Oncol Biol Phys,* 21(6), 1653–1667 (1991).
14. Kikinis R, Shenton ME, Gerig G et al. Routine quantitative analysis of brain and cerebrospinal fluid spaces with MR imaging. *J Magn Reson Imaging,* 2(6), 619–629 (1992).
15. Kohn MI, Tanna NK, Herman GT et al. Analysis of brain and cerebrospinal fluid volumes with MR imaging: Part I. Methods, reliability, and validation. *Radiology,* 178, 115–122 (1991).
16. Kuhn M, Gerristen FA, Ayerdi I et al. COVIRA: Multimodality medical image analysis for diagnosis and treatment planning: COmputer VIsion in RAdiology. In: MJ Ladeira, MF Laires, JP Christensen (Eds.). *Studies in health technology and informatics,* Vol. 24, 138–160. Amsterdam: IOS Press (1995).
17. Minoshima S, Koeppe RA, Frey KA, Kuhl DE. Anatomic standardization: Linear scaling and nonlinear warping of functional brain images. *J Nucl Med,* 35(9), 1528–1537 (1994).
18. Minoshima S, Koeppe RA, Mintun MA et al. Automated detection of the intercommissural line for stereotactic localization of functional brain images. *J Nucl Med,* 34(2), 322–329 (1993).
19. Pavlidis T, Loiw Y-T. Integrating region growing and edge detection. *IEEE Trans Pattern Anal Machine Intelligence,* 12(3), 225–233 (1990).
20. Pelizzari CA, Chen GT, Spelbring DR et al. Accurate three-dimensional registration of CT, PET, and/or MR images of the brain. *J Comput Assist Tomogr,* 13(1), 20–26 (1989).
21. Pietrzyk U, Herholz K, Fink G et al. An interactive technique for three-dimensional image registration: Validation for PET, SPECT, MRI and CT brain studies. *J Nucl Med,* 35(12), 2011–2018 (1994).
22. Robb RA. A software system for interactive and qualitative analysis of biomedical images. In: SM Pizer, KH Höhne, H Fuchs (Eds.). *3D Imaging in medicine,* New York: Springer Verlag Vol. F60 *NATO ASI,* 333–361 (1990).
23. Stiehl SH. 3D image understanding in radiology. *IEEE Eng Med Biol* [Special Issue], 9(4), 24–28 (1990).
24. Talairach J, Tournoux P. *C-planar stereotaxic atlas of the human brain.* New York: Thieme Medical Publications (1988).
25. Vannier MW. Validation of MRI multispectral tissue classification. *Comp Med Imaging Graphics,* 15(4), (1991).
26. Vehkomäki TS. *Image segmentation by contour grouping: Knowledge based search in attributed proximity graph.* Ph.D. thesis, No. 11211. Zurich: Swiss Federal Institute of Technology (1995).
27. Woods RP, Cherry SR, Mazziotta JC. Rapid automated algorithm for aligning and reslicing PET images. *J Comput Assist Tomogr,* 16(4), 620–633 (1992).
28. Woods RP, Mazziotta JC, Cherry SR. MRI-PET registration with automated algorithm. *J Comput Assist Tomogr,* 17(4), 536–546 (1993).

Functional Imaging, edited by
Gustav von Schulthess and Jürgen Hennig.
Lippincott–Raven Publishers, Philadelphia, © 1998.

5

Gamma Rays: Nuclear Medicine

Cyrill Burger
and Gustav K. von Schulthess

INTRODUCTION

From a historical perspective, the use of gamma rays emitted from radioactive isotopes has been at the basis of the evolution of all functional studies. Radioactive isotopes have properties that make them ideally suited for such studies. They are excellent physiologic "spies" to image human functional processes either as such (in the case of iodine in the thyroid) or bound into biomolecules (in almost all other applications) for five main reasons.

1. In an ideal situation such as ^{131}I or ^{123}I, gamma-ray emitters, and ^{11}C, a positron emitter, the corresponding nonradioactive elements occur normally in biomatter: A perfect "spy" can be synthesized.
2. The effect to be measured (one or two gamma rays) stems from a nuclear reaction not involving the electrons: There is no interference with the biochemical properties of the "spy" in use, and therefore, the detection does not interfere with biochemistry. A "spy" like ^{123}I itself or a biomolecule incorporating ^{11}C is not recognized as foreign by the human body.
3. The background level of radiation within the human body is minimal and due only to a little radioactive potassium and some cesium. Hence there is little signal in the image not coming from the radiopharmaceutical. This is very much in contradistinction to the other imaging modalities, where contrast media always produce an effect on top of some existing signal.

C Burger and GK von Schulthess: Department of Medical Radiology, University Hospital, Zurich, Switzerland.

4. Since radioactivity can be detected with very high sensitivity, the result is that even minute quantities of radioactive "spies" can be detected. Nuclear medicine (NM) techniques therefore are and will likely remain the most sensitive techniques to evaluate biochemical processes in vivo. In particular, they are the only suitable agents to detect what we termed *low-concentration, high-affinity receptors* (see Chap. 2).

5. Related to points 2 and 3, NM studies are relatively easy to quantify, particularly positron-emission tomographic (PET) studies, provided that an appropriate physiologic model is available (see Chap. 3).

Therefore, in almost all conceivable situations, the amount of radioactive tracer introduced does not disturb the physiologic process under study. This is also true for laboratory tests, with the still very widely used technique of radioimmunoassay. However, many of the radioimmunoassays have been supplanted by nonradioactive assays using enzymatic amplification and optical detection effects, which are possible in in vitro measurements, while there is no replacement in sight for radioactivity in in vivo imaging. Nuclear medicine imaging procedures are the only ones capable of demonstrating receptor distributions even when these receptors are present in picomolar concentrations. When processes are examined where the molecular concentration involved is not that small (i.e., when looking at sugar metabolism), the quantity of radiopharmaceutical needed for imaging is so small that neither pharmacologic nor physiologic effects have to be expected, which is again of major importance. NM methods are thus not only minimally invasive with regard to patient manipulation but very minimally invasive in terms of interference with the patients' physiology; for practical purposes, the amount of marker substance administered can be considered to be negligible in almost all NM examinations. It is important to recognize that this distinguishes NM studies clearly from MR spectroscopy and MRI studies, where the effects observed are always very small, and a substantial amount of molecules or a sizable effect has to be involved to be observable. Using MRI or MRS to look at receptor interactions therefore will be possible only when studying physiologic phenomena, where the molecular species under scrutiny is present in concentrations that are way beyond the concentrations at which most of the known receptor-ligand systems operate.

As stated, NM data are relatively simple to quantify. This is first and foremost due to the fact that radioactive counts per voxel are measured. All other imaging modalities measure a complicated function of tissue properties, namely, among others, absorption, relaxation properties, or reflexivity. The signal measured is further varied by adding contrast media, which may not produce a linear relation between the parameter measured and the concentration of contrast media given (see Chap. 2). Typical examples are the MR contrast agents where standard compounds have a combined effect on T1 and T2 relaxation at higher doses. Furthermore, in MRI, signal changes are also sensitive to modifications of the pulse sequence, which further complicates the relation between the signal measured and the substances present and responsible for the signal. Hence, provided that an appropriate physiologic model is available, NM data, and particularly those obtained with PET, can be used to extract quantitative information about a physiologic process; for example, is it possible to indicate how much glucose normal brain tissue metabolizes in milligrams per minute per 100 g of brain tissue?

Since the data are easy to quantify and the amount of data obtained is substantially smaller than when using other higher-resolution imaging modalities, NM has already in the early computer days developed a vast array of techniques to analyze the image contents mathematically. Transforming a time—or spatial—series of images into a single image or extracting quantitative information from a time series of images has been standard practice in nuclear medicine for almost two decades. An example is the quantitative wall motion analysis in nuclear cardiology initially described by Adam et al. (1). Many of these techniques now find their way into data-analysis algorithms in other modalities. Hence many concepts of image manipulation and of modeling, devised originally in NM, have been generalized to be used in conjunction with other imaging techniques. This is why these concepts have been introduced in Chaps. 2, 3, and 4 preceding the ones dealing with the various imaging modalities.

Quantitation requires physiologic modeling, which is of paramount importance for NM function imaging, because NM measures counts only but in contradistinction to MRS cannot deduce in vivo to which molecular species the radioisotope is bound. Hence only if we have a simple, quantitative physiologic model for the biochemical reactions in which the originally injected molecule is involved can we deduce the quantities of interest, i.e., reaction constants and molecular species concentrations. The paradigmatic model developed originally for autoradiographic studies by Sokoloff (40) is that for glucose metabolism. It will be discussed in detail toward the end of this chapter.

As a result of the detection physics in NM imaging devices, the spatial resolution of the images obtained is relatively low. Typically, good planar single-photon systems have a spatial resolution close to the camera of 2 to 3 mm; single photon emission computed tomographic (SPECT) systems in clinical use have spatial resolutions in the range of $10 \times 10 \times 10$ mm and positron-emission tomography (PET) systems in the range of $4.5 \times 4.5 \times 4.5$ mm. While there is room for improvement on these numbers, the systems will always be inferior in spatial resolution to the anatomic modalities CT, MRI, and ultrasonography because of the physical limitations discussed below. Since NM studies often contain little anatomic image information anyhow (no physiologic accumulation of the tracer in standard anatomic structures) with the probable sole exception of a bone scan, providing an anatomic backbone for an NM (or other functional) study becomes increasingly important. As a result of this necessity and the fast developments in computer technology, registration of images obtained by CT or MRI with NM images, so-called image fusion, is becoming routine, and so is the use of image fusion for interstudy registration of like data and the registration of functional MRI data with anatomic MRI images. The principles and the techniques used to this end are described in Chap. 4.

PHYSICAL AND TECHNICAL BASIS OF NUCLEAR MEDICINE IMAGING

Nuclear medicine is based on the physiologic "spy" concept, as introduced above. A pharmaceutical is labeled with a radioactive isotope to form what is called a *radiopharmaceutical* (see Chap. 2). Image formation involves the detection of the gamma rays emanating from the radioactive isotope. Grossly, NM procedures are subdivided on the basis of the detection technology used, i.e., planar single photon imaging, SPECT, and PET, but also from a physiologic point of view on the basis of the radiopharmaceuticals used. The radioisotopes are either reactor produced (^{131}I), cyclotron produced (^{123}I, most widely used PET radioisotopes), or generator produced (^{99m}Tc). The first part of this chapter deals with the effects detected and the detection technology. The second part discusses the various methodologies used in NM function studies that have not been discussed yet in Chap. 4.

The Effects and Their Detection

Images in nuclear medicine are obtained by detecting gamma rays resulting directly or indirectly (electron-positron annihilation, Compton scattering) from nuclear decay processes, which are briefly described. Starting from the point of its generation, a gamma ray or photon travels along a straight line until it interacts with matter. In the desired case this happens within the detector outside the body and results in an event that is recorded. However, if the photon interacts with body matter on its way to the detector, it is deflected ("scattered") from its original direction or absorbed. Scattered photons should not be counted in the detector, since it is not possible to deduce where they originated from. Different methods are used either to prevent the detection of these events (mechanical or electronic collimation; see below) or to separate them from the true unscattered events (mathematical scatter corrections). It is only the fraction of unattenuated gamma rays that must be used for generating an image of the radionuclide distribution. Absorbed photons are not counted and therefore do not degrade image quality; however, they prevent the measurement of the true number of photons emitted from a volume element and thus they interfere with quantitation. If quantitative results are desired, absorption correction is also necessary.

Radioactive Decay

Nuclides used to label radiopharmaceuticals must be radioactive. They decay in one or more transitions to reach a more stable configuration. There are several decay modes that are subsequently described. For being useful in radionuclide imaging, it is important that a decay process be accompanied by the emission of gamma rays suitable for detection. They must have enough energy to penetrate the body yet be low enough to be absorbed in detectors.

MODES OF RADIOACTIVE DECAY

The first mode of decay is *isomeric decay*. It occurs if a nucleus exists in an excited state above the ground state. Such excited states are called *isomeric states*. They have half-lives ranging from picoseconds to years. When isomeric states are long-lived, they are referred to as *metastable states* and denoted by an *m,* as in ^{99m}Tc (technetium). The most common isomeric transition from an energetically upper excited state to a lower state or the ground state is by emission of a gamma ray. An alternative transition is the internal conversion process whereby an electron and x-rays are emitted. For ^{99m}Tc, which is used in single photon emission imaging (standard planar imaging and SPECT), 90% of the decays are by gamma-ray emission.

The second type of decay is formed by the family of *beta decays*. Atomic nuclei consist of neutrons and positively charged protons. Whether an atom is in a stable configuration or not is determined by the ratio of protons to neutrons in the nucleus.

For an unstable, neutron-rich nucleus, a beta decay converts a neutron into a proton, an electron, and an antineutrino. After the beta decay, the nucleus may exist in an excited state. In this case, one or more isomeric decays will occur subsequently. This means that beta decays are followed by gamma-ray emissions, if energetically permitted. The beta decay of a nuclide may result in different excited states of the daughter nuclide, as shown for ^{131}I with daughter ^{131}Xe in Fig. 1. In this case, gamma rays of different energies arise from the decays of one radionuclide.

When a nucleus is proton-rich, it can decay either by positron emission or by electron capture. In a *positron-emission decay,* a proton is converted into a neutron, a positron, and a neutrino. The energy difference between the parent and the daughter nuclide must at least be 1022 keV, equivalent to two electron masses in accordance with the famous $E = mc^2$ law of Einstein (energy E equals mass m times velocity of light c squared). One of the masses has to be added to the proton to create a neutron; the other one belongs to the positron. The rest of the energy difference is shared between the neutrino and the positron. Therefore, a positron is emitted with a variable amount of kinetic energy that lies in a continuous range up to a maximum energy (several hundred keV). As the positron passes matter, it is slowed down by ionizations. By the time it has lost almost all its kinetic energy, it interacts with an electron. In this process, called *annihilation,* the mass of the two particles is converted into photons of 511 keV, again according to Einstein's law, which are emitted at a 180° angle.

An alternate possibility for nuclei with an excess of protons to turn into a stable isotope is by *electron-capture decay.* Here an electron from the atom is captured by a proton from the nucleus, forming a neutron and a neutrino. The resulting nuclide may be in an excited state, as in the example of ^{123}I and further decay by internal conversion emitting gamma rays to reach a stable ground state, or it may continue to decay by positron emission or electron capture.

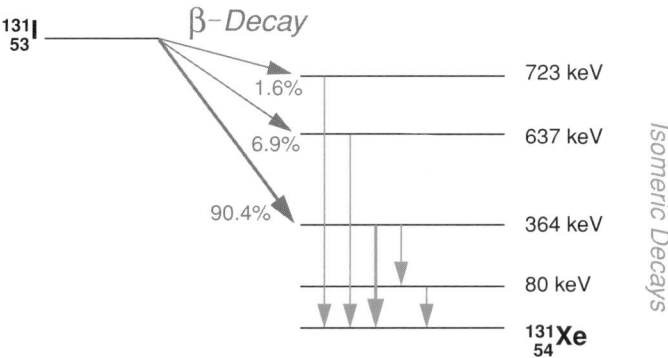

Figure 1. Simplified example of a beta decay resulting in different excited states. Beta decay of ^{131}I yields ^{131}Xe in the states 723, 637, and 364 keV above the ground state (38). While the first two excited states decay directly into the ground state, there is an intermediate excited state at 80 keV that may or may not be reached by the isomeric transition from 364 keV. In 80% of the ^{131}I decays, 364-keV gamma rays will be emitted.

While the types of transitions are different among the decay modes, the rate at which they occur obeys a common law. The decay of a radionuclide is a random process that is independent of its age. If a set of N radionuclides is considered, the decay probability for each of them is only proportional to the duration that is observed. Therefore, the number of decaying nuclides dN in a time interval dt is given by

$$dN(t) = -\lambda N(t)\, dt \tag{1}$$

where the negative sign expresses the decrease in the radioactive nuclides left. The decay constant λ denotes the fraction of radionuclides that disintegrates in a unit of time. For instance, if $\lambda = 0.1 \text{ s}^{-1}$ for a specific radionuclide, 10% of the radionuclides present at a given time have decayed 1 second later. The number of radionuclides left at a specific time can be found by integrating the preceding equation:

$$N(t) = N(0)e^{-\lambda t} \tag{2}$$

The activity A or radioactivity of a sample is given by the number of decays per time:

$$A(t) = -dN/dt = \lambda N(t) = \lambda N(0)e^{-\lambda t} \tag{3}$$

Since the initial activity $A(0)$ is given by $\lambda N(0)$, the activity at a later time point is

$$A(t) = A(0)e^{-\lambda t} \tag{4}$$

which means that the activity decreases in the same way as the number of radionuclides.

Every radionuclide is characterized by its half-life $T_{1/2}$, which is defined by the time required to reduce the activity to one-half. The half-life is related to the decay constant by

$$T_{1/2} = \frac{0.693}{\lambda} \tag{5}$$

Since the initial activity $A(0)$ is reduced by a factor of 2 after each half-life, after n half-lives it will be $A(0)/2^n$. Specifically, after 10 half-lives it is reduced by a factor of 1024, or to about 0.1% of the initial activity.

In radionuclide imaging, the local activity is not reduced by the radioactive decay process alone. Physiologic processes such as fecal or urinary excretion, perspiration, and exhalation simultaneously remove the applied pharmaceutical. Often, pharmaceuticals disappear from an organ according to an exponential law with a half-life T_b, the biologic half-life, or at the decay constant $\lambda_b = 0.693/T_b$. After T_b, half the substance has disappeared from the biologic system. Consequently, labeled substances disappear from a biologic system due to both the physical decay of the radionuclide and the biologic elimination of the radiopharmaceutical. The effective rate λ_e of radioactivity loss is therefore given by

$$\lambda_e = \lambda_p + \lambda_b \tag{6}$$

where λ_p denotes the physical decay constant. It follows that

$$\frac{1}{T_e} = \frac{1}{T_p} + \frac{1}{T_b} \quad \text{or} \quad T_e = \frac{T_p T_b}{T_p + T_b} \tag{7}$$

The effective half-life T_e is always shorter than T_b and T_p. If one of the half-lives is much longer than the other, T_e will be almost equal to the shorter half-life.

The units of radioactivity are the bequerel and the curie. One bequerel (Bq) is defined as representing one disintegration per second (dps). One curie (Ci) was defined historically as the disintegration rate of 1 g of radium with 3.7×10^{10} dps. Thus

$$
\begin{aligned}
1 \text{ kilobequerel} &= 1 \text{ kBq} &&= 10^3 \text{ dps} &&= 2.7 \times 10^{-8} \text{ Ci} \\
1 \text{ megabequerel} &= 1 \text{ MBq} &&= 10^6 \text{ dps} &&= 2.7 \times 10^{-5} \text{ Ci} \\
1 \text{ gigabequerel} &= 1 \text{ GBq} &&= 10^9 \text{ dps} &&= 2.7 \times 10^{-2} \text{ Ci}
\end{aligned}
$$

and

$$
\begin{aligned}
1 \text{ Ci} &= 3.7 \times 10^{10} \text{ Bq} &&= 37 \text{ GBq} \\
1 \text{ mCi} &= 3.7 \times 10^{7} \text{ Bq} &&= 37 \text{ MBq} \\
1 \text{ } \mu\text{Ci} &= 3.7 \times 10^{4} \text{ Bq} &&= 37 \text{ kBq}
\end{aligned}
$$

Labeling of a pharmaceutical with a radionuclide will never be 100% successful. A fraction of the sample will therefore be nonradioactive. If chemical reactions are considered like the ones described in Chap. 3, the unlabeled or "cold" substance will compete with the labeled substance in the reaction being imaged. The resulting concentration of the radioactive atoms in the organs is therefore dependent on the radioactivity per unit mass of the sample, its specific activity. If, for example, a 100-mg sample of a radiopharmaceutical contains 12 GBq of radioactivity, its specific activity is 12 GBq/100 mg = 120 MBq/mg. The concentration of a radiotracer in the target organ is directly related to its specific activity.

Interaction of Gamma Rays with Matter

A radiopharmaceutical used for radionuclide imaging gets distributed in the body, emitting gamma rays (equivalent with photons) at one or more energies. The gamma rays fan out in all directions from the source locations. On their way toward the body surface there is a probability that they undergo interactions with the body tissues whereby some of the photons are absorbed and others are deflected from their original direction, losing a part of their energy. More than 10 different effects are known, the most important ones being Compton scattering, photoelectric absorption, and pair production (35).

In the *photoelectric effect,* the incident photon is absorbed (Fig. 2). It transfers all the energy to an electron of the absorber atom. This electron, called a *photoelectron,* is

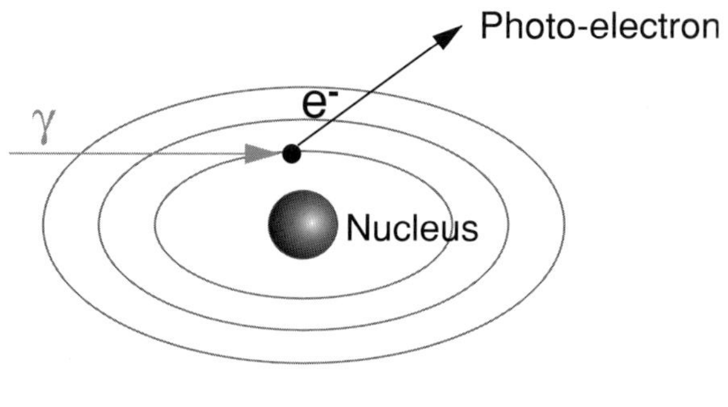

Figure 2. Photoelectric absorption (or photoelectric effect). The incident photon γ is absorbed and transfers all the energy to an electron e^- that is ejected.

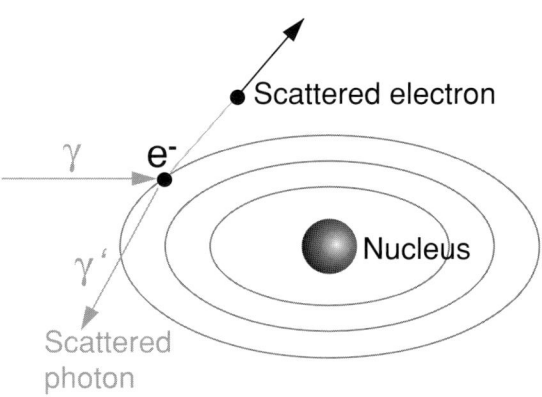

Figure 3. Compton scattering. The photon γ hits an electron e^- that is ejected from the atom and gets itself deflected, continuing with less energy γ'.

ejected from the atom with a kinetic energy equal to the photon energy reduced by the energy with which it was bound to the absorber atom. The electron then interacts with atoms producing secondary ionizations and excited atoms. The photoelectric effect occurs primarily for low-energy photons. In *Compton scattering,* the photon strikes an atomic electron to which it transfers a part of its energy (Fig. 3). The electron is ejected from the atom, and the photon is deflected from its original direction, continuing with less energy. At low photon energies, forward and backward scattering is equally likely; i.e., the direction of the scattered photons is symmetrically distributed about 90° off the original direction. At higher energies, scattering in the forward direction dominates more and more. The electron leaves the site of collision and follows a tortuous path along which it interacts with matter by ionizations and excitations. In a scintillator crystal such as sodium iodide, nuclei are thus excited to such energy levels that visible blue light is emitted as they decay to the ground state. This light flash is used in nuclear medicine to detect photons. The scattering pattern is simply a consequence of the law of conservation of momentum. If the photon energy is larger than twice the electron mass, the photon can be converted into two particles, an electron and a positron. This process, called *pair production,* happens mostly when the pair-producing photon passes the atom close to the nucleus (Fig. 4). In soft tissue the effect is not significant up to energies of 10 MeV. Photoelectric absorption dominates over Compton scattering for photons of low energy and dense absorbers. For the energy range 35 to 511 keV used in nuclear medicine, however, the fraction of photons attenuated due to photoelectric absorption is relatively low. In water, which constitutes most of the human body, it amounts to 5%, 0.7%, and 0.02% for the gamma-ray energies 70, 140, and 511 keV (14). Thus Compton scattering is the predominant mode of interaction with body tissues for the intermediate photon energies used in NM imaging.

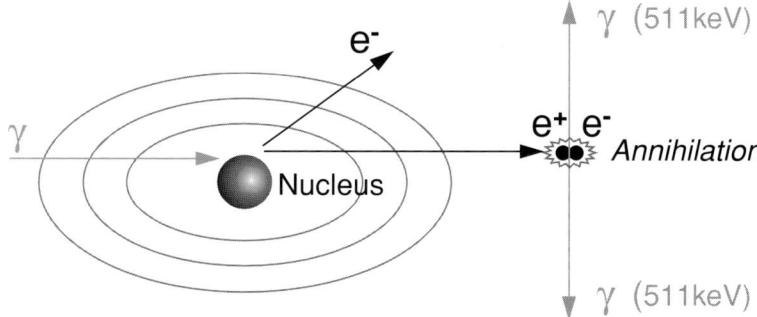

Figure 4. Pair production. A photon with sufficient energy $\gamma > 1022$ keV gets converted into an electron e^- and a positron e^+ (positively charged electron) upon interaction with a nucleus. Later on the positron interacts with an electron in an annihilation, whereby they get converted into two 511-keV photons γ.

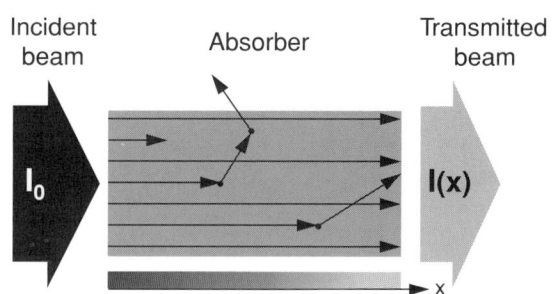

Figure 5. Attenuation of a photon beam in an absorber with linear attenuation coefficient μ. Attenuation describes the fact that some of the photons get absorbed and some get deflected once or several times. The net effect is that the number of photons in a directed beam decreases exponentially with the thickness of the penetrated absorber material.

As the gamma rays pass the body to eventually impinge on an outside detector, they interact with the patient's tissues in the ways described above. The result is that the photon beam from a source location directed toward a detector gets attenuated (Fig. 5). Only a fraction $I(x)$ of the initial intensity $I(0)$ is transmitted:

$$I(x) = I(0)e^{-\mu x} \qquad (8)$$

The fraction $e^{-\mu x}$ is determined by the thickness x and the linear attenuation coefficient μ (cm^{-1}) of the absorber. The attenuation coefficient is dependent on the photon energy and proportional to the density of the absorber (11). To compare the attenuation of different tissues, the latter dependence is removed by dividing μ by the density ρ to form the mass attenuation coefficient μ_m:

$$\mu_m = \mu/\rho \ (\text{cm}^2/\text{g}) \qquad (9)$$

Figure 6 shows a comparison of the attenuation in different body tissues, air, and lead. It illustrates several facts. First, mass attenuation decreases with increasing photon energy. Therefore, radionuclides should emit photons with 100 keV or more so that they have a sufficient probability to exit the body and arrive at the detector. Second, when imaging with x-rays, as discussed in Chap. 5, the tissue absorption itself is the phenomenon that gives contrast; hence appropriate absorption is desirable. Therefore, photons of about 30 keV are optimal for x-ray imaging, since the contrast between different tissues is good, while the penetration is still sufficient.

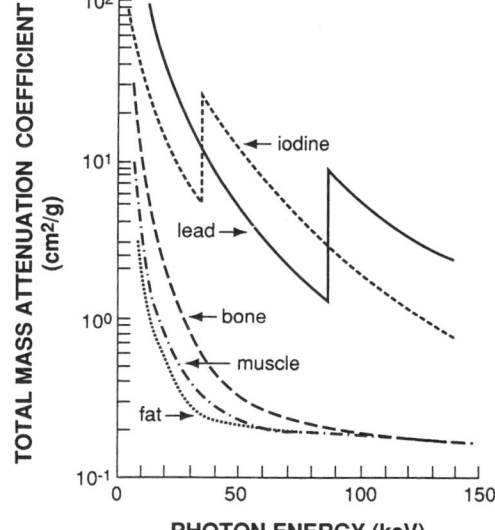

Figure 6. Attenuation coefficients in different body tissues as a function of photon energy. Reprinted with permission from Saha GB: *Physics and radiobiology of nuclear medicine.* New York: Springer (1993).

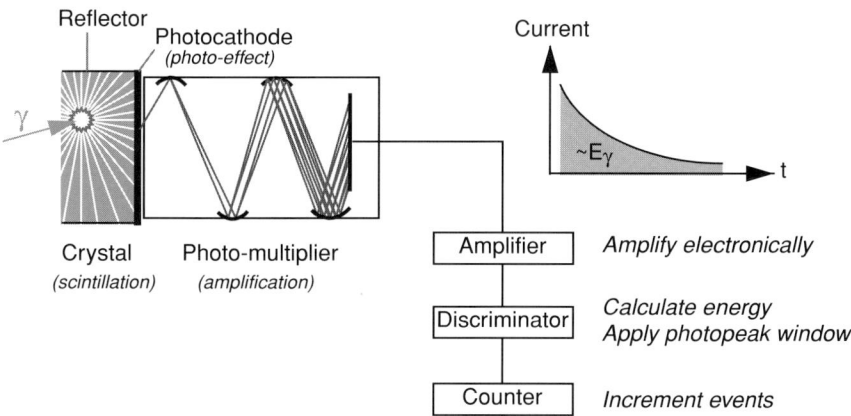

Figure 7. Detection of a photon γ with a scintillation counter. The incident photon produces a light flash in the detector crystal that causes photoelectrons to be released at the light-sensitive surface of the succeeding device, the photomultiplier. It amplifies the number of initial photoelectrons to a current that is proportional to the light flash. The succeeding processing devices convert the current into an energy estimate of the incident photon, and an event is counted if this energy corresponds to the decay process being observed.

Detection of Gamma Rays by Scintillation Counters

While interactions of photons with body matter have the undesired effect of decreasing the observable activity, interaction with a detector material is required to obtain a signal in the detector and thereby count the number of radioactive decays.

There are various types of detectors. The most commonly used detectors consist of an inorganic scintillation crystal coupled to amplification and processing devices. Their principle of operation is shown in Fig. 7. The sequence of processes resulting in a detected event is as follows: A photon of energy $E\gamma$ enters the crystal. It interacts with the crystal atoms until it has lost all its energy. Thus the atoms are raised into excited states. The atoms in the excited states return to the ground state by emitting visible-light photons (fluorescence light). These photons can traverse the crystal, which is transparent to optical photons. The ones reaching the light-sensitive surface of the photomultiplier tube cause a photo effect (see "Interaction of Gamma Rays with Matter" above). This means that electrons are released, which are then multiplied by a cascade of stages in the phototube. As a result, a current leaves the photomultiplier that is proportional to the number of light photons. Due to the linear relation between gamma energy and the number of scintillation photons, the current is proportional to $E\gamma$. After further linear amplification, the current reaches a discrimination unit. There it is mapped to an energy, the measured energy $E\gamma_{meas}$, which is then compared with the gamma-ray energy $E\gamma_{expect}$ related to the decay process to be observed. The discrimination unit decides whether the photon should be counted as a relevant event. If so, the counter is incremented by one.

One important factor determining the quality of the detector system is its energy resolution, which specifies how accurately a gamma energy can be measured. Many of the processes involved in detection, fluorescence, photo effect, and amplification, underly statistical variations. Therefore, the estimated energy also shows a distribution around the true value, known as the *photopeak* (Fig. 8). The photopeak for a certain energy can be obtained by plotting a histogram of the measured energies for an ensemble of incident gamma rays. The broader the peak, the worse is the energy resolution of the detector system. A good energy resolution is important to separate scattered from unscattered photons. Scattered photons have lost a part of their energy and thus result in lower-energy events. By appropriate energy discrimination in the detector system, they can be excluded from being counted. To this end, a lower energy threshold is defined below which detected events are discarded.

With an ideal detector system, each impinging radiation of a specified gamma energy would be counted as an event. Real systems, however, lose a certain fraction of the

Figure 8. Photopeak measured for [99mTc]. It represents the histogram of the energies measured with a scintillation detector. If there were only photons at 140 keV, the photopeak would be Gaussian in shape, representing the energy resolution of the detection system. Due to Compton scattering, however, some of the photons have lower energies. They produce the scatter tail to the left of the photopeak. To separate them from unscattered photons, a discrimination window is centered on the photopeak.

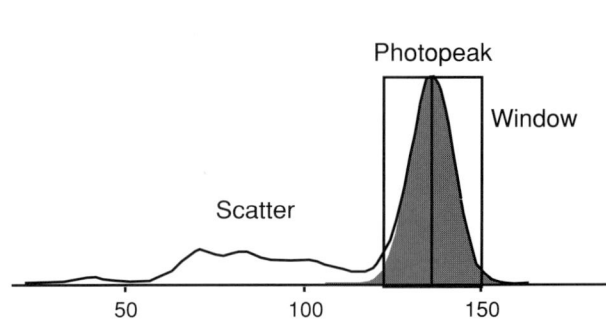

events mainly because not all gamma rays are absorbed inside the detector system. The amount of this sensitivity loss is an important system characteristic. It is described by the detector efficiency, i.e., the fraction of detected photons (counts under the photopeak) to the number of incident photons of a certain energy. The efficiency is affected by many factors, such as the stopping power of the detector (given by the attenuation properties of the detector material and its thickness) and the fraction of photons accepted in the energy discriminator window to all photons under the photopeak curve. Included in the sensitivity are losses due to the finite speed by which the events can be processed by the counter. These losses are separately characterized by the *dead time*. It denotes the time between the moment where a scintillation starts in the crystal to the moment when processing has progressed so far that the next event can be accepted. The dead time depends both on the scintillation characteristics of the crystal and on the layout of the processing components.

SCINTILLATION CRYSTALS

The number of visible photons produced during a scintillation event in a detector crystal varies from a few hundred to a few thousand depending on the scintillation crystal. For NaI(Tl), about 20 to 30 photons per kiloelectronvolt are generated (38). The half-time of the scintillation process describes how fast the light photons are released. It ranges between 0.5 and 300 ns. If a succeeding photon hits the crystal while the scintillation due to a previous event is ongoing, the two scintillations overlap (pulse pileup), resulting in an energy that will be rejected. Hence both photons are lost. A short scintillation decay reduces the probability of pulse pileup. This is particularly favorable in situations where the number of arriving gamma photons per time unit is high (high count rates).

The most frequently used scintillation crystals consist of sodium iodide doped with small amounts of thallium [NaI(Tl)]. These crystals are relatively inexpensive and have physical properties that yield efficient detectors. A disadvantage is their tendency to absorb water, whereby the light transmission properties change. Therefore, NaI(Tl) detectors must be sealed. In PET cameras, where 511-keV photons from positron annihilations are detected, bismuth germanate (BGO) scintillators have been used predominantly. The advantages of BGO over NaI(Tl) are the 50% better stopping power and that it is nonhygroscopic (see Table 1). On the other hand, the light output of BGO is much lower, resulting in an energy resolution that is only half that of NaI(Tl). The decay of the light flash is also somewhat slower, resulting in a longer dead time. Because BGO is very expensive, a recent development of a less expensive PET camera makes use of NaI(Tl) crystals.

Table 1. *Properties of scintillators*

	NaI(Tl)	BGO
Attenuation coefficient at 511 keV (1/cm)	0.34	0.92
Detector efficiency for 3-cm-thick crystal (%)	64	94
Decay time (ns)	230	300
Light output (relative)	100	15
Energy resolution (FWHM) (%)	7	15

From Muehllehner G, Karp JS. Positron emission tomography imaging: Technical considerations. *Semin Nucl Med* 16(1), 35–50 (1986).

Principles of Nuclear Medicine Imaging Systems

In NM imaging, a suitable radiopharmaceutical is applied to the patient. Either it accumulates within a target organ, or it stays within the vascular system. Gamma rays are emitted from the resulting isotope distribution. A fraction of them hits a detector system set up to form an image of the radionuclide distribution. Similar to x-ray examinations, two types of image acquisition are possible: In planar imaging, a projection of the distribution onto a plane is recorded. Thus structures along the projection direction are overlayed much in the same way as in a radiograph. The aim of tomographic imaging is to recover the three-dimensional (3D) radionuclide distribution in the body itself as accurately as possible. To this end, many planar projections in different directions must be collected. They are combined in a reconstruction process to form tomographic images of the radionuclide distribution in body slices.

Planar Imaging

Planar imaging is done with a stationary detector system. It consists of two parts, the collimator and the gamma camera, as illustrated in Fig. 9. The collimator acts as a kind of "lens" that projects an image of the radionuclide distribution onto the gamma camera surface. The gamma camera in turn converts this virtual image consisting of incident gamma rays into an explicit digital image.

Different types of mechanical collimators are described in the following box. While they have different characteristics, such as resolution or efficiency, they share a common operating principle. From within the radionuclide distribution, gamma rays are emitted into all directions. The ones picked up in the detector can only be used in forming the projection image if their incident direction is known. The collimator therefore ensures that each gamma ray impinging on the detector has a well-defined direction. It does so by allowing only gamma rays traveling along specified directions, e.g., vertical to the camera surface, to pass and absorb all the others.

The detection camera most frequently used in NM is the Anger camera, which was invented by Hal O. Anger in the late 1950s. As opposed to a scintillation counter, the camera not only counts the total number of events in the crystal but also records for each event its position of interaction in the crystal. A digital image of the projection is obtained by dividing the crystal area into an array of equal-sized image elements (pixels) and by summing the events falling into each of these pixels. The resulting units are counts per pixel. At the end of the acquisition, the recorded counts are transformed into a gray-level image. For the purpose of event localization, the Anger camera is equipped with an array of photomultiplier tubes that cover the back of the NaI(Tl) crystal (see Fig. 9). Interaction of a gamma ray with the crystal causes light photons to be emitted into all directions equally. On the crystal back face, the number of photons per square centimeter is largest perpendicularly behind the event and decreases in a bell-shaped fashion away from the event. The photomultipliers sample this light distribution. As a consequence, they get an amount of light that depends on their relative position to the event. These light intensities are converted into proportional electric signals and fed into a processing circuit. By averaging the signals with appropriate weights, the centroid of the

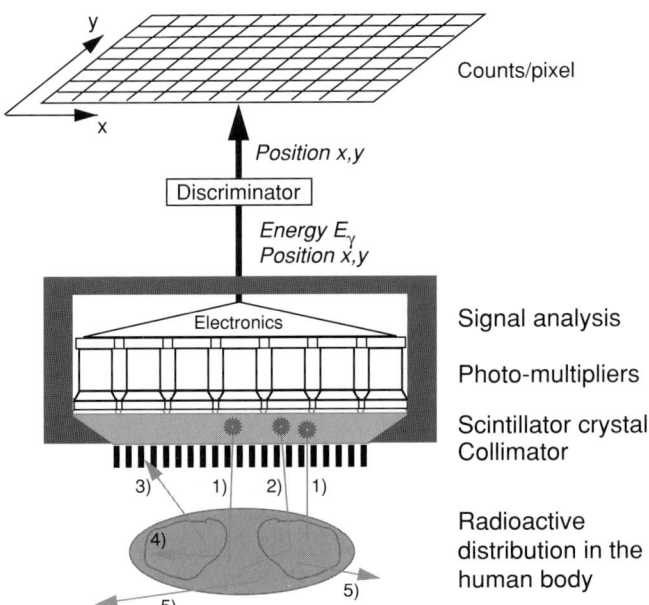

Figure 9. Operation principle of the Anger gamma camera (see text). The photons emitted in the radionuclide distribution have the fate (1) to be detected (true counts), (2) to be scattered in a way that they can pass the collimator and are detected (scattered counts), (3) to be absorbed in the collimator, (4) to be absorbed in the tissue itself, or (5) to miss the detector.

light distribution is calculated, which is supposed to be identical with the event position. The total of the signals recorded from a single light flash in the crystal is related to the gamma photon energy and can therefore be used for energy discrimination, i.e., to reject events not falling into the photopeak of the radionuclide used (see Fig. 8).

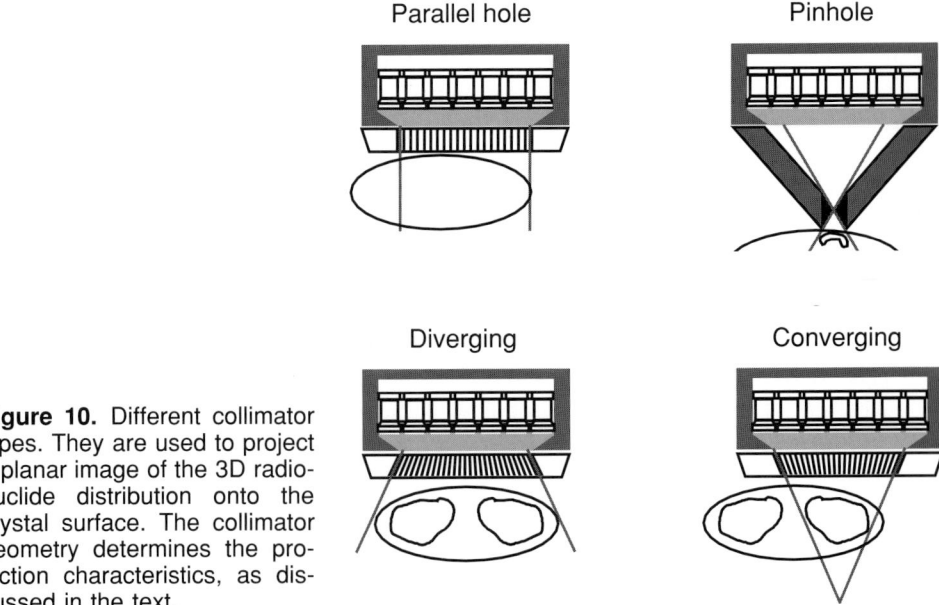

Figure 10. Different collimator types. They are used to project a planar image of the 3D radionuclide distribution onto the crystal surface. The collimator geometry determines the projection characteristics, as discussed in the text.

TYPES OF MECHANICAL COLLIMATORS

A collimator projects an image of the radionuclide distribution onto the scintillation crystal. This is achieved by an array of holes embedded in heavy metal, typically lead. The holes let the photons pass to the detector crystal along the desired directions, while the walls ideally absorb all the photons impinging on the collimator surface from an undesired direction. In practice, however, some of the photons are able to penetrate the walls and contribute to an elevated image background. Four basic collimator types are used in planar imaging, as illustrated in Fig. 10.

The *parallel-hole collimators* have holes perpendicular to the detector surface, separated by walls called *septa*. If round holes are chosen, the collimator has a honeycomb appearance. Parallel-hole collimators provide a one-to-one projected image of the field of view. The sensitivity, i.e., the number of counts measured per unit activity, is almost constant at different distances from the collimator (26). The resolution, however, depends on several collimator design factors and on the object-to-collimator distance. Decreasing the hole diameter or lengthening the septa improves resolution at the cost of a reduced sensitivity. The resolution is best at the collimator surface and deteriorates with increasing distance from it. Therefore, patients should be placed as close to the collimator as possible in clinical examinations (38). The thickness of the septa has to be optimized for the energy of the imaged photons. On one hand, the septa must be thick enough to prevent penetration by oblique gamma rays, which would obscure the image. On the other hand, thick septa reduce the sensitivity because with thick septa the photons impinging on the collimator will see fewer holes and more absorber material if the hole size is kept constant. As a result, fewer gamma rays may pass. Combining the constraints of collimator design with the desire to use photons that pass the human body without absorption but are readily stopped in the scintillation crystal results in an optimal energy for radionuclides of about 50 to 300 keV for use in NM. Below 50 keV most photons are absorbed by body tissue, while above 300 keV it is difficult to build efficient collimators that are able to prevent septal penetration, and the efficiency of the detector crystals decreases. The parallel-hole collimator is the most commonly used collimator.

The *pinhole collimator* is made out of lead or tungsten and is conical in shape with a small aperture at the tip of the conus. The gamma rays must pass through this ''pinhole'' and form an inverted image on the crystal. From each point source in the object only a small fraction of the emitted gamma rays may reach the crystal. The camera principle used is that of the ''camera obscura'' (remember the camera made out of a shoe box during your high school days!). As the object moves closer to the aperture, more gamma rays may pass. Hence the sensitivity is increased. At the same time, the image is enlarged, while the visible part of the body (field of view) is reduced. Due to these characteristics, pinhole collimators are used mainly in imaging small organs such as the thyroid gland or the bones of a hand.

Converging collimators have holes that converge at a point in front of the detector. They are used to provide magnified images of organs. Resolution and sensitivity are better than those of a comparable pinhole collimator.

The *diverging collimators* work the other way around. They are focused toward a point behind the detector to image a large organ such as the lung on a smaller detector. Diverging collimators are rarely used because nowadays detectors with large crystals are widely available. Typically, converging collimators can be turned, and then they function as a diverging collimator.

Tomographic Imaging

All that can be seen from the distribution of an incorporated radiotracer is the radiation leaving the body. We have discussed how this radiation can be collimated, detected, and further processed to form projections of the actual distribution. These projection images are clinically valuable in situations where screening for disease is necessary and whenever data acquisition has to occur fast, as in dynamic imaging.

The aim of tomographic imaging in NM is to assess the three-dimensional (3D) radionuclide distribution itself, if possible in quantitative fashion. The intrinsic problem to solve is that the activity in a unit of volume cannot be measured independently from that of other volume elements. The best that can be done is to direct a collimated detector toward a volume element of interest and to count all events coming from exactly this direction. But all other radioactive decays on this line also will contribute to the recorded counts, and there is no way to relate them to their position along the line. Therefore, a solution has to be found as to how to calculate from such superimposed radiations the underlying activity distribution. The method used is similar to that developed for x-ray CT scanning (see Chap. 6), but the problem is more difficult in radionuclide imaging. Here absorption in the body is an undesired side effect rather than the mechanism of contrast, as in CT. An ideal solution has not yet been found. However, there are approximate solutions with different degrees of accuracy. All of them are based on using many projections acquired with different camera orientations at a 180° to 360° arc perpendicular to the patients' body axis. The total data collected provides enough information to reconstruct an approximation of the activity distribution in a process called *reconstruction from projections.*

In what follows it will be shown what requirements the data acquisition must fulfill and how the measurements are organized in so-called sinograms. Various types of reconstructions that transform the sinograms into images will then be outlined. The images obtained in the way so described suffer from distortions due to attenuation and scatter effects. They result from the self-attenuation of photons in body tissue by scattering and absorption. These effects must be compensated for in order to obtain quantitative images. It is described how attenuation and scatter manifest themselves in the images, and approaches for compensating attenuation are outlined. These principles apply to SPECT imaging and with minor modifications also to PET imaging.

Acquisition and Projection Geometry. To describe the method of data acquisition in emission tomography, we consider an object for which only one section is drawn in Fig. 11. At each location in the object there is some activity that we want to measure. Outside the object there is a detector, drawn as a bar. It is large enough to accommodate the parallel projection of the object as it rotates about the object. At each position the detector measures a whole projection, formed by a set of parallel projection rays that divide the object into strips of equal width. All the activity that decays within a projection ray sends a fraction of the gamma rays along the projection direction toward the detector, where they are counted. Their total forms the projected value of that ray, which is stored in a cell of computer memory (sinogram cell). Each projection ray is defined by its angle θ with the y axis and its distance r from the center of rotation. All rays of a projection share the same angle, while the distance increments in steps equal to the ray width. After one projection measurement has been accomplished, the detector rotates about an angular increment and acquires the next projection. This process continues until projections all around the object have been taken. As a result, a whole set of projections is available for the subsequent reconstruction. The projections are normally arranged in a two-dimensional array called a *sinogram* (see Fig. 11). Each value in the sinogram represents a projection ray. All rays in a projection form a sinogram row. Successive rows represent projections at incremented angles. The minimal number N_θ of angle increments to obtain sufficient information for an adequate reconstruction depends on the number of desired image elements (pixels). It is given by

$$N_\theta = \frac{n\pi}{4} \tag{10}$$

where n is the number of rays (resolution elements) in the projection (4).

Analytical Reconstruction by Filtered Backprojection. The most frequently used reconstruction method is *filtered backprojection.* As the name suggests, it is a combination

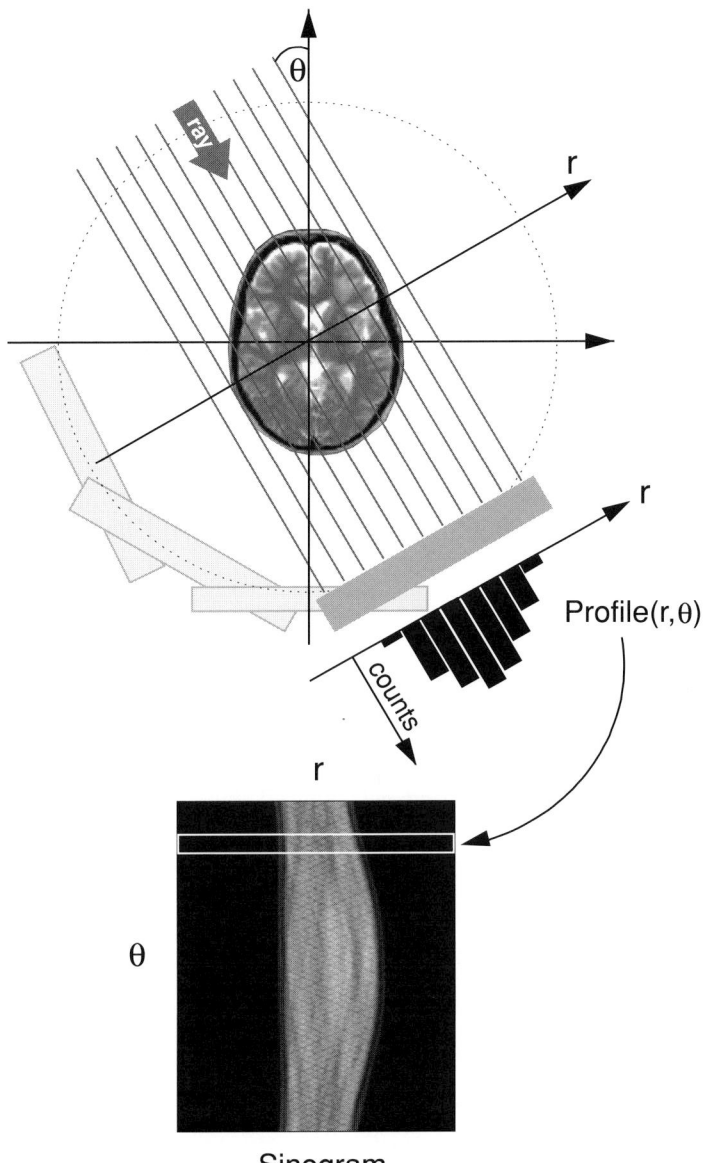

θ

r

Profile(r,θ)

counts

r

r

θ

Sinogram

Figure 11. Acquisition of angled planar projections for radionuclide tomography by rotating a detector around the object. The projection geometry is given by the projection angle θ and the ray width. All decays happening within a ray and sending their gamma rays along θ add one count to the projected value of that ray. At the end of the acquisition for an angle all the projected values together form the projection profile, which is entered into the sinogram. Then the next acquisition is taken at an incremented angle θ + Δθ.

of two mathematical processes. Backprojection is an attempt to reverse the projection inherent in the acquisition physics. However, it does not accurately model the imaging process. Therefore, simple backprojection results in images with a blurring artefact. It can be avoided when applying a filter function to modify the acquired data in a way that blurring components cancel themselves out. By changing the form of the filter, the noise and resolution characteristics of the resulting image can be adapted further.

The basic principle of backprojection is very straightforward. For each projection value it is known that it represents the total activity of all points along the corresponding ray. Since their relative contributions are unknown—for this is the solution to be found—the signal intensity is simply attributed to all of them. If this is done for all the projections while adding the intensities at each point in the field of view, an image is formed that

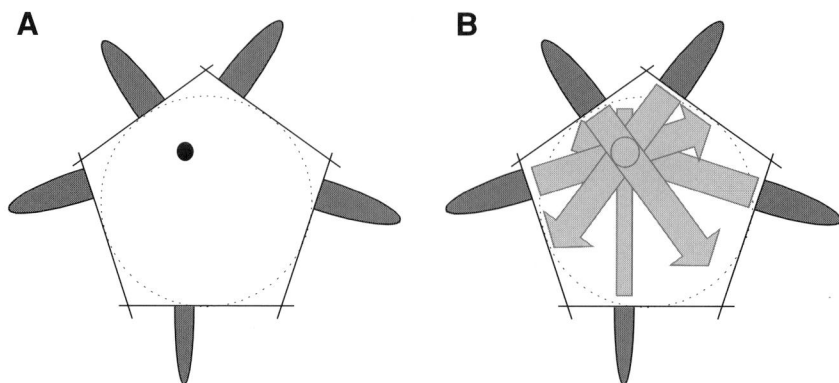

Figure 12. Illustration of projection and backprojection for a homogeneous circular object. (**A**) Five projections are taken with an angle increment of 72° yielding the indicated profiles. (**B**) Simple backprojection of the five profiles. Initially, the image is zero. A profile is backprojected by adding the profile values to the image pixels met along the projection direction θ. The superposition of all five backprojected profiles results in a starlike pattern intersecting at the object location.

is an approximation of the actual body section. The processes involved are illustrated in Fig. 12 for a simple circular object with homogeneous activity concentration. The acquisition yields a set of profiles shown at five different angles. The values of the five projections are then backprojected, forming a starlike pattern intersecting at the location of the circle. This starlike pattern is the most striking artefact of backprojection. If many more projections are used, the pattern gets blurred, but points outside an object still receive some of the backprojected intensity. Furthermore, since points within the object also receive components of neighoring points, subtle differences cannot be assessed.

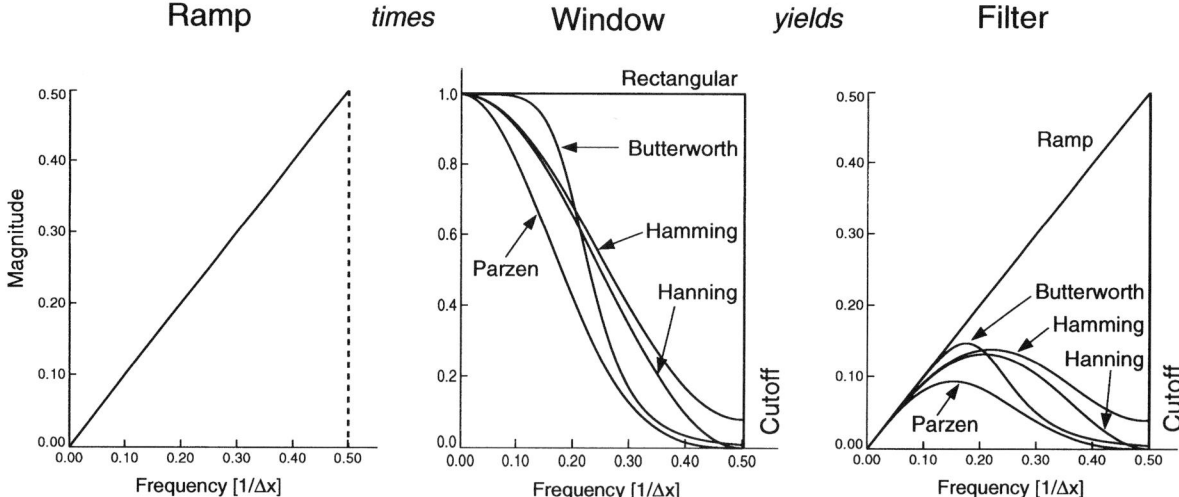

Figure 13. Filters used in image reconstruction by backprojection. The frequency equivalent of the projection profiles is multiplied by one of these filters before being backprojected. The filters are formed by the product of the ramp with a window function. The ramp component compensates for the $1/r$ smearing artefact of backprojection. However, it also amplifies noise in the data toward high frequencies. This effect is reduced by combining the ramp with tapered window functions. The rectangular window only suppresses frequency components that cannot be resolved. Its cutoff is given $\frac{1}{2}\Delta x$, where Δx is the sampling interval along the profiles. The tapered windows decline in different shapes that determine the relation between noise suppression and the entailed resolution loss. For a discussion of the filters mentioned, see Budinger and Gullberg (6). As a general rule, the more the high frequencies are attenuated, the less are both the statistical fluctuations and the resolution in the resulting images.

The nature of the blurring artefact can be described as follows: The activity distribution in the object can be viewed as a set of point sources with superposing emissions. For each point source, its activity is smeared over the whole image by the projection-backprojection process. The contribution thus attributed to a remote image point decreases in proportion with its distance from the point source. When this effect is analyzed mathematically, there exists an easy way to exactly counterbalance it. The projection data can be filtered—a well-defined distortion—such that a backprojection of these modified profiles yields the unsmeared image of the object. The appropriate weighting function is known as the *ramp filter*. This works perfectly for an idealized acquisition with infinitely many projection angles and ideal rays. Hence filtered backprojection gives an analytical solution that can be implemented in a simple and fast computer program. In real situations, however, neither of the idealizations is exactly fulfilled. Rather, the projections are sampled at a limited set of angles, with discrete rather than continuous profiles. As a

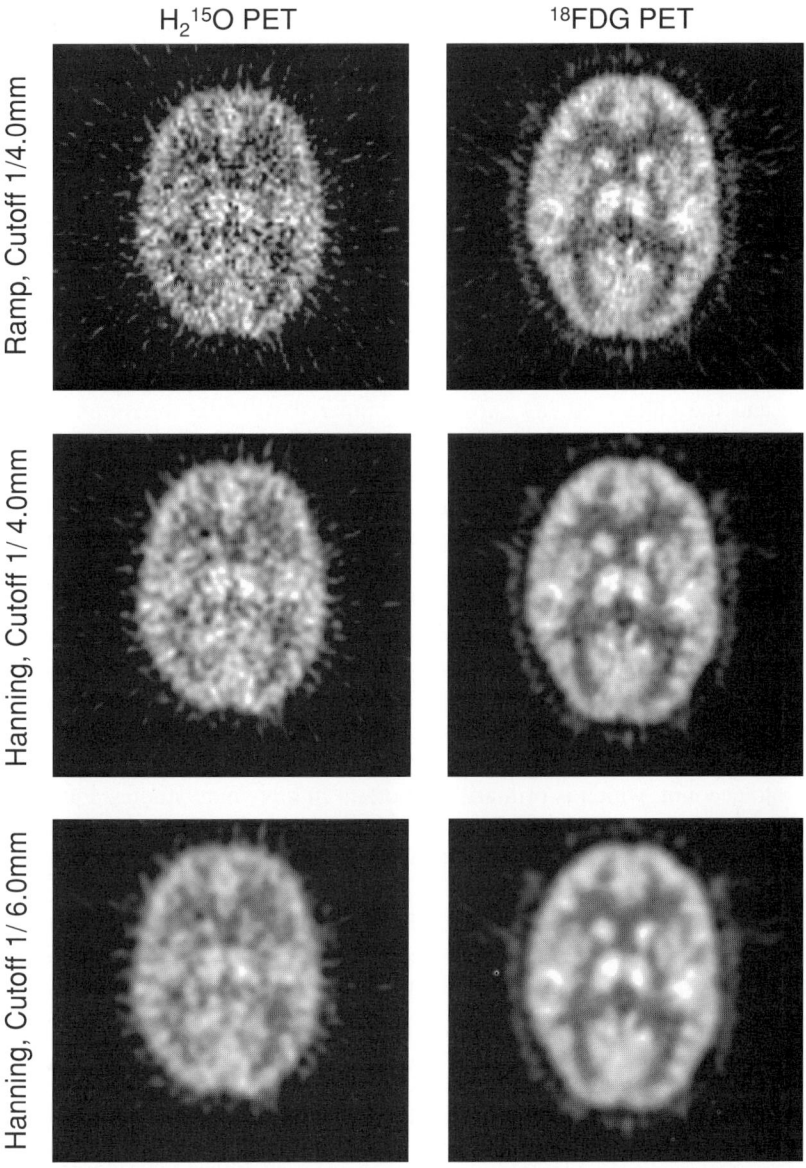

Figure 14. PET images reconstructed with backprojection and different filters. The ramp filter preserves the optimal resolution but amplifies high-frequency noise. The Hanning filter smooths the images, whereby both the noise and the resolution are reduced. Acquisition times were 20 and 1 minutes for the FDG and the H_2O PET acquisitions, respectively.

result, the ramp filter produces a "ringing" artefact with ripples around sharp discontinuities in the image. Furthermore, it amplifies the noise visible in the image. These problems can be reduced at the cost of a resolution loss by modifications of the filter in the way shown in Fig. 13. The more the filter shape flattens out at the end, the better are the noise characteristics in the image. The smoother its termination, the less visible are the ripples. For each study protocol, therefore, the optimal filter shape has to be determined that provides the optimal resolution at a tolerable noise level. Figure 14 illustrates the effect of a smoothing filter on two PET studies with different noise levels.

ALGEBRAIC (ITERATIVE) RECONSTRUCTIONS

Algebraic reconstruction methods take more aspects of the real-world projection physics into account than filtered backprojection. They are therefore potentially able to reconstruct more accurate images. The basic principle is that both the object and the ray are modeled as discrete quantities (Fig. 15). The object is normally decomposed into a set of quadratic elements (pixel), each supposedly being homogeneous with activity a_i (4). The rays have a finite width w typically equal to the pixel size. In this configuration, the projection process easily can be modeled by an algorithm called *projector*. Suppose a projection is to be taken at an angle θ. For each ray the projector determines which pixels intersect the ray area. These pixels contribute to the projected value proportional to both their fractional area f_i in the ray and their activity a_i. The projection value or ray sum at the distance r is therefore simply given by

$$p(r, \theta) = \Sigma_{\text{intersected pixels}}(f_i a_i) \tag{11}$$

Now the idea of iterative reconstruction can be summarized as follows: First, an initial distribution of activities a_i is assumed. It is projected along all measured angles, and the calculated ray sums are compared with the measured projection values. If there is a discrepancy between estimated and true values, the assumed distribution is adjusted in a way that a subsequent projection provides better agreement. The cycle adjust-project-compare is repeated or iterated until the degree of agreement suggests that a likely distribution a_i and hence a reasonable image has been found.

There are many implementations of iterative reconstruction methods. They differ in how much of the projection physics is taken into account, what consistency criterion is used, and according to what strategy the pixel values are updated. A very notable iterative approach is the so-called maximum likelihood (ML) method. These methods lend themselves very nicely to the incorporation of all physical knowledge available (19). Particularly, the Poisson nature of the decay statistics is taken into account, which is primarily important in low-count studies. Furthermore, the estimated activities are guaranteed to be positive. Although an evident restriction, this property is not fulfilled with filtered backprojection and not easily enforced in most iterative algorithms.

While iterative reconstructions are able to calculate more accurate images than filtered backprojection, they also have some drawbacks. A common problem of all iterative algorithms is convergence. First, it has to be ensured that the estimation approaches a reasonable solution, and second, the iteration has to be stopped when the approximation is "sufficiently good." The widely used practical approach is to stop after a prescribed number of iterations. Because of the time-consuming computations involved, the number of iterations must be kept fairly small to ensure acceptable reconstruction times. While the computation times were prohibitive a few years ago, improvements in the hardware and streamlining of the algorithms have brought iterative reconstruction to an initial phase of clinical usability.

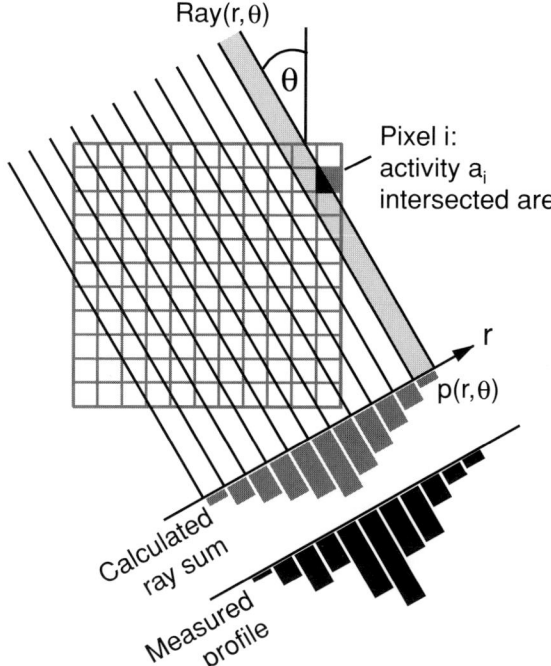

Figure 15. Discrete geometry used for iterative reconstruction methods. The activity distribution is defined in a matrix of quadratic pixels. A projected ray value is calculated as the sum of the contributions from all intersected pixels, as explained in the text. The profiles calculated in this way from an assumed activity distribution are compared with the measured profiles to derive better estimates of the distribution.

Other reconstructions are able to compute more accurate images than filtered backprojection, as discussed in the following box. However, there still remain some advantages unique to filtered backprojection. It has an unbeatable speed, it is able to provide reasonable reconstructions for incomplete data, and it allows one to directly reconstruct a portion of the entire field of view (19).

Effect of Attenuation. It has been outlined so far that reconstructions define a model of the physical effects by which the measured projections are formed and perform an (approximate) numerical reversion of those effects to form an image. While discrete sampling and some portions of the projection geometry are taken into account by the methods described so far, the photon attenuation by the tissue of the object being imaged has been neglected. The example of a ^{99m}Tc brain study shall illustrate the order of this effect. While 86% of the photons emitted at a depth of 1 cm beneath the scalp are able to penetrate the intervening tissue and to leave the body, only 18% do so from the center of the brain (6). An ideal reconstruction without attenuation compensation yields an image reflecting this number of detected counts. Therefore, the activity will be underestimated by 82% in central brain and by 14% at the cortex.

To illustrate the nature of the artefact, let us consider a homogeneous disk with constant activity concentration and attenuation (Fig. 16). As in the unattenuated case, the projection onto the detector is composed of the contributions along rays. However, these contributions are weighted according to the exponential law of attenuation. Since the attenuation is assumed to be constant, the weight of a certain contribution is given by $e^{-\mu d}$ (Eq. 8), where d is the distance that has to be traveled from its origin through attenuating matter. Therefore, the weights exponentially decrease from 1.0 at the border facing the detector to the opposite border. All the weighted contributions must be integrated along the rays to form the projection. In the homogeneous disk case the solution can be derived analytically (6). Figure 16 shows the resulting profiles for different attenuation coefficients. Using these profiles in a reconstruction that assumes them to be unattenuated results in an image with underestimated central activity. In the example configuration the result again can be derived analytically. The profiles through the reconstructed section shown in Fig. 16 illustrate the severity of the artefact.

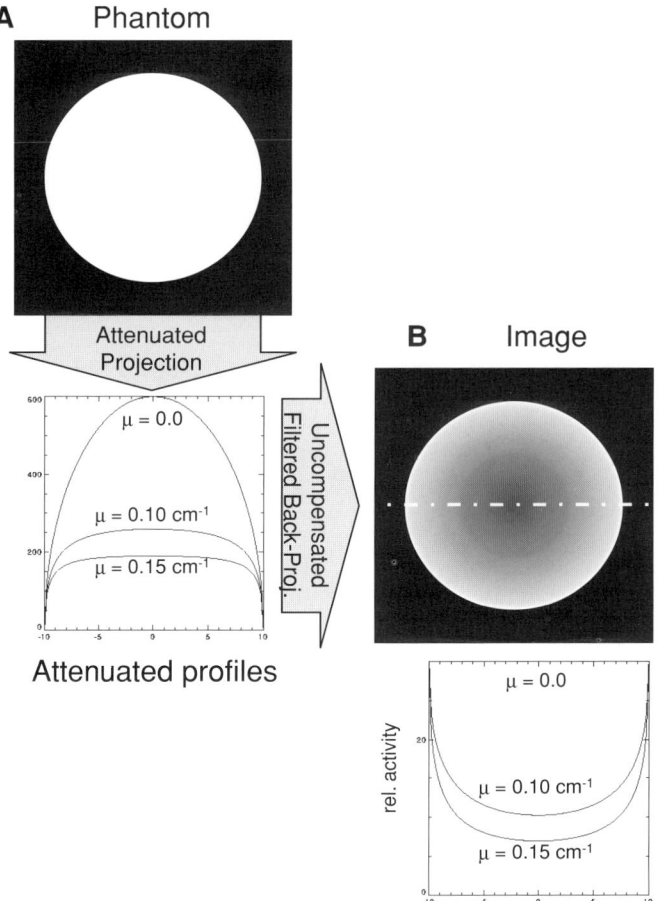

Figure 16. (**A**) Profiles for a homogeneous disk phantom calculated for different attenuation coefficients, as explained in the text. The profiles labeled with $\mu = 0.0$, $\mu = 0.10$, and $\mu = 0.15$ cm^{-1} represent the situation of no attenuation, attenuation of the 511-keV PET photons, and attenuation of the 140-keV photons in ^{99m}Tc SPECT, respectively. (**B**) Resulting image intensities when using the attenuated profiles in an ideal reconstruction. The activity in the center is progressively underestimated. See also Fig. 17.

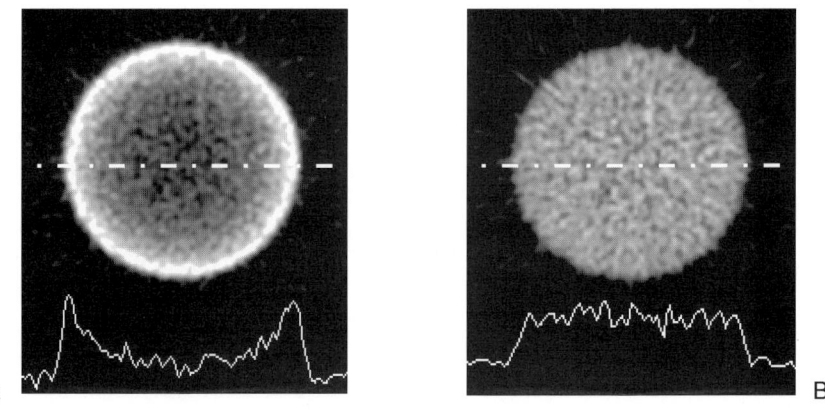

Figure 17. PET images of a cylindrical water phantom containing ^{18}FDG. Section and profile when reconstructing (**A**) without and (**B**) with calculated attenuation compensation. In **B,** the phantom outline could be derived readily by a thresholding process.

ATTENUATION CORRECTION METHODS

The problem of attenuation correction is twofold: The distribution of the attenuation coefficient μ has to be found in the whole field of view, and it must be included into the reconstruction algorithm to compensate for the attenuated photons. Basically, there are two approaches in practical use to obtain the attenuation coefficients. Either they are measured in a simultaneous or separate transmission study (measured attenuation correction), or they are derived using simple assumptions (calculated attenuation correction).

While there are different practical solutions to measured attenuation correction, they share the common principle of transmission computed tomography discussed in Chap. 5. A transmission source is required, which emits photons at a known intensity I_0. It is rotated about the object in the field of view, and the opposing detectors measure the intensity I of the transmitted beam, which is attenuated along the ray source detector (see Figs. 23 related to SPECT and 40 related to PET). In principle, this is the same projection geometry as for radionuclide emission imaging discussed before. The differences are that the location and the activity of the source are known, that it is outside the body, and that it has to be rotated in order to sample all the necessary projections. Furthermore, the interpretation of measured projection values I is also different. It can be shown easily that the logarithm $\ln(I/I_0)$ represents the projections of the linear attenuation coefficient μ. Thus any of the reconstruction methods discussed in the preceding section can be applied to the data of the transmission study or, more specifically, to $\ln(I/I_0)$ to form an image $\mu(x, y)$ of the attenuation coefficient. PET scanners are normally equipped with the necessary hard- and software for transmission measurements (see "Corrections and Processing" below). It is only recently with the evolution of multiheaded cameras that SPECT systems are set up to perform transmission measurements in clinical routine (see below).

All practical realizations of calculated attenuation correction assume a constant and known attenuation coefficient. Hence they are also termed *uniform attenuation corrections*. Many approximate methods have been proposed for calculated attenuation correction. Due to the simplification by uniform attenuation, they are relatively easy to implement, fast, and yield reasonable compensation so long as the underlying assumptions are not violated too much. Their most successful representative is Chang's method (8). Introduced in 1978, it is still predominant in SPECT studies because it combines speed and performance. Its essence can be outlined as follows: Given homogeneous attenuation, the number of counts that a point source contributes to a projection is only dependent on its activity and on its distance from the body surface. Some mathematical transformations of this fact reveal that reconstruction and attenuation correction can be separated. This means that first an uncompensated image is reconstructed by filtered backprojection. A correction factor is then calculated for each image point. It must compensate for the attenuation of that point's activity along all projection directions. Therefore, it is not surprising that it is the reverse of the average attenuation from that point to the body surface in all directions. Multiplication of the image with the correction factors yields the attenuation-compensated image. In order to calculate the correction factors, the distance from each point to the body outline must be known. It can be obtained either by applying a preset threshold value to the attenuated image or from a human observer to which the image is presented and who delineates the contour. While Chang's method is exact for point sources, it deteriorates for extended sources (36). This flaw can be reduced by an iteration of successive correction steps. Due to noise amplification, only one or two iterations are applied in practical situations. In clinical use, this compensation method is quoted for yielding good qualitative information, especially for focal distributions and cold lesions. Figure 17 shows a comparison between the images of a homogeneous disk phantom reconstructed without and with calculated attenuation correction.

The inclusion of attenuation coefficients into reconstruction is different for SPECT and PET. Since it is simplified for PET due to the coincidence principle, we will outline solutions aimed at SPECT in what follows. Chang's method can be adapted to include nonuniform attenuation coefficients known from a transmission study. To this end, the calculation of the correction factors is modified. Thus the differing attenuations of intervening pixels along the projection paths are taken into account when calculating the average attenuation for a pixel activity. Various types of iterative methods are also suitable for including the measured attenuation maps. Here they are used when calculating the projections of an activity distribution estimate, which are then compared with the measured profiles. The resulting error profiles are then backprojected, again taking the attenuation coefficients into account. They represent corrections that are applied to the previous activity estimates to form better estimates.

Although measured attenuation correction represents the best solution to the attenuation problem in theory, several problems exist in its practical application. The transmission study adds radiation exposure to the patient. Unless the emission and transmission studies are done simultaneously, the examination is prolonged at the cost of patient comfort. Noise present in the transmission study propagates into the corrected images. Therefore, the statistics of the transmission study must be good enough to allow for reliable estimation of the attenuation coefficients. Hence the duration of the transmission measurement is comparable with that of the emission study. A further concern raised in separated emission and transmission studies is the potential mismatch of their respective images due to patient movement. In this case, an inadequate attenuation compensation will be applied, resulting in distorted rather than corrected images.

Much can be expected from hybrid compensation methods that are now being explored. They combine the advantages of measured and calculated attenuation compensation. A transmission study is performed, which may be relatively short. However, the attenuation coefficients resulting from the transmission study reconstruction are not used directly for compensation. Rather, the image of attenuation coefficients is first analyzed with the aim to assign each of the pixels to one of a set of predefined tissue types, such as air, lung, or soft tissue. Since the attenuation coefficients are known for these tissues, a new ''segmented'' attenuation map can be formed by replacing the experimental values with the mapped ideal values. The segmented attenuation map, which contains only reasonable attenuation coefficients, is then used for attenuation compensation. This hybrid method in combination with simultaneous transmission and emission measurements promises to make quantitative imaging of the whole body feasible (23).

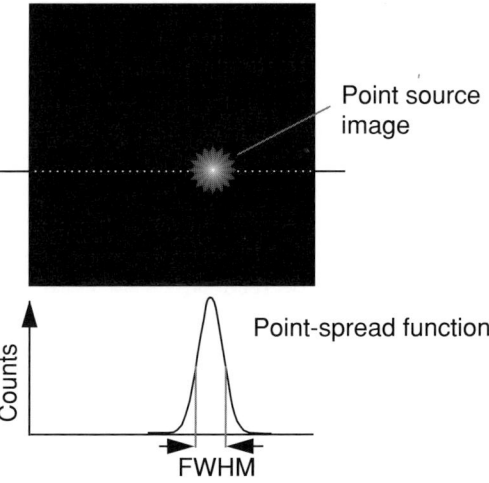

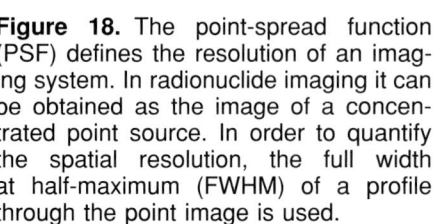

Figure 18. The point-spread function (PSF) defines the resolution of an imaging system. In radionuclide imaging it can be obtained as the image of a concentrated point source. In order to quantify the spatial resolution, the full width at half-maximum (FWHM) of a profile through the point image is used.

Effect of Scatter. A photon that is deflected from its original direction by one or more scatterings is absent from the projection ray it belongs to. If it is lost at all, either because it is completely absorbed, because it misses the detector, or because its energy has fallen below the discrimination level, attenuation compensation will do the required correction. However, if its loss of energy is not severe, and if it reaches a detector in accordance with collimation, it is counted as an event on another than true projection ray. In a typical brain or cardiac SPECT study these ''scattered'' events can amount to 20% to 40% of the total counts (43). Since scattered events would be attributed to wrong locations, they must be removed from the projection data. If not, scatter manifests itself mainly as a high background in the image that deteriorates contrast.

Similar to attenuation, scatter increases with the source depth. In fact, the nature of scatter in a study depends in a very complex manner both on the composition of the body itself and on the acquisition setup, namely, collimator and detector characteristics. Therefore, scatter is a 3D spatially varying phenomenon or, in other words, *nonstationary* (7).

Performance Characteristics of Nuclear Imaging Systems

There are a number of criteria used to describe the performance of imaging systems in NM. The *spatial resolution* gives a measure for the degree of detail the final reconstructed image provides and hence the size of lesions that might potentially be detected. However, in the context of radionuclide imaging, resolution is not the only prerequisite for a clinically useful image. An equally important requirement is *good image statistics.* Since the radioactive decay is a Poisson random process, the number of decays for a given activity concentration is only a statement about the average number of counts expected in a certain time interval. The actual number, however, fluctuates about this average, with the probability given by the Poisson distribution. The higher the average number—representing more activity—the relatively narrower are the fluctuations and the more accurately the activity can be measured. Therefore, as many of the decays in the radionuclide as possible must be detected and reflected in the image. To describe this behavior of the counting statistics, several notions are important, namely, the efficiency, the sensitivity, and the count-rate behavior. Together with the resolution properties, these concepts are important when judging the image content in functional studies.

Spatial Resolution. The *spatial resolution* of an imaging system describes how fine the details are that can be separated. Most common measures of resolution are based on the system's *point-spread function* (PSF). In the case of NM, the point-spread function can be explained as follows: Consider an object consisting of an ideal point source. The image of this object will at least be one pixel wide. Normally, it will rather be a spot of several pixels, brightest in the center and gradually darker away from the center. This image function is the point-spread function. Obviously, the better the resolution, the more concentrated is the spot. If a profile through the spot is plotted, we obtain a one-dimensional PSF, as shown in Fig. 18. Now the resolution can be defined as the width within which the PSF drops to half the maximal value, called *full width at half maximum* (FWHM). The PSF need not be symmetrical, so there may be different spatial resolutions in different directions, as, for example, in PET. If the object consists of two point sources, just the distance FWHM apart, there is a fair chance that they will be separated in the image. Figure 19 shows that this is the case for a Gaussian PSF.

For the evaluation of imaging systems, the spatial resolution is measured in exactly the way described by placing a point source at different places within the field of view and plotting the point-spread function. Often it is convenient to use a thin-line source (pin source) instead of a point source. Then the PSF can be evaluated all along the line, although only orthogonal to the line's extension.

Sensitivity, Dead Time. The *sensitivity* of an imaging system describes how well the radioactive decays in the tracer distribution are exploited to form image counts. It is defined by the number of counts per unit time detected by the device for a unit activity in the source and commonly expressed as counts per second per megabequerel. Put in other words, sensitivity is given by the number of detected counts divided by the number of decays in the source. According to the different stages in the detection process, there

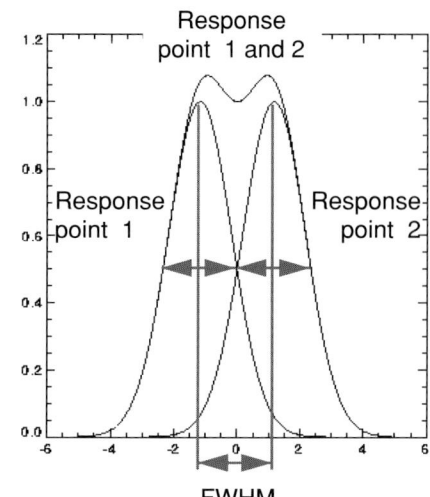

Figure 19. Resolution for a hypothetical system with Gaussian PSF. Two point sources are positioned exactly FWHM apart. They can be differentiated in the resulting image, although with little contrast.

are several components affecting sensitivity. Since a source radiates isotropically into all directions, the first issue is how much of the solid angle around the source is covered by the detector. If a collimator is mounted in front of the camera, only a fraction of the photons defined by the collimator efficiency will reach the crystal surface. Only a fraction of these impinging photons will be absorbed in the crystal, depending on the crystal material, its thickness, and the photon energy. From the resulting events, only a fraction will fall into the photopeak; the others will be rejected depending on the setting of the discrimination window.

Some of the events are also lost because the system is still busy processing a previous event. The probability for this situation increases with higher activities so that relatively more events are lost due to system dead time. In the extreme case, the system can even be saturated (Fig. 20). This means that any further increase in the activity will not increase the detected count rate but may even decrease it. Any effort to quantify the activity must compensate for this behavior, which depends on the actual layout of the system.

Figure 20. The percentage of system dead time denotes the fraction of time during which the system is busy processing and hence misses incoming events. The example given in (**A**) shows its dependence on the activity in the field of view. As a result of dead time, the number of detected counts does not rise linearly with the activity. (**B**) A saturated state may be reached after which further increase of the activity causes a drop in the detected count rate.

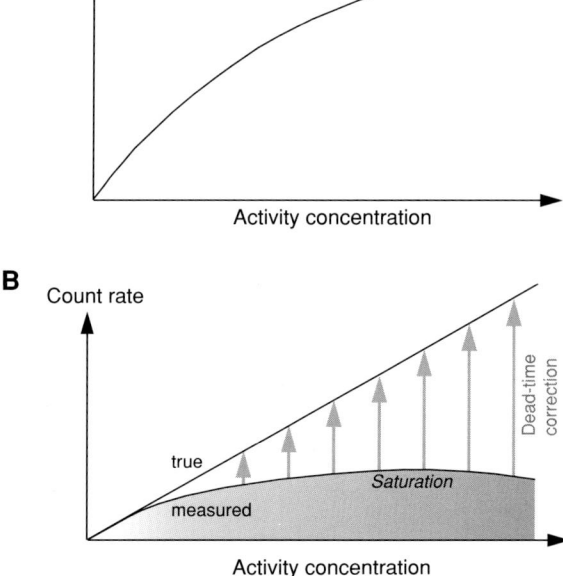

Signal-to-Noise Ratio (SNR). Both the sensitivity and the spatial resolution together constitute the *signal-to-noise ratio,* which is described as the relative strength of the desired information and the noise. The information is the image contrast of a feature such as a lesion. It is defined by the difference in the average pixel value in the lesion and the background divided by the background average (36). If the lesion is small compared with the spatial resolution (FWHM of the PSF), the contrast is reduced because the high lesion activity is blurred into the neighborhood by the detector response.

The derivation of the noise characteristics in a reconstructed image pixel is not straightforward. It is important to note that contrary to what would be expected according to strict Poisson statistics, the noise in an image pixel is not directly related to the square root of the reconstructed counts in that pixel (5). The reason is that the noise at different locations gets correlated by the reconstruction process. However, as a guideline, the following dependencies can be stated for the relative noise (percent root-mean-square noise): It decreases in proportion to the square root of the total number of detected events in the entire slice. Hence four times the counts (or sensitivity) halves the relative noise. Furthermore, it goes up almost linearly with the number of image pixels, but it also depends on the reconstruction algorithm used (41).

Uniformity, Linearity. An obvious requirement for an imaging system is that the image of an object be independent of its position in the field of view. This would be the case if the detector had the same response to a point source throughout the field of view. Real systems, however, do not provide such a uniform response. The most important reasons are variations in the response of the photomultipliers, affecting both the energy estimate and the event localization. As a result of variations in energy output, a different measure of radioactivity is obtained when placing a source at different locations. Nonlinearity in the position detection distorts measurements such as an area or volume of interest. These problems are severe. Even for well-tuned and well-adjusted systems, a nonuniformity of 10% must be expected (38). However, the variations in uniformity can be assessed in calibration measurements and used to derive correction factors. If these are accounted for during image generation, nonuniformity can be reduced to about 3%. Due to the impact of uniformity on image quality, these calibrations, called *normalization* in PET, have to be repeated in regular intervals.

Quantitation

So far the principles have been outlined as to how an image of a radionuclide distribution can be obtained. The question of quantitation, then, is: What does the numerical value attributed to an image pixel really mean? The answer clearly depends on the system specifications, as well as on the acquisition and processing steps taken. With PET and, recently, with SPECT also, absolute quantitation is feasible, as we will see in succeeding sections. *Absolute quantitation* means that each image pixel provides the average activity concentration in the corresponding body tissue. Hence the quantitative image pixel dimension is in megabequerels per milliliter.

The events detected during an acquisition are just a fraction of the true number of events that actually reflect the tracer distribution. For quantitative imaging, therefore, the true number of events must be estimated from the measured events and knowledge of system performance. Each loss in an acquisition step must be counterbalanced exactly by a compensation. Let us take the example of losses due to system dead time. There are basically two methods to estimate dead time, and they must be adapted to each individual system. Either it can be derived from the detected count rate and a model of the processing components, or it can be measured electronically. Then, from knowing the percentage time where the system was not dead and the number of accepted events, the true count rate can be calculated (see Fig. 20).

After all the compensations have been done and the image has been reconstructed, the pixel values are still in counts per second per milliliter and not yet in megabequerels per milliliter. Rather, it first must be scaled by a calibration factor reflecting the efficiency of the whole system. To obtain the calibration factor, a uniform phantom with a known activity concentration is measured and reconstructed with all compensations. The efficiency is then given by the count rate in the image by the known activity, each in a unit volume.

Since absolute quantitation provides absolute concentrations, the results of different studies, even among different subjects, can be compared. This is certainly an advantage, especially for scientific applications. In many clinical questions, however, this capability is not required, and relative quantitation is much more relevant. *Relative quantitation* means that one region can be compared with a reference, be it contralateral tissue in the same study or from a database of normals.

Single Photon Emission Computed Tomography (SPECT)

SPECT systems are able to measure the 3D distribution of a radionuclide. All the theoretical background to understand them has already been discussed. The available commercial systems essentially represent engineering solutions aimed at specific objectives. Therefore, the different components of SPECT systems shall only be presented briefly, pointing out the advantages and limitations of some of the implementations. Then the general limitations of SPECT systems, particularly with respect to quantitation, are summarized.

System Components and Acquisition

SPECT systems use the principle of acquiring planar projections of the body part under investigation at many angles. From the resulting projection data, images of the activity distribution within the body are reconstructed. There are basically two solutions to obtaining the required projections. So-called multidetector systems consist of a closed ring or polygon of detectors into which the body section of interest is placed. To date these systems are dedicated to brain studies and not in widespread use. The favored solution is a gantry with one or more movable heads. In fact, apart from the mobile systems, practically all gamma cameras nowadays are capable of SPECT acquisition.

Acquisition Overview. Let us go through the different steps of a SPECT study with a multicamera system, as shown in Fig. 21. In the preparation phase, a collimator is

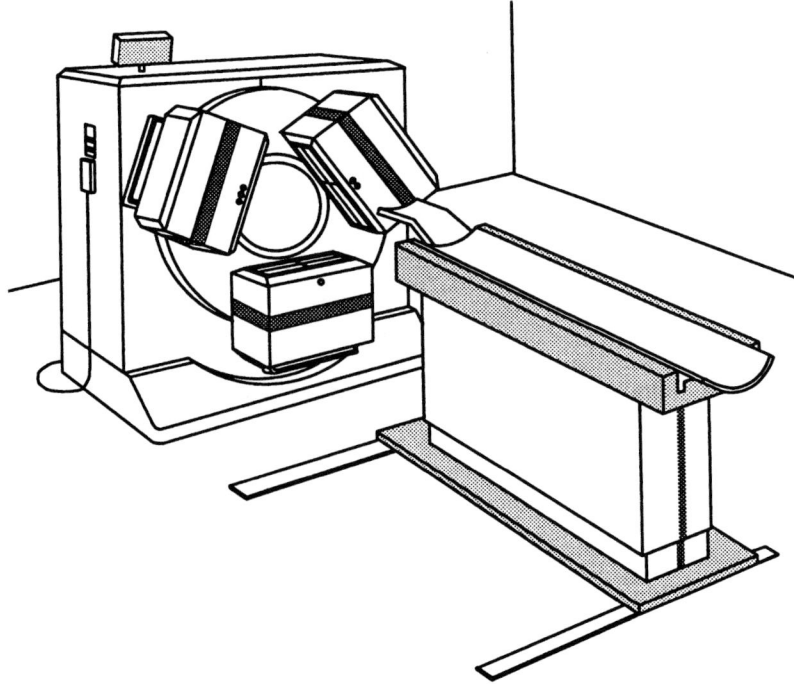

Figure 21. A SPECT camera with three detector heads (Picker Prism 3000).

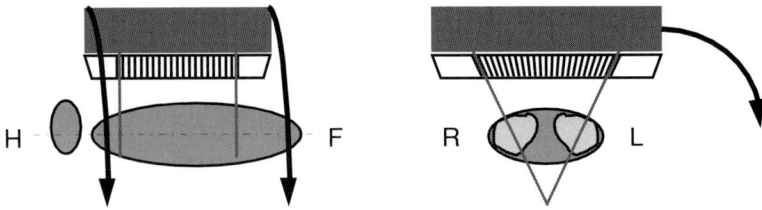

Figure 22. Fan-beam collimator with a focused geometry that increases the sensitivity for small objects. Fan-beam collimators are used mainly for cardiac and brain SPECT studies.

mounted onto each of the camera heads. Its characteristics must be adapted to the study performed. Before—or in parallel—the radiopharmaceutical is administered. The patient is placed on a movable bed and positioned appropriately so that the body section to be investigated lies in the field of view of the system. Since the camera heads must be moved around the body in order to acquire the projections, their orbit is specified. The photopeak of the detected photons is measured, and the discrimination window is adjusted to sort out the scattered photons by their reduced energies. Then the acquisition is started. The heads move along the prescribed orbits and measure projections at the angular positions defined by the acquisition protocol. The projection data are corrected for system imperfections by applying compensation maps generated in a system calibration for each collimator-detector pair. After all projections have been acquired and corrected, images can be reconstructed for body slices orthogonal to the detectors. Some of the system components mentioned as well as special acquisition protocols are discussed in what follows.

Collimators. Several criteria must be observed for the choice of the optimal collimator. The septal walls must be thick enough to prevent penetration by oblique photons. Hence they must be adapted to the photon energy of the radionuclide used. At the low end of the energies used ($\leq$140 keV), the collimator septa may be so thin that they can hardly be manufactured (LE = low-energy collimator) (26). At high energies ($>$300 keV), the septa must be so thick that it is difficult to design collimators that are not visible in the image (HE = high-energy collimator). At the same time, the collimator geometry must compromise between sensitivity and spatial resolution. It can either favor high resolution (HR) or high sensitivity (HS). Today it is well-established practice to favor high-resolution collimation with SPECT (22). In an attempt to minimize the sensitivity loss that occurs at high-resolution collimation, specialized SPECT collimators were developed using convergent rather than parallel holes. Notable examples are cone-beam and fan-beam collimators, the latter of which is illustrated in Fig. 22. They typically increase the sensitivity by 50% to 100% at the same spatial resolution (43). Data acquired with these collimators require dedicated reconstruction algorithms taking into account the special projection geometry. Since convergent collimators have a reduced field of view, they are most suited for brain and cardiac imaging.

Orbits and Acquisition Angles. There are two issues related to the camera orbit around the body, namely, its shape and the extent of the angular sampling (360° or 180°). In order to understand the impact of the orbit shape, it is important to recall that the spatial resolution is best at the collimator face and deteriorates linearly with increasing distance, an effect that is less pronounced for thicker collimators. It is therefore obvious to expect a resolution gain when minimizing the collimator-to-body distance along the orbit. To this end, modern cameras offer not only the smallest circle orbit around the body but also elliptical orbits, which are more adequate in most studies except for the head, and even orbits following closely the body contour. These approaches require both sophisticated and robust hardware and adapted reconstruction algorithms. It is still debated under what conditions image quality is really improved by noncircular orbits, since artefacts may arise due to the spatially variant detector response (36).

With regard to the angular sampling, it is interesting to note that transmission CT only requires 180° acquisition because the "back" 180° is equivalent to the "front" 180°

data. With SPECT, however, factors such as variations in tissue attenuation and detector resolution cause significant differences in the front- and backprojections. Therefore, it is commonly assumed that complete angular sampling is required for accurate reconstruction. Nonetheless, it has been found that in some cases SPECT images with better contrast can be obtained by using only 180° data. This protocol is commonly applied for cardiac studies, where the posterior projection data would be attenuated severely (22).

Step-and-Shoot and Continuous Acquisition Modes. Most SPECT systems acquire the projections in a "step-and-shoot" fashion as they orbit the patient. The camera moves to a projection angle, stops, measures, then moves about the angular increment, stops, measures again, and so on. The time of moving takes 2 to 4 seconds, during which the counts are lost. Continuous acquisition allows one to avoid this sensitivity loss. Thus the camera rotates continuously and slowly while always acquiring counts, which are rebinned into an appropriate number of projections. This approach, of course, introduces a blurring, smaller blurring if more projection angles are used.

A guideline can be given for the least number N of required angles, depending on the camera resolution Δx and the size of the patient D, namely,

$$N \geq \frac{\pi D}{\Delta x} \tag{12}$$

for 360° acquisition (36). If fewer projections are used, radial streak artefacts may occur in the periphery of the reconstructed image. The image pixel size should be smaller than $\Delta x/2$.

Dual-Isotope Studies. A scintillation detector is able to measure the energy of the incident photon. This property can be exploited in several ways for radionuclide imaging. As we have seen, it can be used to separate "good" from "bad," namely, scattered, counts by setting an energy window around the photopeak of the radionuclide being imaged. Other applications are in scatter and attenuation compensation, as discussed later, and in dual-isotope imaging. Thus two radiopharmaceuticals tracing different processes are applied simultaneously. They must be labeled with distinct radionuclides with their photopeaks at sufficiently separated energies. In this situation, an energy window can be placed over each of the photopeaks, and every count is either rejected or attributed to one of the tracers. The acquisition results in two data sets, which when reconstructed provide two aligned image sets. A problem that has to be considered in dual-isotope studies is the so-called crosstalk. This means that a fraction of the photons originating from the higher-energy nuclide lose sufficient energy by scattering and are erroneously detected in the photopeak of the lower-energy nuclide. These photons cause an elevation of the background in the reconstructed image of the low-energy nuclide. However, there are compensation methods that try to estimate what the fraction of these scattered photons is, thus allowing one to recover the unscattered fraction and to avoid the high background level.

Transmission in the Presence of Emission. The most important application of the dual-isotope principle in SPECT is simultaneous emission and transmission imaging. While scientific implementations have been reported for some time, commercial solutions are now being introduced, usually as multiheaded systems. Let us consider a typical three-head camera system, as illustrated in Fig. 23. One of its detectors is (nonexclusively) used for the transmission measurement (9). This transmission detector is equipped with a fan-beam collimator, in the focus of which a thin line source is mounted. It is collimated in a way that the unscattered photons are not able to reach the emission detectors. Exploiting the high sensitivity of the converging collimator, this arrangement allows transmission measurements with relatively low activities. The collimators of the emission detectors may be parallel or also convergent. During the acquisition, both the transmission and the emission photons are measured simultaneously as the heads rotate about the body. After completion, first the attenuation coefficients are reconstructed from the transmission data; they are then used in an iterative reconstruction to calculate attenuation-compensated emission images.

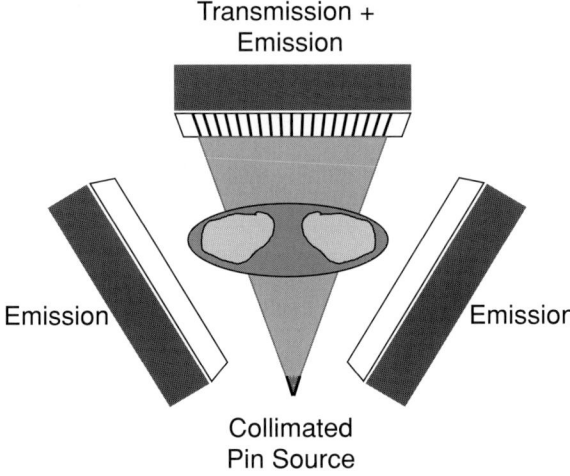

Figure 23. Simultaneous acquisition of emission and transmission data with a triple-headed camera, as described in the text. The transmission data are reconstructed into attenuation coefficients. These are used in an iterative reconstruction to compensate for attenuation in the emission data.

This simple description of transmission in the presence of emission should not suggest that it is easy to implement. Several issues have to be coped with. One is the crosstalk between the emission and the transmission measurement. Due to the detector arrangement, the emission photons can freely enter the transmission detector. The unscattered ones can be sorted out directly, provided that the photopeaks of the nuclides in the transmission source and the tracer are sufficiently separated (Fig. 24). On the other hand, photons from the transmission source may be scattered to eventually hit an emission detector. Crosstalk occurs in the direction from the higher to the lower energy. Hence there may be crosstalk from transmission to emission, the other way around, or even in both directions if a nuclide has more than one photopeak, such as thallium (^{201}Tl, 135- and 167-keV photons plus x-rays at 68.9 to 82.6 keV), depending on the two nuclides used. The amount of crosstalk can be estimated from the acquired data and approximately be compensated for. A further problem is that the reconstructed attenuation map of the transmission study does not exactly represent that of the emission study because photon attenuation is energy dependent. The common solution is to assume that attenuation varies linearly between the emission and transmission energies and to interpolate for the emission attenuation coefficients. While the assumption is justified for most tissues (heart, lungs, thorax), a poor approximation must be expected for bone (12).

Scatter Compensation. As mentioned earlier, scattering is an important effect that significantly affects the quantitative accuracy of the generated images. Any compensation scheme must try to estimate the scatter fraction within the detected events for a projection ray and subtract it. In SPECT studies, the way to obtain information about scattering is to monitor the energy of the photons arriving at the detector. They show a spectrum such as the one shown in Fig. 25. The energies of the scattered photons cover a broad range,

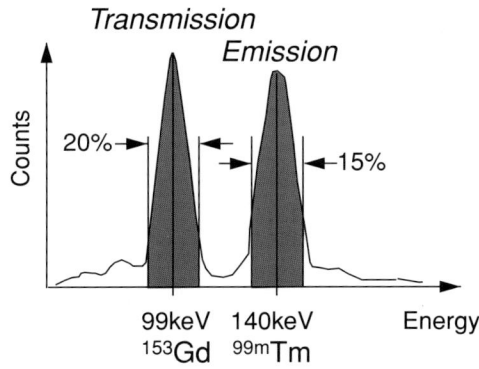

Figure 24. Example dual-isotope energy spectrum in the camera head that detects emission and transmission photons in Fig. 23. The radiopharmaceutical was labeled with ^{99m}Tc, while the line source was filled with ^{153}Gd. The respective photopeaks are sufficiently separated to distinguish emission and transmission counts.

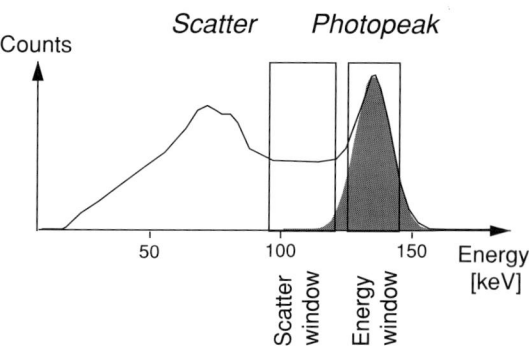

Figure 25. Dual-energy window technique for scatter correction in SPECT. The number of scatter counts in the photopeak window is assumed to be proportional to that in the scatter window. The factor must be determined experimentally for each study type.

extending from the photopeak down to low energies. The unscattered photons are distributed mainly within the photopeak, which should be Gaussian in shape according to the energy resolution of the system. What can be sampled in a specific energy window is the superposition of the scattered and the unscattered contributions. Today, most compensation algorithms use data acquired in two different energy windows, the width and position of which depend on the correction strategy. Their essence shall be illustrated by a brief outline of the most straightforward one, the dual-window technique. In this technique a ''scatter'' window is selected in a region below the photopeak, and it is assumed that its counts solely originate from scatter. It is furthermore assumed that the scatter in the photopeak is proportional to that in the scatter window with a proportionality factor k, which must be determined experimentally. Then the scatter compensation simply consists of subtracting the fraction k of the counts in the scatter window from the counts in the photopeak. Typical values of k range between 0.4 and 0.6 (36).

The drawbacks of dual-window compensation are obvious. Dependence of scatter on the source distribution, the composition of the scattering tissue, and on the detection geometry is neglected. While the obtained images have significantly better contrast, they cannot be considered to be quantitative (7). There are many more refined approaches, ranging to full simulations of the physics within the scattering tissue and the detector. While they are still mainly used in scientific settings, they promise future improvements in quantitative accuracy of clinical SPECT studies.

Limits of Detection and Quantitation in SPECT Systems

There are several limiting factors in SPECT imaging. The minimal acquisition time is relatively long due to the mechanical movements for sampling the required projections. Acquisition times down to 1 minute may be feasible (22), but in clinical studies the durations are rather on the order of 20 minutes to attain the required signal-to-noise ratio. In order to avoid blurring artefacts, it has to be ensured that the changes in the tracer distribution are small compared with the acquisition time. Hence dynamic scanning of tracer uptake is very difficult to perform. Rather, a tracer is applied, and a period is waited until it has reached a relatively stable distribution.

Another issue is spatial resolution, which depends on the collimator and the camera but also on the reconstruction procedure. As a consequence, general figures can hardly be stated. Under the most favorable conditions, a spatial resolution down to 5 mm FWHM is reported (brain imaging with a multidetector system) (36), but in most of the studies it is in the range of 10 to 15 mm. In general, higher resolution entails lower sensitivity. Between these two image characteristics a compromise has to be found. Both together constitute the signal-to-noise ratio. A decrease in sensitivity directly affects the statistical quality of the image, because if fewer counts are detected, the pixel values obtained are relatively less certain.

The signal-to-noise ratio is linked to image quality. When measuring the image quality by the ability of a viewer to discriminate a ''hot'' spot from the background, it has been found that a small improvement in SPECT resolution is equivalent to a large increase in sensitivity (22, 25). This fact guides the use of modern SPECT systems, which have higher sensitivity due to multiple detector heads and lower dead time. Rather than completing a study in a shorter time at the same resolution, the acquisition time is maintained, but higher-resolution collimators are used.

It has been discussed before that there are many effects that distort a reconstructed SPECT image if not properly taken care of. On the one hand, the effects must be minimized by an adequate system design. Examples are collimators optimized for specific study types or the ability of a system to perform transmission measurements. On the other hand, the remaining effects require reconstruction algorithms that include them into the estimation process to provide compensations. Examples are the compensation of attenuation and scatter and the depth dependence of spatial resolution. These techniques, while computationally demanding, improve both quality and quantitative accuracy of SPECT images. However, their effect on clinical diagnosis must still be evaluated.

Positron-Emission Tomography (PET)

PET scanners are designed to assess the distribution of tracers labeled with positron-emitting nuclides such as carbon-11 (^{11}C), nitrogen-13 (^{13}N), and oxygen-15 (^{15}O). Since each positron emission is followed by an annihilation process that produces two 511-keV photons, the SPECT approach described above can be applied to detect the escaping 511-keV photons and to reconstruct images of the tracer distribution. In this approach, however, a large fraction of the photons escaping from the body is absorbed in the mechanical collimator. The problem is especially severe in the situation of PET because high-energy collimators with thick walls are required to stop the 511-keV photons. Luckily, the existence and properties of the two photons per annihilation in PET allow for a much more efficient "electronic" collimation. Its principle, as shown in Fig. 26, is very straightforward: The two 511-keV photons depart almost colinearly from the location of annihilation. Due to their high speed, they almost simultaneously reach two detectors placed at opposite ends of that line. There they cause two events that are practically coincident. Put the other way around, the principle is: If we observe coincident events in two opposing detectors (a "coincidence"), we assume that an annihilation took place somewhere between them on the "line of response" and add a count to that projection ray.

Electronic collimation has several advantages. Most important is its higher sensitivity. Projections in many directions can be acquired simultaneously provided that detectors coupled by coincidence logic cover a large fraction of the solid angle around the patient. Furthermore, electronic collimation makes attenuation correction much easier. The reason

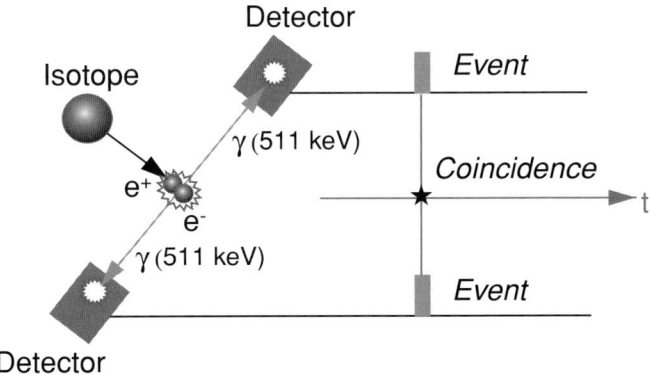

Figure 26. Coincidence principle in PET. The two photons resulting from a positron-electron annihilation travel collinearly. In practical imaging situations they hit the two detectors almost simultaneously, since a path-length difference of 15 cm results in an arrival-time difference of only 1 ns.

is that both photons of an annihilation pair must reach the detectors to create a coincidence event. Hence the total absorber material between them must be penetrated such that attenuation is independent of the position where along the line between the detectors the annihilation happened. On the other hand, electronic collimation also has some disadvantages. Two unrelated photons cause a "random coincidence" if they happen to arrive at the same time in two detectors coupled by coincidence logic. Furthermore, both photons of an annihilation pair must be stopped by the detectors. Thus, if each of the detectors has 80% efficiency of photon detection, the combined efficiency for annihilation detection is only 64%.

Due to electronic collimation, the components of PET system hardware as well as the data-processing steps are somewhat different from the ones used in SPECT imaging. These issues are outlined next.

System Components and Acquisition

Acquisition Overview. In order to introduce the components of a typical PET scanner, let us describe the phases of a simple static PET study with a tracer at equilibrium. First, the positron-emitting radiopharmaceutical is administered to the patient lying on the table. The table is moved such that the organ to be investigated becomes centered in the sensitive volume of the scanner. It is defined by one or several detector rings that are housed in a gantry. Positron-electron annihilation photons leave the body in all directions. Once the acquisition is started, the photons interacting with a detector trigger a whole sequence of processing steps (see Fig. 33). Similar to a gamma camera, the location of the event in the detector and the energy of the incident photon are determined, and an energy window placed around 511 keV is applied in order to exclude scattered photons. If the photon is accepted, it is a likely candidate for an annihilation photon, so it is recorded with its interaction time as a "single" event. Now the coincidence logic tries to find the other photon belonging to the same annihilation. It must have been recorded at almost the same time in one of the opposing detectors. Exact coincidence of the two related events, however, cannot be expected mainly due to statistical components in the detection and processing timing. Therefore, an appropriate time window τ must be defined within which two events are regarded as being "simultaneous." It is normally in the range of 10 to 20 ns (10). If the coincidence logic finds two simultaneous singles, it rates them as a coincidence and passes them to the next processing step. Here, the line on which the annihilation happened is calculated by using the position information of the singles. Since the line belongs to a projection ray, the number of detected emission counts of that projection ray is incremented by one, or stated otherwise, its sinogram value is incremented. It is important to note that there are active projection rays at many angles because the detectors enclose the patient body in a 360° circle (Fig. 27). Conse-

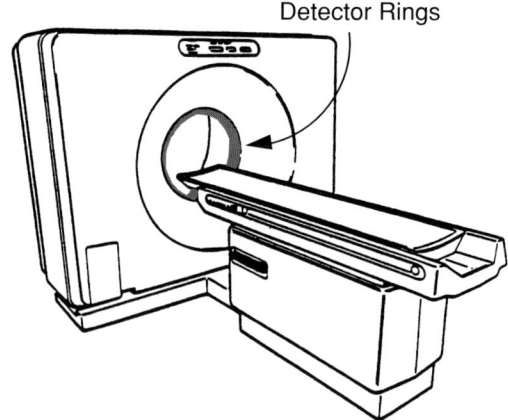

Detector Rings

Figure 27. A whole-body PET system with the detector rings indicated. They represent the sensitive volume within which the organs to be investigated must be positioned.

quently, sufficient projections for a reconstruction are acquired simultaneously. After enough counts have been collected and some corrections have been applied, the projection data are reconstructed yielding transversal images of the tracer distribution.

In order to obtain quantitative images showing activity per volume, the PET system must be calibrated thoroughly. To this end, a set of quality-control procedures must be performed regularly. Furthermore, an attenuation correction must be included in the reconstruction process. As has been discussed in ''Attenuation Correction Methods'' above, the required correction factors can be obtained in a transmission measurement or calculated from the contours of the organs in the field of view.

PET DETECTION AND COINCIDENCE SYSTEM

The most widely used design of the PET detection system is to employ several adjacent rings of BGO scintillation crystals. This design will be discussed briefly, while alternative designs are mentioned in a separate section (see below). The aim of the detection system is to detect each incident 511-keV photon and attribute it to that crystal where it interacted. To this end, the crystals are optically coupled to photomultipliers that convert the scintillation light into electric pulses. Since the phototubes are significantly larger than the crystals used in PET, one photomultiplier normally covers the back of several crystals simultaneously, as shown in Figs. 29 and 30. The pulses of the photomultipliers are used by a position-decoding logic much in the same way as in the Anger camera to estimate the interaction location

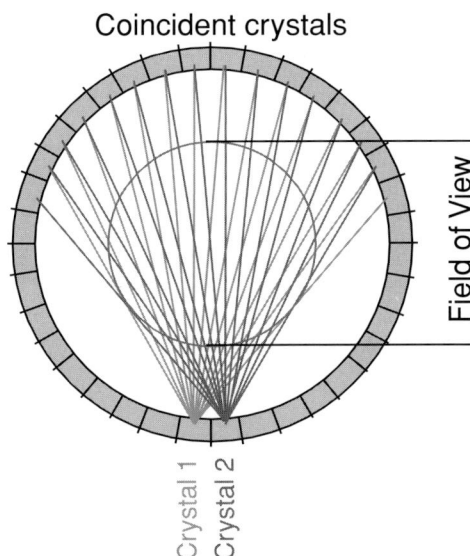

Coincident crystals

Crystal 1
Crystal 2

Field of View

Figure 28. Schematic diagram of a BGO crystal ring used in PET. The coincidence logic relates each crystal to a set of opposing crystals in a treelike structure. Only two of these trees are drawn.

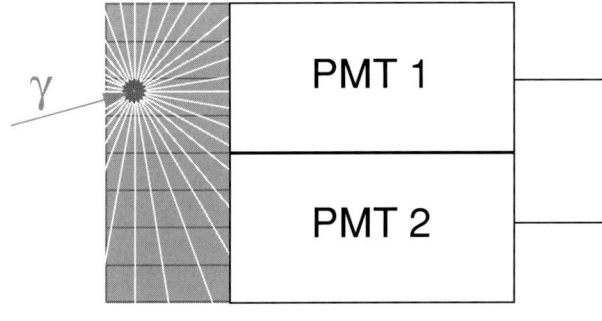

Crystals Photo-multipliers

γ

PMT 1

PMT 2

Figure 29. Formation of detector blocks out of BGO crystals and photomultipliers. Most designs use a many-to-one relationship between the crystals and the PMTs. The scintillation light penetrates from the event location into neighboring crystals. Anger logic is used to locate the crystal where the event happend out of the PMT signals.

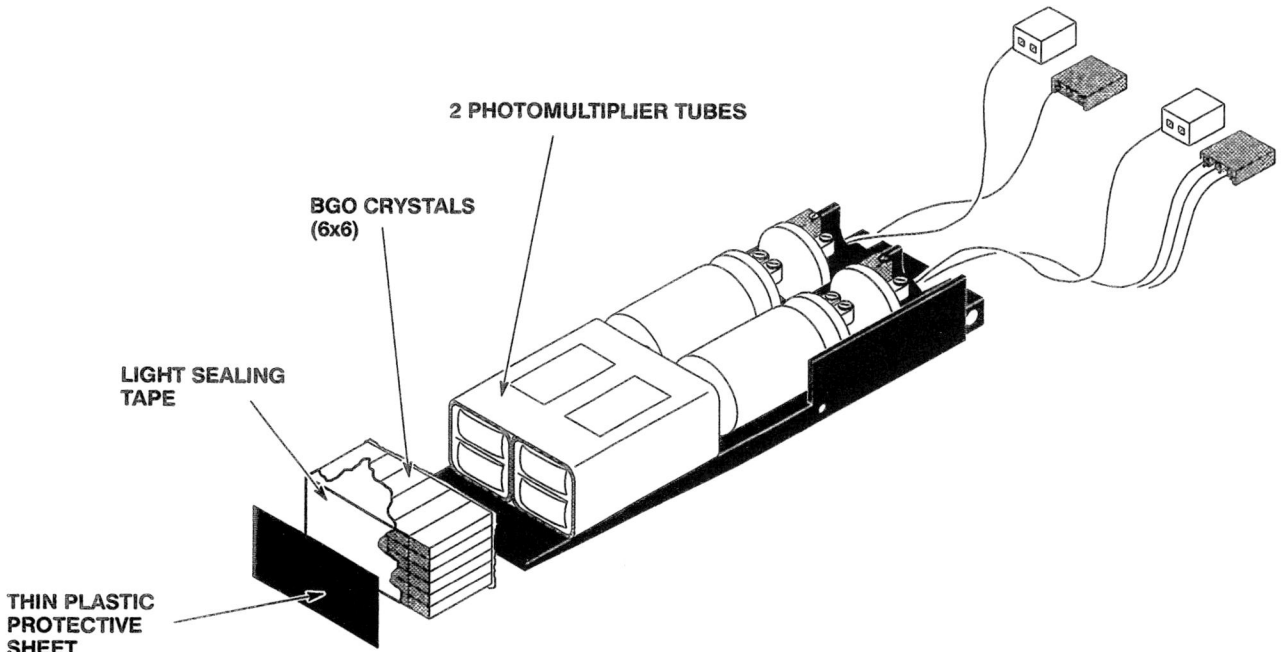

Figure 30. Detector block as employed in the General Electric PET Advance system (2). The crystal dimensions are 4 × 8 × 30 mm in the transaxial, axial, and radial directions.

in the crystals. From the location thus calculated, it is then possible to derive the crystal where the photon most likely entered. It is clear that the localization of an event is more precise if smaller crystals are used. Thus the spatial resolution in the reconstructed image is also improved. If other deteriorating factors are disregarded, the image resolution is approximately equal to half the crystal width (28).

The coincidence logic relates each crystal with a set of opposing crystals, thus defining the lines of response, as shown in Fig. 28. When the coincidence logic is fed by a single event detected in a crystal, it looks for a simultaneous event at the other end of one of the lines of response. More specifically, both events must have happened within the coincidence timing window. In this case, the number of counts is incremented for the projection ray corresponding to that line of response.

A system operating in 2D mode in principle images transaxial planes of the investigated part of the body independently. As indicated in Fig. 31, direct planes and crossplanes can be distinguished. The *direct planes* are defined by the crystal rings, and their images are formed by coincidences among crystals belonging to one ring. The necessity for the *crossplanes* can be seen as follows: Imagine a positron source located close to the axial position of a septum. Only photons emitted strictly vertical to the axial direction will result in a coincidence within a ring. Any inclination will result in two single events belonging to different rings; hence they will not be counted for the direct plane. In contrast, for a source located midway between two septa, there is a certain solid angle within which the photons do not leave the ring. These considerations show that sensitivity is highest in the center of a direct plane and drops toward the plane edge following a triangular shape. Therefore, the crossplanes sample the regions centered at the septal positions by detecting coincidences between crystals of adjacent rings. From Fig. 31 it is clear that the sensitivity profile for these planes is different from that of the direct planes. The rings are separated by tungsten septa that ensure that photons traveling at angles larger than occurring in crossplanes are absorbed. Such photons would increase the load on the detection system without contributing useful information, since coincidences between rings far apart are not considered in 2D mode.

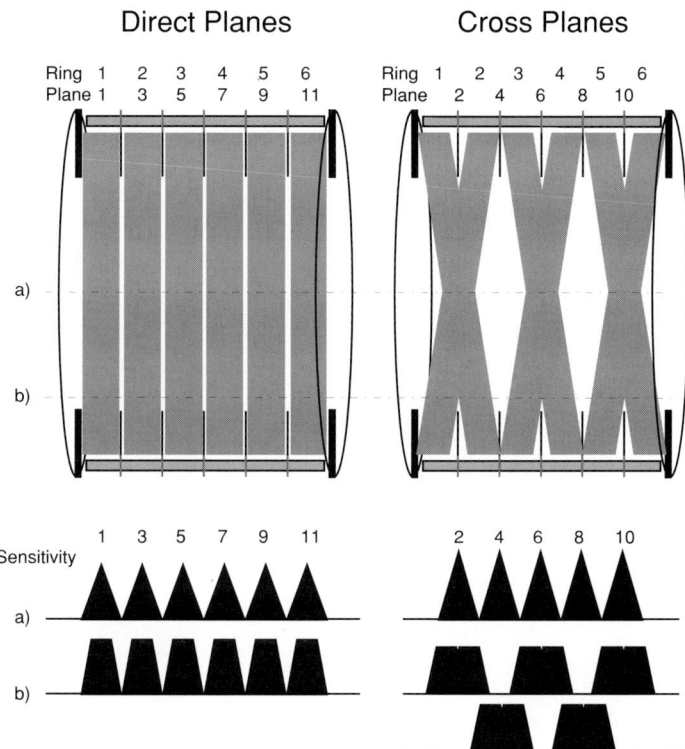

Figure 31. Slice definition of a multiring PET system operating in 2D mode, as described in the text. In high-sensitivity mode, additional coincidences between more distant rings also can be accepted. For instance, coincidences between rings 1 and 3 also would be counted for direct-plane 2.

Corrections and Processing

In order to be quantitative, PET requires careful calibration and correction procedures. All the different degrading effects during the acquisition process must be assessed and compensated for. The overall flow of acquisition and processing is schematically outlined in Fig. 32. This figure shows that three types of data are involved: calibration data describing the static characteristics of system components, correction data describing system performance during the acquisition, and the projection data themselves.

The calibration data are assessed at the time of system setup and at different stages of the quality-control procedures. They include the characteristics of the crystals and the photomultipliers needed in correction steps during event localization and energy discrimination, a "blank scan" used in attenuation correction, and calibration factors to account for differing sensitivities among the slices.

Single events are processed in several steps, and the coincidence events found are collected in the projection data, as summarized in Fig. 33. An acquisition results in the projection data, which are one sinogram per image slice in 2D mode, plus the correction data. In the reconstruction process, several corrections are applied successively to the detected counts per projection ray (Fig. 34). The aim is to recover the true number of counts that would have been detected if there were no degrading effects. It is noteworthy that there are not only effects reducing the number of detected counts such as dead time or attenuation but also effects that erroneously increase them. These are *random coincidences* caused by two unrelated photons hitting two detectors sensitive for coincidences by chance within the coincidence timing window (Fig. 35) and *scattered coincidences,* whereby one annihilation photon has been scattered so that the event is attributed to a wrong line of response (see Fig. 37).

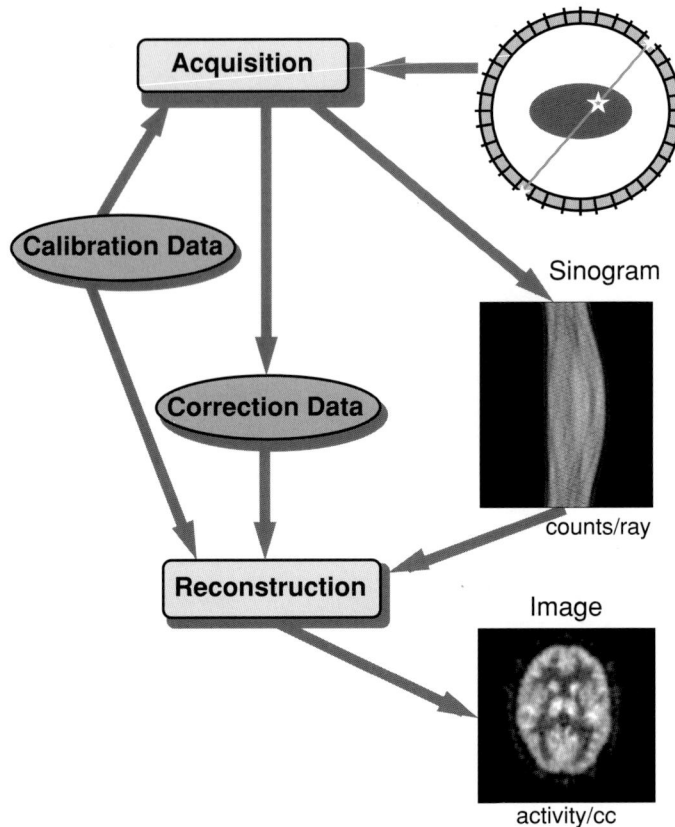

Figure 32. Overall data flow during PET acquisition and processing.

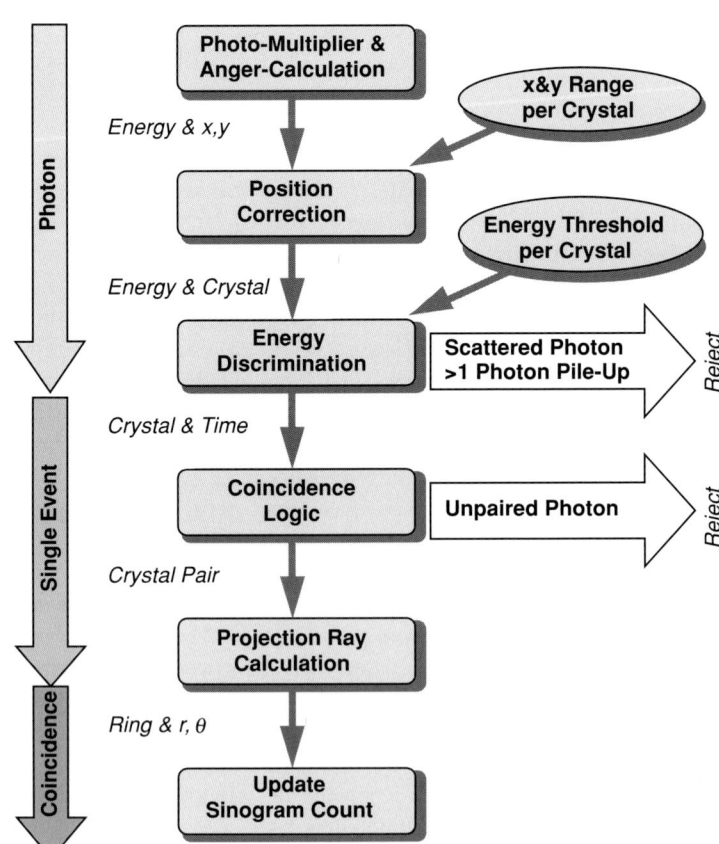

Figure 33. Processing on detection of a single event. The detector block calculates the photon energy and the (*x, y*) position in the crystal array. The position is corrected to account for differences in crystal and PMT characteristics, and the crystal where the event happened is then determined. If the energy is not within the photopeak around 511 keV, the event is discarded. Otherwise, a coincident event is looked for along all relevant lines of response. An unpaired event is discarded, and a coincident pair is forwarded to projection ray calculation, which results in incrementing the corresponding sinogram cell.

CORRECTIONS FOR PET

Figure 34 shows the different stages of corrections and processing of PET coincidence data.

Random Subtraction

If random coincidences (see Fig. 35) are not subtracted, they manifest themselves as a uniformly elevated background level, reducing the image contrast (10). Basically, there are two methods to determine the fraction of random coincidences, either by measurement or by estimation.

The rate of random coincidences can be measured using a second ''delayed'' coincidence circuit in addition to the undelayed, ''prompt'' coincidence circuits (Fig. 36). The prompt circuit yields true plus random coincidences; the delayed circuit yields only random coincidences. It does so by using the same events, but

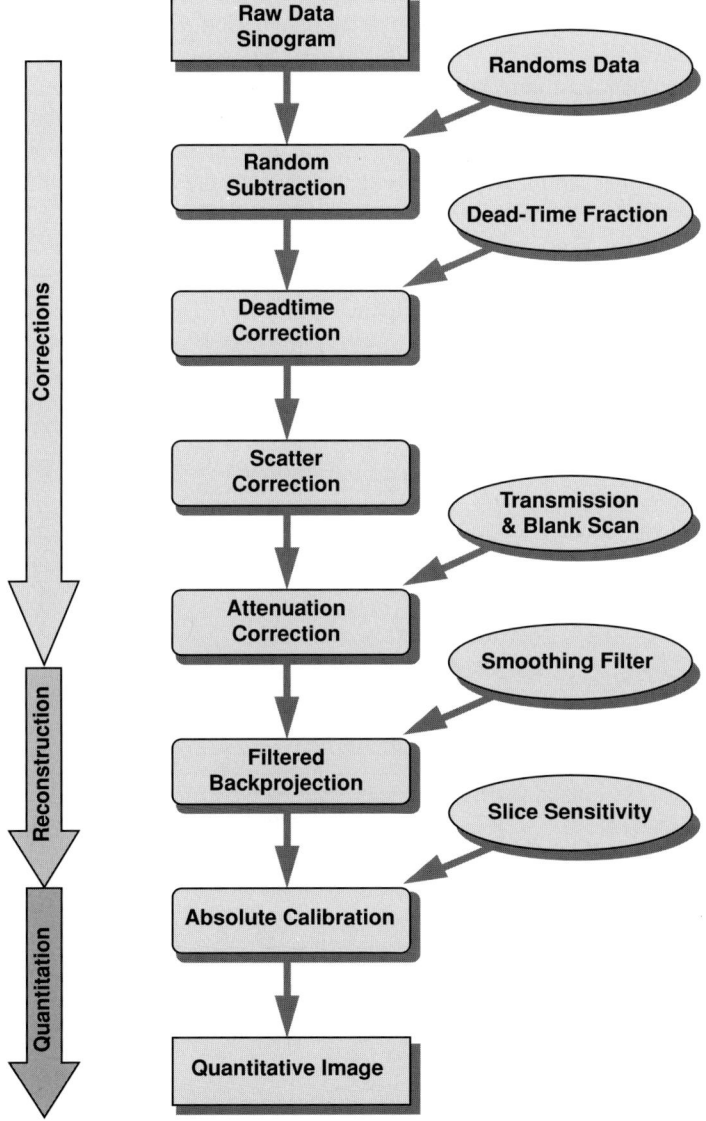

Figure 34. Summary of the processing steps needed to calculate quantitative images out of the coincidence sinograms. All the stages are discussed in the text.

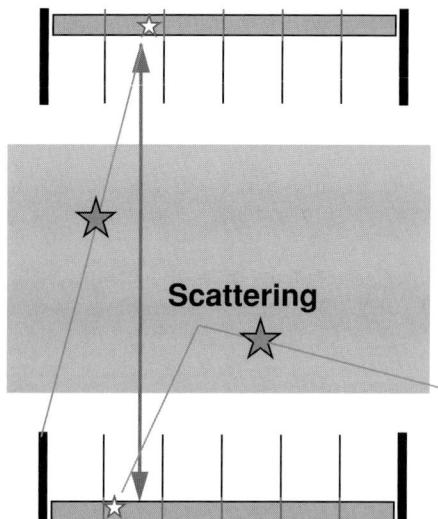

Figure 35. Origin of random coincidences. Two unrelated 511-keV photons hit crystals related by the coincidence logic within the coincidence timing window. Sources are photons that have undergone Compton scattering or which stem from outside the field of view.

with a shifted time tag for one of the detectors sharing a line of response. The time shift is several coincidence windows long, so true coincidences are avoided, and all the coincidences found are by chance. While the randoms thus found in the delayed circuit are not exactly the ones occurring in the prompt circuit, the rate at which they happen is equal for both. Subtraction of the delayed events from the prompts over the acquisition time will therefore yield a good approximation for the number of true coincidences.

The rate of the random coincidences R on a coincidence line also can be estimated. It depends on the rate of the single events in the two related detectors S_1 and S_2 and the duration of the coincidence window τ. The random coincidence rate is then given by the expression

$$R = 2\tau S_1 S_2 \tag{13}$$

Dead Time

The detection system is broken up into different processing units, depending on the actual system layout. These units can operate in parallel. For reasons of space

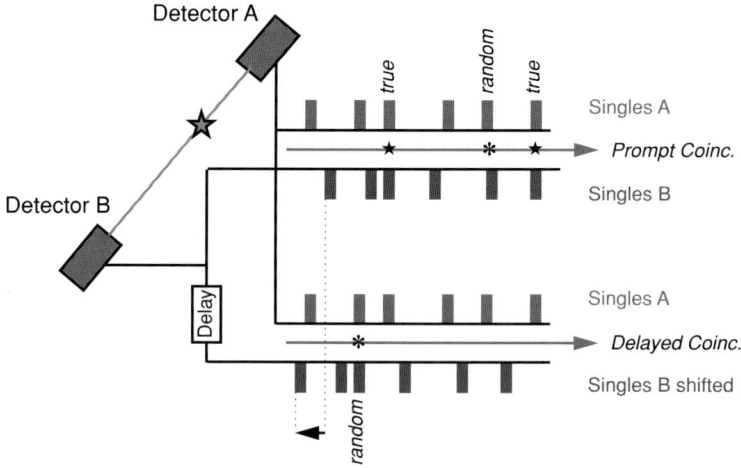

Figure 36. Measuring the rate of random coincidences. Coincidences in the delayed coincidence line are always random; hence they provide an estimate for the random rate in the prompt line (see text).

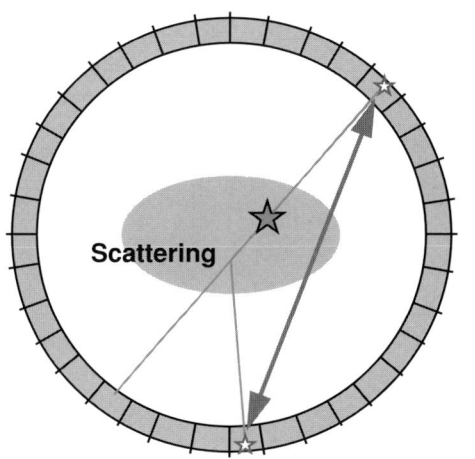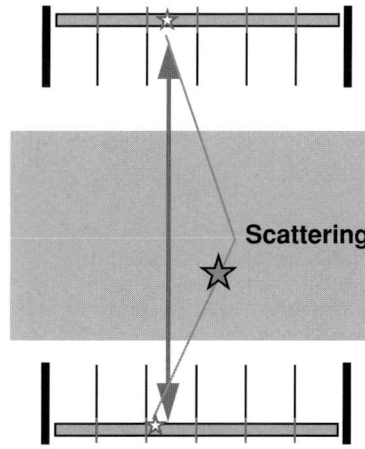

Figure 37. Origin of scattered coincidences. If both annihilation photons are detected, although one has been scattered, the event is localized on a wrong line of response.

and cost, a processing unit normally handles the impulses originating from many crystals. Events in different units therefore can be accepted simultaneously. Within a unit, however, only one event at a time can be processed. If the next event arrives before the processing unit is ready again, the event must be discarded. The fraction of events lost due to system dead time depends on the system layout and the activity in the field of view, i.e., the count rate of the singles (see Fig. 20).

As with random correction, dead-time correction is accurate and can be based on actual measurements or on estimates. To measure the dead time, impulses are injected at regular intervals into the front-end electronics, and the number of accepted events is monitored. The percentage of lost events then reflects the system dead time. For the estimation of dead time, a model of the system behavior as a function of the singles rate is required that must be adequate for the actual system configuration.

The accuracy of the randoms and the dead-time corrections decreases with increasing activity level. At the same time, these events also affect the statistical noise in the reconstructed images. Therefore, the optimal dose of activity administered to a patient must be assessed for a study protocol. It should be in a range where the statistical improvement of higher activities still outweighs the degradation caused by the corrections. In any case, it is recommended that the activity be such that the dead-time losses and the random coincidences remain below 50% (10).

Scatter Correction

Scattered coincidences cannot be distinguished from true coincidences. By definition, they are generated by annihilations for which one of the emitted photons is deflected by Compton scattering but keeps enough energy not to be rejected by energy discrimination (Fig. 37). The fraction of scattered events is high, ranging between 15% and 20% with septa and between 50% and 70% without septa of the total events detected in a study (14). To avoid image distortions, the scatter fraction therefore must first be estimated and then subtracted. There are two reasons for the high level of scatter in PET. One is the limited energy resolution of the detectors, which ranges between 10% and 20%, meaning that the FWHM of the energy determined for the incoming 511-keV photons is 50 to 100 keV. Hence the lower energy threshold is usually set at 300 to 380 keV for BGO detectors and at 400 to 450 keV for NaI(Tl) detectors. The second reason is that 511-keV photons scatter mainly at small angles, thereby only losing a little energy. From all the scattered

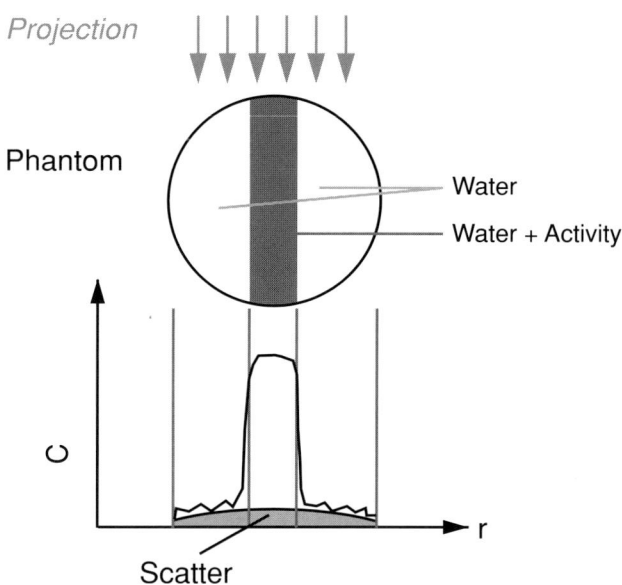

Figure 38. Illustration of the scatter correction by interpolation between scatter tails. The projection profile of the phantom shows counts outside the known border of the activity distribution that originate from scatter. Interpolation between the two tails gives an estimate for the number of scattered counts within the activity. Subtracting the interpolation curve from the profile yields a scatter-corrected profile.

photons, 73% have energies above 350 keV, and 52% have energies above 450 keV (10). This explains why most scattered events are accepted as valid events.

While there is no exact method for estimation of the scatter fraction, several approximate compensation schemes have been described. Only the most simple one shall be described here. It is based on the assumption that scatter is almost constant throughout the object and larger than outside the object. Counts detected outside the body contour represent scatter counts. By interpolating between the two scatter tails on both sides of the body, the scatter within the body therefore can be estimated (Fig. 38). This operation can be performed directly on the sinogram data. It removes 80% to 90% of the scatter events without the danger of subtracting true events and is thus acceptable for most studies (14).

Attenuation Correction

In PET, attenuation reduces the number of counts coming from the center of the body by a factor of 20, and even in head studies, the average reduction is still a factor 4 to 5 (14). Correction for this high loss is therefore desirable, although the images may still be qualitatively interpretable without. Photon attenuation and correction approaches for emission computed tomography have already been discussed.

In PET, however, accurate attenuation correction is much easier to attain. The reason lies in the coincidence principle by which the PET counts are detected and collimated. Let us consider different annihilations happening on a coincidence line and sending their photons along that line (Fig. 39). The photons are either attenuated, i.e., absorbed or scattered, or they are recorded in the detector. Only if both photons pass is an event counted. The probability that a photon reaches the detector depends on the attenuating media between its origin and the detector. If for a moment we assume a constant attenuation coefficient μ and a distance d_1 to penetrate, then the probability of penetration is $e^{-\mu d_1}$. The probability of a coincidence event given an annihilation equals the joint probability that both annihilation photons penetrate. Hence it is given by the product of the individual probabilities:

$$p(\text{coincidence}) = p(\text{single}_1)\, p(\text{single}_2) = e^{-\mu d_1} e^{-\mu d_2} = e^{-\mu D} \qquad (14)$$

where d_1 and d_2 are the path lengths of the two photons in tissue and D is the total

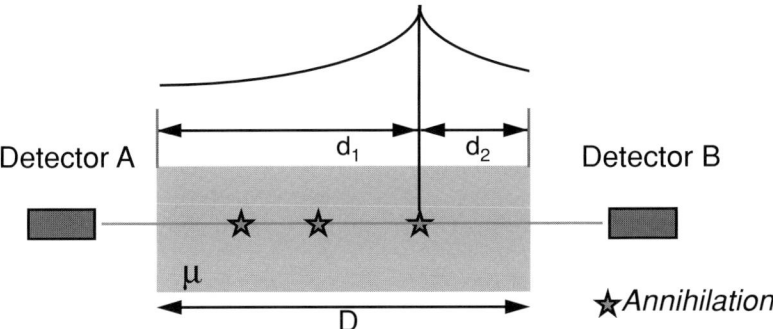

Figure 39. In PET, attenuation is constant along a line, contrary to SPECT. Because both annihilation photons must penetrate, the only quantity that matters for attenuation is the total absorber material between the two detectors (see text). Hence the attenuation is $e^{-\mu D}$.

absorber thickness. This result means that attenuation is only determined by the total absorption along a coincidence line and that it is independent of the position on the line where the annihilation happens. It is important to note that this is a general result that holds exactly in the stated way even if the attenuation coefficient is not constant.

As we have just shown, the number of counts detected on a coincidence line is reduced by the factor $e^{-\mu D}$. Attenuation correction therefore means to determine $e^{-\mu D}$ and to multiply the count number by $e^{\mu D}$, the *attenuation correction factor* (ACF). With measured attenuation correction, these factors—one for each coincidence line—are obtained by two acquisitions, a *blank scan* and a *transmission scan.* The blank scan is performed routinely in the morning before patient scans start. It is a transmission scan without an object in the field of view. In this way, one or more transmission sources are rotated about the field of view, and the coincidences for all lines of response are collected (Fig. 40). For a specific coincidence line, the (unattenuated) number of resulting counts is N_0. The same measurement is repeated in the transmission study, with the only difference that now the patient body to be investigated by the emission study is in the field of view. In this case, the number of collected counts is reduced by the same attenuation that will be effective during the emission study, so what is measured is given by $N_0 e^{-\mu D}$. Division of blank by transmission counts therefore yields the ACF. To obtain all the desired ACFs

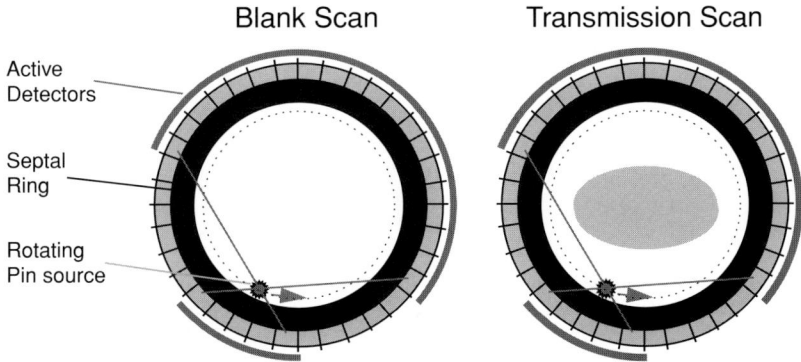

Figure 40. Measured attenuation correction in PET requires two acquisitions. In a blank scan a pin source is rotated around the field of view, and the unattenuated coincidences are measured. In the transmission measurement the attenuated coincidences are acquired with the organ in place that is to be investigated in an emission study. The ratio of blank-to-transmission coincidences provides the correction factors needed to correct the emission coincidences for self-attenuation within the patient tissue.

at once, the sinograms of the blank scan [blank(r,θ)] are divided by those of the transmission scan [transmission (r,θ)]:

$$\mathrm{ACF}(r,\ \theta) \ = \ \frac{\mathrm{blank}(r,\ \theta)}{\mathrm{transmission}(r,\ \theta)} \tag{15}$$

Attenuation then simply amounts to multiplying the emission sinograms by the ACF sinograms.

Absolute Calibration

After all corrections have been performed and the resulting sinograms have been reconstructed, usually by filtered backprojection, images of the reconstructed counts in transverse slices are obtained. They are transformed into images of the average count rate (in counts per second) by dividing the count numbers by the acquisition duration. These images are almost quantitative. The only missing correction is for the differing sensitivities of the slices, meaning that the same activity concentration produces differing count rates when imaged in different slices. Due to the different number of coincidence lines, it is obvious that the sensitivity differs for the direct and the cross slices (see Fig. 31), but there are also differences among the slices of either type. In order to compensate for this behavior, the reconstructed counts within each slice are multiplied by a corresponding calibration factor. These factors can be obtained in a system calibration acquisition using a homogeneous phantom of known activity concentration and geometry. It is reconstructed with all corrections. Since the geometry of the phantom is known, an accurate calculated attenuation correction can be applied. The calibration factor per slice is then given by the activity concentration in the phantom (MBq/cc) by the average count rate within the slice.

3D Acquisition

The situation is different for multiring PET systems operating in 3D mode without septa for restricting the angles of the incident photons. Here, coincidences between other than neighboring rings are also accepted to exploit as much information as possible. As Fig. 41 illustrates, the 3D approach has a potential for many more lines of response and hence coincidences. As a consequence, the sensitivity and axial sampling are improved. On a typical system, the number of true coincidences increases by a factor 5 to 8. The improvement is largest in the center of the axial field of view, dropping toward the edge. At the same time, however, the number of scattered coincidences also increases by a

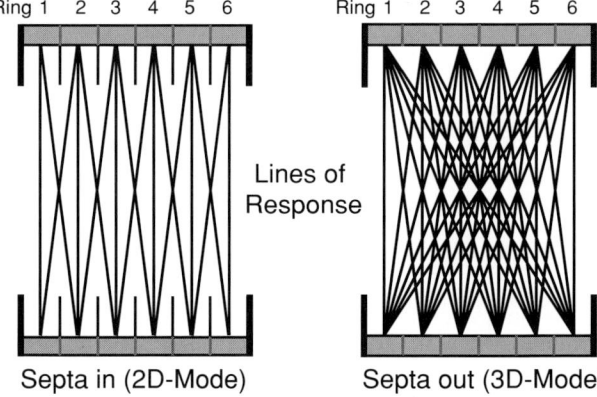

Figure 41. Lines of response (LOR) of a multiring PET scanner in 2D and 3D modes. As the septa are retracted, the number of LORs increases drastically. The effect is largest in the center of the axial field of view and disappears toward the edges.

Table 2. *Properties of positron emitters*

Isotope	$T_{1/2}$ (min)	d (mm)	FWHM (mm)
^{11}C	20.4	4.1	0.28
^{13}N	10	5.4	0.39
^{15}O	2.1	8.2	1.05
^{18}F	109.7	2.4	0.22
^{68}Ga	68.3	~10.0	1.4
^{82}Rb	1.3	>20	2.6

factor of about 3 because there are no septa absorbing angled photons. In the outermost planes the signal-to-noise ratio therefore may be degraded, because the number of co-incidence lines and hence the true events is not increased but the number of wrong coincidences is (10).

Evaluation of the performance of a system operating in 3D mode shows the following behavior (20). In the central half of the axial field of view the transaxial spatial resolution is as good as in 2D mode. Toward the end of the field of view it worsens by about 10%. Axially, the resolution is quite homogeneous in all three directions of the field of view but about 20% worse than with high-sensitivity 2D. The high level of scatter, 50% to 70% relative to the true coincidences, makes scatter correction a major concern in 3D acquisition.

Limits of Detection and Quantitation in PET Systems

Resolution. There are two fundamental processes that limit the resolution obtainable with PET: the range of the positrons between emission and annihilation and the deviation from exact collinearity of the two emitted annihilation photons (28). The distance that a positron travels from the emitting nucleus to the point of annihilation depends on its kinetic energy. The maximum range traveled is characteristic for a positron emitter. As seen in Table 2, this range is smallest with 2.4 mm for ^{18}F and goes up to more than 20 mm for ^{82}Rb. Because the positron's way is not straight, the resolution loss is much smaller than the maximal range, namely, between 0.22 and 2.6 mm FWHM. When the positron meets the electron, it is still moving. Therefore, a momentum is transferred to the electron-positron system that is maintained by the annihilation pair. As a consequence, the angle between the two 511-keV photons is not exactly 180°. The angles show an almost Gaussian distribution with an FWHM of about 0.5°. It is clear that a deviation from 180° causes the annihilation to be located on a wrong line. The resulting resolution loss increases with the diameter D of the detector ring. It can be calculated by

$$\Delta x = 0.5D \tan 0.25° \qquad (16)$$

where Δx is the resolution loss in the center of the ring (28). For a whole-body scanner with 100-cm diameter, noncollinearity causes a resolution loss of 2.2 mm. Hence the fundamental resolution limit of PET is about 3 mm.

To date, the detection system of commercial scanners is not able to maintain the optimal resolution, but a resolution of 4 to 6 mm at the center of the field of view can be expected. The degradation depends on the actual system design. It is noteworthy that the resolution is far from being constant throughout the whole field of view. For a scanner with crystal rings, the resolution within a transaxial plane can be decomposed into a radial and a tangential component, as illustrated in Fig. 42. The radial resolution degrades significantly from the center toward the border of the field of view, whereas the tangential resolution degrades only slightly. The reason is the following effect: A photon penetrates into the crystal until it is stopped and interacts. The interaction depth shows a statistical variance. Therefore, an obliquely entering photon may or may not penetrate into a neighboring crystal before interacting. If it does, a wrong radial localization of the annihilation results. The tangential location, on the other hand, is not much affected by erroneously

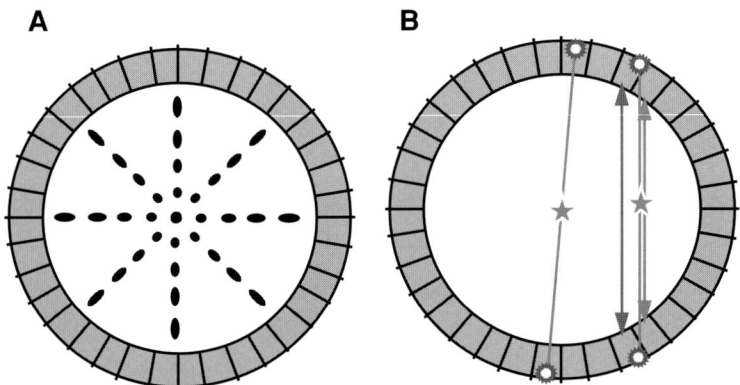

Figure 42. (**A**) Degradation in spatial resolution for a ring scanner when moving out of the center. The radial component is much more affected than the tangential one. The reason is shown in **B**. The photons of tangential LORs at the border of the field of view enter obliquely into the crystal. They may penetrate into the neighboring crystal before interacting. In this case the event is counted on a radially offset line of response.

selecting a neighboring rather than the true line of response. The situation outlined does not arise for photons coming from the ring center because they always hit the crystal perpendicularly, but it becomes increasingly likely when moving out of the center.

Sensitivity. The sensitivity of a PET scanner is limited by the solid angles at which coincidences are accepted. For these geometric reasons, a scanner in 2D mode will only be able to see less than 5% of the annihilations, even disregarding attenuation effects (10). Only 25% to 64% of these will be detected due to the finite detector efficiencies, which ranges between 50% and 80% for 511-keV photons. Therefore, only 1% to 3% of the annihilation events can be detected with a 2D scanner. The actual sensitivity of a system, furthermore, depends on several design factors such as the detector size, the ring diameter, the septa, and the axial acceptance window, i.e., the number of rings between which coincidences are allowed for. Favoring sensitivity often means that another system characteristic gets compromised. For instance, if the septa are removed for 3D imaging, the number of true coincidences increases by a factor 5 to 8. At the same time, however, the scatter fraction is also increased by a factor 3, whereby the accuracy of scatter correction becomes much more important.

Alternative PET System Designs

Modern BGO multiring scanners cover an axial field of view of about 15 cm using 18 to 24 crystal rings. Due to the high cost of the detector units, they are expensive devices. Different approaches therefore have been pursued to make PET more affordable for clinical applications, especially in oncology. Three approaches are outlined in what follows. The first approach relies on the BGO multicrystal design proven in multiring scanners but reduces the number of detectors. The second approach employs a hexagonal arrangement of six large NaI(Tl) detectors. Both systems operate in 3D mode to optimize sensitivity, which is inherently less than that of a full-ring BGO scanner. The third approach is to upgrade SPECT cameras such that imaging of positron-emitting radionuclides is also supported.

Rotating BGO PET Scanner. The principle of the rotating PET scanner developed by Townsend et al. is shown in Fig. 43 (42). Basically it has the same design as a conventional BGO multiring scanner, but instead of the full 360° angle, it covers only twice 60° by two rotating detector buckets. Only one-third of the detectors are thus required, resulting in a significant cost reduction. At the same time, however, the sensitivity is also reduced. To counterbalance the sensitivity loss, the system operates in 3D acquisition

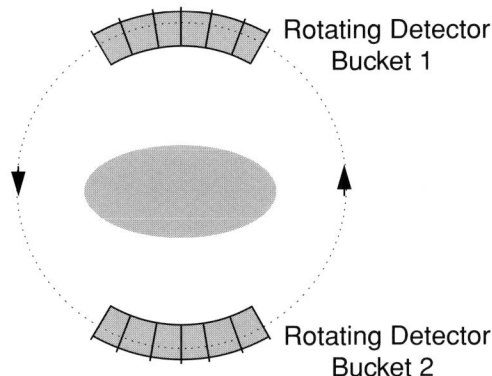

Figure 43. Principle of the rotating BGO PET scanner (Siemens/CTI ECAT ART). Two detector blocks orbit the field of view continuously to sample all projections. By operating in 3D mode, the sensitivity loss is compensated for. Reducing the required detectors to one-third results in substantial cost savings.

mode. By this means the sensitivity recovers, but the scatter fraction also increases from about 12% to 35% and must be compensated for by sophisticated scatter-correction procedures.

This design has matured into a commercial product, the Siemens/CTI ECAT ART. In this scanner, the detector banks rotate continuously at 30 revolutions per minute. Thus the minimal acquisition duration is 2 seconds, and continuous dynamic frames are supported at a rate of one frame per 10 seconds. The detectors sweep 24 rings, yielding 47 transaxial slices over a 16.2-cm axial field of view. The spatial resolution in the center is 5.2 mm, and the sensitivity exceeds that of the comparable full-ring scanner in 2D mode by almost a factor 2 (30).

Hexagonal NaI(Tl) PET Scanner. The idea behind the PENN-PET scanner developed by Muehllehner et al. (16, 27) was to design a less complex system with more cost-effective detectors yet with optimal performance. NaI(Tl) rather than BGO therefore was used as the scintillator material and a few large crystals instead of many small ones. Six rectangular crystals were hexagonally arranged as shown in Fig. 44. Each crystal is optically coupled to an array of square photomultipliers that covers the entire surface. Upon interaction of a photon in a crystal, the output of the photomultipliers is used for position calculation. Either all the outputs can be considered or only the ones lying next to the scintillation site in a local centroid calculation. The system operates in 3D mode, accepting coincidences over a large axial acceptance angle.

This design has several advantageous features, partly from using NaI(Tl) and partly from using continuous detectors. As Table 1 shows, NaI(Tl) has a high light output combined with a short decay time. These properties allow use of a short coincidence timing window, thereby reducing the number of random coincidences and allowing a

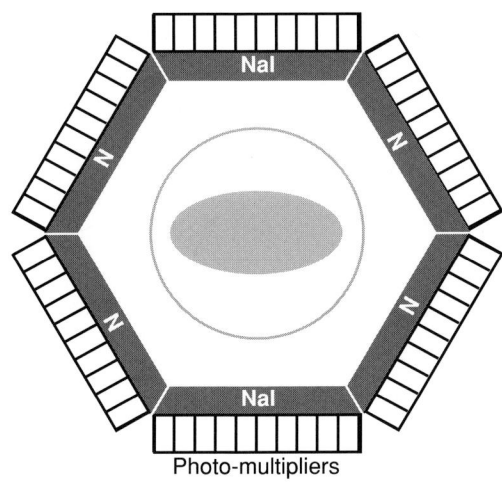

Photo-multipliers

Figure 44. Principle of the hexagonal NaI(Tl) PET scanner (General Electric Quest). Six large NaI(Tl) detectors operating with an optimized Anger approach are used to enclose a large axial field of view. Sophisticated hardware and software approaches are required to measure at moderate to high count rates. Advantages are continuous slice definition and reduced cost due to avoidance of the expensive BGO detectors.

good spatial localization. The high-energy resolution allows for an effective rejection of scattered events. The use of continuous detectors ensures high sampling along all three axes, resulting in good spatial resolution. Since the slice thickness is not determined by a ring structure, it can be varied almost continuously depending on the study. The design also has disadvantages: Due to the detector gaps at the crystal interfaces, there are missing projection data that have to be compensated for in the reconstruction algorithm. NaI(Tl) has a lower efficiency than BGO, meaning that fewer entering photons are stopped. Since all photons interact in a few large detectors, they must be able to handle high count rates, requiring special hardware and software techniques.

This system also has evolved into a commercial product, General Electric's Quest scanner, noteworthy for its large axial field of view of 25 cm.

Use of SPECT Cameras for PET Imaging. SPECT systems conventionally operate with mechanical collimation. While this is required for single-photon studies, it represents a poor solution when imaging 511-keV annihilation photons. Using coincidence collimation instead provides much higher sensitivity and better resolution. Currently, most SPECT systems can be equipped with adapted high-energy collimators for PET studies, while coincidence systems are only emerging very recently. These systems in principle represent the combination of the previously described designs, namely, a rotating system with large NaI(Tl) detectors. Obvious disadvantages relative to the state-of-the-art PET scanner are the reduction in sensitivity due to both geometry and detector efficiency and the required mechanical motion. The reported resolution obtainable with these systems lies at 5 mm or below and is hence comparable with that of a typical PET scanner. Compared to 511-keV SPECT with mechanical collimation, they offer a sensitivity gain of factor 10 to 15 (21). These figures indicate that with such upgraded SPECT systems some types of PET studies that are not critical with respect to sensitivity may become just another NM procedure if FDG distribution sites become more widespread.

METHODOLOGY FOR NUCLEAR MEDICINE FUNCTIONAL STUDIES

In principle, all NM studies are functional studies because the radiopharmaceuticals used employ a physiologic or pathophysiologic mechanism to make evident disease. In the earlier days, NM examinations were unique in providing even some anatomic information such as making visible brain tumors or the thyroid gland; however, the radiologic cross-sectional imaging modalities have replaced this type of NM study since the early eighties. Nowadays, anatomic information is never the principal information sought when ordering an NM examination, but anatomy is still important because it permits one to spatially localize the process detected and thereby detect regional variations in organ function. While some NM studies provide sufficient anatomic detail to appropriately direct the clinician to the site of disease, this is not true in many circumstances. Anatomically appropriate information is frequently obtained in bone, lung, kidney, thyroid, and heart studies, while in brain studies and studies for tumor detection, be it with standard NM or PET techniques, the anatomic information may be insufficient. Fusion of NM and PET images with images obtained by CT and MRI are thus most helpful and start to enter into clinical routine. Techniques of image fusion were discussed in Chap. 4.

As pointed out in Chap. 3, most clinically used NM studies are qualitatively interpreted, and semiquantitative or quantitative analysis often is not contributory. Still, most quantitative methods currently used in medical image analysis originated in NM. The NM data lend themselves most easily to quantification because in the simplest case of an inert substance the measured counts are proportional to the substance present in the region examined. Deriving absolute values from NM data is nevertheless quite involved. As discussed in the earlier sections of this chapter, quantitation is achieved most readily with PET systems, but there are some newer developments that permit quantitative data extraction with SPECT systems as well. Many of the fundamental methods used in analyzing functional image data were treated in Chap. 3 because they are being used increasingly in conjunction with other imaging methods or are likely going to have some relevance for other methods in the future.

A survey of the most widely used methods for quantification shows that the most reliable methods base themselves on a comparison of paired organ structures, such as region-of-interest (ROI) analysis of activities measured on bone scans or lung or brain studies. Other studies determine uptake ratios between an ROI and an appropriately defined reference or background ROI, deriving criteria on when such ratios are normal and when they are pathologic. More sophisticated methods use curve-fitting algorithms on paired organs to derive relative function as in renal function studies or algorithms to derive regional volume changes in the heart. The latter make use of edge-detection algorithms and methods to find the center of gravity of the organ under study, i.e., the heart. These methods have been introduced even for the quantification of x-ray ventriculography obtained during cardiac catheterization. Extraction of some sophisticated information from cardiac perfusion studies also has been achieved, but the improvement in clinical value by such methods is not large enough so that no single methodology has won out over others. Analysis of perfusion curves using arterial input deconvolution techniques was en vogue in nuclear cardiac and brain perfusion studies, but the lack of accurate first-pass data obtained and the ready availability of ''chemical'' microspheres such as thallium, Tc-MIBI, Tc-HMPAO, and Tc-ECD for evaluation of perfusion with NM methods prevented widespread use of such techniques in clinical practice.

PET imaging, however, which provides quantitative data relatively easily and at a high enough temporal resolution, has seen extensive and sophisticated quantification. Input sampling of arterial or arterialized venous blood is standard even in some clinical PET studies, and curve fitting using compartment modeling to derive data on perfusion, blood volume, oxygen extraction, and metabolite and receptor-ligand kinetics is used widely. This does not mean that PET images have to be quantified at all times. Recent clinical experience with whole-body PET in oncology suggests that in this case unquantified data can be interpreted very much like bone scans to yield highly relevant clinical data.

It is the aim of this section to outline some of the methods specific to NM image data quantification. In doing this we will heavily draw on the results presented in Chap. 3 and specify the results obtained there to NM methodology here. Hence we will follow the same order as used in Chap. 3 and start with the discussion of tissue perfusion measurements and then discuss the determination of blood volume and oxygen extraction fraction and end with the quantitative characterization of fluorodeoxyglucose (FDG) metabolism.

NM Studies of Tissue Perfusion

It was defined in Chap. 3 what characteristics substances must have that they can serve as good tissue perfusion markers. The key is that they are either extracted as much as possible during first pass, that they are freely diffusible throughout the tissue, or that they stay completely intravascular. Good examples of the first type are mechanical or chemical microspheres, although mechanical microspheres do not truly enter the tissue. An excellent chemical microsphere is ammonia labeled with ^{13}N for the heart. Good examples of freely diffusible substances are water or carbon dioxide labeled with ^{15}O and radioactive xenon gas for all organ systems. Most standard contrast media used in x-ray or MRI studies stay completely intravascular in the brain as long as the blood-brain barrier is intact. Similar compounds used in NM such as Tc-DTPA or Tc-glucoheptonate have the same properties. These compounds pose difficulties, however, for quantitative data analysis as soon as there is extravasation into the surrounding tissue. This occurs whenever there is a breakdown of the blood-brain barrier or in all other organs where such a barrier does not exist. Then tissue uptake has to be modeled, which makes data analysis much more complex, as already noted in Chap. 3. Better intravascular markers are Tc-labeled albumin or red blood cells (RBCs) and carbon monoxide labeled with ^{15}O, which stays intravascular because it is tightly bound to the hemoglobin inside the RBCs. Qualitative perfusion imaging is widely used in clinical NM practice and relies either on absolute defects observed in regions where perfusion is detected (lung scanning) or on the comparison of paired organ structures or neighboring tissues (heart and brain perfusion scanning). The most sophisticated methodology used is ROI analysis and computational manipulations with the data obtained from measuring counts in the ROIs. In the ensuing section we are going to revisit quantitative perfusion scanning as applicable to NM methods.

The point of departure for all tissue perfusion experiments in NM is Eq. (4) in Chap. 3, which relates the concentration of substance measured with the imaging system $C_t(t)$ to the arterial input function $C_a(t)$ measured in megabequerels per milliliter, the so-called wash-out constant k, and the perfusion flow f:

$$C_t(t) = C_t(0)e^{-kt} + fe^{-kt} * C_a(t) \tag{17}$$

$C_t(t)$ is measured in megabequerels per gram, and f is the perfusion per unit tissue mass measured in units milliliters per minute per gram. The wash-out constant $k = f/P$, where P is the partition coefficient of the tracer substance between tissue and blood and incorporates the solubility of the tracer in the tissue relative to blood. The asterisk denotes the convolution operation. This equation is the point of departure for all tissue perfusion measurements and is modified according to the experimental setup used.

The Microsphere Approach

This approach has been discussed in full detail. The method bases itself on the following equation, which was derived as Eq. (7) in Chap. 3:

$$f = C_t(\infty)F/m \tag{18}$$

This formula relates tissue flow f in milliliters per minute per gram to the following quantities, which are determined experimentally:

• The tissue concentration of microsphere tracer radioactivity $C_t(\infty)$ measured in megabequerels per gram, where (∞) denotes a time that is late enough after injection that virtually all microsphere radioactivity has been cleared from the bloodstream.
• A constant flow F measured in milliliters per minute with which blood is drawn from an arterial line, for example, in the radial artery for long enough that the microspheres have virtually disappeared from the circulation.
• m, which is the total radioactivity in megabequerels measured in the total sample drawn.

This method is experimentally quite simple to perform. Absolute values of $C_t(\infty)$ are obtained by calibration against a phantom with known activity per gram, and m is measured in a counter.

While mechanical microsphere methods are the "gold standard" when perfusion experiments have to be validated, they are not practical because their use requires injection of tracer spheres into the left ventricle for all organs except the lungs. The same Eq. (18) approximately applies for ammonia perfusion studies (32). There $C_t(\infty)$ is measured by the PET camera and F and m again by acquiring a blood sample that is drawn at a constant flow rate F for long enough. Imaging measurements typically start 10 minutes after injection of [^{13}N]ammonia. Ammonia is quickly extracted as it is transferred into the glutamine pool by glutamine synthetase. Since ^{13}N has a half-life of 9 minutes, correction of tracer decay has to be performed to obtain the quantitative data. The method to quantify ammonia is so simple that it is used widely.

Other chemical microspheres are not completely extracted because at higher flows the extraction fraction is smaller than 1 (see Figs. 8 and 20 in Chap. 3). If the extraction fraction of the tracer has been determined by calibrating it against microsphere flow, then flow can be determined also using this particular tracer with the help of Eq. (8) in Chap. 3. This method has been applied with rubidium (^{82}Rb) (29) because this tracer can be provided to PET sites that have no cyclotron (39).

Perfusion Measurements Using Equilibrium Tracer Inhalation

Equilibrium determination of perfusion has been applied in PET imaging but has been supplanted largely by bolus techniques mainly because of issues regarding radiation hygiene, since the bolus techniques expose the patient to substantially smaller radiation doses. As will be seen in the quantitative analysis, the equilibrium technique works only with radioactively decaying tracers that have half-lives comparable with the time it takes the blood to reach the organ of interest from the point of arterial input. The only available tracer for such experiments is ^{15}O, which with its 2-minute half-life satisfies this condition.

The imaging measurement is performed with the patient in the PET camera while he or she is connected to a delivery system of radioactive carbon dioxide gas $[C^{15}O_2]$. After providing the gas at a constant flow and activity, a steady state is reached. This obviously means that the rate of change in the tissue concentration of the marker substance measured is zero; the maker substance input to the tissue must equal the marker substance output. The quantitative analysis expanded in the following box shows that tissue perfusion can be obtained by measuring the tissue concentration with the tomographic scanner and that it suffices to measure a single arterial sample to calibrate the measurement. The carbon dioxide gas, which is inhaled by the patient, is completely and instantly transformed into H_2O by the carbonic anhydrase reaction on contact with the blood in the lungs. The tissue concentration measured C_{tm} in the scanner equals the true tissue concentration C_{tt} times the correction for the radioactive decay.

In a steady-state situation, Eq. (2) in Chap. 3 simplifies to

$$0 = dC_t/dt = f(C_a - C_t/P) = f/P(PC_a - C_t)$$

and therefore

$$C_t = PC_a \qquad (19)$$

Hence the tissue concentration equals the arterial input multiplied by the partition coefficient. From Eq. (19) it is obvious that perfusion flow f cannot be measured with inert substances because the equation becomes independent of the quantity f.

The situation is different when using an isotope like ^{15}O with a very short half-life of $t_{1/2} = 0.693/\lambda$ of 120 s and the decay constant λ of 0.35 min^{-1}. In this setting, a decay correction has to be introduced to describe the measurement adequately, because radioactive decay occurs between the arterial input of radioactivity and the time C_t is measured. Hence the true tissue concentration C_{tt} of the tracer, as it arrives in the organ, is higher than the measured concentration C_{tm}. Their relation is simply given by the decay law of radioactivity: $C_{tm} = C_{tt}e^{-\lambda t}$ (Eq. 1). The true tissue concentration has to be corrected upward by $C_{tt} = C_{tm}e^{\lambda t}$. The number of counts measured per unit time has to be constant under steady-state conditions; hence $dC_{tm}/dt = 0$. Noting that $dC_{tt}/dt = d(C_{tm}e^{\lambda t})/dt = dC_{tm}/dt \exp(\lambda t) + \lambda C_{tm}e^{\lambda t}$, Eq. (2) in Chap. 3 can be rewritten for a steady-state perfusion situation:

$$0 = dC_{tt}/dt = dC_{tm}/dte^{\lambda t} + \lambda C_{tm}e^{\lambda t}$$
$$= f/P(PC_{am} - C_{tm})e^{\lambda t} \qquad (20)$$

Solving this equation for the tissue concentration C_{tm} and tissue perfusion f, we find

$$C_{tm} = \frac{C_{am}fP}{f + \lambda P} \qquad \text{and} \qquad f = \frac{\lambda C_{tm}P}{PC_{am} - C_{tm}} \qquad (21)$$

where P can be set equal to 1 for water. While C_{tm} is measured with the PET camera after proper calibration, C_{am} is obtained from an arterial blood sample measured in a well counter. A PET image can thus be calibrated directly to represent a perfusion map or perfusion functional image by computing the preceding expression on a pixel-by-pixel basis.

The arterial concentration C_{am} is constant almost right from the beginning; thus Eq. (20) can be readily integrated (obviously early on $dC_{tt}/dt \neq 0$):

$$C_{tm} \approx C_{tm0}\{1 - e^{-(f+\lambda)t}\} \qquad (22)$$

The equilibrium state C_{tm0} is accordingly reached with a time constant $f + \lambda$, and (as a lower limit, because arterial equilibration was ignored) it takes approximately $3/(f + \lambda)$ minutes for the tissue to reach 95% of the equilibrium value. With $\lambda = 0.35$ min^{-1} for ^{15}O and typical cerebral flow values of 0.7 to 1 min^{-1}, a critical appraisal of the equilibrium method is possible (44).

- It will take several minutes (at least more than 3 minutes) for the equilibrium state to be reached, and a shorter half-life isotope than ^{15}O would even be preferable (Eq. 22) to increase the decay constant. If tissues with lower perfusion values are measured, the time to equilibrium becomes even longer.
- At higher flow values, the measurement of tissue perfusion flow f becomes less accurate due to the nonlinearity between f and C_{tm} in Eq. (21). From this point of view, it also would be desirable to have a shorter half-life isotope than ^{15}O. If the half-life were longer and thus the decay constant λ smaller, it is obvious that the method would not work because Eq. (21) becomes independent of flow, as stated at the outset of this discussion.

Dynamic Perfusion Measurements: Wash-out Techniques

These methods were discussed at full length earlier because they not only bear relevance to NM experiments but also have applications in CT and potentially MRI experiments to measure, for example, cerebral perfusion. It should suffice here to reiterate that the method works best when at a given point in time the arterial input of tracer suddenly drops to zero because then the second term in Eq. (17) becomes zero, that is,

$$C_t(t) = C_t(0)e^{-kt} \qquad (23)$$

or in integrated form

$$f = kP = PC_t(0) \left/ \int_0^\infty C_t(t)\, dt \right. = PC_t(0)/A$$

A measurement of the tissue radioactivity at time zero and at some points in time later permits one to obtain $k = f/P$ by fitting the data to a straight line on a semilogarithmic plot. Alternatively, the tissue time activity is integrated, which is the simpler experimental approach in NM, since data acquisition can just be continued to the point where there is no major change in tissue radioactivity any more. The initial radioactivity is then divided by this quantity to yield tissue flow. Note that the partition coefficient P for a freely diffusible tracer equals 1. For strictly intravascular tracers, the regional blood volume rBV has to be known, since $P = rBV$.

Notice that in NM freely diffusible tracers are preferred for perfusion measurements, since their transit times through the tissues of interest are substantially longer than those of intravascular agents. Hence temporal resolution of the measuring instrument is not as critical. The quantitative description of wash-out techniques as discussed earlier can be applied without modification when using intracarotid radioactive xenon injections, while the systemic administration of a gas by ventilation or venous injection requires the full use of Eq. (17) because the condition of immediate drop to zero of the arterial input is no longer met.

Dynamic Perfusion Measurements: Bolus Techniques

Bolus techniques are currently the preferred method of obtaining tissue perfusion information using PET systems and intravenous injection of ^{15}O-labeled water. There are two methods to acquire and quantitate the data, which both rely on Eq. (17) (or Eq. (4) from Chap. 3). They are suitable to calculate brain perfusion on a pixel-by-pixel basis and hence allow one to generate functional maps showing absolute perfusion in milliliters per gram per minute.

The autoradiographic approach (13, 34) does not try to resolve the temporal behavior of the tissue activity. Rather, it provides a formulation of the problem that allows one to calculate perfusion from the total activity seen in a tissue element during the passage of the bolus. The experimental procedure is as follows: An $H_2{}^{15}O$ bolus is injected intravenously. Upon arrival of the bolus in the brain (raise of count rate), the PET scanner starts the acquisition and accumulates the counts due to the instantaneous tissue activity $C_t(t)$ during a period T_1 to T_2 (40 to 60 seconds). At the same time blood is drawn from an arterial line and measured in a well counter to obtain the arterial activity concentration $C_a(t)$, the input curve. To derive the operational equation, we apply the fact that the PET scanner simply integrates the activity during the acquisition period. Assuming that the initial brain activity was zero, we integrate Eq. (17) accordingly and obtain

$$ C_{\text{PET}} = \int_{T_1}^{T_2} C_t(t)\, dt = f \int_{T_1}^{T_2} C_a(t) * e^{-f/Pt}\, dt \tag{24} $$

Given experimental values for C_{PET} and the time course of $C_a(t)$, and assuming a fixed value for the partition coefficient P, this equation can be solved analytically or numerically for perfusion f.

This autoradiographic model is based on various assumptions that may not be exactly fulfilled in practical experiments. The impact of such deviations on the accuracy of the derived perfusion values has been investigated. Notable results are that the solution for f is unique (13), and that timing errors between the blood curve and the PET curve cause large estimation errors (13, 18).

In the dynamic approach, the time course of $C_t(t)$ is monitored by acquiring short frames of typically 10 seconds' duration. As a result, a time-activity curve is available for each image pixel. It can be analyzed using the nonlinear methods of compartment modeling. However, a computationally much more efficient method has been given by Alpert et al. (3). The operational equation can be derived as follows: Both sides of Eq. (17) are multiplied by a time-dependent weighting function $W(t)$ and integrated over the total acquisition duration. This process is done for two different weighting functions $W_1(t)$ and $W_2(t)$, and the ratio is formed, yielding

$$ \frac{\displaystyle\int_{T_1}^{T_2} W_1(t) C_t(t)\, dt}{\displaystyle\int_{T_1}^{T_2} W_2(t) C_t(t)\, dt} = \frac{f \displaystyle\int_{T_1}^{T_2} W_1(t) C_a(t) * e^{-f/Pt}\, dt}{f \displaystyle\int_{T_1}^{T_2} W_2(t) C_a(t) * e^{-f/Pt}\, dt} \tag{25} $$

The weighting functions are chosen to minimize bias and variance of the resulting perfusion estimates. Originally, 1 and t were proposed as W_1 and W_2, but simulations have show slightly superior performance of $1/\sqrt{t}$ and $\sqrt{t}$ (18). The computational procedure is to initially tabulate the ratio by evaluating the right side of the equation for the expected range of f/P values, yielding the so-called r table. Then, for each time-activity curve, the left side is evaluated, and the ratio obtained is compared with the r table, resulting in that f/P value which produces such a ratio on the right side. In a second step, f itself is calculated. This can be achieved by inserting f/P into the expression

$$ f = \frac{\displaystyle\int_{T_1}^{T_2} W_1(t) C_t(t)}{\displaystyle\int_{T_1}^{T_2} W_1(t) C_a(t) * e^{-f/Pt}\, dt} \tag{26} $$

which represents the upper part of Eq. (25) resolved by f. Finally, an estimate for the partition coefficient P can be obtained from f and f/P. This dynamic approach has been demonstrated to perform nearly as well as standard nonlinear least-squares techniques, but at a dramatic improvement in computation speed (17). It has a clear advantage over the autoradiographic method because no fixed value for the partition coefficient over the entire brain must be assumed.

Determination of Blood Volume

As discussed above, blood volume determinations can be made using either an equilibrium or a dynamic approach. The equilibrium situation can be attained with labeled albumin or red blood cells in NM and with $C^{15}O$ in PET (31). The relevant formula to apply is Eq. (21) from Chap. 3:

$$rBV = \frac{C_t(t)}{drC_v(t)} \tag{27}$$

Remember that rBV is the fraction of the tissue volume that consists of vessels. r is a correction factor, typically on the order of 0.85, which accounts for the fact that the hematocrit in capillaries is lower than in the large vessels. Obviously, this correction has only to be made when the "tracer" is red cell bound. d is the density of organ tissue in grams per milliliter. Since $C_t(t)$ is measured in counts per gram and $C_v(t)$ in counts per milliliter, rBV is dimensionless. Tissue concentration also can be measured directly as counts per milliliter, in which case $d = 1$.

In the dynamic approach, the basic idea is that whatever substance goes into the organ has to come out again eventually. Hence, for any substance not metabolized in a given tissue, we can determine rBV as

$$rBV = \frac{\int_0^\infty C_t(t)\,dt}{\int_0^\infty C_a(t)\,dt} = \frac{\int_0^\infty C_t(t)\,dt}{rd\int_0^\infty C_v(t)\,dt} \tag{28}$$

Integration of the data obtained from an arterial input curve and from a tissue curve yields the desired results. The correction factor r and the density d introduced in Eq. (27) are needed as in the equilibrium approach.

Oxygen Consumption Measurements

The model used to describe the events occurring during oxygen delivery to tissues was shown in Fig. 17 in Chap. 3. When ^{15}O is inhaled, it is transported by the hemoglobin located in the red blood cells to the organ under consideration. There it enters the cells and is transformed immediately and completely into $[^{15}O]$water ($H_2{}^{15}O$) by oxidative phosphorylation so that it may be fairly assumed that the tissue contains no ^{15}O in the form of oxygen. The $H_2{}^{15}O$ produced by oxidative phosphorylation is a freely diffusible substance, as already assumed when analyzing the problem of tissue perfusion. Hence it is in equilibrium with the venous bloodstream through which it leaves the cells and recirculates. The total ^{15}O radioactivity in the tissue compartment C_{tO} is thus a sum of the $H_2{}^{15}O$ generated by the conversion of $^{15}O_2$ and of recirculating $H_2{}^{15}O$. Conservation of substance applied to the $H_2{}^{15}O$ compartment requires that the difference in the flux of substance into and out of the tissue compartment equals the rate of change of the substance within the compartment. The flux into the compartment is the sum of the fraction of the oxygen converted into water by the metabolic conversion of $^{15}O_2$ into $H_2{}^{15}O$ in the tissue and the recirculating $H_2{}^{15}O$. The flux leaving the tissue is equal to the tissue concentration C_{tH_2O}, which again is presumed to be in equilibrium with the venous concentration divided by the tissue–blood partition coefficient for water P. As for perfusion, the oxygen extraction fraction OER can be measured under steady-state conditions or using the bolus injection approach. In both steady-state and dynamic approaches it may be deemed necessary to correct the final result for the oxygen activity bound intravascularly to hemoglobin. Such a correction requires a blood volume measurement in addition to the measurement of tissue flow and oxygen extraction.

Equilibrium Determination of the Oxygen Extraction Fraction

The equilibrium approach to determine the oxygen extraction fraction is comparable with the one used to determine perfusion. Rather than giving the patient $C^{15}O_2$ to inhale, $^{15}O_2$ is given (15). The analysis bases itself on the model described in the preceding section and requires solving of the conservation of mass equation for labeled $H_2^{15}O$, which is generated during oxidative phosphorylation in the cells. Hence, while we consider the $H_2^{15}O$ compartment again, $H_2^{15}O$ is generated by the cells rather than being produced in the lung by conversion of $C^{15}O_2$. Since flow enters as an important variable in the equation for $H_2^{15}O$ generation, it has to be obtained by measurement of the tissue flow f, as discussed in Chap. 3. Depending on the accuracy of the measurement desired, a determination of blood volume also has to be performed.

If a fraction OER of the arterial oxygen is extracted and—by model assumption—completely converted into water in the tissue, the flux of labeled $^{15}O_2$ into the $H_2^{15}O$ compartment is $f(C_{aH_2O} + OERC_{aO_2})$, where f is the blood flow and C_{aH_2O} and C_{aO_2} are the concentrations of radioactivity in the arterial blood present in the form of $H_2^{15}O$ and $^{15}O_2$, respectively. The conservation of mass equation (Eq. (1) in Chap. 3) states

$$dC_{tH_2O}/dt = \underbrace{f(C_{aH_2O} + OERC_{aO_2})}_{\text{Arterial influx}} - \underbrace{fC_{tH_2O}/P}_{\text{Venous outflux}} \qquad (29)$$

where P is the blood-water partition coefficient. For a general description, this linear differential equation has to be integrated.

In a steady-state situation, the change in tissue concentration of labeled water is zero. In analogy to "Equilibrium Model of Constant Tracer Inhalation" in Chap. 3, a correction for the radioactive decay of $^{15}O_2$ has to be introduced. Then the preceding equation can be rewritten:

$$d(C_{tH_2O}e^{\lambda t})/dt = \lambda C_{tH_2O}e^{\lambda t} = f/P(PC_{aH_2O} + POERC_{aO_2} - C_{tH_2O})e^{\lambda t}$$

$$\text{or} \qquad (\lambda + f/P)C_{tH_2O} = fC_{aH_2O} + fOERC_{aO_2} \qquad (30)$$

where $dC_{tH_2O}/dt = 0$ (steady-state condition) was used. Solving for the measured tissue concentration of labeled $H_2^{15}O$, we find

$$C_{tH_2O} = \frac{fC_{aH_2O} + fOERC_{aO_2}}{\lambda + f/P} \qquad (31)$$

While C_{tH_2O} is measured by PET and C_{aH_2O} and C_{aO_2} from the arterial blood, f has to be determined by a second measurement, namely, that of perfusion according to "Perfusion Measurements Using Equilibrium Tracer Inhalation" above. Using the same notation for the concentrations determined in the equilibrium perfusion measurement by carbon dioxide inhalation, i.e., C_{am} and C_{tm} for the arterial and tissue concentrations, a combination of Eqs. (21) and (31) yields an expression for the oxygen extraction fraction OER:

$$OER = \frac{C_{am}C_{tH_2O}/C_{tm} - C_{aH_2O}}{C_{aO_2}} \qquad (32)$$

C_{tH_2O} and C_{tm} are measured by the respective PET experiments, while C_{am} is measured from an arterial sample in the perfusion experiment. We are left with determining the quantities C_{aH_2O} and C_{aO_2}, which are the whole-blood concentra-

---

tions of the recirculating water and the arterial oxygen in the $^{15}O_2$ inhalation experiment. This is done as follows: If we measure the radioactivity in whole blood and in plasma in both experiments in well counters, we obtain the quantities C_{apH_2O} and $C_{a(H_2O+O_2)}$, because only the erythrocytes in the whole-blood fraction contain radioactive oxygen. If the same measurements were made during the perfusion experiment, the corresponding quantities $C_{am} = C'_{aH_2O}$, C'_{apH_2O}, and their ratio $A = C'_{aH_2O}/C'_{apH_2O}$ can be obtained. The quantities needed for obtaining OER *in the preceding equation are* C_{aH_2O} *and* C_{aO_2}. C_{aH_2O} *is obtained by multiplying* C_{apH_2O} *by A,* since the ratio of water of whole blood to plasma must be the same in both experiments:

$$C_{aH_2O} = AC_{apH_2O}$$

The concentration of oxygen in whole blood C_{aO_2} is obviously the difference between the total radioactivity in whole blood $C_{a(H_2O+O_2)}$ and the water radioactivity C_{aH_2O} in whole blood, as calculated above. Hence

$$C_{aO_2m} = C_{a(H_2O+O_2)} - AC_{apH_2O}$$

The cerebral metabolic rate of oxygen CMRO$_2$ is simply OERfC_{aO_2}.

While the steady-state approach yields adequate results, there are two major problems with it. First, it requires two steady-state measurements, which as stated earlier require prolonged equilibration and hence prolonged inhalations of radioactive gases with relatively high concomitant radiation exposure to the lungs and the trachea. Second, the scanner and cyclotron are used for a relatively long time to perform the measurements, which, with scan time on an expensive instrument being costly, is not optimal.

Dynamic Determination of the Oxygen Extraction Fraction

For both reasons, a dynamic approach to determine OER has been proposed by Mintun et al. (24). The compartment model presented in Fig. 17 in Chap. 3 remains the same as that for the steady-state situation, but the analysis of the dynamic approach also requires a description of the dynamic fluxes in the ^{15}O compartment, since the total radioactivity measured C_{tot} in a PET experiment is the sum of water- and oxygen-bound ^{15}O, and the latter contribution cannot be neglected compared with the former through the entire course of the experiment. In fact, when the bolus arrives in the tissue, not much oxygen has been transformed into water yet. However, the assumption that all the oxygen entering the cells is converted into water still holds so that, as in the equilibrium case, oxygen can be assumed to stay in the intravascular compartment. While oxygen is present in the arteries with a concentration C_{aO_2}, the venous concentration is reduced by what has been extracted by the perfused tissue, and the capillary concentration is assumed to be the mean between the arterial and venous concentrations.

In the dynamic approach we have to use the integral form of the flux equation (Eq. 29), which is obtained using standard integrating methods such as when obtaining Eq. (3) from Eq. (1) in Chap. 3, and use the quantities labeled in correspondence to Eq. (29). The total radioactivity in a volume V is the sum of that in the oxygen and the water compartments, which are assumed to have respective volumes V_1 and V_2. The radioactivity per unit time q_{H_2O} in the volume V_2 of the water compartment equals the water volume times the concentration C_{tH_2O} and is given by

$$q_{H_2O} = V_2 C_{tH_2O} = V_2 f C_{aH_2O} e^{-kt} + V_2 f OER C_{aO_2} e^{-kt} \qquad (33)$$

where it should be noted that the first term, describing the initial conditions under which the differential equation is solved, was left out because there is no substance present initially; thus $C_{tH_2O}(0) = 0$. Furthermore, as above, we use the definition of the wash-out constant $k = f/P$.

The fluxes in the $^{15}O_2$ compartment have been qualitatively described above. The venous concentration of oxygen is given by $C_{vO_2} = C_{aO_2}(1 - OER)$, and assuming that the capillary concentration is the average of the arterial and venous concentrations, $C_{cO_2} = C_{aO_2}(1 - OER/2)$. To be able to compare radioactive counts, we have to multiply all concentrations by their respective volumes with $V_a + V_v + V_c = V_1$. The total radioactivity per unit time in the oxygen compartment q_{O_2} is thus

$$q_{O_2} = V_a C_{aO_2} + V_v C_{vO_2} + V_c C_{cO_2} = C_{aO_2}[V_1 - OER(V_v + V_c/2)] \quad (34)$$

The total radioactivity time-activity curve measured is that in the oxygen plus that in the water compartment q_{tot}:

$$q_{tot} = q_{O_2} + q_{H_2O}$$
$$= C_{aO_2}[V_1 - OER(V_v + V_c/2)]$$
$$+ V_2 f C_{aH_2O} e^{-kt}) + V_2 f OER C_{aO_2} e^{-kt}$$

The PET experiment measures the radioactivity over a given time, that is,

$$Q_{PET} = \int_{T_1}^{T_2} q_{tot} \, dt$$

where T_1 and T_2 are the start and stop times of the PET scan. Inserting the preceding expression into the integral and solving for OER yields

$$OER = \frac{Q_{PET} - V_2 f \int C_{aH_2O} e^{-kt} \, dt - V_1 \int C_{aO_2} \, dt}{V_2 f \int C_{aO_2} e^{-kt} \, dt - (V_v + V_c/2) \int C_{aO_2} \, dt} \quad (35)$$

Determination of the volumes V_v and V_c is not possible in vivo independently, and therefore, literature values have to be taken (37). In the brain, the ratios V_v/BV and V_c/BV are 0.83 and 0.01, where BV is the total blood volume. Since oxygen resides in the red cells, effects of small-vessel hemodilution have to be taken into account by multiplying rBV by a ratio r corresponding to the small to large vessel hematocrit. This takes care of the hematocrit dilution at the tissue level so that $r \cdot rBV$ corresponds to V_1 in Eq. (35). The local rate of oxygen consumption $CMRO_2$ is obtained by multiplying the concentration with the flow and the oxygen extraction ratio:

$$CMRO_2 = OER f C_{aO_2}$$

The quantitative analysis of the problem to determine OER shows that its determination is relatively involved. Not only do we need to perform a dynamic acquisition to obtain the quantity Q_{PET} of tissue radioactivity after the injection of $^{15}O_2$ together with arterial blood measurements to obtain the time-activity curves for $^{15}O_2$ and $H_2^{15}O$ in arterial blood as well as total arterial oxygen, but two additional measurements are needed to determine regional blood flow f and blood volume rBV.

An Important Example of Compartmental Modeling to Evaluate Tissue Metabolism

Many systems have been analyzed using modeling concepts as outlined in Chap. 3. The aim is always to obtain information on the rate constants describing the system that determine the essential properties of the system examined. Remember that modeling is required because NM studies measure radioactivity and hence cannot assign the measured signal to a given compound, as is possible for some entities by using MR spectroscopy. The only model with wide relevance is the model describing cellular metabolism of fluorodeoxyglucose originally developed by Sokoloff et al. (40).

The Fluorodeoxyglucose Model

The most widely used molecule in PET is [^{18}F]fluorodeoxyglucose (FDG), which has proven to be an excellent marker of metabolism as an ideal analogue of glucose. While the brain is an obligatory user of glucose, the heart can use either glucose or free fatty acids, acetate, and other substrates. Furthermore, much evidence has accumulated over the last years that FDG is an excellent marker of malignancy, since malignant tumors tend to exhibit a much elevated glucose uptake. Additionally, FDG is taken up into foci of acute inflammation. Hence it appears to be a highly sensitive but not a completely specific marker of malignancy. FDG is excreted through the kidneys, and the general biodistribution is shown in Fig. 45. FDG is an ideal marker molecule because it possesses

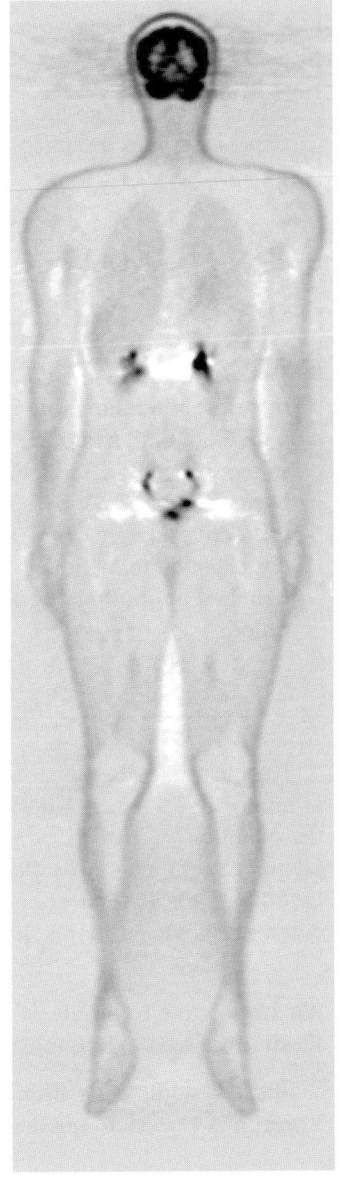

Figure 45. Coronal image of a whole-body ^{18}FDG PET study showing physiologic tracer distribution at the time of acquisition. Glucose uptake is prominent in the brain and in the urinary tract. The acquisition was started 40 minutes after injection. It consisted of 13 transaxial field of views with 15-cm thickness that were imaged successively during 5 minutes. No attenuation correction was performed. As a consequence, the body contour and lungs show exaggerated uptake.

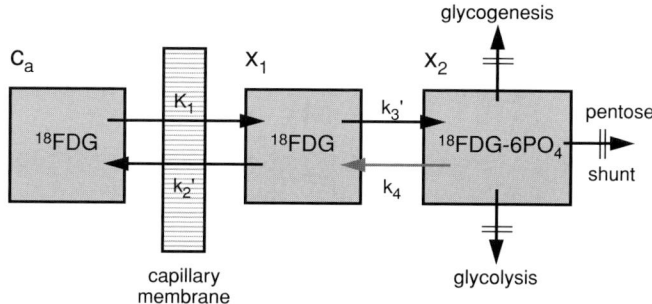

Figure 46. Compartment model for FDG. The three compartments are the intravascular space and the interstitial and intracellular spaces combined containing FDG and FDG-6PO$_4$. The relevant rate constants are K_1, k_2', and k_3'. Note that the backreaction k_4 can be neglected for times up to approximately 1 hour.

the same kinetics as glucose insofar as uptake into the tissue and 6-phosphorylation by the enzyme hexokinase is concerned. However, FDG participates neither in glycogenesis nor in glycolysis or the pentose phosphate shunt (Fig. 46), since for these further steps of glucose metabolism the FDG molecule is too different from glucose proper. The key to the overwhelming success of FDG as a glucose analogue is the fact that hexokinase is the rate-limiting enzyme; i.e., hexokinase is "turned on" when glycolysis is active and "turned off" when metabolism of glucose proceeds only at a low level. FDG uptake is increased when demand of normal cells is increased, while in tumors it appears that additional glucose transporter proteins enhance transport into the malignant cells. No glucose analogue behaving in a similar way as FDG is known thus far that would be suitable for single-photon imaging; hence there is no good marker of glucose metabolism for conventional NM imaging.

As a result of the phosphorylation reaction, FDG-6PO$_4$ accumulates in the cells, which at the concentrations used in PET imaging is physiologically irrelevant. In fact, there is only a slow decay of the molecule back into FDG by hydrolysis. This backreaction can be ignored for approximately the first hour after FDG administration. As a result, a three-compartment model, as depicted in Fig. 46, using the three rate constants K_1, k_2', and k_3' is adequate to quantitatively describe glucose metabolism, and k_4 has to be incorporated only when FDG behavior beyond 1 hour of injection is to be modeled (here we have stayed with the notation of "Two-tissue Compartment Model" in Chap. 3). The structure labeled "capillary membrane" in Fig. 46 is different in the brain than in the other tissues. In the brain the resorption of glucose or FDG through the capillary membrane is very slow compared with the passage of the molecules from the interstitium into the cells; hence the physiologic space corresponding to compartment x_1 in Fig. 46 is the combined extracellular and intracellular fluid space except the vasculature. In other organs where there is no blood-brain barrier, this exchange proceeds more quickly.

Using the results of the compartmental analysis in Chap. 3, we note that the total activity measured with the PET camera corresponds to the activities coming from all three compartments. The activity in blood plasma is given by $C_a(t)$ multiplied by the regional blood volume rBV, and the tissue activities are multiplied by $(1 - \text{rBV})$, yielding

$$C_t(t) = \text{rBV}C_a(t) + (1 - \text{rBV})(x_1 + x_2) \tag{36}$$

$$\approx \text{rBV}C_a(t) + x_1 + x_2 = \text{rBV}C_a(t) + C_{\text{tiss}}(t)$$

where it was assumed that $\text{rBV} \ll 1$. For early times t, i.e., when dynamic experiments are being performed, the first term cannot be neglected because a large fraction of FDG is still present in the intravascular compartment, but if late FDG uptake is to be modeled, $\text{rBV} = 0$ is acceptable. The quantity was given in Eq. (42) in Chap. 3, and by modeling the data with the function given in the following box, one derives the rate constants K_1, k_2', and k_3' and, if necessary, rBV.

The full quantitative description of FDG kinetics is given by the expression below, where use has been made of Eq. (42) from Chap. 3.

$$C_t(t) = \text{rBV}C_a(t) + C_{\text{tiss}}(t) = \text{rBV}C_a(t) + x_1 + x_2 \tag{37}$$

$$= \text{rBV}C_a(t) + [K_1/(k_2' + k_3')][(k_3' + k_2')e^{-(k_2' + k_3')t}]C_a(t)$$

Thus kinetic data on $C_t(t)$ and the arterial input function $C_a(t)$ can be modeled using K_1, k_2', and k_3' as free parameters. If in a dynamic measurement rBV is also used as a fourth free parameter, rBV can be determined directly as well. Note again that K_1 has the dimensions of ml/(g/min) rather than just min^{-1} and is thus written in capital letters.

From the kinetic constants determined by modeling, one can obtain the regional metabolic rate of glucose (MR$_{\text{Glc}}$) (33):

$$\text{MR}_{\text{Glc}} = \frac{c_{\text{Glc}}K_1 k_3'}{\text{LC}(k_2' + k_3')} \tag{38}$$

Here, c_{Glc} is the glucose concentration in blood plasma, and LC is an experimentally determined constant, the so-called lumped constant that contains the differences in transport and phosphorylation kinetics of FDG as compared with normal glucose metabolism. MR$_{\text{Glc}}$ is a quantity that measures at what rate glucose is transformed into glucose-6-phosphate and thus a measure of the regional efficiency of glucose metabolism. Note that when k_2' is small compared with k_3', that is, when virtually no backdiffusion of glucose takes place, MR$_{\text{Glc}}$ becomes independent of k_2' and k_3' and is only determined by the uptake of glucose into the cells, that is, by K_1.

This determination of MR$_{\text{Glc}}$ requires dynamic PET and the determination of the rate constants. However, there is a simpler way to determine MR$_{\text{Glc}}$ from a single PET measurement assuming that we can take the rate constant values from a set of normals. This is certainly acceptable when normal tissue with altered metabolism is examined but becomes problematic if MR$_{\text{Glc}}$ of other structures such as tumors is to be determined (Table 3) because there is a wide range of MR$_{\text{Glc}}$ values possible. MR$_{\text{Glc}}$ from a single measurement is determined by using the formula (33, 44)

$$\text{MR}_{\text{Glc}} = \frac{c_{\text{Glc}}}{\text{LC}} (c_{^{18}\text{F}} - c_{\text{FDG}})/A_b \tag{39}$$

The total amount of FDG-6P generated up to a time point t is equal to the total measured activity of ^{18}F ($c_{^{18}\text{F}}$), which is determined by PET, minus the concentration of free FDG in tissue c_{FDG}, which can be determined by the arterial input function and the constants

Table 3. *FDG rate constants in human brain tissue*

Normal brain	K_1	k_2'	k_3'	MR$_{\text{GLc}}$
White matter	0.057	0.123	0.041	17.3
Cerebellum	0.091	0.142	0.046	28.6
Cortex	0.083	0.136	0.069	35.8
Thalamus	0.089	0.133	0.064	36.8
Nucleus caudatus	0.088	0.138	0.082	40.9
Pathologic brain	K_1	k_2'	k_3'	MR$_{\text{GLc}}$
Infarct	0.065	0.131	0.037	17.3
Alzheimer	0.066	0.132	0.047	20.8
Tumor (active)	0.075	0.135	0.102	49.2
Tumor (inactive)	0.06	0.14	0.035	18.1

From Wienhard K, Wagner R, Heiss WD. *PET Grundlagen und Anwendungen der Positronen-Emissions-Tomographie.* Berlin: Springer-Verlag (1989).

as determined from the model (see Table 3). A_b represents the total amount of FDG that has entered the tissues up to time t, which is the integral of the plasma concentration of FDG up to time t reduced by a correction factor that is due to the delay in which FDG gets into tissues from plasma. Multiplication with the plasma glucose concentration c_{Glc} and divided by the lumped constant to correct for the fact that we use FDG rather than glucose as a tracer explains the preceding formula.

REFERENCES

1. Adam WE, Bitter F, Geffers H, Garvie NW. Regional evaluation of the left ventricular wall motion by radionuclide ventriculography. *Br J Radiol,* 55(650), 120–124 (1982).
2. *Advance PET imaging system: Description and specification.* General Electric Company (1994).
3. Alpert NM, Eriksson L, Chang JY et al. Strategy for the measurement of regional cerebral blood flow using short-lived tracers and emission tomography. *J Cereb Blood Flow Metab,* 4(1), 28–34 (1984).
4. Brooks RA, Di Chiro G. Theory of image reconstruction in computed tomography. *Radiology,* 117, 561–572 (1975).
5. Budinger TF, Derenzo SE, Greenberg WL et al. Quantitative potentials of dynamic emission computed tomography. *J Nucl Med,* 19(3), 309–315 (1978).
6. Budinger TF, Gullberg GT, Huesman RF. *Emission computed tomography.* In: GT Herman (Ed.). *Image reconstruction from projections.* Berlin: Springer (1979).
7. Buvat I, Benali H, Todd Pokropek A, Di Paola R. Scatter correction in scintigraphy: The state of the art. *Eur J Nucl Med,* 21(7), 675–694 (1994).
8. Chang L-T. A method for attenuation: Correction in radionuclide computed tomography. *IEEE Trans Nucl Sci* 25(1), 638–643 (1978).
9. Datz FL, Gullberg GT, Zeng GL et al. Application of convergent-beam collimation and simultaneous transmission emission tomography to cardiac single-photon emission computed tomography. *Semin Nucl Med,* 24(1), 17–37 (1994).
10. Daube-Witherspoon ME. *Positron emission tomography (PET): Operational guidelines.* In: HN Wagner, Z Szabo, JW Buchanan (Eds.). *Principles of nuclear medicine.* Philadelphia: Saunders (1995).
11. Fercher AF. *Medizinische physik,* 1st ed. Wien: Springer (1992).
12. Ficaro EP, Fessler JA, Rogers WL, Schwaiger M. Comparison of americium-241 and technetium-99m as transmission sources for attenuation correction of thallium-201 SPECT imaging of the heart. *J Nucl Med,* 35(4), 652–663 (1994).
13. Herscovitch P, Markham J, Raichle ME. Brain blood flow measured with intravenous $H_2{}^{15}O$: I. Theory and error analysis. *J Nucl Med,* 24(9), 782–789 (1983).
14. Jaszczak RJ, Hoffman ED. *Positron emission tomography (PET): Scatter and attenuation.* In: HN Wagner, Z Szabo, JW Buchanan (Eds.). *Principles of nuclear medicine.* Philadelphia: Saunders (1992).
15. Jones T, Chesler DA, Ter Pogossian MM. The continuous inhalation of oxygen-15 for assessing regional oxygen extraction in the brain of man. *Br J Radiol,* 49(580), 339–343 (1976).
16. Karp JS, Muehllehner G, Mankof FD et al. Continuous-slice PENN-PET: A positron tomograph with volume imaging capability [Comments]. *J Nucl Med,* 31(5), 617–627 (1990).
17. Koeppe RA, Holden JE, Ip WR. Performance comparison of parameter estimation techniques for the quantitation of local cerebral blood flow by dynamic positron computed tomography. *J Cereb Blood Flow Metab,* 5(2), 224–234 (1985).
18. Koeppe RA, Hutchins GD, Rothley JM, Hichwa RD. Examination of assumptions for local cerebral blood flow studies in PET. *J Nucl Med,* 28(11), 1695–1703 (1987).
19. Lange K, Carson R. EM reconstruction algorithms for emission and transmission tomography. *J Comput Assist Tomogr,* 8(2), 306–316 (1984).
20. Lewellen TK, Kohlmyer SG, Miyaoka RR et al. *Investigation of the performance of the General Electric advance positron emission tomograph in 3D mode.* In: *IEEE MIC.* San Francisco: (1995).
21. Lewellen TK, Miyaoka RS, Kaplan MS et al. *Preliminary investigation of coincidence imaging with a standard dual-headed SPECT system.* In: *Annual meeting.* Minneapolis: Society of Nuclear Medicine (1995).
22. Links JM. Multidetector single-photon emission tomography: Are two (or three or four) heads really better than one? *Eur J Nucl Med,* 20(5), 440–447 (1993).
23. Meikle SR, Bailey DL, Hooper PK et al. Simultaneous emission and transmission measurements for attenuation correction in whole-body PET. *J Nucl Med,* 36(9), 1680–1688 (1995).
24. Mintun MA, Raichle ME, Martin WR, Herscovitch P. Brain oxygen utilization measured with O-15 radiotracers and positron emission tomography. *J Nucl Med,* 25(2), 177–187 (1984).
25. Muehllehner G. Effect of resolution improvement on required count density in ECT imaging: A computer simulation. *Phys Med Biol,* 30(2), 163–173 (1985).
26. Muehllehner G, Colsher JG. *The scintillation camera.* In: DE Kuhl (Ed.). *Radionuclide imaging.* New York: Pergamon Press (1983).
27. Muehllehner G, Karp JS. A positron camera using position-sensitive detectors: PENN-PET. *J Nucl Med,* 27(1), 90–98 (1986).
28. Muehllehner G, Karp JS. Positron emission tomography imaging: Technical considerations. *Semin Nucl Med,* 16(1), 35–50 (1986).
29. Mullani NA, Goldstein RA, Gould KL et al. Myocardial perfusion with rubidium-82: I. Measurement of extraction fraction and flow with external detectors. *J Nucl Med,* 24(10), 898–906 (1983).
30. Myers M, Bailey DL, Bloomfield PM et al. *ECAT ART: A low cost BGO PET camera using rotating detectors.* In: *Annual meeting.* Minneapolis: Society of Nuclear Medicine (1995).

31. Phelps ME, Huang SC, Hoffman EJ, Kuhl DE. Validation of tomographic measurement of cerebral blood volume with C-11-labeled carboxyhemoglobin. *J Nucl Med,* 20(4), 328–334 (1979).

32. Phelps ME, Huang SC, Hoffman EJ et al. Cerebral extraction of N-13 ammonia: Its dependence on cerebral blood flow and capillary permeability—surface area product. *Stroke,* 12(5), 607–619 (1981).

33. Phelps ME, Huang SC, Hoffman EJ et al. Tomographic measurement of local cerebral glucose metabolic rate in humans with (F-18)2-fluoro-2-deoxy-D-glucose: Validation of method. *Ann Neurol,* 6(5), 371–388 (1979).

34. Raichle ME, Martin WR, Herscovitch P et al. Brain blood flow measured with intravenous $H_2{}^{15}O$: II. Implementation and validation. *J Nucl Med,* 24(9), 790–798 (1983).

35. Rohrer RH. *Nuclear Physics and radiation.* In: HN Wagner, Z Szabo, JW Buchanan (Eds.). *Principles of nuclear medicine.* Philadelphia: Saunders (1995).

36. Rosenthal MS, Cullom J, Hawkins W et al. Quantitative SPECT imaging: A review and recommendations by the Focus Committee of the Society of Nuclear Medicine Computer and Instrumentation Council. *J Nucl Med,* 36(8), 1489–1513 (1995).

37. Rushmer RF. *Cardiovascular dynamics,* 4th ed. Philadelphia: Saunders (1976).

38. Saha GB. *Physics and radiobiology of nuclear medicine.* New York: Springer (1993).

39. Schwaiger M, Muzik O. Assessment of myocardial perfusion by positron emission tomography. *Am J Cardiol,* 67(14), 35d–43d (1991).

40. Sokoloff L, Reivich M, Kennedy C et al. The [14C]deoxyglucose method for the measurement of local cerebral glucose utilization: Theory, procedure, and normal values in the conscious and anesthetized albino rat. *J Neurochem,* 28(5), 897–916 (1977).

41. Soussaline F. *The single photon tomograph.* In: DE Kuhl (Ed.). *Radionuclide imaging.* New York: Pergamon Press (1983).

42. Townsend DW, Wensveen M, Byars LG et al. A rotating PET scanner using BGO block detectors: Design, performance and applications. *J Nucl Med,* 34(8), 1367–1376 (1993).

43. Tsui BM, Zhao X, Frey EC, McCartney WH. Quantitative single-photon emission computed tomography: Basics and clinical considerations. *Semin Nucl Med,* 24(1), 38–65 (1994).

44. Wienhard K, Wagner R, Heiss WD. *PET Grundlagen und Anwendungen der Positronen-Emissions-Tomographie.* Berlin: Springer-Verlag (1989).

Functional Imaging, edited by
Gustav von Schulthess and Jürgen Hennig.
Lippincott–Raven Publishers, Philadelphia, © 1998.

6

Functional Imaging with X Rays

Willi A. Kalender and Christoph Suess

FLUOROSCOPY AND COMPUTED TOMOGRAPHY: AN OVERVIEW

Functional imaging has met with great scientific interest in the past few years. It is often associated with functional magnetic resonance imaging (MRI) and positron-emission tomography (PET), which are discussed in depth in Chaps. 5 and 8 of this book. These imaging modalities offer impressive insight into the function of the brain, for example. Responses to stimuli of various origin—sensory, motoric, pharmacologic, or others—have been documented and discussed in many publications and even in the popular press. Thus functional imaging is on everybody's mind, but it is very rarely associated with x-ray imaging modalities. We do not want to question the leading role of PET or MRI and their vast potential, which has not even been fully explored. Yet we feel that there is more than enough work and results using x rays that fall into the category of functional imaging. Some of these efforts should not go unmentioned for reasons of scientific rigor and completeness; some are highly topical and of clinical relevance nowadays.

Perfusion imaging, predominantly of the brain, is the one well-known dynamic computed tomographic (CT) procedure to be discussed. Nevertheless, we will look here at functional imaging in a broader sense and include additional procedures. They all have in common that we do not limit ourselves to the original images, which present a more or less truthful representation of anatomy and morphology. We will look at all those procedures which make use of a series of images, obtained as a function of time, space, or energy, that are used to calculate tissue parameter images associated with some organ or body function. This is not done with the claim to present the method of choice in each case, but rather to give a more or less complete overview and to stimulate thinking.

WA Kalender and C Suess: Institut für Medizinische Physik, Universität Erlangen-Nürnberg, Erlangen, Germany.

Using such a broad definition of functional imaging, there may be enough reasons to include applications in fluoroscopy and digital subtraction angiography as well. In fact, such procedures have been used over decades to examine functions of different body parts and organs, such as, for example, the motility of joints, the acts of swallowing or excreting, the determination of coronary blood flow, or in particular, angiocardiography. Although the advent of digital technology had a positive influence, it appears that no significant new developments of conventional x-ray methods are to be expected. Fluoroscopy can only offer superposition images and thereby has a significant drawback as compared with the slice imaging modalities CT, MRI, and PET. A number of reviews on x-ray imaging have just been published in connection with the one-hundredth anniversary of the discovery of x-rays; these offer both a historical overview and an assessment of recent capabilities, as, for example, in the volume edited by Rosenbusch, Oud-

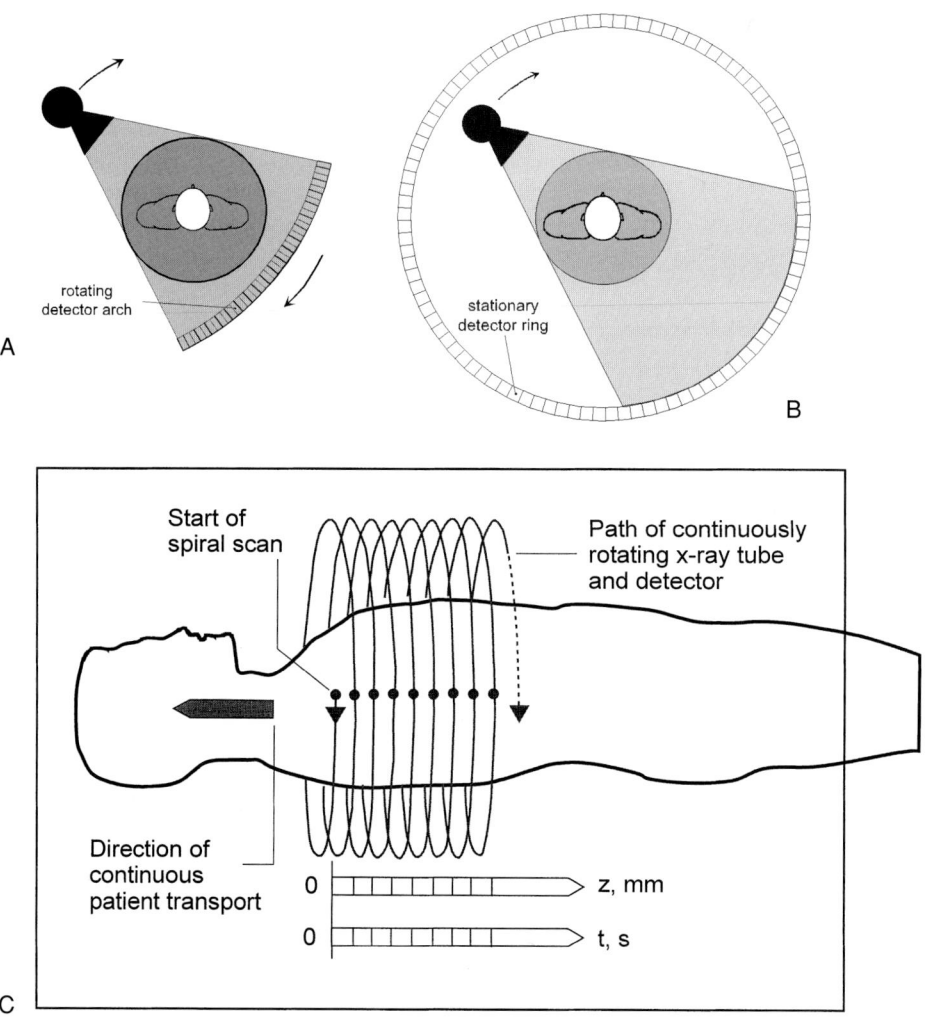

Figure 1. Data acquisition in computed tomography. **(A, B)** Today's standard scanners operate with the x-ray tube rotating around the patient and a fan beam that covers the complete patient cross section. There are designs with rotating detector **(A)** and designs with stationary detector rings **(B)**. **(C)** When continuous data acquisition over many rotations is combined with continuous patient transport, a spiral scan results that allows imaging of complete organs in typically 20 to 60 seconds.

kerk, and Ammann (27). The interested reader is referred to such sources for functional studies by classic x-ray imaging.

The present chapter will focus solely on x-ray computed tomography, starting with a short review of the principles and technical developments and hints to recent developments, in particular to efforts at fast volume imaging. The biggest part of the chapter is dedicated to different approaches to determine perfusion in the brain and body organs. These presently bear the highest clinical relevance and promise for future work. In addition, various other techniques, such as ventilation measurements, that may potentially gain importance in the future are included in an additional section.

STATE OF THE ART IN THE COMPUTED TOMOGRAPHY

CT was introduced by G. N. Hounsfield in 1972; it constituted the first powerful slice imaging modality at that time. CT scanning was slow initially, but it reached a mature technical status within only 10 years, with scan times of typically 2 to 5 seconds. Due to the advent of MRI and improvements in PET instrumentation, there were many forecasts that CT had reached saturation and that it would be largely substituted by MRI within a few years. The advent of spiral CT, a volume imaging mode described below, has changed this situation; a renaissance of CT was observed in the nineties. Today, there is renewed interest and efforts to improve the technology, image-reconstruction algorithms, and clinical applications. Fast-volume scanning is the declared aim. Even new and alternative technical designs are under discussion again.

Conventional CT Scanning

The principle of CT scanning is well known and established. Typically, data are acquired for a single slice over a range of 360°. The x-ray tube is rotated around the patient; the detector is either moving along (Fig. 1A; third generation) or is built up as a stationary ring encircling the patient (Fig. 1B; fourth generation). Today, only minor performance differences are observed between these two designs. Image quality is more than adequate. Scan times per slice are in the range of 0.5 to 2 seconds, such that patient motion is rarely a problem. A range of slice thicknesses between 1 to 10 mm and a wide variety of scan parameters is offered. Some typical values are assembled in Table 1, which also indicates the impressive increase in performance over time. The increased speed became available due to the introduction of slip-ring technology into CT in the late eighties: slip rings are used to transmit the necessary electrical power to the rotating x-ray tube during

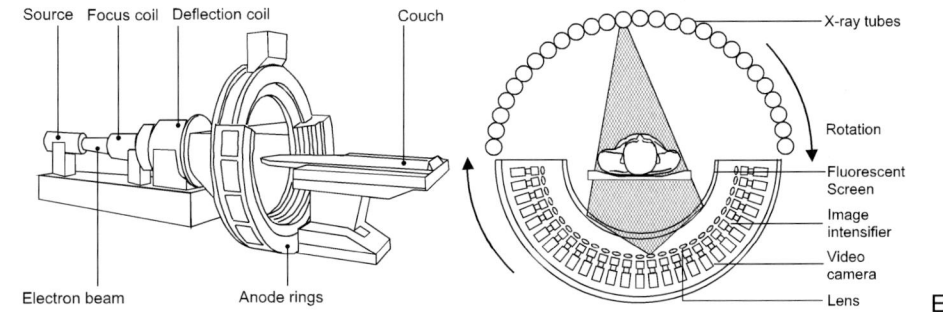

Figure 1. *(continued)* **(D)** In electron-beam CT, there are no moving parts involved. An electron beam is swept across a semicircular anode ring, which allows scanning of single slices in typically 50 to 100 ms. **(E)** The dynamic spatial reconstructor was a unique design with area detectors in an effort to cover complete volumes within 1 second or less.

Table 1. *Performance characteristics of CT: 1972–1995*

	1972*	1995*
Minimum scan time	300 s	0.5–1 s
Data per scan	57.6 kbyte	2 Mbyte
Image matrix	80 × 80	1024 × 1024
Power	2 kW	60 kW
Section thickness	13 mm	1–10 mm
Spatial resolution	3 lp/cm	15 lp/cm
Contrast resolution	5 mm/5 HU/50 mGy	3 mm/3 HU/30 mGy

* Typical values.

the scan; they make cable connections obsolete. As a result, data can be acquired over many 360° rotations without a stop. This has boosted the dynamic capabilities of CT and has provided the possibility to scan continuously or in very fast succession with defined intervals. Continuous scanning up to typically 60 seconds is possible on modern scanners; flexible series of scans with arbitrary preprogrammed interscan delays are available just the same.

Spiral CT

Spiral CT has become possible due to the advent of slip-ring technology and the possibility to acquire data continuously. It was presented for the first time in 1989 (9) and has since gained general acceptance as the scan mode of choice for most standard applications. The basic idea is relatively simple: When the patient is moved through the gantry in synchrony with the continuous data acquisition, the x-ray tube's focus describes a spiral path relative to the patient (Fig. 1C). It allows one to scan complete organs or body sections in very short time intervals of 20 to 60 seconds. Repeated scans are also possible for dynamic studies, mostly undertaken to monitor contrast medium kinetics. Spiral CT has decisive practical advantages due to the short examination time, which allowed for the development of CT angiography, for example. It also offers improved three-dimensional (3D) spatial resolution due to the fact that many overlapping images can be reconstructed retrospectively from the volume data. Also, dose can be reduced significantly, since the table speed can be chosen up to a factor of 2 higher than the slice collimation. Some typical performance parameters are summarized in Table 2; a more technically oriented review can be found in Goldman and Fowlkes (4).

While spiral CT has increased the speed of volume scanning tremendously and thereby has redefined the role of CT in radiology, it has not improved dynamic capabilities to the same degree. The scan time per 360° rotation is the same in a conventional scan mode as in a spiral scan mode. When high temporal sampling is required, spiral scanning offers no significant improvement. Only for applications where complete volumes are to be scanned repeatedly at larger time intervals (see "Xenon-enhanced Dynamic CT" below, for example) or where high 3D spatial resolution is required (see "Biomechanical

Table 2. *Scan and reconstruction parameters unique to spiral CT**

Spiral scan time	24–100 s
Table feeder 360° rotation	1.0–20.0 mm
Table speed	1.0–26.0 mm/s
Number of revolutions	20–60
Scan range	30–1500 mm
z-Interpolation algorithms	Various, mostly 360° or 180° linear interpolation
Reconstruction increment	0.1–5 mm

* Typical values.

Assessment of Bony Structures'' below, for example) is there an indication for spiral CT. This lack of dynamic volume scanning capabilities has stimulated efforts to look into alternative CT designs.

Alternative Technical Developments

Alternative designs that were proposed in the past above all aimed at higher scan speed. One of the most innovative and successful approaches was developed at the University of California at San Francisco (2) and was later commercialized by Imatron Corp. In this design (Fig. 1D), an electron beam is swept across semicircular targets that encircle the patient. Due to the absence of mechanical motion, very fast scanning is possible. The scanner operates typically at 50 to 100 ms per slice; there are about 50 installations worldwide. While image quality is slightly reduced as compared with conventional scanners, its particular strength has been proven in cardiac imaging, in both morphologic and functional applications. The scanner is now being developed further to adapt it to the needs of volume imaging. With respect to the time needed per volume imaged, it does not offer the same advantage with respect to time needed per slice. Nevertheless, its dynamic capabilities exceed those of conventional scanners in this respect also.

A further design that did not aim at subsecond slice scanning but at dynamic volume scanning is the Dynamic Spatial Reconstructor (26). It was a unique installation at the Mayo Clinic in Rochester, and it was used heavily for functional studies on animals. It consisted of a huge ring carrying 14 x-ray tubes with intensifying screens opposite them (Fig. 1E). The principal idea of using area detectors instead of a single or dual row of detector elements is considered up-to-date again today, since it may be the best and most economical way to scan volumes fast. Technologic and algorithmic problems will have to be solved, but fast-volume scanning by CT can be considered a realistic goal.

Dose Considerations

Concern about patient dose in x-ray procedures has always been high and is increasing further as alternative imaging modalities such as MRI and ultrasound, which do not use ionizing radiation, steadily improve in their performance. It often appears that dose issues receive more attention than performance issues; i.e., the focus is solely on the risk but not on the benefit. To enter a discussion of risk versus benefit, it is important to get an estimate of the doses and of the risks involved. This is not a trivial task.

CT scanners operate efficiently today, and dose specifications have to be provided by all manufacturers. Phantom measurements that are useful for scanner comparisons do not give an immediate clue to patient dose, however. In particular, special effort and know-how are required to determine organ and whole-body equivalent effective dose values. Respective values are compiled in Table 3 for some typical examinations in a standard male using a kerma in air value of 14.6 mSv per 100 mA as specified for the Siemens

Table 3. *Dose values in some typical spiral CT examinations*

Anatomic region	Head	Chest	Abdomen	Pelvis
Scan range, mm	160	320	300	160
Slice width, mm	5	10	5	3
Scan time, s	32	32	40	40
Tube current, mA	210	165	210	165
Organ of interest	Eye lens	Lung	Liver	Bladder
Organ dose, mSv	28.1	18.3	16.4	13.3
Effective dose, mSv	1.1	5.3	5.5	2.7

Somatom Plus at 120 kVp. It is understood that dose values will vary strongly with the selection of scan parameters, in particular with the chosen mA value, and with the type of scanner used. But the tabulated values should indicate the orders of magnitude involved in volume scanning in a realistic way. In particular, they allow a crude comparison with other exposures and risks. The natural background radiation level of about 2.4 mSv per year offers the most useful point of orientation.

For repeated scanning of volumes, the respective dose values increase according to the number of repetitions. It is obvious that this may become prohibitive. It is important to limit the volume scanned and the number of temporal samples. This is done in almost all protocols, as described below. For example, when three slices are scanned eight times each in a xenon perfusion measurement, this corresponds in effective dose approximately to a volume scan of 24 slices, which constitutes a typical examination.

TISSUE PERFUSION STUDIES WITH DYNAMIC CT

Dynamic CT allows one to monitor temporal changes of contrast medium concentration in tissues with high sensitivity and high spatial resolution. The sampling rate of 1 to 1.5 images per second in conventional CT and up to 20 images per second in electron beam CT provides high temporal resolution as well. Therefore, it is well suited to detect an indicator's time-density curve and to assess tissue perfusion with the basic approaches of indicator dilution methods used in nuclear medicine (see Chap. 5).

Indicators for CT have to fulfill several requirements: They must provide a sufficient x-ray attenuation, and they must be tolerated by humans in relatively high concentrations. Common approaches use two different types of contrast media. The first is stable xenon gas, which is washed into blood and slowly diffuses into all types of tissues after continuous inhalation (diffusible tracer), and the second is isotonic solutions of elements with high atomic number, mainly iodine, that are injected into vessels and stay within the body's blood pool (nondiffusible tracers).

Dynamic CT studies with stable xenon measure the slow tissue enhancement of the physically dissolved noble gas over a period of several minutes. The method was established clinically during the last decade; it is used mainly to quantify cerebral blood flow. Only a few studies applied the method to quantify blood flow in other organs such as, for example, the kidneys.

Studies with nondiffusible tracers detect and evaluate the contrast enhancement in vessels and parenchyma after injection of a fairly compact contrast bolus. For these tracers, only the first pass of the bolus can be used, and data-acquisition times are limited to several seconds. Different methods evolved in the past, but none of them has gained wide clinical acceptance yet. A new, rather basic approach of data evaluation looks very promising and proved clinical relevance in acute infarct patients already.

Xenon-Enhanced Dynamic CT

In 1977, Winkler et al. demonstrated that xenon, just like iodine, could serve as a contrast agent for dynamic CT; they reported first results on studies of the brain. Following these first trials, the method of measuring cerebral blood flow with stable xenon and CT was further investigated and developed by several research groups in the late 1970s and the early 1980s. In the mid-1980s, all major CT manufacturers started to offer this method as add-on equipment to standard CT scanners (5). Meanwhile ''xenon CT'' has gained clinical acceptance for cerebral blood flow (CBF) measurements with several hundred installations worldwide (30).

Physiologic Model for Diffusible Tracers

Blood flow determination using diffusible tracers is based on the Fick principle (see Chap. 3). This principle simply states the conservation of matter, i.e., the amount of

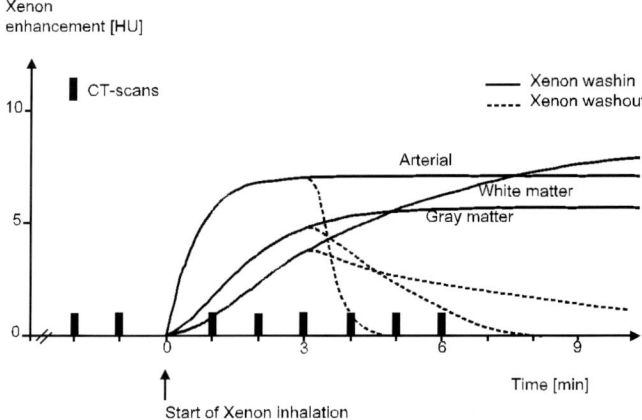

Figure 2. Xenon enhancement patterns in arterial blood and in typical gray and white matter during inhalation of 30% xenon in oxygen and typical timing of CT scans. Curves show enhancement for the wash-in method *(solid lines)* and the wash-in/wash-out method *(dashed lines)* after 3 minutes of inhalation.

indicator in a tissue region, is given by he amount supplied by arterial blood minus the amount drained by venous blood. The concentration in venous blood needs not to be known if equilibrium, i.e., instantaneous diffusion, between capillary blood and surrounding tissue is assumed. Following this concept, Kety (13) derived the relationship between the local cerebral blood flow f and the concentrations of tracer in tissue $C(t)$ and arterial blood $C_a(t)$ [Eq. (3) of Chap. 3]:

$$C(T) = \sum_i w_i f_i \int_0^T C_a(t) e^{-k_i(T-t)} \, dt \qquad (1)$$

The index i in Kety's equation represents the tissue compartments with different flow f_i and k_i, with the sum of the weights w_i adding up to 1. The solubility of tracer in tissue, the so-called brain-blood partition coefficient λ, is hidden in the enhancement parameter k. For instantaneous equilibrium, which is generally assumed in xenon CT, the partition coefficient is given by $\lambda = f/k$. Imperfect tracer diffusion, e.g., in regions with very high flow rates, would lead to a correcting factor m, with $\lambda = mf/k$. Basically, two parameters have to be measured as a function of time in xenon CT to calculate the flow f and λ for a tissue region: the arterial xenon concentration $C_a(t)$ and the uptake of xenon in the respective tissue $C(t)$.

Brain parenchyma consists of two different compartments, gray matter with high flow values in the range of 50 to 80 ml/min/100 g of tissue and a small partition coefficient λ of 0.7 to 0.9 and white matter with low flow rates of 10 to 30 ml/min/100 g and a partition coefficient of 1.2 to 1.6. The uptake of xenon in gray matter with the preceding flow rates reaches saturation after about 6 minutes of continuous xenon inhalation, while in low-flow white matter regions the contrast will increase over up to 25 minutes (Figs. 2 and 3A).

Technical Approaches

Although the speed, stability, and image quality even of early days' CT scanners can be regarded sufficient for measuring the xenon enhancement in brain tissue, detecting the arterial concentration of xenon cannot be accomplished easily. There were several direct and indirect methods established in the past. All direct procedures, e.g., scanning of arterial blood samples or monitoring the partial pressures of CO_2 and O_2 in blood samples of denitrogenated patients, are cumbersome and somewhat invasive and therefore

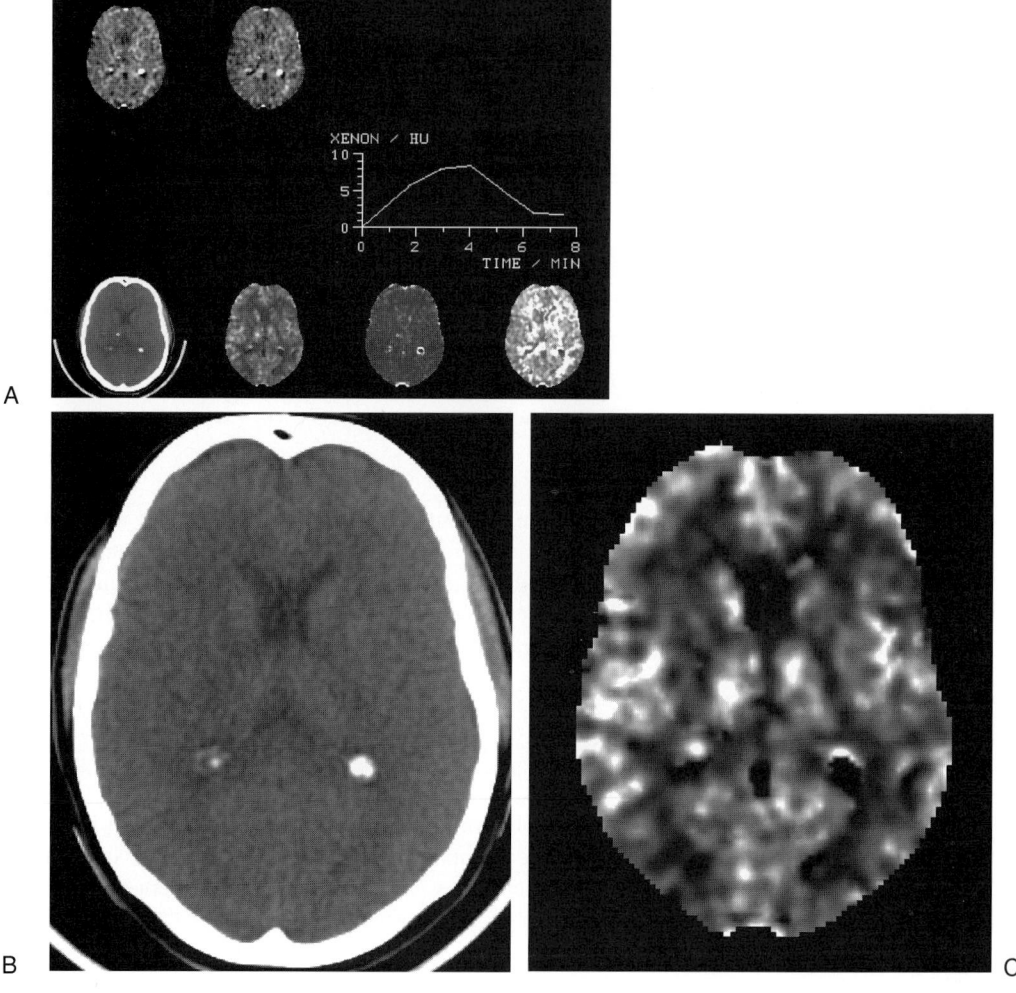

Figure 3. Xenon-enhanced CT provides images of tissue perfusion calculated from a series of scans. **(A)** Series of contrast images after background subtraction. **(B)** Original CT image. **(C)** CBF map in ml/min/100 g of tissue.

not widely used. The indirect methods are based on the assumption that the arterial gas concentrations are in equilibrium with the alveolar air, which was validated in several studies and holds true except for patients with severely impaired gas exchange. Therefore, the time-dependent arterial xenon concentration can be monitored as the concentration of gas in the end-tidal air. Several types of monitors were used in the past; while direct mass spectrometry and gas chromatography appeared to be inconvenient for clinical routine studies, measurement by thermal conductivity cells or setups with radionuclide and photomultiplier tubes can be regarded state of the art now. While the thermal conductivity principle is very easy to handle and cost-effective, it has a rather slow response and exhibits cross-sensitivity to CO_2. The gamma-ray absorption method is more accurate but necessitates the use of radioisotopes.

All indirect methods require conversion of the end-tidal xenon concentrations $C_{Xe}(t)$, measured as a percentage, into arterial enhancement $C_a(t)$ given in Hounsfield units (HU). The conversion is based on the patient's hematocrit value Ht, because the solubility of xenon in blood Θ_{Xe} significantly differs for blood cells and plasma, and on the scanner and object-dependent mass attenuation coefficients for water $(\mu/\rho)_w$ and xenon $(\mu/\rho)_{Xe}$:

$$C_a(t) = \frac{5.15\Theta_{Xe}}{(\mu/\rho)_w/(\mu/\rho)_{Xe}} C_{Xe}(t) \tag{2}$$

with

$$\Theta_{Xe} = 0.0011\text{Ht} + 0.10 \tag{3}$$

Mass attenuation coefficients for xenon and water can be either calculated or determined in experimental setups. Both methods demonstrate large variations of $(\mu/\rho)_{Xe}$ for different x-ray tube voltages and object attenuations, mainly influenced by the effective ray path through soft tissues and bone and the amount of xenon dissolved in tissue. Particular care is requested in determining the specific mass attenuation coefficients and the patient's hematocrit value.

With respect to stable xenon inhalation techniques, two different principles were established in the past. Rather simple and easy-to-handle "open" systems work with a container of premixed xenon-oxygen gas and release exhaled gas into room air; the more complex "closed-loop" systems offer selectable xenon and oxygen concentrations and reuse the exhaled xenon in a closed breathing circuit. Both systems have their specific advantages. The closed systems are more complex and costly but preferable for economic use of the expensive xenon gas and for individual selection of adequate inhaled xenon concentrations. Whatever inhalation unit one employs, it should provide an accurate xenon monitor for the exhaled gas and a reliable data-reduction software to extract true end-tidal xenon concentrations. An on-line link to the CT computer is recommended for transfer of the data and, even more important, for reliable temporal correlation of the xenon curve and the series of CT scans to avoid bias by timing errors.

Data Processing and Functional Images

Calculation of parameter images from a series of xenon-enhanced CT scans and the end-tidal xenon curve within reasonable time requires some basic mathematical background and extensive computing power (see Fig. 3). CT images usually are displayed and stored in matrix size 512 × 512. Every picture element (*pixel*) of the digital image represents a volume element (*voxel*) in brain, and for every voxel, the time-dependent xenon enhancement curve, sampled at five to eight points in time, i.e., by five to eight CT scans, has to be fitted to Eq. (1). In xenon CT it is generally accepted to simplify Kety's equation with respect to the amount of different compartments in one voxel. Assuming only two compartments in every voxel, the six unknowns in Eq. (1), f_1, f_2, k_1, k_2, w_1, and w_2, would be underdetermined by the five to eight data points. A reasonable fit can only be expected for the two parameters of a single compartment. The very limited volume of a single voxel justifies this approximation. Kety's equation for a single compartment can thus be rewritten as

$$C(T) = f \int_0^T C_a(t)e^{-k(T-t)}\, dt \tag{4}$$

Various mathematical approaches are described for least-squares fitting of the parameters f and k in Eq. (4). The straightforward iterative method used initially was replaced by several more effective and less time-consuming techniques. Some of these approximate the arterial curve $C_a(t)$ by mono- or biexponential functions or use lookup-table techniques to limit the calculation times to less than a minute for a set of parameter images.

The basic problem of all fit procedures lies in the relatively poor signal-to-noise ratio (SNR) of the xenon-CT method. Even with optimized CT parameters and inhaled xenon concentrations beyond 30%, the CT enhancement will not significantly exceed 10 HU and pixel noise levels will be in the range of 3 to 6 HU, depending on the applied dose per scan. Therefore, the original CT images have to be smoothed to some degree to improve the SNR and the quality of parameter images. In general, smoothing is achieved by reducing the matrix size and/or applying digital filters with different size and weighting characteristics to the images. However, the balance between the increase in SNR and the loss of spatial resolution must be kept adequate for the specific diagnostic application. Simulations for a typical flow study with one precontrast and six contrast scans during a 6-minute wash-in of xenon in an arterial concentration of 10 HU demonstrate that the noise in flow images strongly increases with CT noise levels above 0.6 to 1.0 HU depending on the specific flow rates.

The parameter image calculation usually produces a flow image with values scaled to milliliters per minute per 100 ml and a ''confidence image'' with a scaling reasonably adapted to the appearance of the flow image. The confidence image displays the errors of the curve fitting, the ''reduced chi-squared.'' The diagnostic interpretation of flow images should always be based on the quality of the fit, given by the confidence image.

Most implementations of xenon CT do not provide lambda images, although all parameter image calculations are based on both flow and lambda calculation. Main reasons for omitting this information are the relatively high noise levels of λ values for the rather short protocols with inhalation times of 3 to 6 minutes, which have meanwhile become clinical routine, and also the questionable diagnostic value of the partition coefficient λ. Whenever this coefficient is of specific interest (19), the inhalation times must be extended significantly, close to the point of xenon saturation.

Clinical Protocols

Scanners with integrated xenon-CT options offer optimized scan parameters, especially a low tube voltage to improve the xenon signal, high tube currents for low noise images, and user-defined preprogrammed protocols allowing one to select several scan levels in the brain and a variety of scan sequences. Modern scanners with short scan times may examine up to five levels in one study and scan all levels in a 1-minute interval. The main advantages of these programmable and automated protocols are given by user comfort and, even more important, by improved and more reliable timing of CT scans. Many aspects will influence the choice of adequate clinical protocols: (a) xenon concentration should be selected as high as tolerable to improve the radiographic signal, (b) an increased dose per scan will reduce the noise in CT images and further improve the SNR, (c) xenon inhalation time should be as short as possible to avoid xenon side effects and possible flow activation due to xenon gas, and (d) the duration of the entire study should be as short as possible to reduce the probability of patient motion.

The concentration of inhaled xenon gas can be varied only within a small range, i.e., for routine examinations between 28% and 35%. At concentrations below 28%, the low contrast enhancement limits the accuracy of flow patterns; at levels higher than 35%, xenon may cause side effects that are generally transient but may impair the success of the study. Meanwhile, most clinical protocols work with a concentration of 30% xenon as a standard. An increased radiation dose per scan will increase the SNR; however, tube load and overall patient dose have to be considered. Depending on exposure factors, the dose per scan ranges from 20 to 40 mGy per CT image, adding up to dose values of 100 to 300 mGy per level examined. Although these overall dose rates are rather high, they are comparable with those of other radiographic procedures, e.g., cerebral angiography, and are believed to be clinically acceptable. Because the brain is assumed to be less sensitive to radiation exposure than other organs, the risk of damage due to a xenon-CT study is relatively low. In any case, CT slices should be selected in a way to minimize the radiation exposure to the eye lens.

The duration of xenon inhalation, as well as the entire study time, has to be adapted to the clinical application. Whenever lambda images are of specific interest, the inhalation time has to be extended significantly to achieve reliable values. For routine xenon-CT applications, flow images are of primary diagnostic interest, and examination times can be as short as 4.5 to 6 minutes. While in standard protocols the wash-in of xenon is detected during the entire duration of the study (wash-in method; see Chap. 3), the recently developed wash-in/wash-out protocols allow one to further reduce the time of xenon exposure. This method has the distinct advantage of shorter xenon exposure and therefore a reduced risk of side effects, in particular a reduction in the probability of patient motion artefacts. Also, lower noise levels in flow images are achieved as compared with wash-in studies with the same overall patient dose. In addition to these principal advantages, wash-in/wash-out protocols have gained acceptance due to significantly improved patient handling with fewer side effects and, consequently, equivalent or better quality of clinical flow images (24).

Discussion

Several factors may influence the accuracy of CBF measured by xenon CT. The drift or instability of CT scanners might have the most severe impact. Although most modern scanners provide excellent stability, the reproducibility of CT values over a certain period should be monitored, e.g., by scanning a water phantom and subtracting images, before starting xenon-CT studies on an unknown type of CT unit. The effects of CT noise and tissue heterogeneity can be controlled to a high degree by selecting adequate scan parameters and size of voxels for evaluation. As discussed before, severe limitations of accuracy may be caused by errors in estimating the arterial xenon concentration and the arrival time of xenon in the brain. Control of these parameters requests some care by the responsible operator. Especially response time and calibration of the end-tidal xenon monitor, accurate hematocrit values, and perfect timing of xenon inhalation and start of the scan sequence are essential prerequisites for a successful xenon-CT study. All these effects may add up to an error of up to 100% for a single voxel of approximately $1 \times 1 \times 5$ mm^3; however, in practice, the overall errors can be limited to an acceptable value of 20% or less when looking at volume elements with a size exceeding $8 \times 8 \times 10$ mm.

Despite these limitations, the xenon-CT technique offers several advantages over other comparable CBF-measuring approaches. It is easily available on most CT scanners and can be combined with a standard CT examination, it provides excellent anatomic correlation facilitating the diagnosis (see Fig. 3B, C), and as a methodologic advantage, it uses the true tissue-specific partition coefficient instead of a fixed standard value. These aspects helped the xenon-CT method to establish itself during the last decade in many hospitals as a routine tool for investigating a variety of cerebral disorders.

In the future, the technical progress achieved by new and faster computational approaches, more reliable inhalation devices, and new clinical protocols will support clinical progress. Standard examinations such as, for example, CBF measurements before and after acetezolamide application to study the flow reserve activation in patients with cerebrovascular disease are expected to further increase the clinical acceptance of the method. The latest developments toward volumetric CT, i.e., above all spiral CT, offer new perspectives for functional imaging with CT. Entire volumes can be examined in a short 6-minute study. This would overcome the limitation to a few single slices and offer the possibility to correct for patient motion. Despite all these positive prospects, xenon CT will continue to suffer from the complex inhalation and gas-analysis apparatus used and from the special demands on patient handling.

Iodine-Enhanced Dynamic CT

The application of iodine in CT scanning started in the early days of CT to enhance the contrast of highly vascularized tissues and lesions. Since then, the role of iodinated contrast media in this area has increased rapidly and by now covers a wide range of examinations. In the beginning of dynamic CT, the evaluation of bolus dynamics was used mainly to optimize contrast protocols for routine scanning. With the development of fast, powerful scanners, however, the detection of time-density curves with high quality has become feasible.

Compared with xenon-enhanced dynamic CT, the iodine-based approach offers several distinct advantages. The necessary technical equipment, mostly a power injector, is readily available, and most modern CT scanners offer the required speed and dedicated dynamic scan acquisition modes. The total scan time and examination time are very short and allow examination of even less than cooperative patients. However, the measured volume is usually limited to a single axial slice of up to 10 mm thickness, unless a multislice setup can be used.

Iodine as a nondiffusible tracer passes the vascular system very quickly, and after the first passage of a contrast bolus through the capillaries, the tracer rapidly develops an equilibrium concentration in blood (Fig. 4) until it is slowly excreted via the kidneys. Therefore, the perfusion information must be acquired during the first bolus passage, and the bolus time-density curve (TDC) must be sampled with the highest temporal resolution available on the scanner.

Physiologic Models for Nondiffusible Tracers

Iodine-based dynamic studies measure the first pass of a contrast bolus in vessels and tissues. The basic physiologic model was first formulated by Meier and Zierler (18). Data analysis is usually based on the mean transit time method (Eq. 15 in Chap. 3), which assumes that an instantaneous bolus of tracer can be delivered to a defined volume of blood and is subsequently washed out by the circulating blood. In this case, the blood flow per volume can be expressed as one over the tissue's mean transit time. These theoretical assumptions, however, are hardly approximated in iodine-enhanced CT with intravenous injection and continuous recirculation of tracer. Leon Axel modified the basic model for TDCs measured by dynamic CT. He applied corrections for recirculation fitting a gamma-variate function and deconvolved the tissue TDC with the arterial input function (1). The arterial curve of a very compact bolus can in most cases not be monitored adequately by CT; a wider arterial TDC, however, implies larger errors and makes it more difficult to quantify the tissue's response function. The mean-transit-time methods in iodine-enhanced CT have to correct for recirculation, and they require several assumptions on the shape of the deconvolution function. These manipulations limit accuracy and reliability of the method and thereby its acceptance and clinical relevance.

A different approach, suggested by Miles et al. (20), was derived from microsphere theory. They adapted a nuclear medicine data-processing technique to CT data, which was originally developed by Peters et al. (23) for isotope tracers not completely extracted by the investigated organ. Their argumentation starts with the basic assumption that the organ blood flow (OBF) as a fraction of total cardiac output (CO) can be measured as the amount of tracer in the respective organ (M_0) divided by the total amount of tracer applied (M_{tot}):

$$\frac{\text{OBF}}{\text{CO}} = \frac{M_0}{M_{tot}} \tag{5}$$

In studies with radiolabeled microspheres (see Chap. 3), the amount of tracer M_0 corresponds to the maximum count rate, i.e., the height H, of the organ's time-density curve multiplied by a scaling factor a to relate the measured counts per second to the actual mass of the tracer:

$$\frac{\text{OBF}}{\text{CO}} = \frac{H \cdot a}{M_{tot}} \tag{6}$$

Because the TDCs of those tracers which are not completely absorbed in the organ will not reach the maximal height, they further derived equations to calculate flow from the maximal slope of time-density curves. Considering an integrated arterial time-activity curve without recirculation described by a gamma-variate function, its shape will be the same as the one obtained with microspheres, but the plateau will be reached at a value

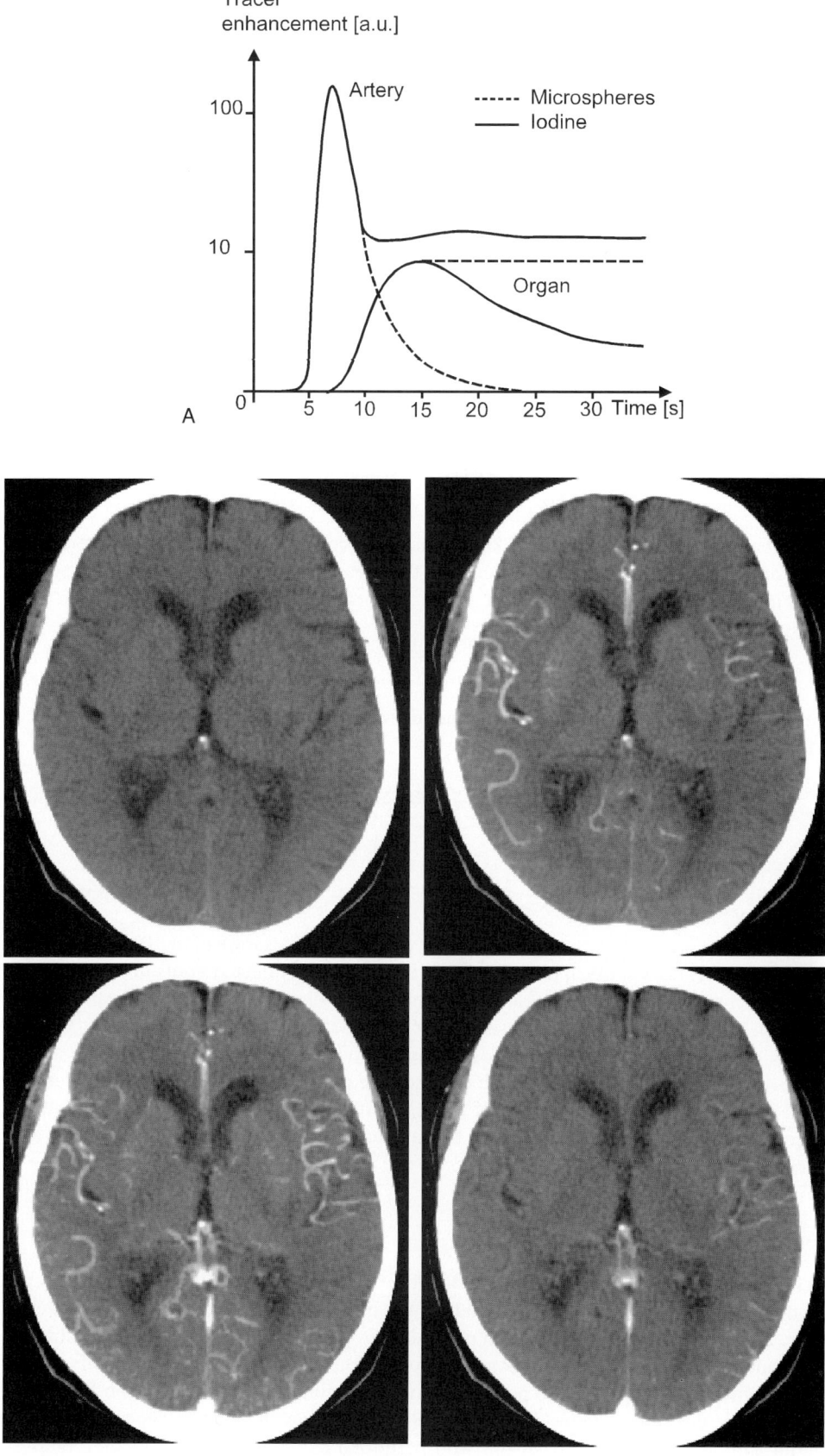

Figure 4. Principle of iodine-enhanced dynamic CT. **(A)** Typical enhancement curves for arterial blood and organ parenchyma. **(B)** Four images of a dynamic series during bolus passage.

A (counts) with a maximal slope $g_{arterial}$ (counts/s). The integrated arterial curve and the organ curve will be related as follows:

$$\frac{g_{organ}(counts/s^2)}{g_{arterial}(counts/s)} = \frac{H(counts/s)}{A(counts)} \qquad (7)$$

A also reflects the area under the arterial curve before integration, and $g_{arterial}$ will be its maximum height. Using Eqs. (6) and (7) to substitute H, the height of the tissue TDC, we get

$$\frac{OBF}{CO} = \frac{A}{M_{tot}} \cdot \frac{g_{organ}}{g_{arterial}} \cdot a \qquad (8)$$

In dynamic CT, the integral A is measured in Hounsfield units times seconds. The correction factor a corresponds to the scaling of the CT enhancement expressed in HU per milligram of iodine per milliliter. The factor depends on the type of CT scanner and mainly on the tube voltage setting. It can be omitted if the amount of tracer M_{tot} is expressed in Hounsfield units times milliliters:

$$\frac{OBF}{CO} = \frac{A(HU \cdot s)}{M_{tot}(HU \cdot ml)} \frac{g_{organ}(HU/s)}{g_{arterial}(HU)} \qquad (9)$$

From other dynamic CT studies it is known that the cardiac output CO can be determined as the amount of injected tracer divided by the area under the arterial curve, corrected for recirculation:

$$CO = \frac{M_{tot}(HU \cdot ml)}{A(HU \cdot s)} \qquad (10)$$

Combining Eqs. (9) and (10), the organ blood flow per milliliter of tissue, i.e., the tissue perfusion, can be written as

$$OBF = \frac{g_{organ}(HU/s)}{g_{arterial}(HU)} \qquad (11)$$

g_{organ} can be determined as the maximum slope of the tissue TDC, and $g_{arterial}$, the maximum slope of the integrated arterial curve, is equivalent to the peak height of the arterial TDC before integration.

Both curves are readily available from a dynamic CT examination. But one has to consider to what degree the application of an intravenously injected bolus of iodine meets the requirements of the physiologic model and allows one to quantify the organ's blood flow. The maximal slope of the tissue's TDC will definitely not be affected by venous outflow of tracer so long as the passage time of tracer through the organ, the so-called *tracer retention,* is long compared with the rise time of the arterial TDC. This requirement can be fulfilled only with very compact injections of a relatively small amount of contrast material. The injection technique has to be adapted to the specific organ's flow rates and tracer retention characteristics.

Clinical Application

The maximum-slope method described above was applied clinically by several groups, and the respective authors reported good results in abdominal organs as well as in brain tissue. Miles et al. measured perfusion of the kidneys and succeeded in separating cortical and medullary flow rates; data on splenic perfusion also were included in this report (20). A further study on hepatic perfusion, including functional images of the liver, was published by the same group (21). The quality of data even allowed separation of the arterial and portal phases of perfusion and permitted parameter images for both phases. Pancreatic perfusion also was assessed successfully (22).

Further studies used this technique for cerebral perfusion imaging. First results on

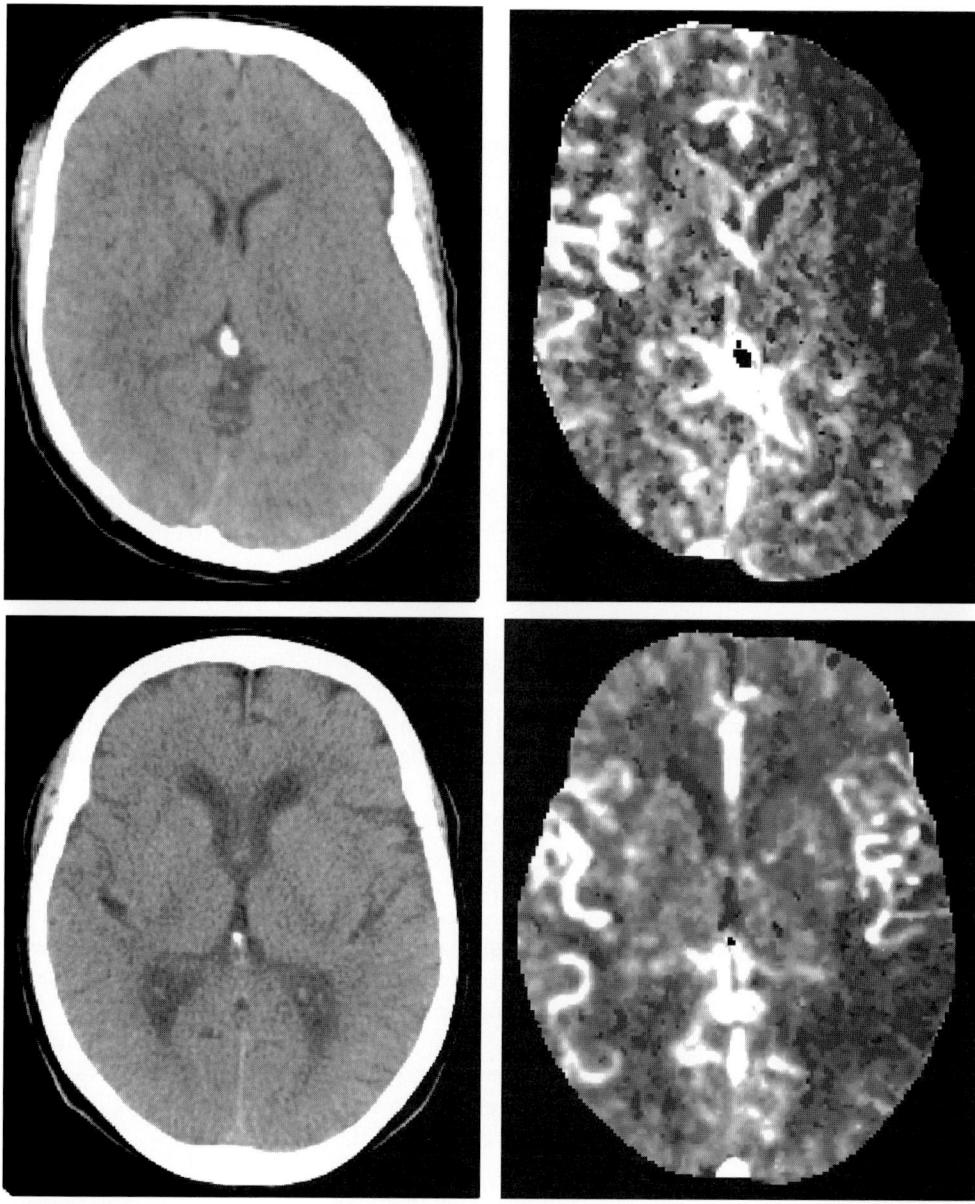

Figure 5. Brain perfusion measurement in patient with a fresh infarct due to occlusion of the medial and anterior cerebral artery *(upper row)* and the posterior cerebral artery *(lower row)*. These studies were performed with minimal technical requirements within a few hours after the infarct occurred.

patients with fresh brain infarcts were reported recently by different groups (14, 17). They applied a compact bolus of 50 ml by manual intravenous injection and achieved an image quality comparable with that of optimal xenon-CT studies (Fig. 5).

Discussion

While most iodine-enhanced dynamic CT studies suffer from basic limitations in the physiologic model and the need for corrections and approximations, the novel approach that only evaluates the height of the arterial curve and the maximum slope of the tissue's TDC promises a wider clinical acceptance. The method only uses information about the tracer's wash-in, and therefore, it only needs to sample the TDCs until the maximum enhancement in tissue is reached. In this short period of usually 15 to 25 seconds the scanner's highest sampling rate can be applied to monitor the TDCs with adequate temporal resolution.

Evaluation of larger regions of interest (ROIs) allows one to reduce the pixel noise significantly and to calculate flow values with high reliability. With respect to calculating functional images, the basic problems are very similar to xenon CT. The noise in pixel-based CT data is in the range of the expected tracer signal of 5 to 10 HU. Image processing again requires several steps of noise reduction, like a reduced matrix size and image filtering, and more sophisticated algorithms to estimate the maximal slope of noisy tissue TDCs. The first results, however, look very promising, and further improvements in data processing are likely. The maximum-slope method or variations of it may well become the most successful application of CT to functional imaging.

Myocardial Perfusion Studies by Electron-Beam CT

Many imaging techniques have been used to assess regional myocardial perfusion, but to date there is no clinically accepted noninvasive method. Single-photon-emission CT suffers from poor spatial resolution, and it does not provide quantifying methods for precise evaluation of ischemic areas. Positron-emission tomography proved to be useful for the study of myocardial perfusion and metabolism; however, PET scanners are not readily available and offer only poor spatial resolution in cardiac imaging. Contrast-enhanced echocardiography was applied to measure myocardial perfusion, but it requires an invasive intracoronary injection and will not gain wide clinical acceptance. Functional MRI offers many promising applications and may be applied to myocardial measurements in the future. Up to now it is still in an experimental stage for this application.

Ultrafast CT with scan times of typically 50 ms, be it electron-beam CT with a multislice modality or a device similar to the Dynamic Spatial Reconstructor at the Mayo Clinic, have the potential to produce 3D images of the heart throughout the cardiac cycle. Combined with contrast material injection, it can be used to measure the tracer's time-density curves in myocardium. Following the basic principles of indicator dilution methods, ultrafast CT allows assessment of myocardial perfusion. A review on myocardial perfusion studies was given recently by Georgiou et al. (3).

The physiologic model for a single tissue compartment with a single entrance and exit is described by the Fick equation (Eq. 2 in Chap. 3): The input flow F_i times the input concentration C_i at time t is equal to the change in the amount of indicator dQ in the compartment per time increment dt plus a constant F_0 times C_0:

$$F_i C_i(t) = \frac{dQ}{dt} + F_0 C_0(t)$$

For constant flow and if there is no loss of indicator, the equation can be solved for the concentration of the indicator:

$$F_i \int_0^\infty C_i(t) \, dt = Q \tag{12}$$

where Q represents the total amount of tracer in the volume V_m with concentration C_m and $Q = V_m C_m$. The flow per unit volume can therefore be written as

$$\frac{F_i}{V_m} = \frac{C_m}{\displaystyle\int_0^\infty C_i(t) \, dt} \tag{13}$$

If recirculation can be corrected for, the area of the input curve is inversely proportional to cardiac output and can be measured anywhere in the central blood pool $[C_{bp}(t)]$, e.g., in the ventricle. The basic formula, used in most ultrafast CT studies, states that the flow per volume can be measured by the height of the tissue TDC (ΔHU) over the area of the input TDC:

$$\frac{F}{V} = \frac{\Delta \text{HU}}{\displaystyle\int_0^\infty C_{bp}(t)\ dt} \tag{14}$$

Several assumptions of the model may limit the application to myocardial perfusion studies. Recirculation of the indicator has to be corrected for. This can be achieved by fitting a gamma-variate curve to the TDCs of larger tissue regions with reduced noise in enhancement data (Fig. 6). The model requests an appropriate coronary input function, which generally can be provided for normal and low flow. For high flow rates, the venous outflow of tracer before reaching the maximal myocardial enhancement will in general cause underestimation of flow values. Finally, the indicator density has to be measured accurately; for this purpose, just as in conventional CT studies, the tracer is quantified after image subtraction, which requires perfect matching of images. Reliable ECG triggering of scans is an essential prerequisite.

Several groups investigated the ultrafast CT myocardial perfusion method in flow phantom setups or in canine models. Ludman et al. (16) measured flow in a vessel and tissue model to validate results for continuous and pulsatile flow. They concluded that cardiac output and tissue perfusion can be quantified accurately if the local iodine attenuation value, which varies inter- and also intraindividually up to a factor of 2, is known. Studies in dogs, as done by Rumberger et al. (28), Gould et al. (6), and Wang et al. (32), for example, compared ultrafast CT and microsphere perfusion measurements. The different groups found fairly good to excellent correlation for normal and low flow rates but a significant underestimation of high perfusion values due to the early venous outflow of tracer. They concluded that the myocardial flow can be well quantified with an intra-arterial contrast injection, but the noninvasive intravenous injection requires correction for early tracer outflow. The suggested mathematical models, however, did not yield a satisfactory correction, and therefore, their application to humans was very limited.

Recently, Wolfkiel and Brundage (33) developed a different algorithm to correct for early tracer outflow in CT data and have achieved a linear correlation to microsphere data for flows up to 8 ml/min/g. These promising results show the potential of the method to determine myocardial perfusion with ultrafast CT in an accurate and reproducible way. The method could help to study the organ's flow reserve and the hemodynamic relevance of coronary artery stenoses.

VARIOUS FUNCTIONAL IMAGING APPROACHES WITH CT

Ventilation Studies of the Lungs

X-ray computed tomography (CT) traditionally has been used for high-resolution morphologic assessment of the lung but very rarely for quantitative or functional examinations. This appears possible, however, if appropriate methodology is provided. We have developed means for spirometric triggering, for xenon inhalation, and for dedicated evaluation to allow for ventilation measurements. Similar to xenon-CT perfusion measurements, stable xenon gas serves as a tracer and contrast medium.

Control of the patient's inspiratory status is a prerequisite for reproducible quantitative evaluation of lung parameters. We have extended the concept of spirometric control and triggering (11); control of the patient's inspiratory status, real-time display of breathing curves, and generation of signals to close the breathing valve and to trigger the CT scan are done via PC. Xenon-oxygen mixtures are provided to the patient by a dedicated inhalation system with an integrated spirometer. Two xenon-oxygen concentrations are offered, 75% Xe and 25% O_2 and 33% Xe and 67% O_2, for single breath and for continued breathing, respectively (Fig. 7A). The patient is instructed to breathe normally

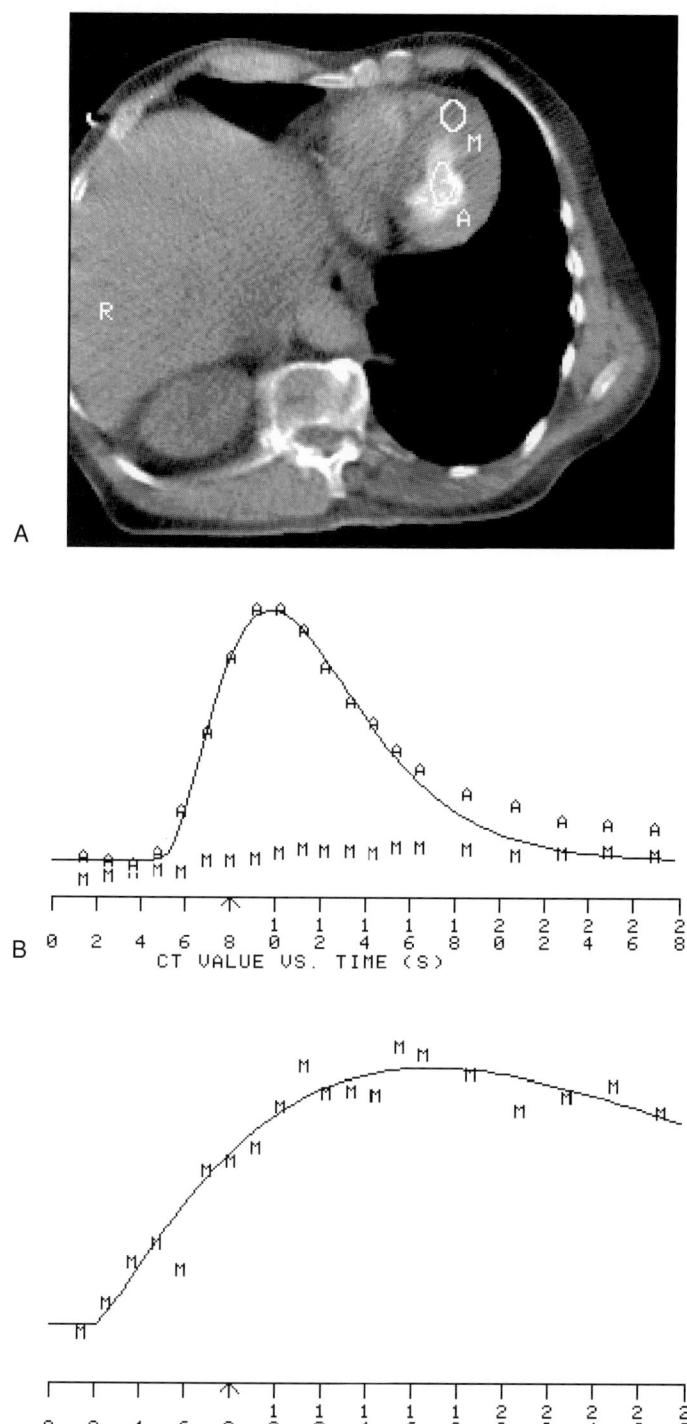

Figure 6. Myocardial perfusion measurement with electron-beam CT and 50-ms scan time. **(A)** One image of a four-level study with 20 scans each triggered at 40% of the RR interval. **(B, C)** Enhancement data for the left ventricle (*A*) and the myocardium (*M*) fitted to a gamma-variate curve for quantification of perfusion.

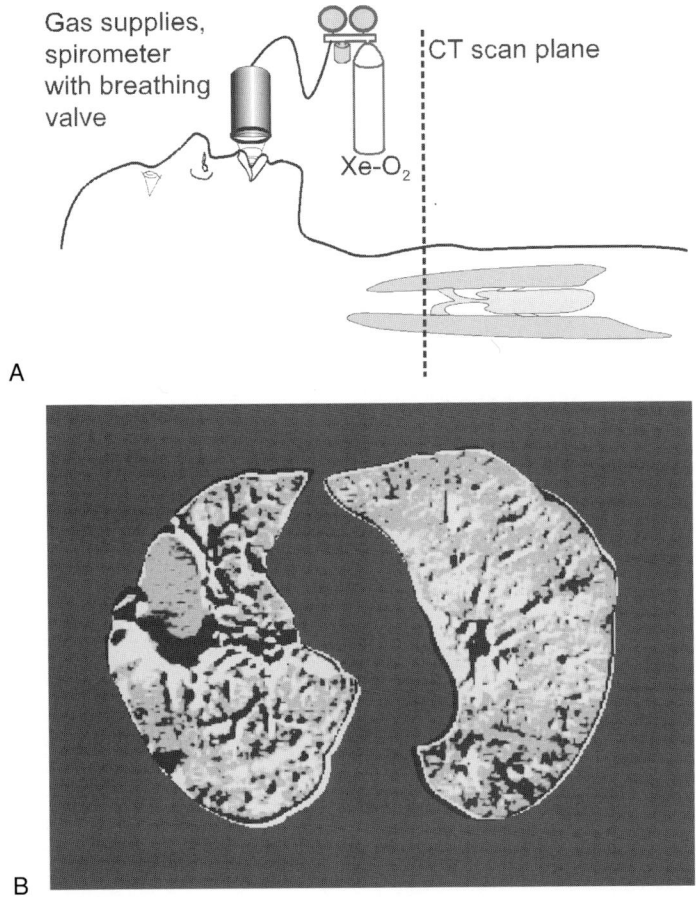

Figure 7. Assessment of lung ventilation with stable xenon gas and dynamic CT. **(A)** The patient inhales xenon under spirometric control. **(B)** The distribution of lung ventilation is obtained by image subtraction with a number of corrections applied or by using physiologic models.

through the spirometer. After a vital capacity measurement has been taken, he or she exhales completely—whereupon the supply is switched from room air to the Xe-O_2 mixture—and then inhales deeply. When a chosen volume is reached, e.g., 80% of vital capacity, the valve is closed and a series of CT measurements triggered. For evaluation purposes, automated segmentation of the lung is done prior to the calculation of ventilation maps. Subtraction images provide the information on local xenon concentration and can be regarded as a first estimate of the distribution of ventilation. Quantification of true ventilation values based on physiologic models demands knowledge of additional parameters, e.g., residual volume, arterial concentration, etc. So far this has only been approached in animal studies (29).

Simplified models suitable for clinical studies are presently under investigation using subtraction and corrections for residual volume and patient breathing motion. Xenon enhancement of typically 50 HU was obtained for the single-breath technique with the possibility of evaluating wash-out dynamics. Ventilation maps of single lung sections were generated for 30 volunteers and for 20 patients so far in a first clinical study (Fig. 7B) (31). They were diagnostically useful in several cases, but breathing motion and registration between the prexenon and the xenon scans remained a problem. The success rate of dynamic studies has to be improved further by design of apparatus and study protocols and, more promising, by extension to spiral volume scans and software efforts for reregistration after patient motion. Work in this direction appears promising.

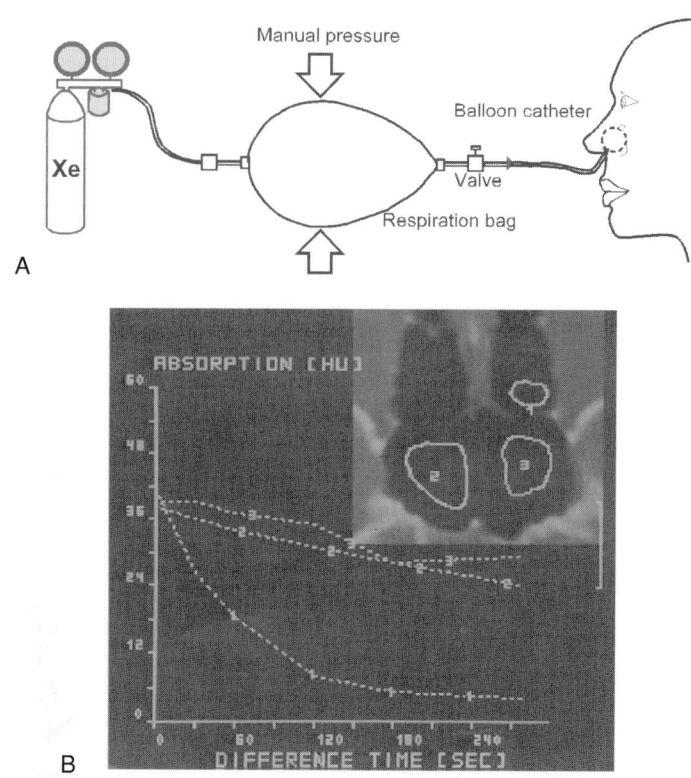

Figure 8. Measurement of paranasal sinus ventilation with stable xenon gas and dynamic CT. **(A)** Xenon is pumped manually into the sinus system via the nostrils. **(B)** The wash-out of xenon is measured at arbitrary locations. Here, poor ventilation of both sphenoid sinuses is demonstrated in direct comparison to the ethmoidal cells.

Ventilation Studies of the Paranasal Sinus System

While the assessment of lung ventilation by dynamic CT has gained the interest of several research groups, the assessment of ventilation in the paranasal sinus system by CT is admittedly a rare topic. Ventilation of the paranasal sinuses plays an important role in the etiology of acute and chronic sinusitis, however. The CT method is of interest because there are no easy and noninvasive alternatives. The known invasive approaches are associated with considerable discomfort to the patient, and they are limited to the maxillary and frontal sinuses, which can be cannulated to insert different devices. Consequently, they are rarely performed. Dynamic CT may offer an alternative (10).

One to two liters of xenon are blown into the sinus system via a balloon catheter in one nostril, with the other nostril blocked by a second balloon (Fig. 8A). CT scans are started about 20 seconds after the end of xenon insufflation to allow for removal of the balloons so that the patient can breathe normally and comfortably. Only a few CT scans are necessary to monitor wash-out of xenon over typically 5 minutes. Enhancement values of typically 30 to 100 HU are observed with this technique. The resulting images or mean values for regions of interest are submitted to a fit procedure; we used a monoexponential fit to determine the mean gas exchange time t_m as a measure of ventilation (10):

$$C(t) = C_0 e^{-t/t_m} \qquad (15)$$

t_{90}, the time at which 90% of the xenon is washed out, can be calculated from this. Results of the studies performed so far agreed well with clinical findings, with gas exchange determined for all sinuses (Fig. 8B). The procedure can be done fast and at relatively low cost. The lack of general acceptance of this technique may be due to either of two reasons: (a) it is not known, or (b) there is no sufficiently urgent clinical demand for this information. It is not clear which reason predominates. As yet, dynamic CT is the only noninvasive quantitative method for the determination of the ventilation of all paranasal sinuses.

Kidney Clearance Studies

Renal function analysis is traditionally done by nuclear medicine methods, predominantly by [^{131}I]hippuran clearance tests. Dynamic CT may offer an interesting alternative. The following procedure has been proposed: After intravenous injection of a contrast medium bolus, enhancement of CT values in the aorta and the kidneys is measured at the height of the kidney hili for 5 to 10 minutes. Standard iodinated contrast media distribute rapidly in plasma and are excreted by the kidneys up to 99%; the excretion rate is directly dependent on the glomerular filtration rate. The enhancement curves are plotted versus time, and the difference between aortic and kidney enhancement is taken as a measure of renal concentration capability. Separate clearance values for the left and the right kidneys can be estimated by determining the areas under the respective curves and by subtracting the aortic values. A simple model was proposed (12) as

$$\text{CT clearance} = \left(\text{AUC}_{\text{right}} \times \frac{1.73}{BSA} - \text{AUC}_{\text{aorta}} \times \frac{1 - \text{Hct}}{1 - 0.4} \right)$$
$$+ \left(\text{AUC}_{\text{left}} \times \frac{1.73}{BSA} - \text{AUC}_{\text{aorta}} \times \frac{1 - \text{Hct}}{1 - 0.4} \right)$$

where *AUC* represents the area under the curve for right and left kidneys and aorta, respectively (Fig. 9); correction for the individual's size by body surface area *(BSA)* and for hematocrit (Hct) are included. CT clearance, here measured in Hounsfield units times seconds, has been shown to correlate strongly with clearance values measured by [^{131}I]hippuran (12). Normal or reference values have to be established, yet a standard examination and evaluation protocol must be done just the same. A particular problem

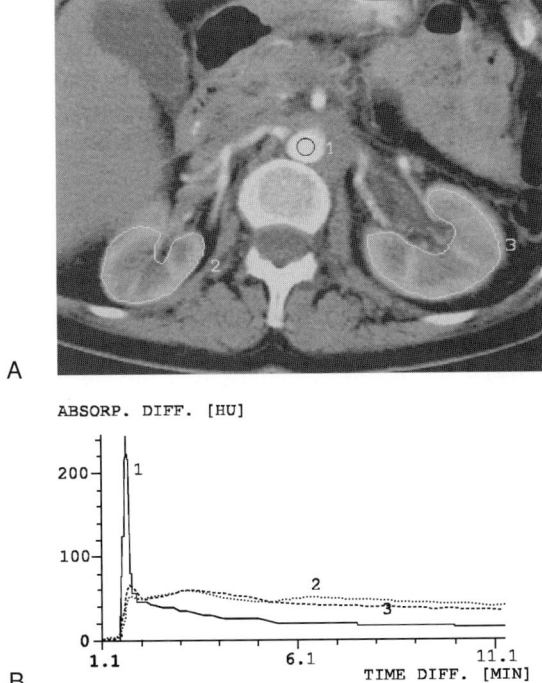

Figure 9. Kidney clearance measurement by dynamic CT. **(A)** Iodine excretion by the kidneys over time serves as a measure of glomerular filtration capacity. **(B)** Enhancement curves in arterial blood and in kidney parenchyma over the first 10 minutes after injection are evaluated to generate quantitative estimates of kidney clearance.

is given by the fact that different contrast media may have different pharmacokinetics. Nevertheless, the procedure is fast and easy to perform, and it provides all the morphologic information of CT in addition to functional information.

Biomechanical Assessment of Bony Structures

The yet unsolved question of how to estimate bone strength in vivo is gaining importance to the same degree as osteoporosis, an age-related bone disease, is gaining importance as a disease of epidemiologic dimension. The inspection of biomechanical parameters of bony structures can be viewed as an effort to estimate the mechanical rigidity of bone in critical locations and thereby its function and the likelihood of fracture. This can be done in either an integral approach, e.g., by calculation of a stress-strain diagram for a whole bone, or specifically, by searching locations of outstanding strain under given stress conditions. Both questions are relevant in osteoporosis research, which is concerned with the estimation of the patient-specific fracture risk.

CT-based bone mineral density measurements are an excellent tool for this purpose: In vitro experiments clearly showed the dependency of bone mineral density and ultimate load that causes the failure of bone (15). Because mainly the femur and the lumbar vertebrae are affected by osteoporosis, these bones lie in the focus of interest. As a prerequisite for functional assessment, bone mineral density values must be known throughout the complete volume of the bone in question. These can be determined easily by a spiral scan (Fig. 10A) and subsequent mapping of CT values to density values. They then serve as a basis to estimate rigidity and elasticity in volume elements of bone on a microscopic level. These two parameters allow for calculation of the biomechanical performance of the whole bone under a simulated load with the aid of finite-element analysis tools (7, 8, 25). The analysis also will reveal the stress distribution within the bone (Fig. 10B).

Although the capacity of modern computers has made it possible to analyze bone in a very detailed way, finite-element analysis of a single bone still requires major efforts due to high computational demands and the necessity of user interactions. Hence the described procedure is not established in clinical work. Also, the insufficient knowledge of the dependency of the microscopic mechanical properties on bone mineral density has to be acknowledged. The situation is further complicated by the difficult question of how the physical condition of the patient, i.e., muscles, ligaments, mobility, etc., influence the overall stability of the bone site. Nevertheless, this is an interesting and promising field of research that may add to clinical diagnosis.

SUMMARY

A number of traditional functional radiographic examinations are still in use, today mostly done by digital subtraction angiography, which were not discussed in detail here. The potential for extended functional imaging with x rays is associated with computed tomography. Measurements of tissue perfusion by dynamic CT using either xenon inhalation or bolus injection of contrast media are the well-known and well-established procedures. Xenon CT is used today in many centers for preoperative evaluation of patients with cerebrovascular complications. Iodine-enhanced dynamic CT is used for the investigation of acute brain infarct patients, for cardiac perfusion measurements, and in a number of research projects. Other CT applications involve ventilation studies of the lungs and the paranasal sinus system, kidney clearance studies, and biomechanical assessment of bone. All these procedures have in common that they can be done relatively fast, easily, and at low cost. The only potential risk involved is the exposure to ionizing radiation. The exposure levels and the risks associated with them can be considered as moderate, however; they are definitely negligible when compared with the problems in the patient populations to be considered. While the potential risks exclude CT from basic functional imaging studies on volunteers, it may become the method of choice in several

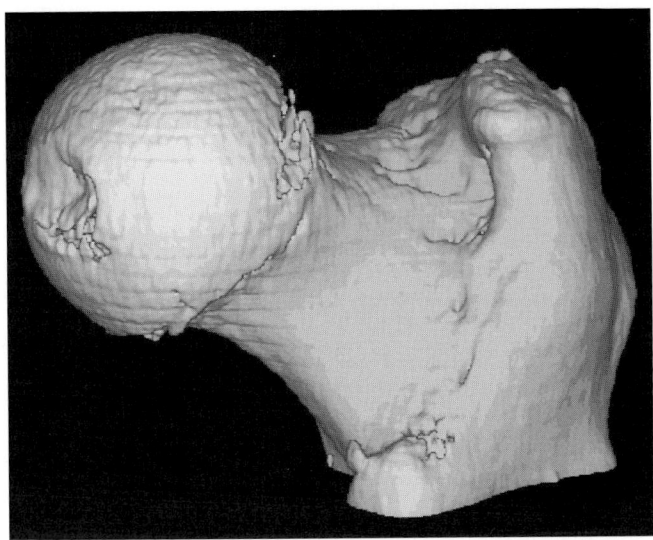

A

B

Figure 10. Estimate of bone strength by finite element analysis. **(A)** Volume scans of bone serve to determine the 3D distribution of bone mineral. **(B)** Fracture risk is assessed by finite-element analysis, which yields zones of excessive strain under given stress conditions. Major interest relates to the femoral neck, which is one of the most critical fracture sites in osteoporotics.

applications due to its ease of use and low cost. The trend toward volume imaging that can be performed in a dynamic way also may further augment the role of CT in assessing function.

REFERENCES

1. Axel L. Tissue mean transit time from dynamic computed tomography by a simple deconvolution technique. *Radiology,* 18, 94–99 (1983).
2. Boyd D, Lipton MJ. Cardiac computed tomography. *Proc IEEE,* 71, 298–308 (1983).
3. Georgiou D, Wolfkiel C, Brundage BH. Ultrafast computed tomography for the physiological evaluation of myocardial perfusion. *Am J Cardiac Imaging,* 8, 151–158 (1994).
4. Goldman LW, Fowlkes JB. *Medical CT and ultrasound: Current technology and applications.* Madison, WI: Advanced Medical Publishing (1995).
5. Gur D, Yonas H, Good W. Local cerebral blood flow by xenon-enhanced CT: Current status, potential improvements, and future directions. *Cerebrovasc Brain Metab Rev,* 1, 68–86 (1989).
6. Gould RG, Lipton MJ, McNamara MT. Measurement of regional myocardial blood flow in dogs by ultrafast CT. *Invest Radiol,* 23, 348–353 (1988).
7. Heitz M, Coman J, Prevrhal S, Kalender WA. Evaluation of femoral mineral density and strength using volumetric CT and anatomical coordinate systems. *Medizinische Physik* 1995, Jahrestagung der Deutschen Gesellschaft fuer *Medizinische Physik,* 74–75 (1995).

8. Jensen KS, Mosekilde L. A model of vertebral trabecular bone architecture and its mechanical properties. *Bone,* 11, 417–423 (1990).

9. Kalender WA, Seissler W, Klotz E, Vock P. Spiral volumetric CT with single-breath-hold technique, continuous transport, and continuous scanner rotation. *Radiology,* 176, 181–183 (1990).

10. Kalender WA, Rettinger G, Suess C. Measurement of paranasal sinus ventilation by xenon-enhanced dynamic computed tomography. *J Comput Assist Tomogr,* 9, 524–529 (1985).

11. Kalender WA, Rienmüller R, Seissler W et al. Measurement of pulmonary parenchymal attenuation: Use of spirometric gating with quantitative CT. *Radiology,* 175, 265–268 (1990).

12. Kaltenborn H, Klose K. Eine Nierenfunktionsanalyse durch die Computertomographie. *Fortschr Röntgenstr,* 156, 517–522 (1992).

13. Kety SS, Schmidt CF. The nitrous oxide method for the quantitative determination of cerebral blood flow in man: Theory, procedure and normal values. *J Clin Invest,* 27, 476–483 (1948).

14. König M, Klotz E, Luka B et al. Perfusions-CT des Gehirns: Erste klinische Erfahrungen in der Akutdiagnostik des cerebralen Infarkts im Vergleich zur SPECT. *RÖFO,* 164 (Suppl I), 150 (1996).

15. Lotz JC, Hayes WC. The use of quantitative computed tomography to estimate risk of fracture of the hip from falls. *J Bone Joint Surg,* 72, 689–700 (1990).

16. Ludman PF, Darby M, Tomlinson N et al. Cardiac flow measurements by ultrafast CT: Validation of continuous and pulsatile flow. *J Comp Assist Tomogr,* 16, 795–803 (1992).

17. Mayer TE, Baranczyk J, Brückmann H et al. Perfusion imaging in hyperacute stroke. *Proc 34th Annu Meet Am Soc Neuroradiol,* 211 (1996).

18. Meier P, Zierler KL. On the theory of indicator-dilution method for measurement of blood flow and volume. *J Appl Physiol,* 6, 731–744 (1954).

19. Meyer JS, Imai A, Ichijo M et al. Local cerebral blood flow and local lambda values change with normal advancing age. In: H Yonas (Ed.). *Cerebral blood flow measurement with stable xenon-enhanced computed tomography,* New York: Raven Press (1992).

20. Miles KA. Measurement of tissue perfusion by dynamic computed tomography. *Brit J Radiol,* 64, 409–412 (1991).

21. Miles KA, Hayball MP, Dixon AK. Functional images of hepatic perfusion obtained with dynamic CT. *Radiology,* 188, 405–411 (1993).

22. Miles KA, Hayball MP, Dixon AK. Measurement of human pancreatic perfusion using dynamic computed tomography with perfusion imaging. *Brit J Radiol,* 68, 471–475 (1995).

23. Peters AM, Brown J, Hartnell GG et al. Non-invasive measurement of renal blood flow with 99mTc DTPA: A comparison with radiolabelled microspheres. *Cardiovasc Res,* 21, 830–834 (1987).

24. Polacin A, Kalender WA, Eidloth H. Simulation study of cerebral blood flow measurements in xenon-CT: Evaluation of washin/washout procedures. *Med Phys,* 18, 1025–1031 (1991).

25. Rietbergen van B, Weinans H, Huiskes R, Odgaard A. A new method to determine trabecular bone elastic properties and loading using micromechanical finite-element models. *J Biomech,* 28, 69–81 (1995).

26. Robb R, Hoffmann E, Sinak LJ et al. High-speed three-dimensional x-ray computed tomography: The dynamic spatial reconstructor. *IEEE,* 71, 308–319 (1983).

27. Rosenbusch G, Oudkerk M, Ammann E. *Radiology in medical diagnostics: Evolution of x-ray applications 1895–1995.* Oxford, UK: Blackwell Science (1996).

28. Rumberger JA, Fiering AJ, Lipton MJ. Use of ultrafast computed tomography to quantitate regional myocardial perfusion: A preliminary report. *J Am Coll Cardiol,* 9, 59–69 (1987).

29. Tajik JK, Tran BQ, Hoffmann EA. Xenon enhanced CT imaging of local pulmonary ventilation. *Proc SPIE,* 2709, 40–54 (1996).

30. Tomonaga M, Tanaka A, Yonas H. *Quantitative cerebral blood flow measurements using stable xenon/CT: Clinical applications.* Armonk, NY: Futura Publishing (1995).

31. Trappe F, Suess C, Blank M et al. Quantitative functional diagnosis of lung diseases by dynamic xenon CT. *Medizinische Physik* 1995, Jahrestagung der Deutschen Gesellschaft fuer *Medizinische Physik,* 72–73 (1995).

32. Wang T, Wu X, Chung N. Myocardial blood flow estimated by synchronous multislice high-speed computed tomography. *IEEE Trans Med Imaging,* 8, 70–77 (1989).

33. Wolfkiel CJ, Brundage BH. A new method for the measurement of elevated myocardial blood flow by ultrafast CT with intravenous contrast medium. *Clin Res,* 38, 450A (1990).

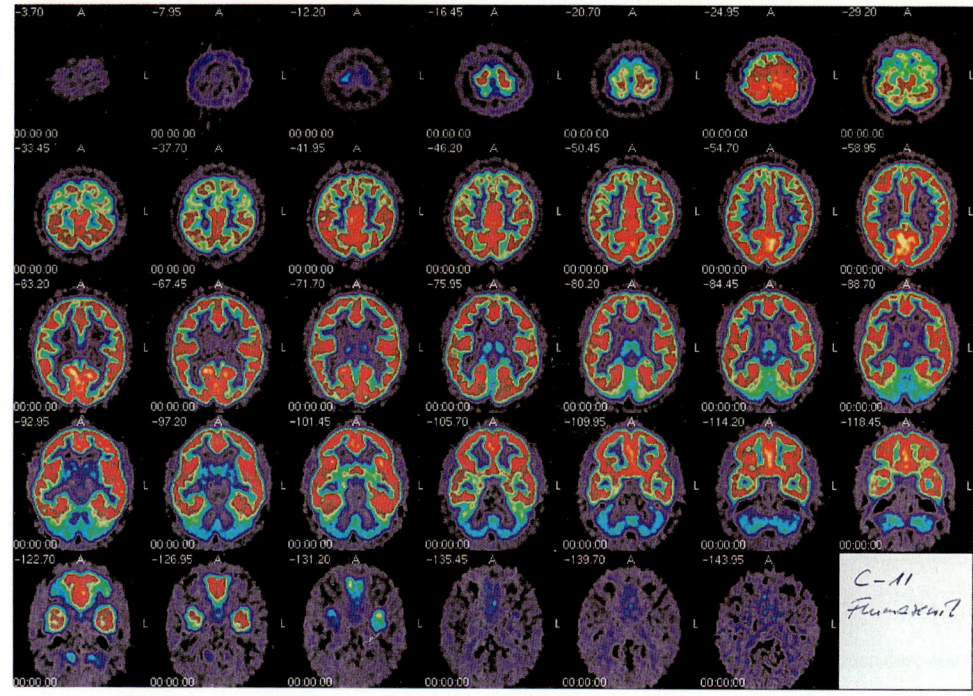

Color Plate 1. [^{11}C]Flumazenil distribution 30 to 60 minutes following injection. Note that the pattern matches the known distribution of the benzodiazepine receptors, with the highest concentration in the occipital and frontal cortex and lower values in cerebellum, basal ganglia, thalamus, cerebellum, and pons.

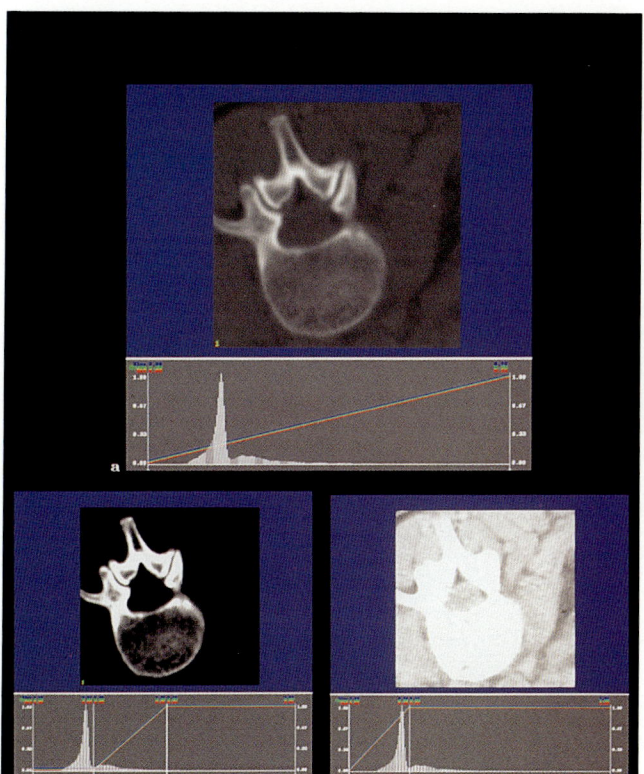

Color Plate 2. Manual adjustment of the brightness transfer function (windowing).

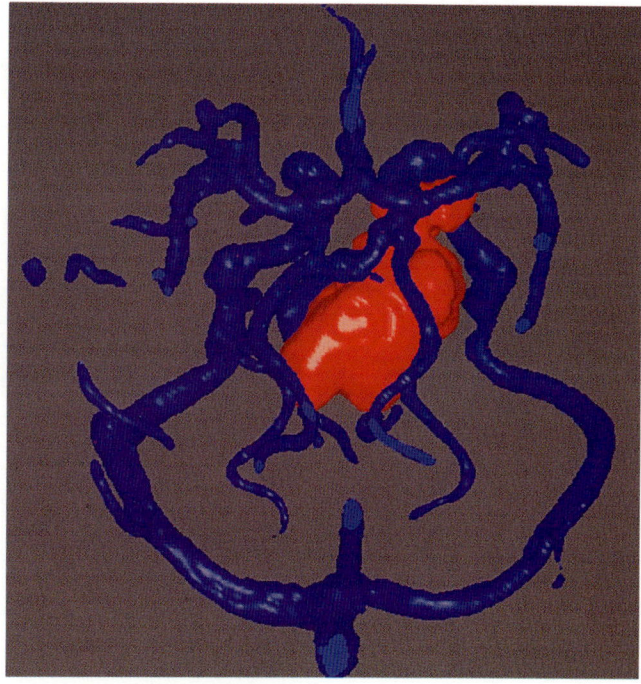

Color Plate 3. Surface rendering of a tumor with the surrounding vascularity obtained from a Gd-enhanced MRA acquisition.

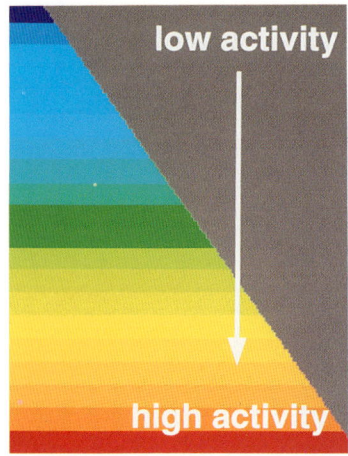

Color Plate 4. Mapping of functional activation strength to color.

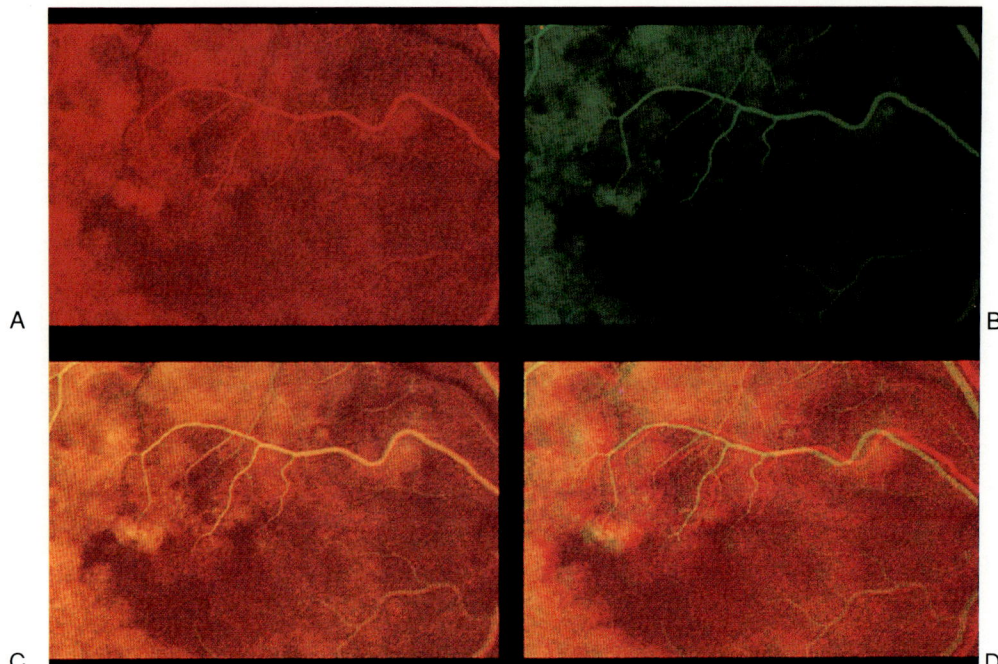

Color Plate 5. Combination of misaligned retinal images for visual registration. Images **A** and **B** show the images to be aligned in red and green. They are combined as color channels to a single color image as demonstrated in images **C** (aligned) and **D** (misregistered).

Color Plate 6. Examples of constrained interactive search. (*Top row*) The original CT image of the pelvis is transformed into a contour image using standard edge detection. (*Middle row*) A precomputed graph of contour fragments and possible links guides the interactive segmentation. A user selects a start point (left image, point 1) and additional control points (points 2–4). The procedure calculates an optimal closed path (right image) based on the precomputed contour fragments and shape criteria. The thin lines indicate structures evaluated as potential paths during the search. The three results shown in the bottom row are obtained by different users and nicely demonstrate the robustness and reproducibility of the procedure, which is not sensitive to the location and number of control points.

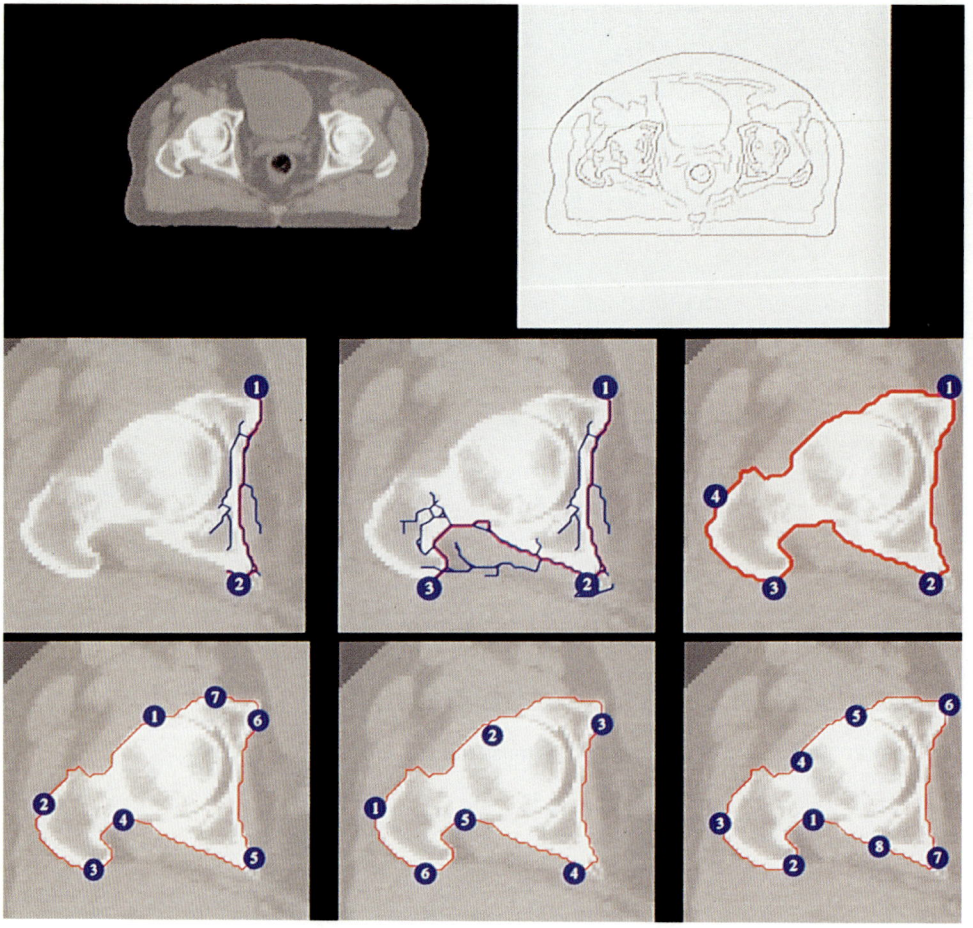

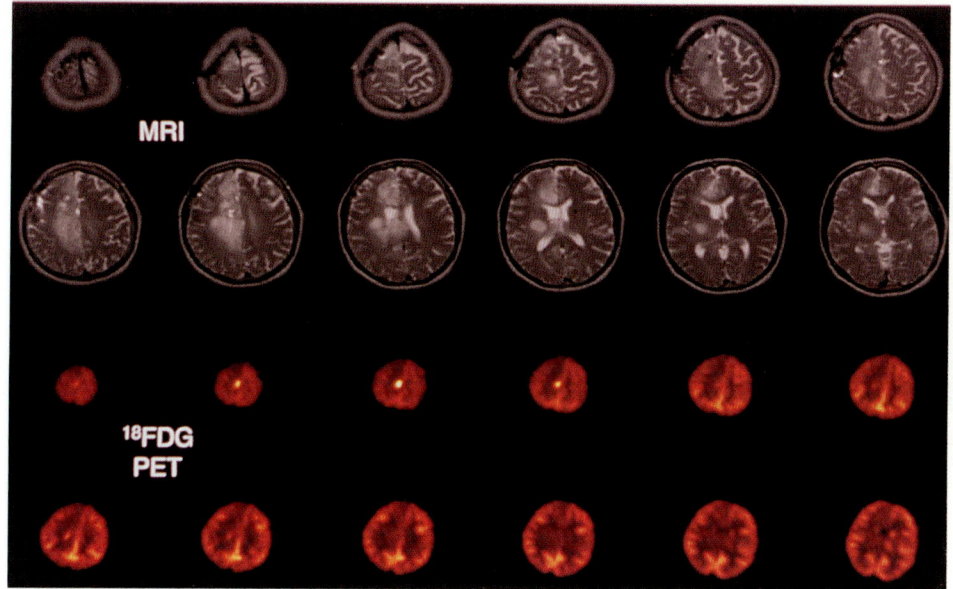

Color Plate 7. Typical situation in correlative imaging. The tissue structures in PET appear oriented and reduced relative to those in MRI due to different patient positioning and field of view. Accurate anatomic localization of the lesion visible in PET is therefore difficult.

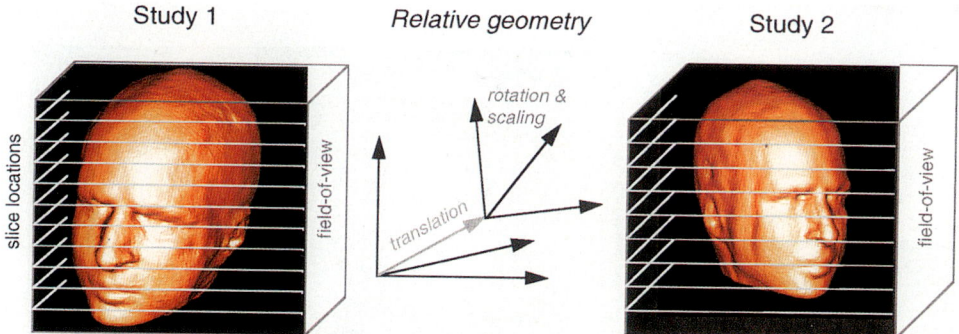

Color Plate 8. The problem posed in rigid image registration. The same head is imaged in two different acquisitions. Its position and orientation within the field of view differ. Therefore, the brain structures in the two image sets share the following relations: The center of the head is dislocated by δ_x, δ_y, δ_z; it is rotated about the angles ϕ, θ, ψ; and the lengths of the pixel edges differ by scale factors s_x, s_y, s_z. While the scale factors are normally known from the acquisition setup, the other six parameters making up the differences in the acquisition geometry must be estimated by an image registration procedure. Then one data set can be transformed into the coordinate space of the other data set and resliced along those slice positions. As a result, the tissue structures in both image sets are aligned.

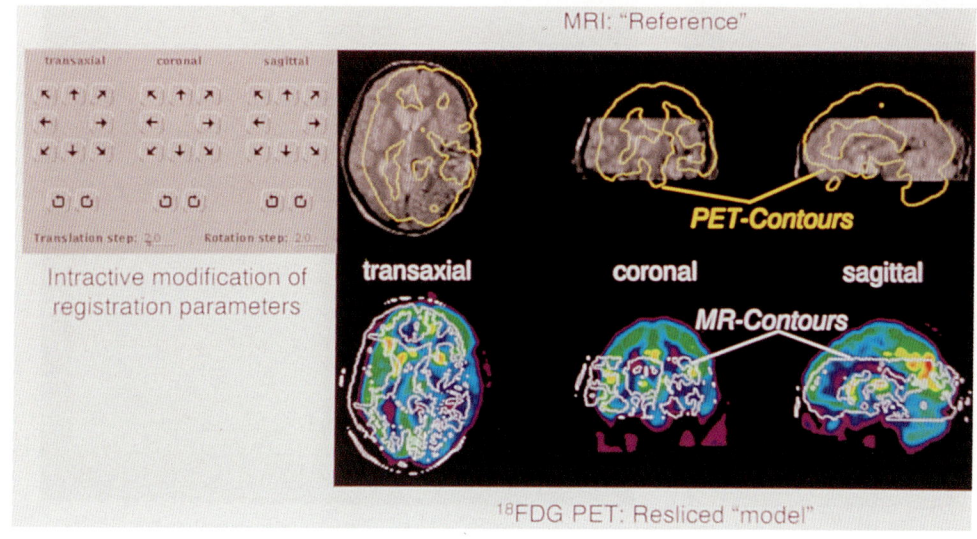

Color Plate 9. Purely manual image registration by an experienced user. Button presses update the transformation parameters and trigger reslicing of the model study. The exchanged contours allow one to evaluate the match visually. The user shifts and rotates the model volume until he or she is satisfied with the alignment.

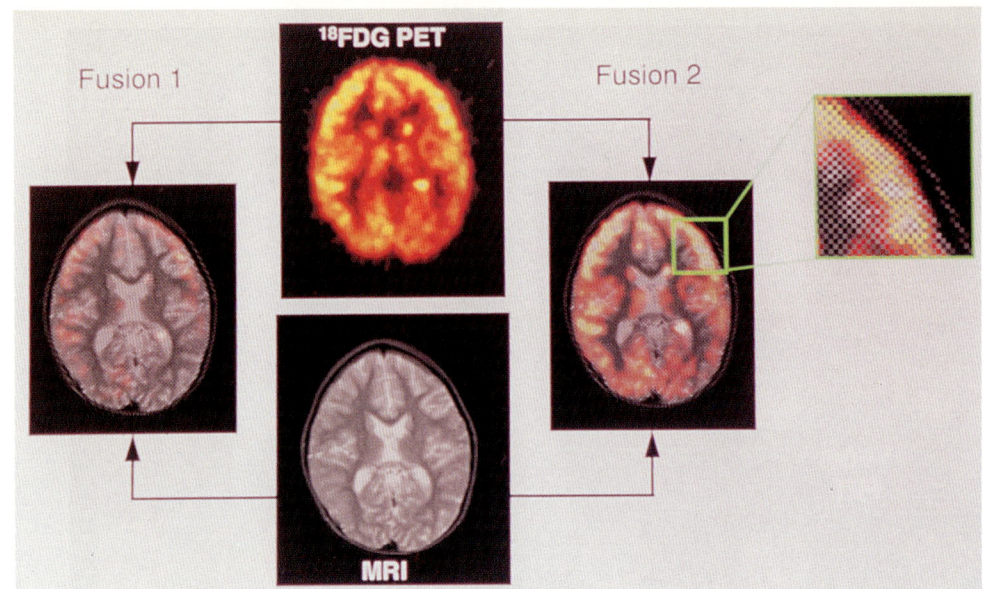

Color Plate 10. Fused image presentation using alternating pixels. In this example a fused image contains MRI information in gray and PET information in color. The color tables can be modified separately during interactive evaluation. Two of the resulting fused images are shown to the left and the right of the original images.

Color Plate 12. Example of a functional MRI acquisition (**A–F**) and the result of its evaluation by subtraction of accumulated images (**G–H**).

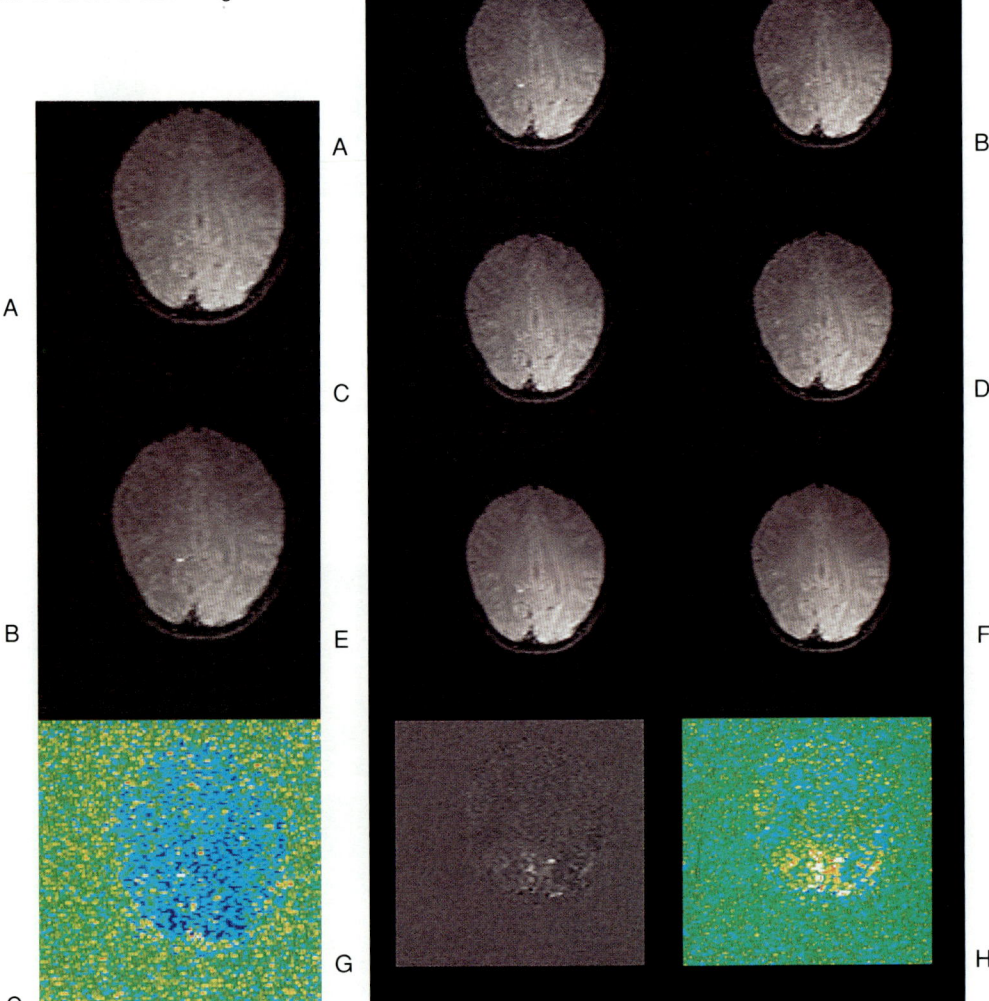

Color Plate 11. The result of direct subtraction of functional MRI images. Images **A** and **B** show the acquired images without and with visual stimulation. The result of the subtraction is color coded on image **C** (growing from blue—negative—to red—positive—values).

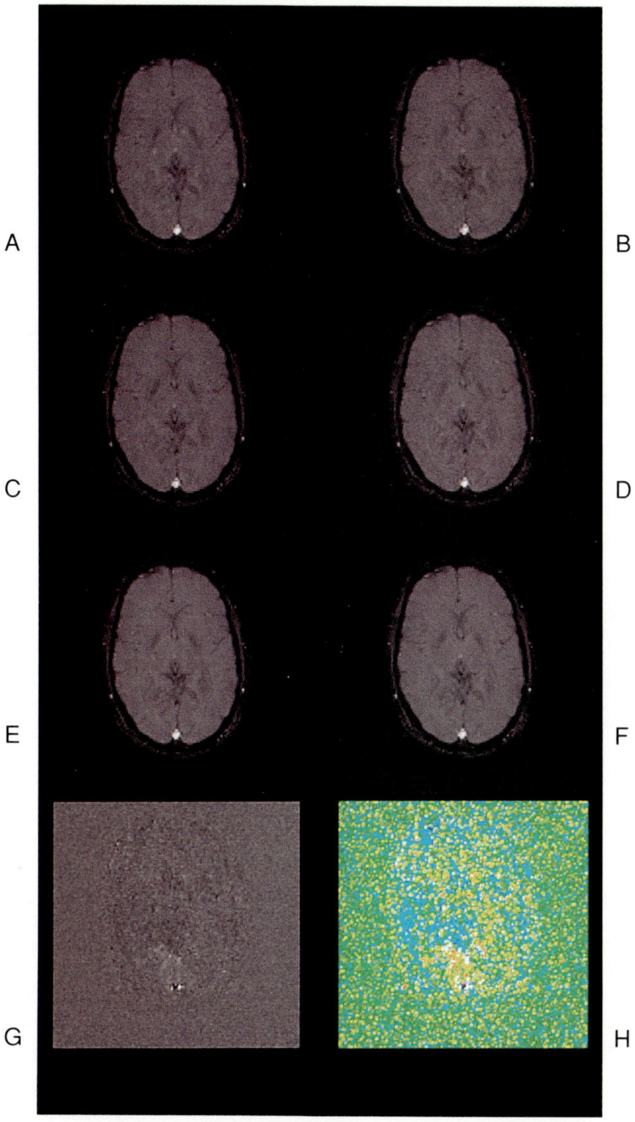

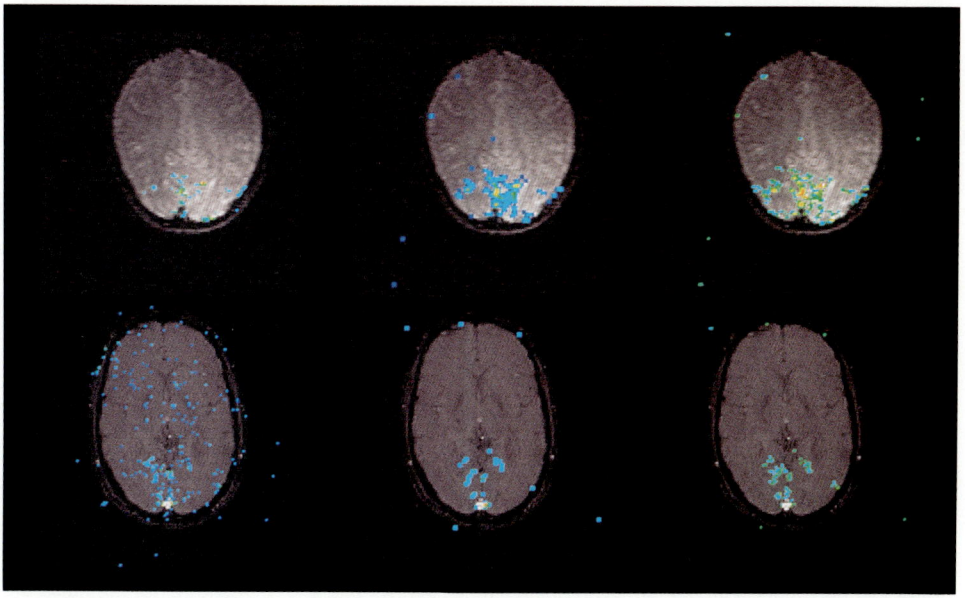

Color Plate 13. Example of another functional MRI acquisition (**A–F**) and the result of its evaluation by subtraction of accumulated images (**G–H**). For this sequence, data accumulation does not provide a satisfactory solution for the detection of activated brain regions.

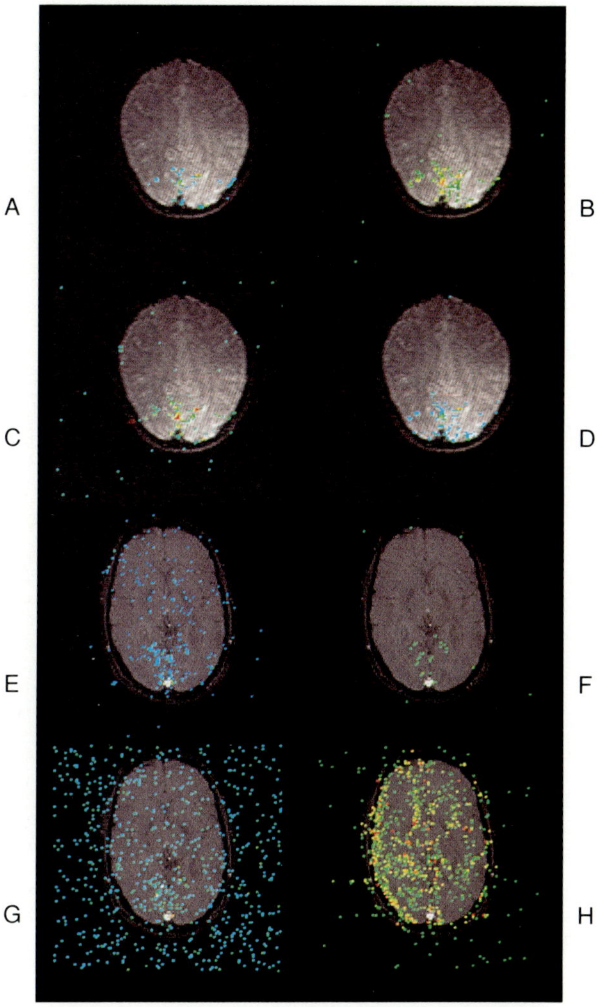

Color Plate 14. Evaluation results on the two previously presented functional MRI data sets. The activation map generated by subtraction (**A, E**), correlation analysis (**B, F**), bandpass filtering (**C, G**), and principal component analysis (**D, H**) were thresholded and overlayed as a color-coded activation map onto the acquired images.

Color Plate 15. Effects of postprocessing on the two previously presented functional MRI data sets. The overlayed activation map is shown for simple thresholding, thresholding of the Gaussian blurted activation map, and hystheresis thresholding (*left* to *right*).

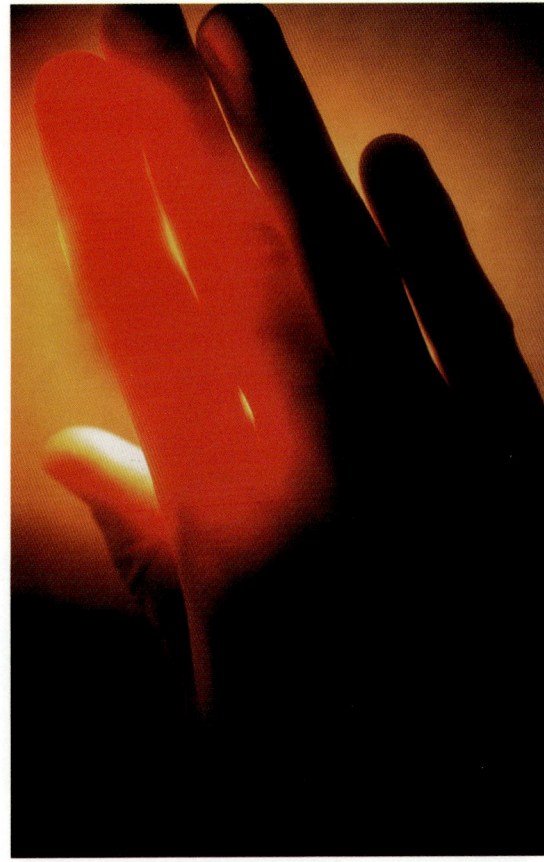

Color Plate 16. Penetration of light through biologic tissue illustrated by illuminating a hand with white light. Penetration is best for long-wavelength red light.

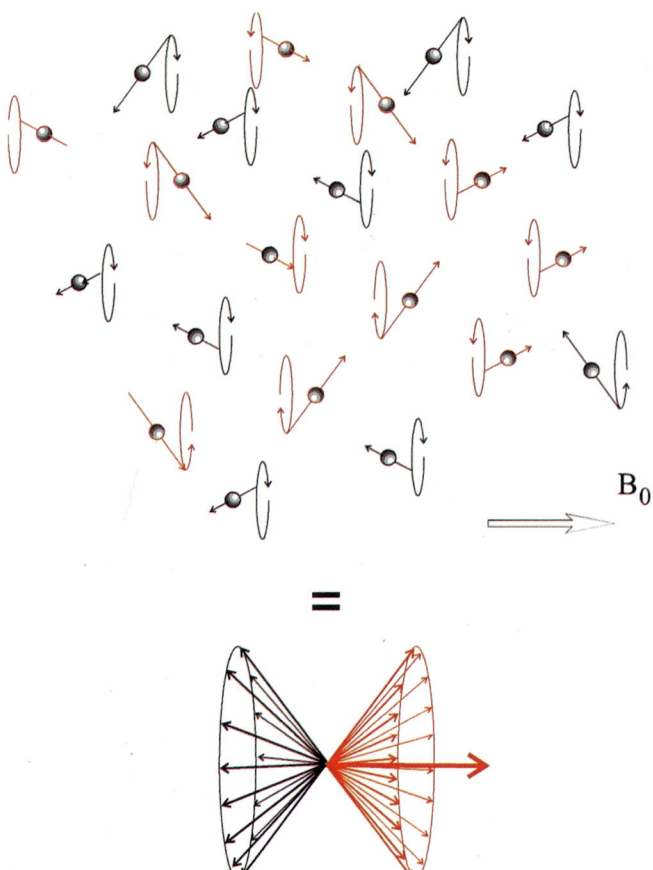

Color Plate 17. The total magnetization is the sum of all spin vectors that precess either parallel (*red*) or antiparallel (*black*) to the outer field. After vector addition, all contributions orthogonal to B_0 will cancel out due to the random orientation of the vectors. The resulting macroscopic magnetization vector will thus be aligned parallel to B_0, reflecting the slight excess of protons with parallel orientation in thermal equilibrium.

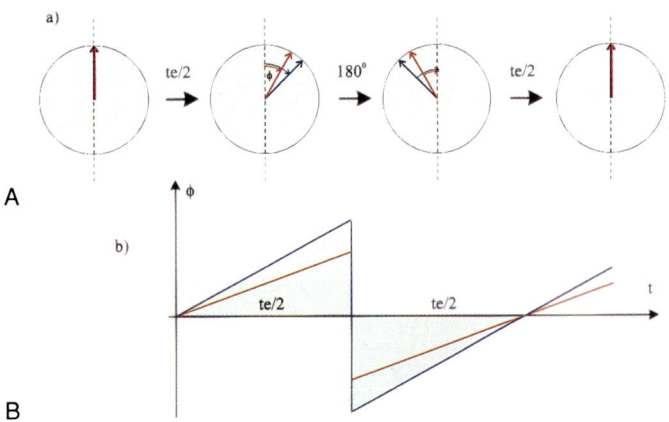

A

B

Color Plate 18. Spin echo with phase diagram. Two spins with slightly different Larmor frequencies will precess by a slightly different angle ϕ during a time $t_e/2$ after excitation. If the vectors are rotated by 180° by an appropriate additional rf pulse, the faster spin (*blue*) will lag behind. After another time interval $t_e/2$, both spins will again be parallel, and an echo is formed (**A**). The accumulated phase angle of the spins also can be represented in a phase diagram (**B**).

Color Plate 19. Decomposition of magnetization vectors. The extended phase graph. Any magnetization vector generated by applying a 1–90° pulse to magnetization that has precessed by *f* can be decomposed into four parts: one part *f*, which is parallel to the vector before the pulse; one part *f**, which is symmetrical to *f* around the *x* axis and thus behaves as if a 180° pulse had taken place; and two vectors f_z and f_z' in the *xz* plane, which represent *z*-magnetization. After this decomposition, the formation of the various echoes easily follows from the extended phase graph. Spin-echo formation follows

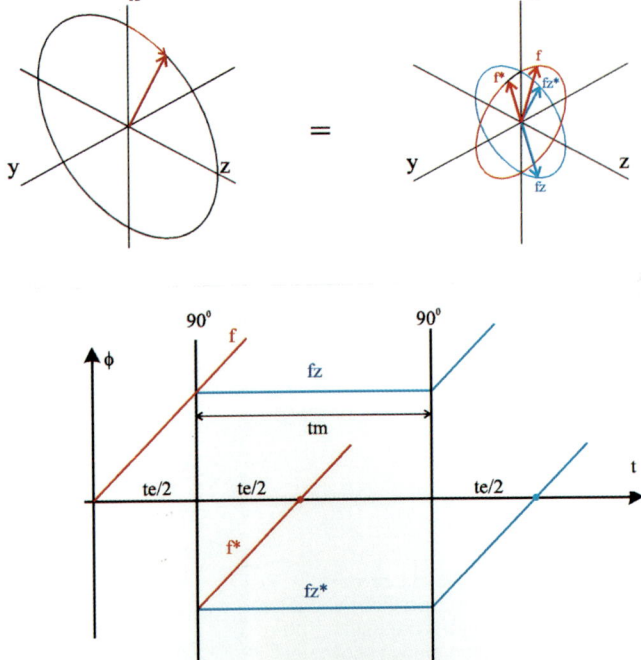

from the phase graph of *f** after the first refocusing pulse (*red*). The second pulse converts f_z' into *f**, which then forms the stimulated echo (*blue*) no matter where the (*red*) graphs of the initial *f* and *f** magnetizations have gone to meanwhile.

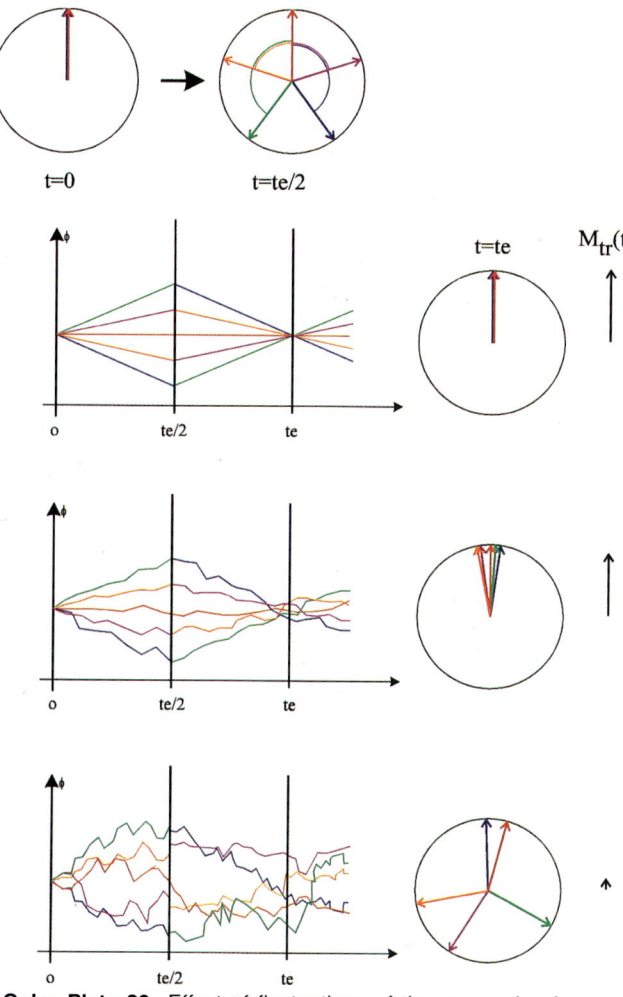

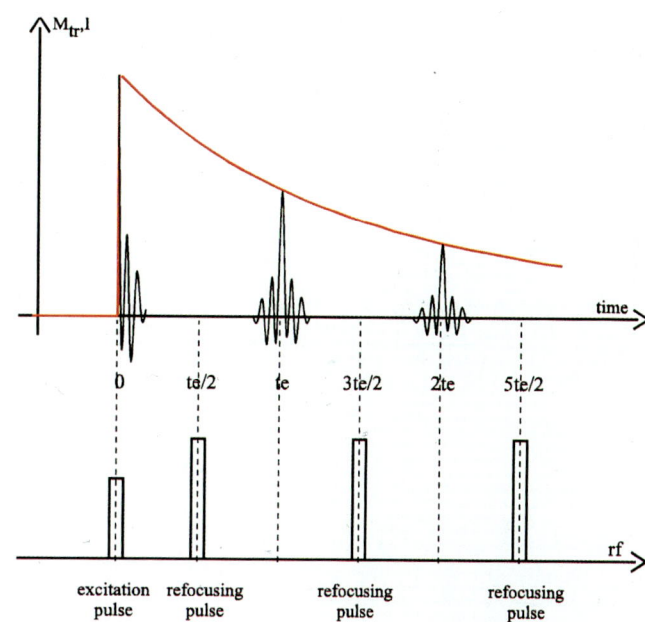

Color Plate 21. Principle of multiecho T2 measurement. Application of equidistant refocusing pulses leads to the formation of an echo train at times t_e, $2t_e$, $3t_e$, etc.

Color Plate 23. Principle of phase encoding. The dephasing of spins will be proportional to their distance along the phase-encoding gradient (*top left*). It will also be proportional to the strength of the gradient (*top right*). If the amplitude of the gradient is changed from one acquisition to the next, the signal phase will thus increase linearly, where spins closer to the center show a smaller slope than those further out (*bottom left*). A linearly varying phase is equivalent to a constant frequency, whereas a steeper slope corresponds to a higher frequency. Frequency analysis will thus generate signals whose frequencies correspond to the locations of spins (*bottom right*).

Color Plate 20. Effect of fluctuations of the precession frequency on the measured T2 relaxation. Three cases are shown that are all categorized by coherence at $t = 0$ and an even distribution of magnetization vectors at the time $t_e/2$ of application of the refocusing pulse but with varying temporal fluctuations of the Larmor frequency of the observed spins as a consequence of, for example, motion in an inhomogeneous field. See text for further details.

Color Plate 22. Principle of spatial encoding with constant gradient. If a linearly varying magnetic field (= constant magnetic field gradient) is applied across a body, the Larmor frequency will vary linearly across the body. See text for further details.

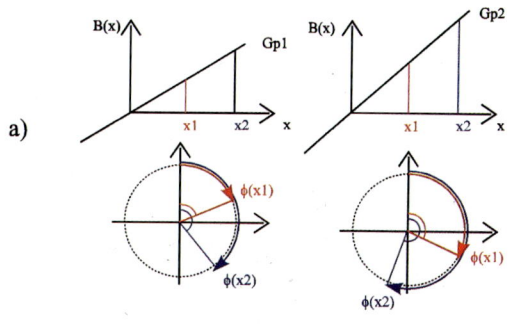

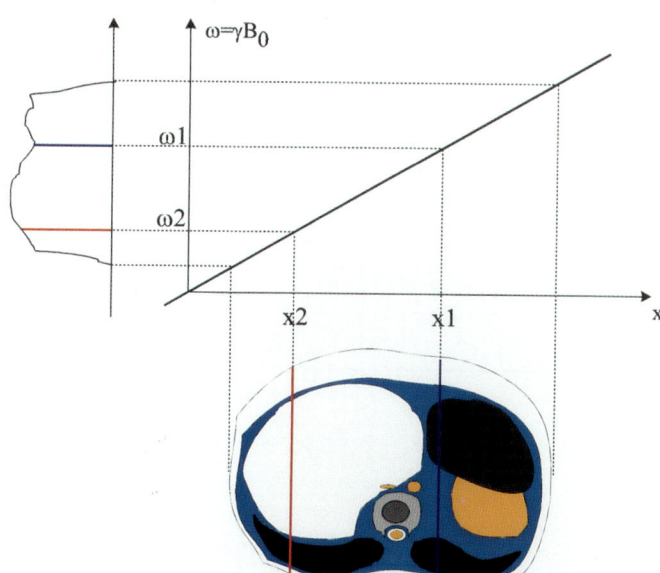

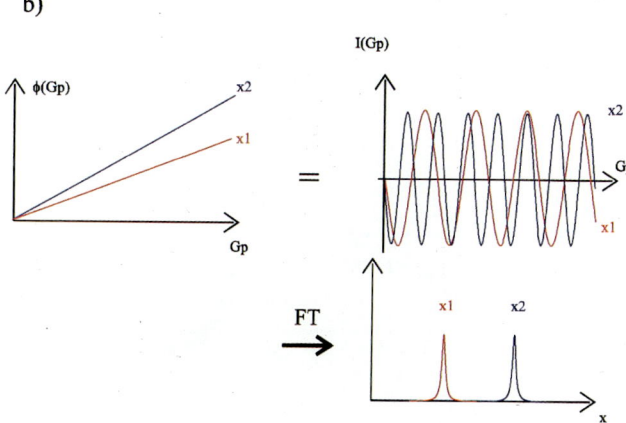

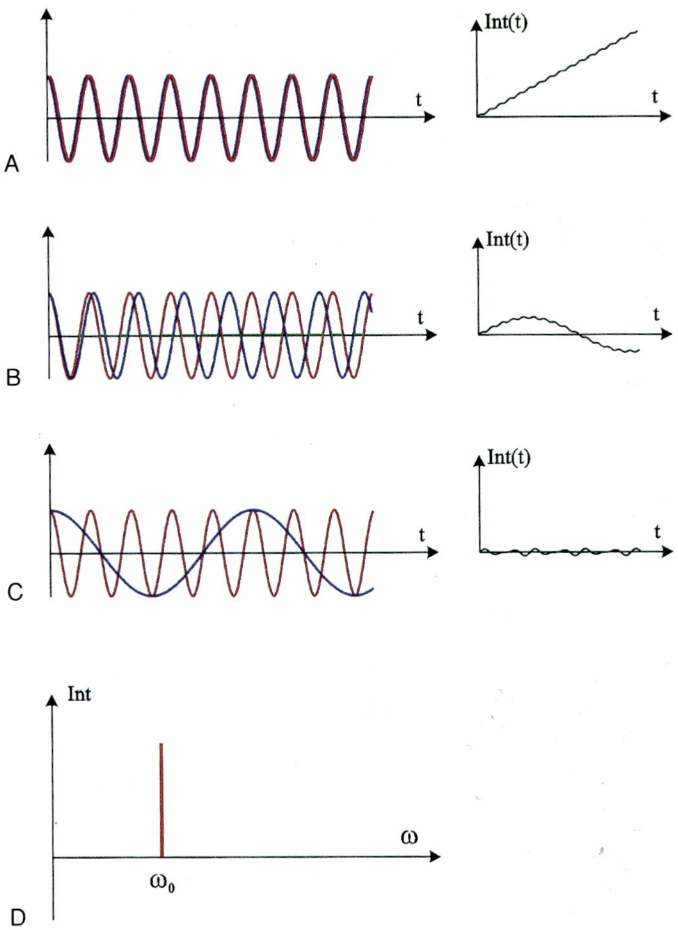

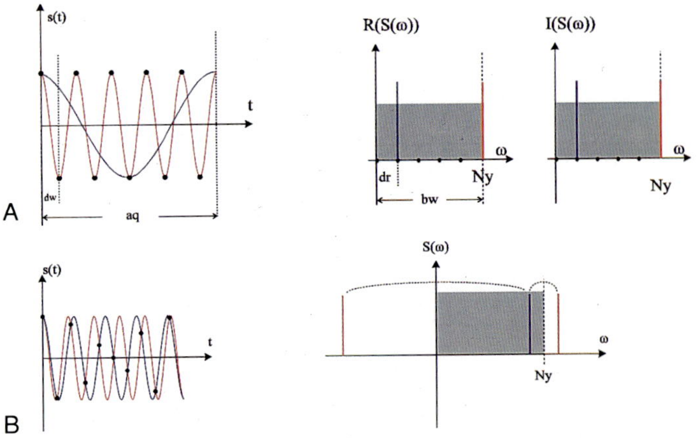

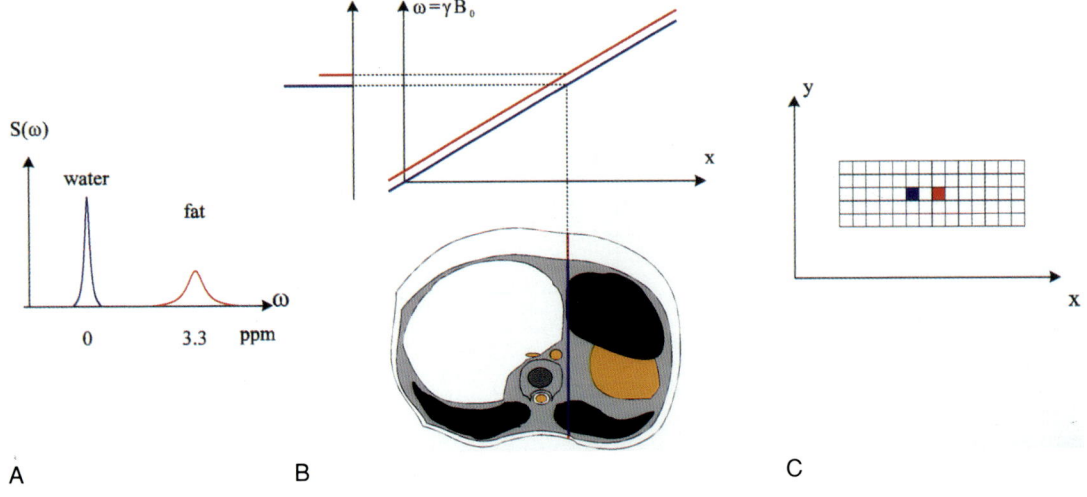

Color Plate 25. The Nyquist frequency and aliasing. For discrete sampling of the (real) time function with a dwell time *dw*, the highest detectable frequency for discrete frequency (*red* in **A**). A higher frequency (*red* in **B**) will have identical values at the discrete sampling points than a frequency that is mirrored back at the Nyquist frequency (*blue* in **B**). By symmetry, folding back also occurs with respect to the zero point of the spectrum. The first nonzero frequency in the discrete frequency domain defines the spectral resolution *dr*. Its time function contains one frequency period over the acquisition window *aq* (*blue* in **A**).

Color Plate 24. Principle of Fourier transformation. The concept of frequency analysis by Fourier transformation uses the calculation of the running sum of the product of the function to be measured (*red*) with sinusoids with varying frequencies (*blue*). Only when both frequencies match will the two signals stay in phase and their running sum Int(*t*) grow arbitrarily (**A**). Even for a slight mismatch of the two frequencies, signals eventually will get out of phase, and their running sum oscillates around zero (**B**). For larger frequency mismatch, the running sum will stay very close to zero. The longer time is left running, the larger will be the ratio of the linearly growing on-resonance value to the off-resonance oscillations (**C**). Extrapolated to infinite time, the resulting scaled spectrum will show a nonzero value only at $\omega = \omega_0$ **(D).**

Color Plate 26. Chemical-shift misregistration. The proton signals from fat and water are separated by about 3.3 ppm **(A)**. This chemical-shift frequency adds to the gradient-dependent Larmor frequency. Fat (*red*) and water (*blue*) spins from the same position will thus be slightly displaced in the spectrum measured under the gradient **(B)** and thus appear shifted in the final image **(C)**.

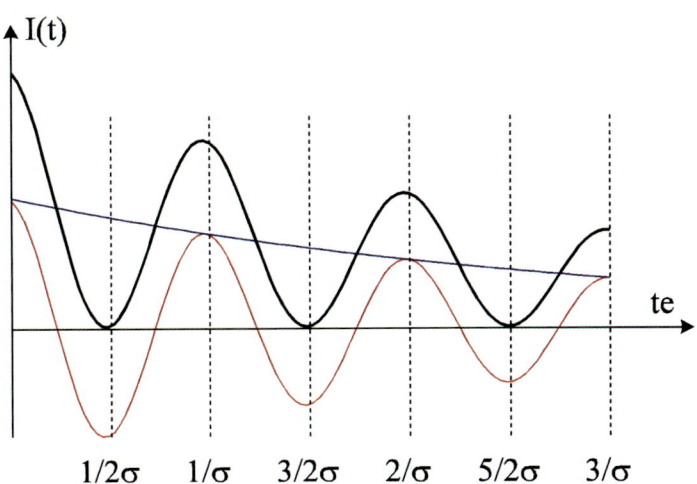

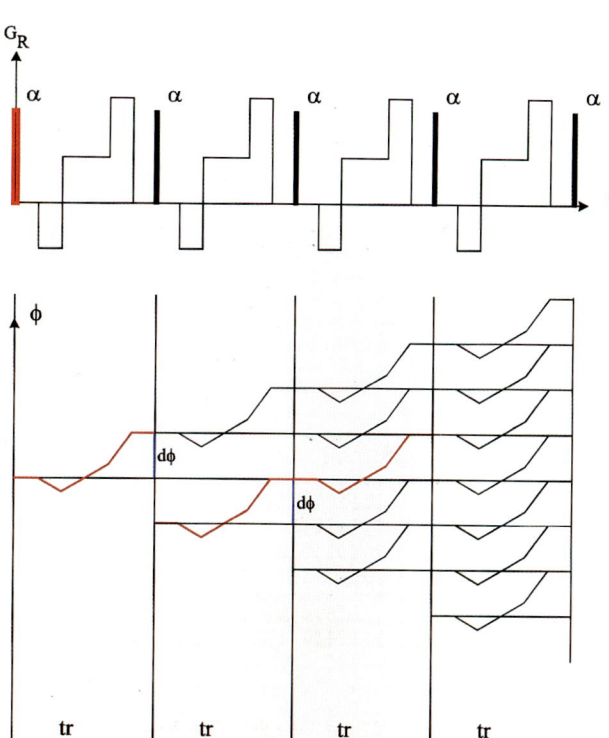

Color Plate 27. In-phase and out-of-phase effects of chemical shift. The on-resonance signal of water (*blue*) decays with T2* when measured with a gradient-echo sequence. Signal from fat (*red*) in addition shows a chemical-shift-dependent signal modulation. In tissue compartments with equal contributions of fat and water (*black*), this leads to a periodic modulation of the signal amplitude with a period of $1/\sigma$, where σ is the chemical-shift difference between fat and water.

Color Plate 28. Extended phase graph of unspoiled FLASH. The phase graph shows the fate of transverse magnetization that is generated by the leftmost (*red*) excitation pulse. It is demonstrated that signal contributions (zero crossings in the phase graph) occur whenever the gradients and thus the dephasing $d\phi$ within each t_r interval remain constant. The red graph corresponds to spin-echo formation leading to even-echo refocusing.

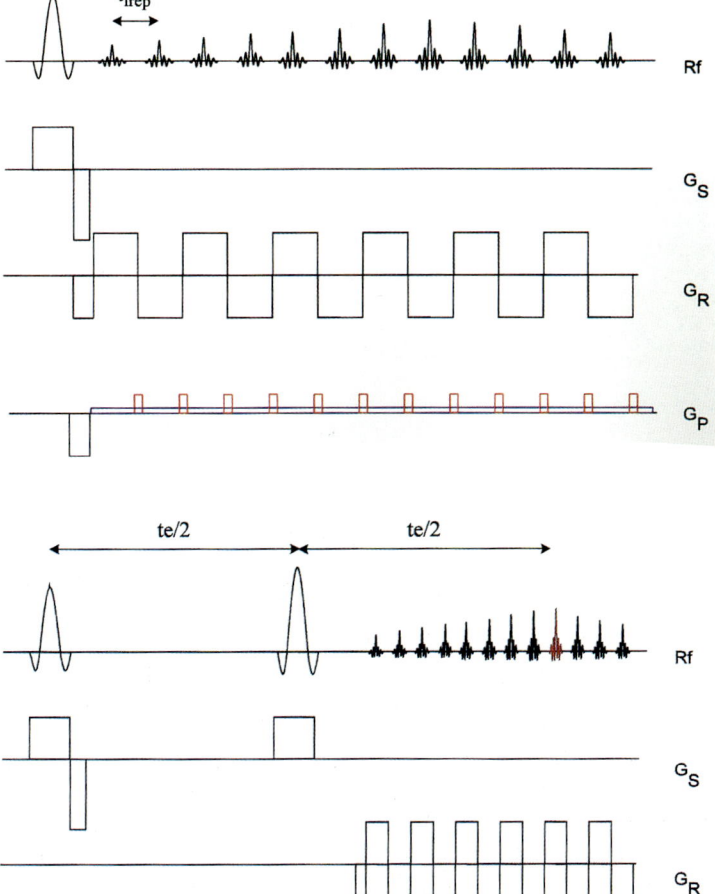

Color Plate 29. Pulse sequence for echo planar imaging (EPI). A long echo train is generated by repetitive reversal of the readout gradient *GR*, whereas the phase encoding-gradient *GP* is applied either continuously (*blue*) or in short "blips" during the reversal of *GR*. The negative gradient lobe in *GP* directly after the excitation pulse serves as a "prewinder" in order to bring the phase-encoding zero point into a later echo.

Color Plate 30. Spin-echo EPI. Signal is generated as a spin echo by applying an excitation pulse followed by a refocusing pulse. The resulting spin echo is then multiplexed by repetitive reversal of the readout gradient *GR*. Note that only one signal (*red*) will occur at the proper refocusing time t_e and thus be properly refocused, whereas the others will carry T2* effects depending on their time interval from t_e.

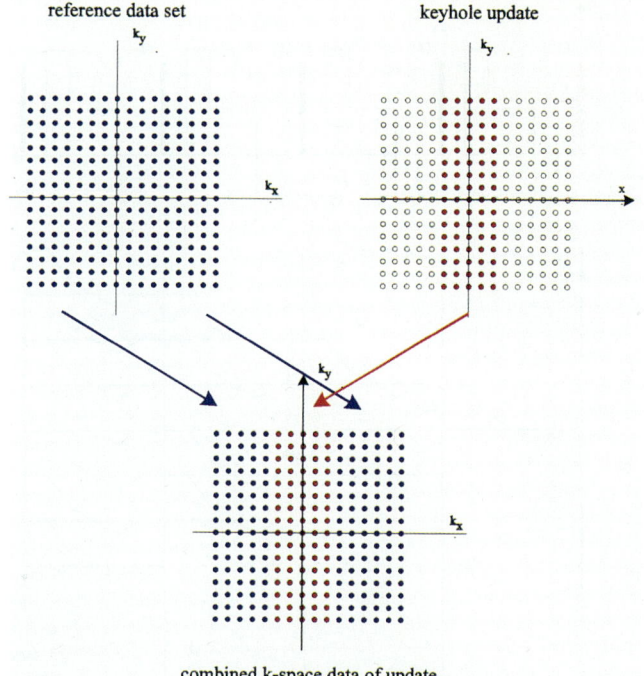

reference data set

keyhole update

combined k-space data of update

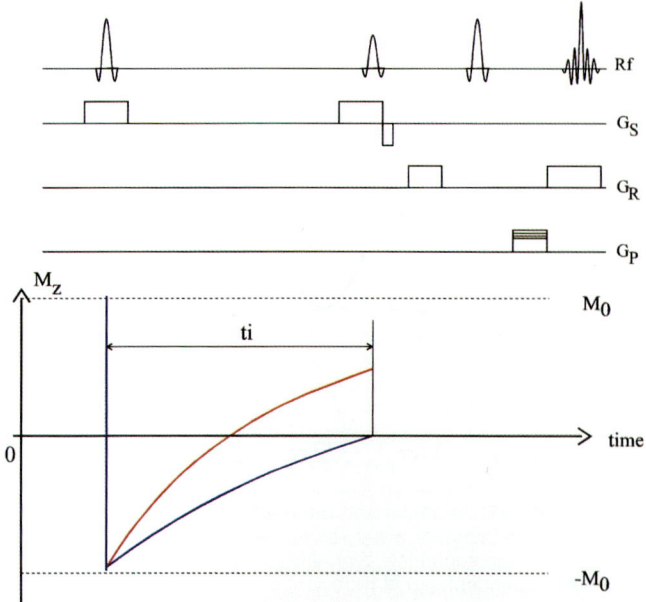

Color Plate 32. Inversion recovery nulling of signal. If the inversion time t_i is chosen such that the longitudinal relaxation of spins with an appropriate value of T_1 is just at its zero crossing (*blue*), then no signal will be generated from those spins.

Color Plate 31. Principle of keyhole imaging. First, a fully resolved reference data set is acquired (*blue*, *top left*). The update images are then acquired with considerably reduced (typically 32) phase-encoding steps normally sampled at the center of k-space (*red*, *top right*). Images are then reconstructed after supplementing the missing k-lines in the updated data sets from the reference data (*bottom*).

Color Plate 33. Principle of tagging sequence. The image-acquisition sequence (here a spin-echo experiment) is preceded by two rf pulses with flip anges of 90°. In the time $t_2 - t_1$ between these pulses a gradient in the readout direction is applied such that spins that are in phase at the time t_1 after the first pulse acquire a position-dependent phase along this gradient at time t_2 of the second pulse. The second pulse will then generate a sinusoidal variation of the z-magnetization along G_x that will show up as an intensity variation across the images. This basic recipe can be modified to tag spins in both image directions as well as to improve the sinusoidal signal variation in order to yield a better defined tagging grid.

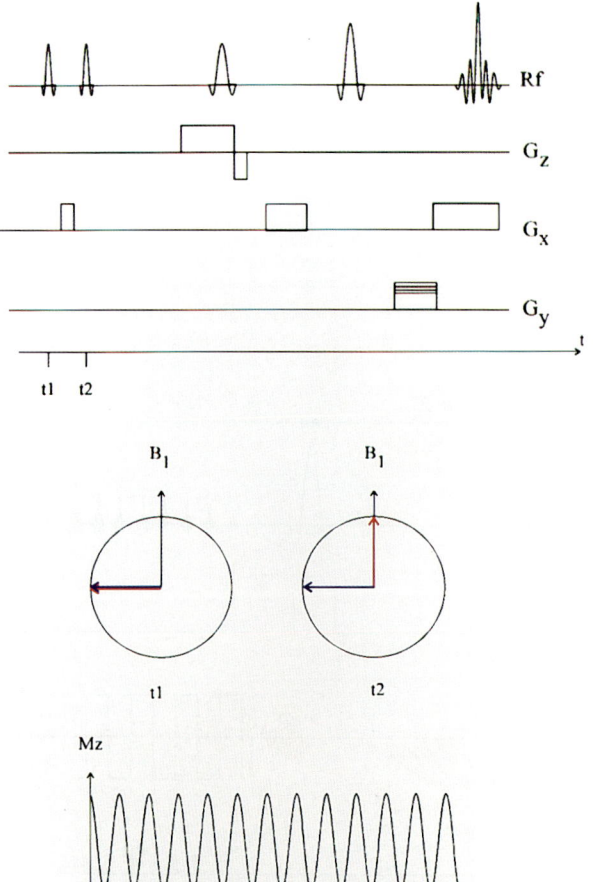

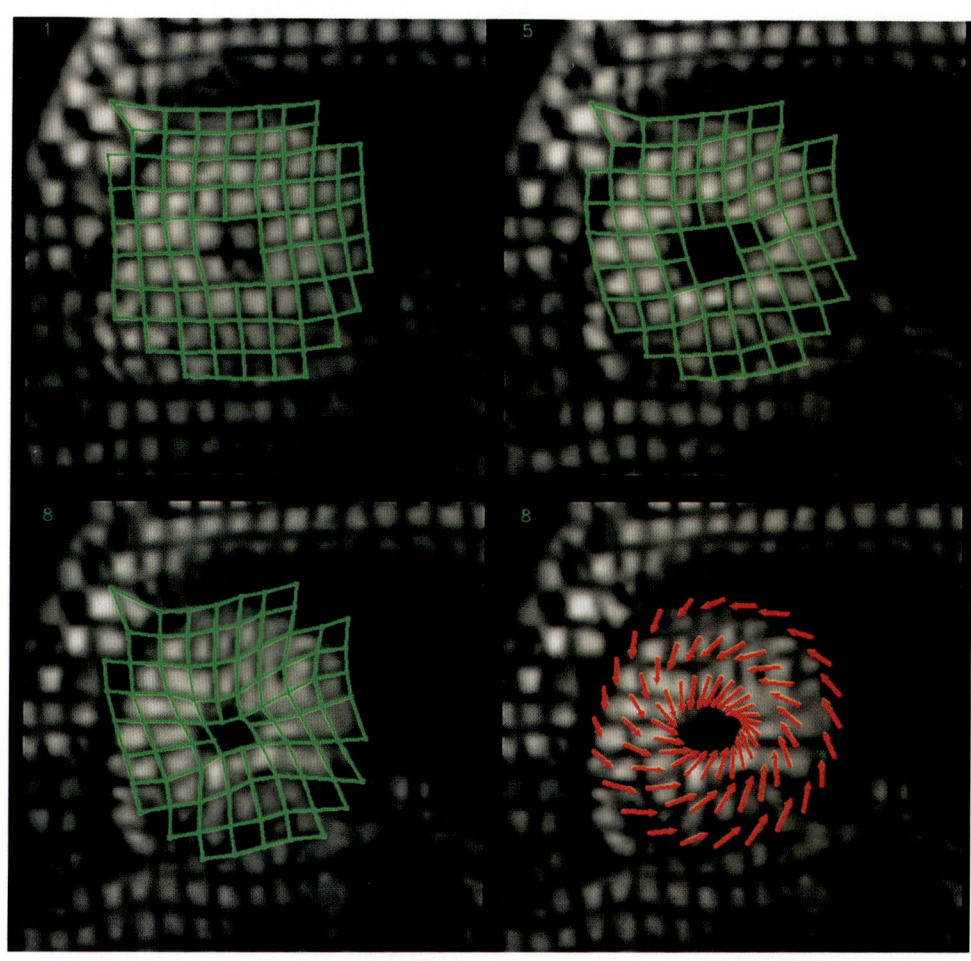

Color Plate 34. Tagging images of the heart acquired with a modified (C-SPAMM) tagging sequence. The grid-lines that are superimposed on the heart are identified (*green*). From the motion of the intersection points on the grid, local velocity vectors (*red lines*, *bottom right*) can be reconstructed. *(Courtesy of K.Boesiger, Institute for Biomedicine, Zurich, Philips 1.5 T.)*

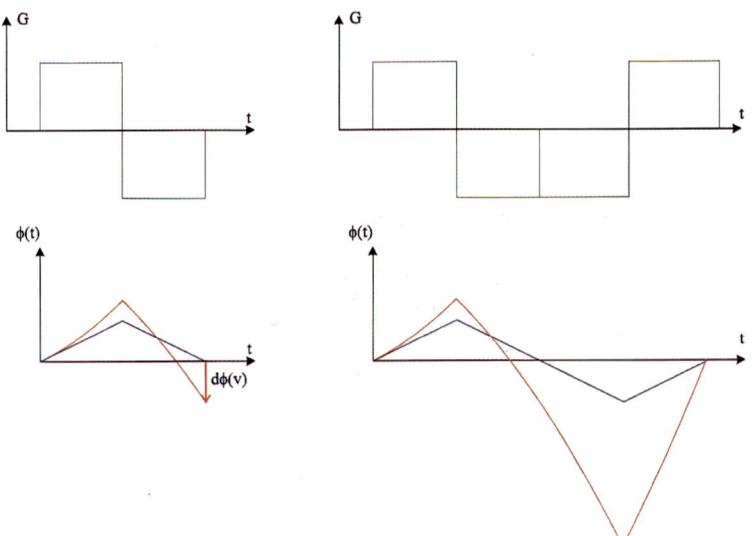

Color Plate 35. Principle of flow compensation. A bipolar gradient that generates no dephasing of stationary spins (*blue*) will show a quadratic phase graph (*red*) for flowing spins leading to a velocity-dependent phase shift $d\phi(v)$. By symmetry, this phase shift can be compensated by adding a time-reversed copy of the bipolar gradient to the sequence (*right*).

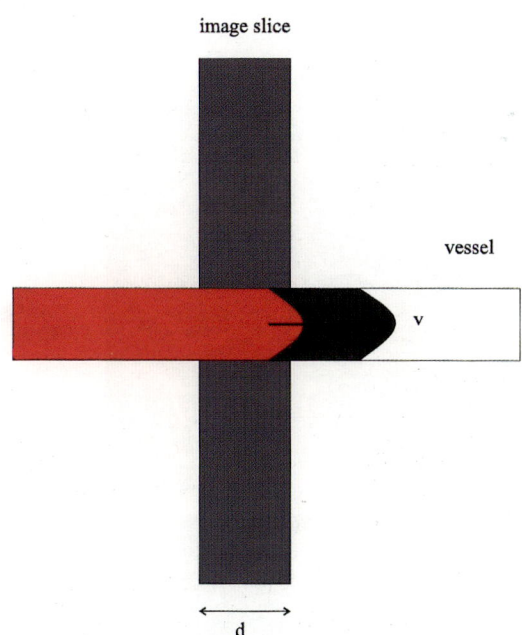

Color Plate 36. Principle of TOF angiography. Unsaturated spins flow into the slice under examination and thus produce high signal intensity (*red*), whereas stationary spins will give low signal with a heavily T1-weighted gradient-echo sequence.

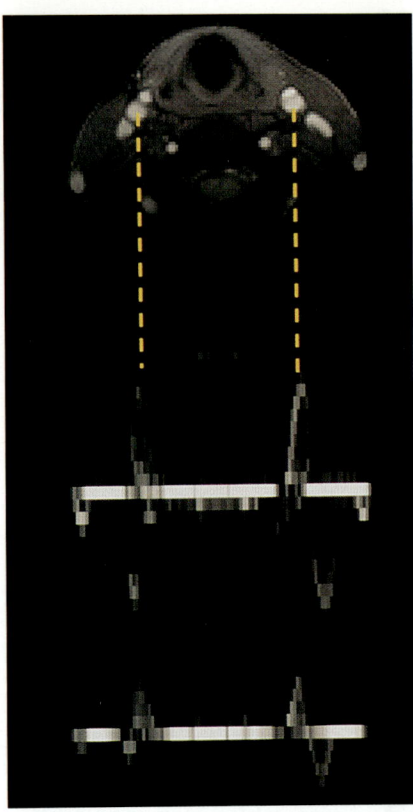

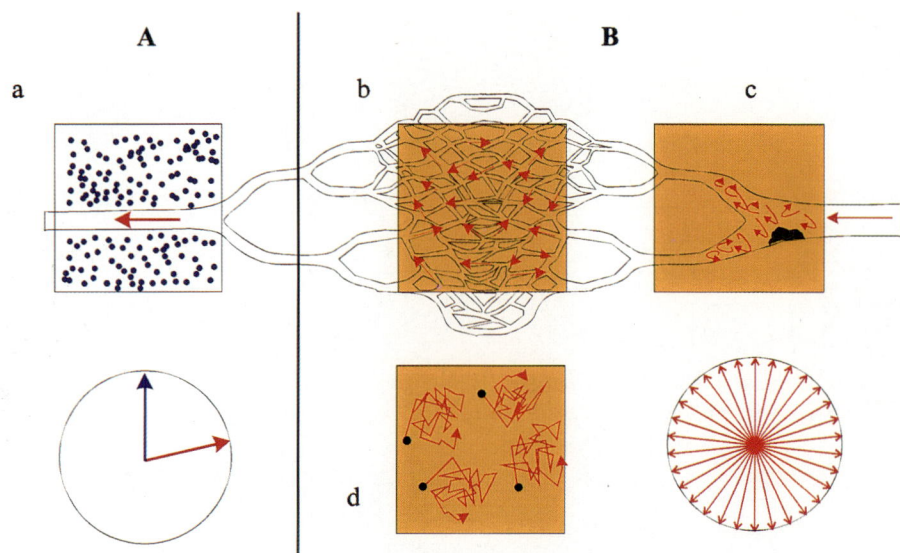

Color Plate 38. Different effects of flow and motion within a voxel (square box in **a–d**). Constant flow will lead to an observable phase difference of flowing spins (*red*) as compared with stationary signal (**A**). Intravoxel flow in capillaries (**b**) as well as turbulent flow around an obstacle (**c**) as well as molecular diffusion (**d**) will all lead to incoherent phase effects and thus to amplitude reduction of the observed signal (**B**). In terms of an MR experiment, these types of motion are thus equivalent in principle and can only be distinguished by their different inherent velocities. Dephasing around a turbulence is much faster compared with capillary perfusion, which again is faster than molecular motion.

Color Plate 37. ECG-gated fast Fourier flow images during diastole (*bottom*) and on arrival of the systolic pulse wave (*middle*) displaying flow velocities orthogonal to the transverse section through the neck of a volunteer shown at the top. The flow profiles in veins (*downward*) and arteries are demonstrated. Vessel profiles can be attributed by projection onto the anatomic image (*yellow lines*).

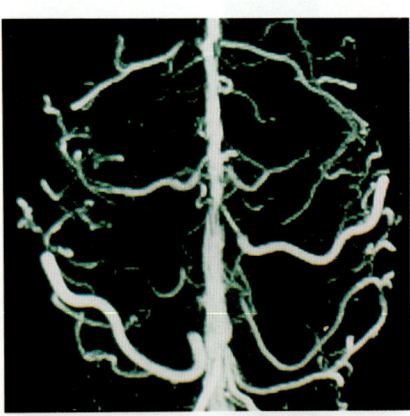

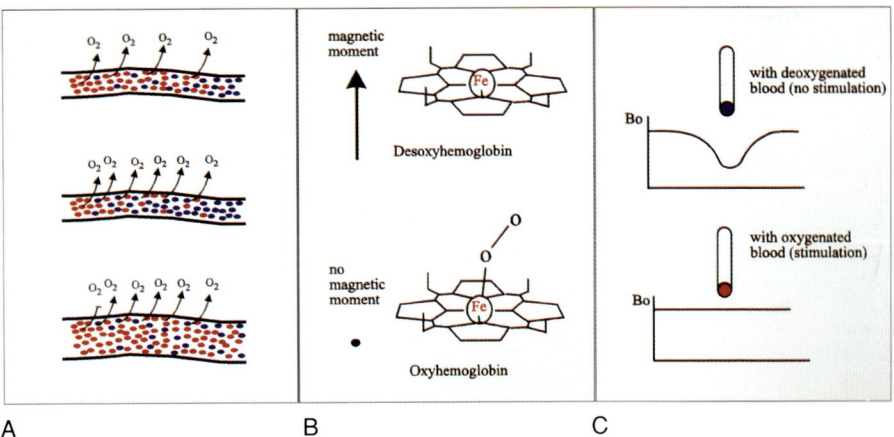

Color Plate 39. Principle of BOLD mechanism used for brain activation studies. (**A**) The increased energy consumption on stimulation leads to an increased blood supply such that the concentration of oxygenated blood (*red dots* in **A**) is increased compared with deoxygenated blood (*blue dots* in **A**). The increased consumption is thus overcompensated. (**B**) Deoxyhemoglobin has a strong magnetic moment due to free electrons at the iron center. This magnetic moment is quenched by adding an oxygen molecule such that oxyhemoglobin has no magnetic moment. (**C**) The magnetic moment of deoxygenated blood will lead to a strong susceptibility effect in the surroundings of a vessel with a high content of deoxyhemoglobin, whereas no such effect will be observed around vessels filled with oxyhemoglobin. Upon activation, the susceptibility effect around capillary vessels will thus change, which can be observed with appropriate susceptibility-dependent measurement sequences.

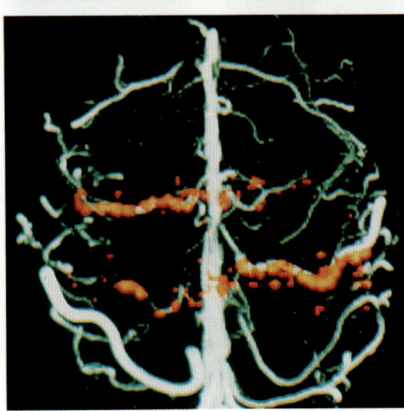

Color Plate 40. Changes in the signal intensities of draining veins as demonstrated by time-of-flight angiography in two volunteers using a paradigm for stimulation of the primary motor areas. The image at the top shows the MR angiogram prior to stimulation; at the bottom an overlay of the stimulation angiogram (*red*) is shown on the reference image. (From Belle V, Delon-Martin C, Massarelli R et al. Intracranial gradient-echo and spin-echo functional MR angiography in humans. *Radiology*, 195, 739–746 [1995].)

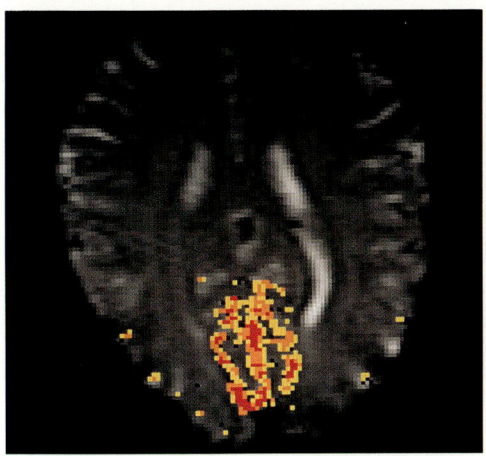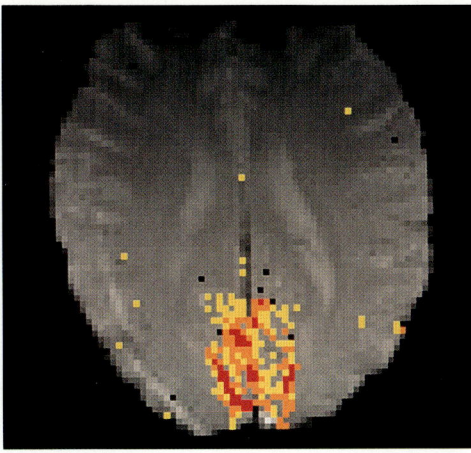

Color Plate 41. Stimulation images derived by cross-correlation on the time scores in regions of interest that appear bright in the difference images between stimulated and nonstimulated periods. For evaluation, the same data sets were used as those leading to the difference images shown in Figs. 96 and 97. The correlation maps are color encoded and superimposed on one image of the time series in order to show the anatomic correlation of activated areas.

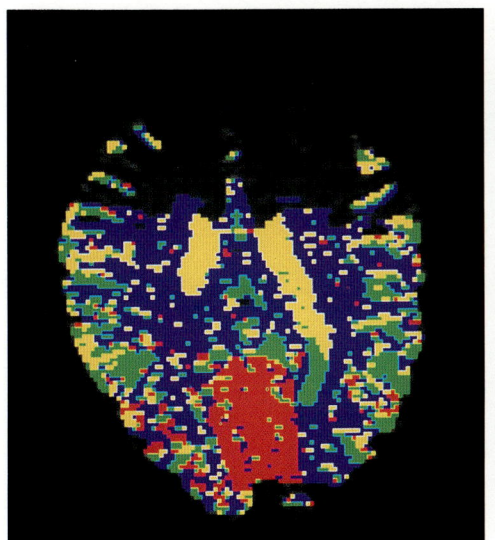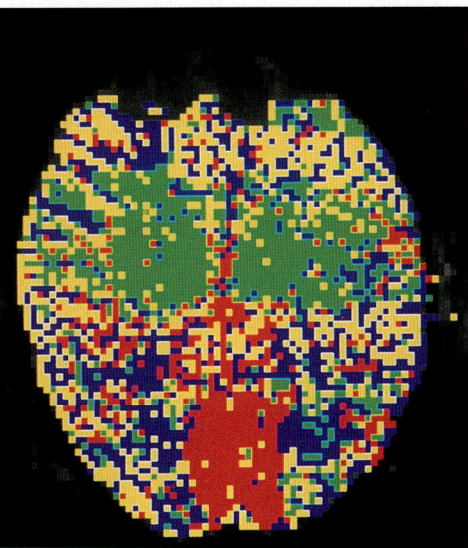

Color Plate 42. Results of cluster analysis of the data sets used for Fig. 102 (and Color Plate 41). Pixels are color encoded according to their membership in different classes found by the algorithm. Note that the activated areas (*red*) are identified, although the algorithm did not use any prior knowledge about the course of the stimulation.

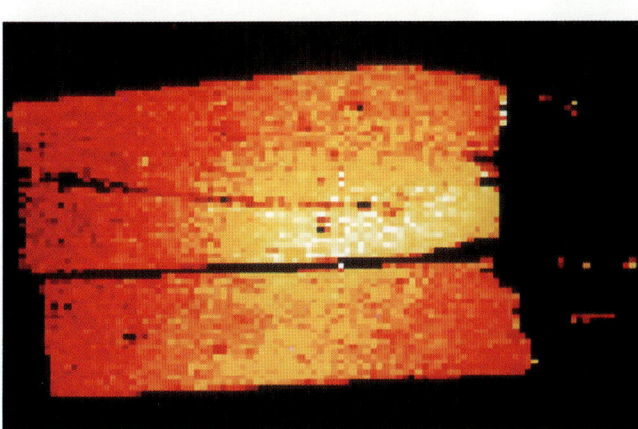

Color Plate 43. Color-coded image of the diffusion coefficient of a gel phantom heated by an rf probe shown as a curved dark line at the center of the phantom. The temperature gradient as measured with a thermocouple ranged from 45°C (*white*) to 25°C (*dark red*).

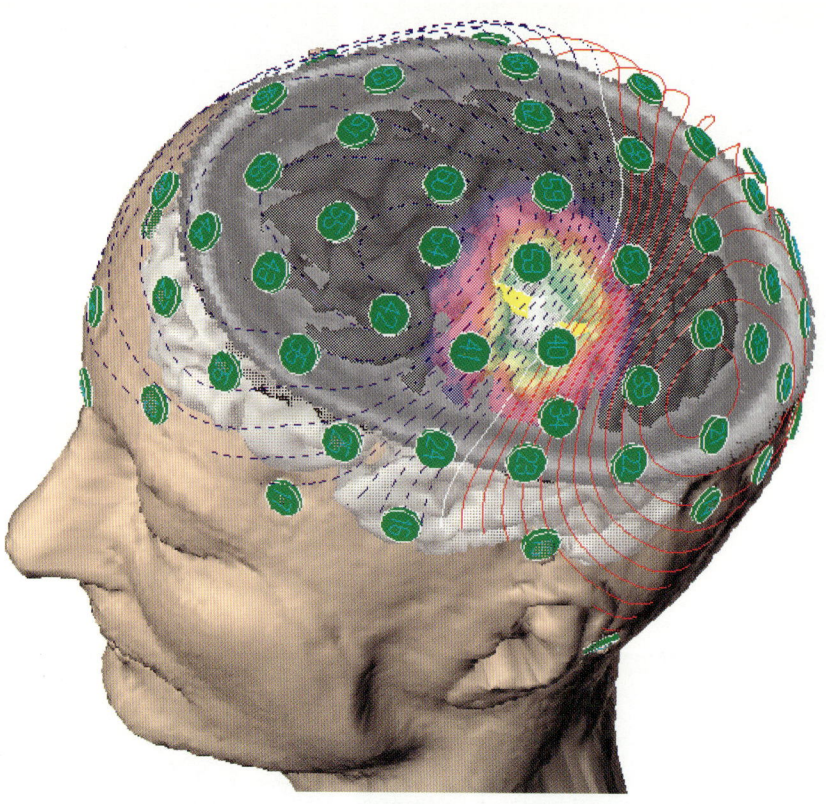

Color Plate 44. Source reconstruction. Somatosensory evoked potential after electric stimulation of the right hand's median nerve, measured with 65 electrodes. Skin and cortex surface were segmented from T1-weighted MRI data. The dashed blue and red lines represent equipotential lines at 20 ms after the stimulus (N_{20}); the yellow arrow underneath electrode 53 represents the fit of a single equivalent moving dipole. (From CURRY, Philips Research, Hamburg.)

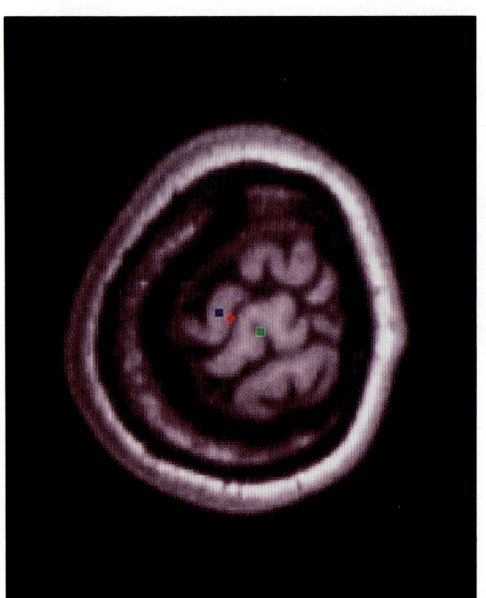

Color Plate 45. Laterally tilted transverse slice of the left hemisphere of one subject of the MEG–functional MRI comparison. Anterior is up, left is medial. The blue square shows the location of the motor cortex dipole; the green square shows the position of the sensory cortex dipole. The red cross shows the location of the functional MRI center, lying directly within the central sulcus.

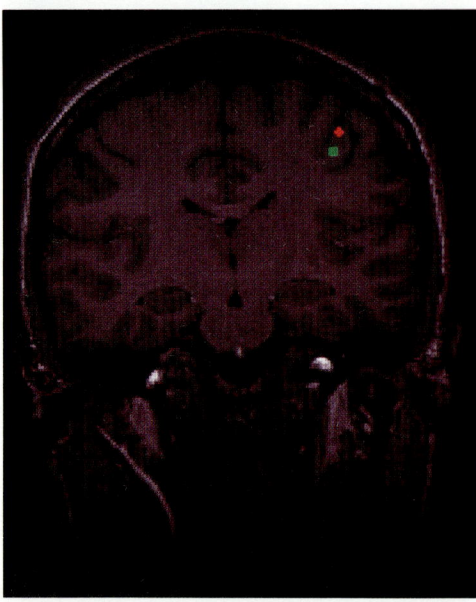

Color Plate 46. Coronal section of the same subject. Up is up, left is right. Here the mean MEG localization (calculated as the mean of the motor and sensory cortex dipole locations) is shown (*green square*). The center of the functional MRI response is shown by the red cross.

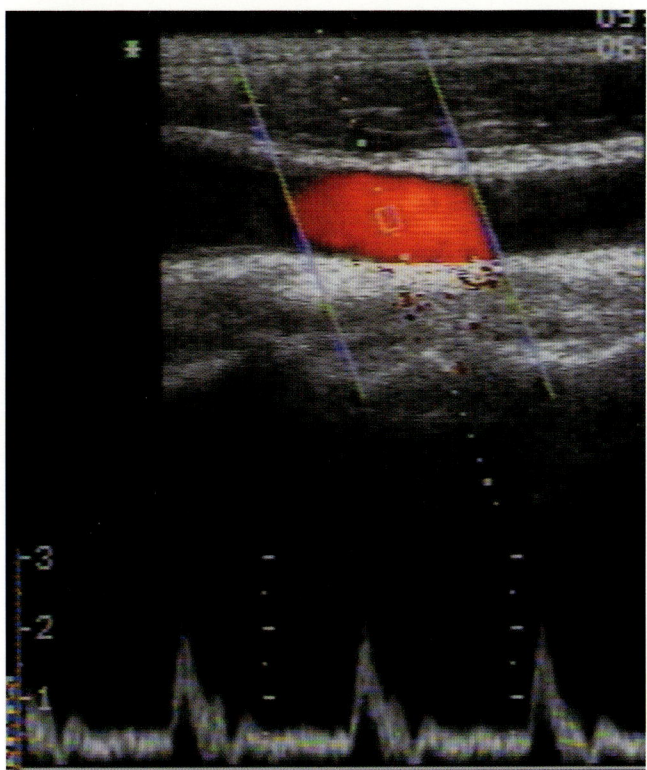

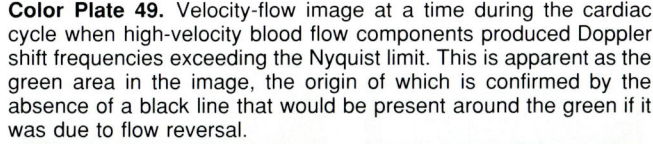

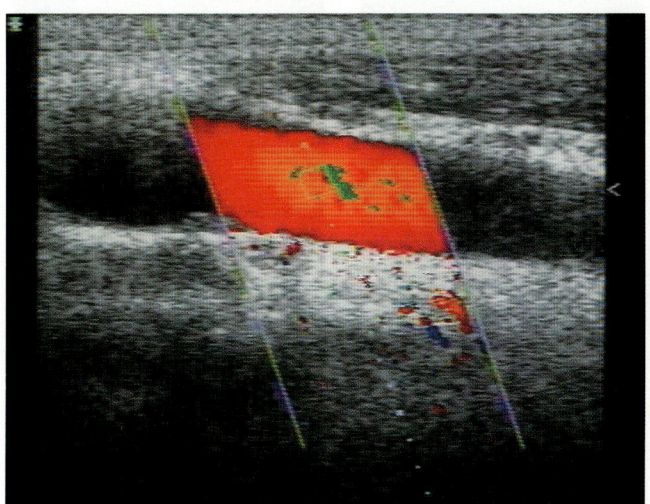

Color Plate 47. Display of information obtained by duplex scanning. In this example, a color-flow image of a normal common carotid artery (coded according to velocity) is shown in the upper part of the display; the dotted line shows the beam direction for acquisition of Doppler signals from the sample volume, the position and size of which are indicated by the superimposed yellow box. The lower part of the display shows the Doppler frequency spectrum over about six cardiac cycles. (Courtesy of M. Halliwell.)

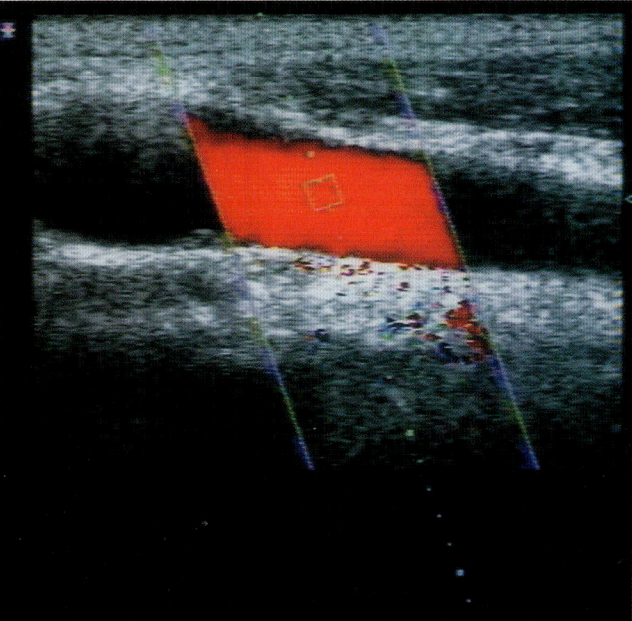

Color Plate 48. Color plates 48, 49, and 50 are examples of Doppler color-flow scans of a normal common carotid artery. A linear-array scanner was used, with the beam directed at an angle of about 65° to the flow direction. Blood flow was toward the probe. Velocity-flow image. The thin black line that can be seen between the color-coded area and the vessel wall, particularly closer to the probe, is due to the highpass filter that suppresses artefacts due to the large-amplitude, low-frequency Doppler signals from the vessel wall.

Color Plate 50. Power-flow image, in which flow direction information is absent but which has fewer artefacts and higher sensitivity than the corresponding velocity flow image. (Courtesy of M. Halliwell.)

Color Plate 49. Velocity-flow image at a time during the cardiac cycle when high-velocity blood flow components produced Doppler shift frequencies exceeding the Nyquist limit. This is apparent as the green area in the image, the origin of which is confirmed by the absence of a black line that would be present around the green if it was due to flow reversal.

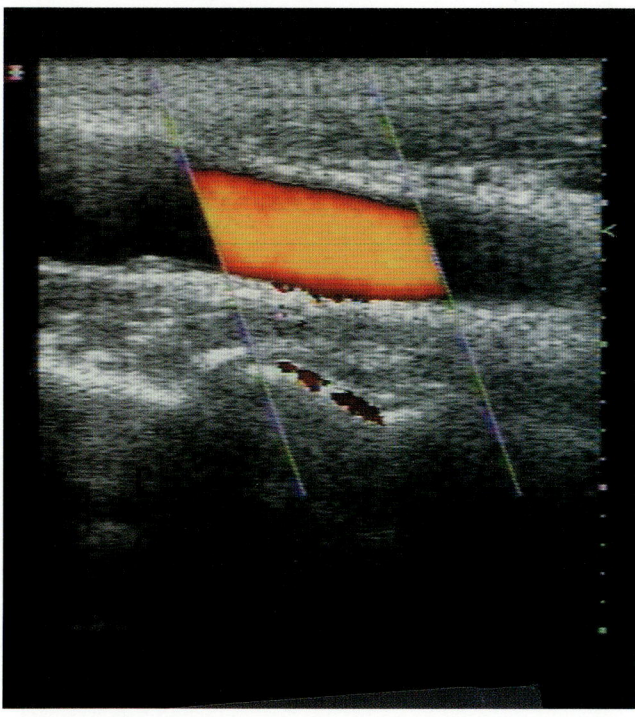

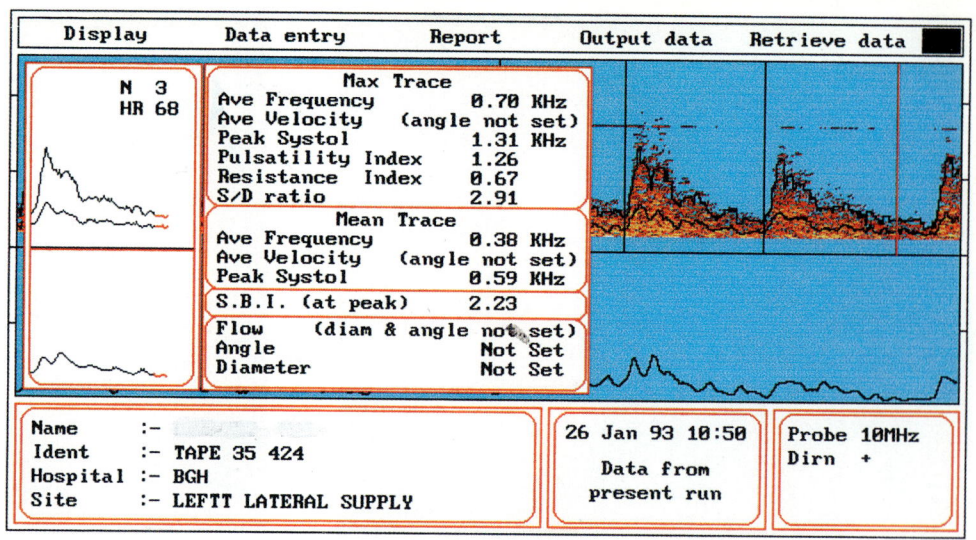

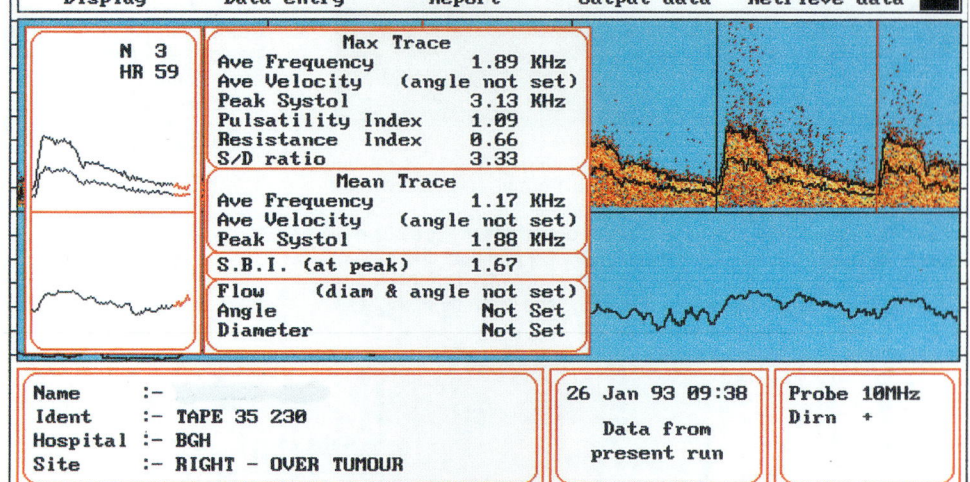

Color Plates 51 and 52. Examples of Doppler frequency spectra obtained from (*top*) a breast tumor and (*bottom*) the contralateral site in the same patient. The results of typical calculations performed by the Doppler frequency analyzer are presented on the display. Note the different frequency scales on the two panels; the markers on the right-hand side of each display are at intervals of 1 kHz. (Courtesy of M. Halliwell.)

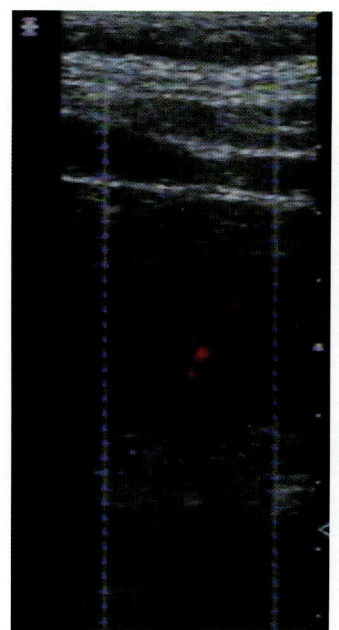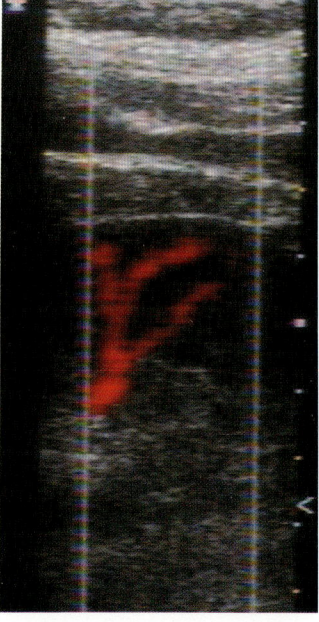

Color Plates 53 and 54. Examples of color-flow scans of small vessels in the kidney. (*left*) Velocity-flow image. (*right*) Power-flow image demonstrating greater sensitivity of this method for visualizing low-velocity, low-volume flow. (Courtesy of M. Halliwell.)

Functional Imaging, edited by
Gustav von Schulthess and Jürgen Hennig.
Lippincott–Raven Publishers, Philadelphia, © 1998.

7

Assessment of Tissue Function Using Optical Methods*

Arno Villringer

INTRODUCTION AND DEFINITIONS

As we know by our own experience, light can be used effectively for image formation. Beside the natural approaches of animal and human eyes, technical approaches include light microscopes, photocameras, video devices, etc. In medicine, such devices are frequently employed for structural *assessment* of tissues or organs. Examples include inspection of patients' skin by dermatologists, endoscopic visualization of morphologic alterations, or light microscopic evaluation of histologic sections. In addition, *functional* information about the state of the tissue or organ also can be obtained. Paleness of a patient may indicate a decrease in the local concentration of blood cells that may be due to anemia, blue coloring of a patient may indicate decreased hemoglobin saturation, and yellow coloring of the sclera may indicate an elevated concentration of bilirubin in the blood due to liver dysfunction.

These examples illustrate one important approach by which light may be used for functional assessment of tissues or organs: A change in light absorption due to the presence of certain substances, such as oxygenated and deoxygenated hemoglobin or bilirubin, may allow the assessment of the concentration of those substances, which in turn gives indications for underlying functional disturbances.

---

* This chapter is dedicated to Britton Chance, pioneer of the optical method.

A Villringer: Division of Neuroimaging, Neurological Clinic, Charité, Humboldt University, Berlin, Germany.

PRINCIPLES

Photons that interact with tissue may undergo

1. Absorption, which may lead to
   a. Radiationless loss of energy to the medium
   b. Fluorescence or delayed fluorescence
   c. Phosphorescence
2. Scattering
3. Doppler shifts due to moving articles in the tissue

Analysis of each of these interactions of light with tissue may give important information about the functional state of the respective tissue.

Measurement of Light Absorption Changes

The concentration of a certain light-absorbing molecule in a tissue may be determined by measuring the extinction of light passing through the tissue. The substance may be an endogenous component of the tissue, or it may be an exogenously administered contrast agent. Important endogenous components include oxygenated hemoglobin (oxy-Hb), deoxygenated hemoglobin (deoxy-Hb), and cytochrome-C-oxidase (Cyt-O_2, Cyt a/a3). These chromophores have characteristic absorption spectra in the range of visible and near-infrared light regions (Fig. 1). The basic approach to determine concentration of such substances is analogous to the determination of concentrations in a photometer. The ratio of the intensity of incident light to the intensity of detected light is related to the concentration of an absorber by the Lambert-Beer law.

It is important to note that this law assumes infinitely small concentration and no scattering in the media. *This assumption does not hold for biologic tissue, which usually is a highly scattering medium. Therefore, L does no longer reflect the true path length of photons, which is prolonged significantly.* In order to obtain the mean path length of photons under those circumstances, L has to be multiplied by an experimentally deter-

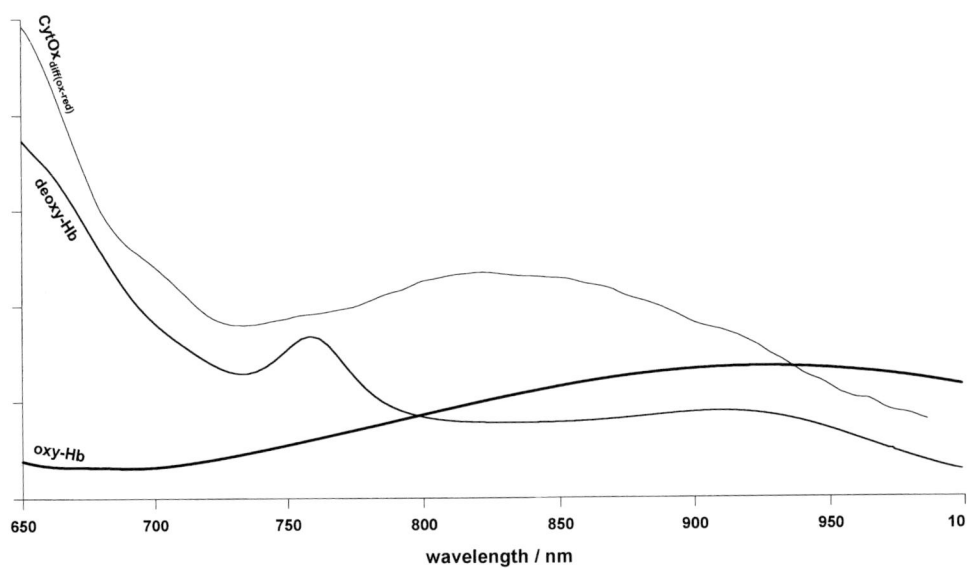

Figure 1. Absorption spectra of oxygenated hemoglobin (oxy-Hb), deoxygenated hemoglobin (deoxy-Hb), and cytochrome oxidase (difference between oxygenated and deoxygenated forms, CytoOx$_{diff}$).

LAMBERT-BEER LAW

$$\log I_0/I = \alpha c L$$

where I_0 = incident light intensity
I = detected light intensity
α = absorption coefficient of the chromophore
c = concentration of the chromophore
L = distance between the points where light enters and leaves the tissue (cm)

---

mined mean differential path length factor (DPF, B in subsequent equation). The subsequent modified Lambert-Beer law describes optical attenuation in a highly scattering medium.

MODIFIED LAMBERT-BEER LAW

$$\log I_0/I = \alpha c L B + G$$

where I_0 = incident light intensity
I = detected light intensity
α = absorption coefficient of the chromophore
c = concentration of the chromophore
L = distance between the points where light enters and leaves the tissue (cm)
B = differential path length factor (DPF)
G = constant attenuation factor related to the optical properties and geometry of the tissue

---

Under certain circumstances, if measurements are made of the *changes* in attenuation, then L, B, and G may be assumed to be constant, and changes in chromophore concentration may be calculated from

$$\Delta c = \frac{\Delta \text{OD}}{\alpha L B}$$

Ideally, the differential path length factor (DPF) should be determined in each experiment; however, technology to do this, though existing (31, 104, 143), has not been available in commercial optical devices so far. It has been suggested that for certain tissues, DPF values are within a certain relatively narrow range, and therefore, values from the literature may be taken as a reasonable estimate. Such DPFs have been measured with either time-resolved or phase-modulated near-infrared spectroscopy (NIRS) for various tissues illuminated at various wavelengths. In a recent study, at a wavelength of 807 nm, DPF values for the adult arm were 4.16% ± 18.8%, for the adult leg 5.51% ± 18% and 6.26% ± 14.1% (31). In addition, algorithms that determine concentration from changes in light attenuation may consider the fact that concentration changes themselves influence mean path length of photons, since increased light absorption tends to preferentially multiply scattered photons and hence reduces the mean photon path length. This interrelationship can be taken into account by including a concentration-dependent factor in the DPF term.

Measurement of Fluorescence, Delayed Fluorescence, and Phosphorescence

Shortly ($<10^{-8}$ s) after a photon is absorbed by a molecule, the molecule may emit a photon that usually has a *longer wavelength* than the absorbed photon. This phenomenon is called *fluorescence*. If the phenomenon occurs within 10^{-8} s and 10^{-6} s, it is called *delayed fluorescence.* When the delay is greater than 10^{-6} s, it is called *phosphorescence.*

In measurements of fluorescence or phosphorescence phenomena, the sample is usually irradiated with light of a certain frequency at which the substance shows high absorbance, and light emitted from the tissue at a *longer wavelength* is observed. In order to measure fluorescence or phosphorescence light, the main task is to minimize the collection of reflected light that has the same wavelength as the exciting light and to maximize the collection of the fluorescent light that usually has a *longer* wavelength. This is usually achieved by a special filter design that tries to separate these two lights by their different wavelengths. For example, to measure fluorescence of the substance fluorescein, one may irradiate the probe at a wavelength of 488 nm and subsequently collect only light at wavelengths higher than 515 nm.

Fluorescent light intensity is related to the concentration of the fluorescent substance by the following relationship:

$$I_{\text{fluor}} = I_0 \phi \epsilon c L$$

where I_{fluor} = fluorescent light intensity
I_0 = irradiated light intensity
ϕ = quantum yield (measure of the efficiency of fluorescence)
ϵ = extinction coefficient
c = concentration of the fluorescent molecule
L = light path

Under the assumption of constant irradiating light intensity (I_0) and constant ϕ, ϵ, and L, there is a linear relationship of I_{fluor} to the concentration of the fluorescent substance.

Measurement of Light Scattering Changes

Whereas for the determination of substance concentrations from light absorbance the path length of light is just a necessary "scaling factor" to be put correctly into the equation, some data (especially on brain tissue) suggest that under certain circumstances *the main or only change* in optical property of tissue that occurs during functional alterations may be in light scattering (52). *Under these circumstances,* path length itself may become a parameter of tissue function. Scattering originates from light traveling through regions of mismatched refractive indices within brain tissue; this may be, for example, the boundary between the intra- and extracellular space or the boundary of organelles within the cell. Changes in the ratio of extra- and intracellular space as they occur, for example, during epileptic seizures may therefore induce changes in scattering properties of tissue. In contrast to changes in, for example, the concentration of oxy- and deoxy-Hb, such scattering changes may more closely reflect electrical activity of neurons, since they do not depend on neuronal-vascular coupling. Hence, whereas optical measurements of oxygenated and deoxygenated hemoglobin in brain tissue measure the vascular response to tissue activity in a fashion comparable with positron-emission tomography (PET) or functional magnetic resonance imaging (MRI) (169), optical methods also may measure events that are more directly related to the electrical activity of neurons comparable with other functional neuroimaging approaches such as magnetoencephalography (MEG) or electroencephalography (EEG). It is clear from these considerations that in order to assess changes in DPF and separate them from absorption changes, methods have to be employed that can separate contributions from absorption and scattering. There are several approaches to determine the path length of light traveling through tissue: The most straightforward approach is to employ ultrashort laser pulses (picosecond duration) as light source and to measure the time the photons need for passage through the tissue using, for example, a streak camera. Path length is the product of the velocity of light and the "time of flight" of the photons (143). Another approach to measure path length uses frequency-modulated light as a light source and compares the phase of the modulation after light has passed through the tissue with the phase of a reference. From the phase shift, a mean path length can be calculated (31, 52). A third approach employs the measurement of an entire light spectrum in the near-infrared light range, including the water absorption peak at 975 nm (105). Assuming a constant water concentration in tissue, a term for path length changes may be derived by measuring the height of this peak.

Measurement of Doppler Shift (156)

Alterations in tissue function frequently are associated with changes in blood flow. These changes in blood flow are accompanied by changes in the concentration of red blood cells and red blood cell velocity.

Photons that interact with tissue are scattered by both stationary tissue and moving blood cells. Scattering by a moving blood cell results in a Doppler frequency shift, whereas light scattered by stationary cells remains unshifted. The average number of Doppler shifts per photon (related to the ac/dc ratio of the obtained signal) is proportional to the red blood cell (RBC) concentration. The mean frequency shift is a measure of blood cell velocity. The product of RBC concentration and RBC velocity is a measure of blood cell flow. Laser-Doppler devices measure blood flow of exposed tissue; hence the technique is usually referred to as *laser-Doppler flowmetry* (LDF) (119).

METHODOLOGIC APPROACHES

Penetration of light into biologic tissue is wavelength dependent. Whereas ultraviolet (UV) light penetrates tissue probably less than 100 μm, penetration depth increases with increasing wavelength, and Fig. 2 illustrates that within the visible light range, best tissue penetration is achieved by the long-wavelength red light (see also Color Plate 16).

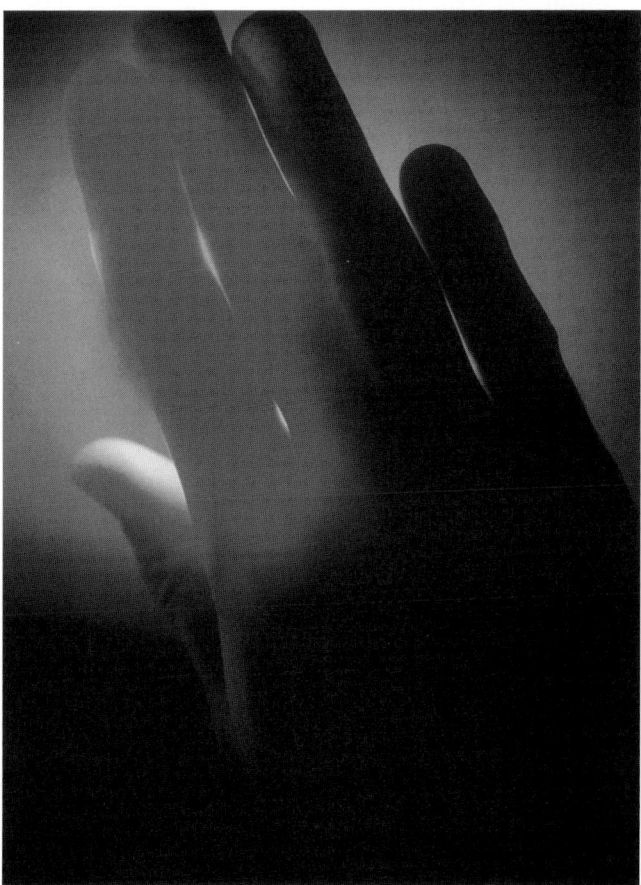

Figure 2. Penetration of light through biologic tissue illustrated by illuminating a hand with white light. Penetration is best for long-wavelength red light (see also Color Plate 16).

Optical Methods

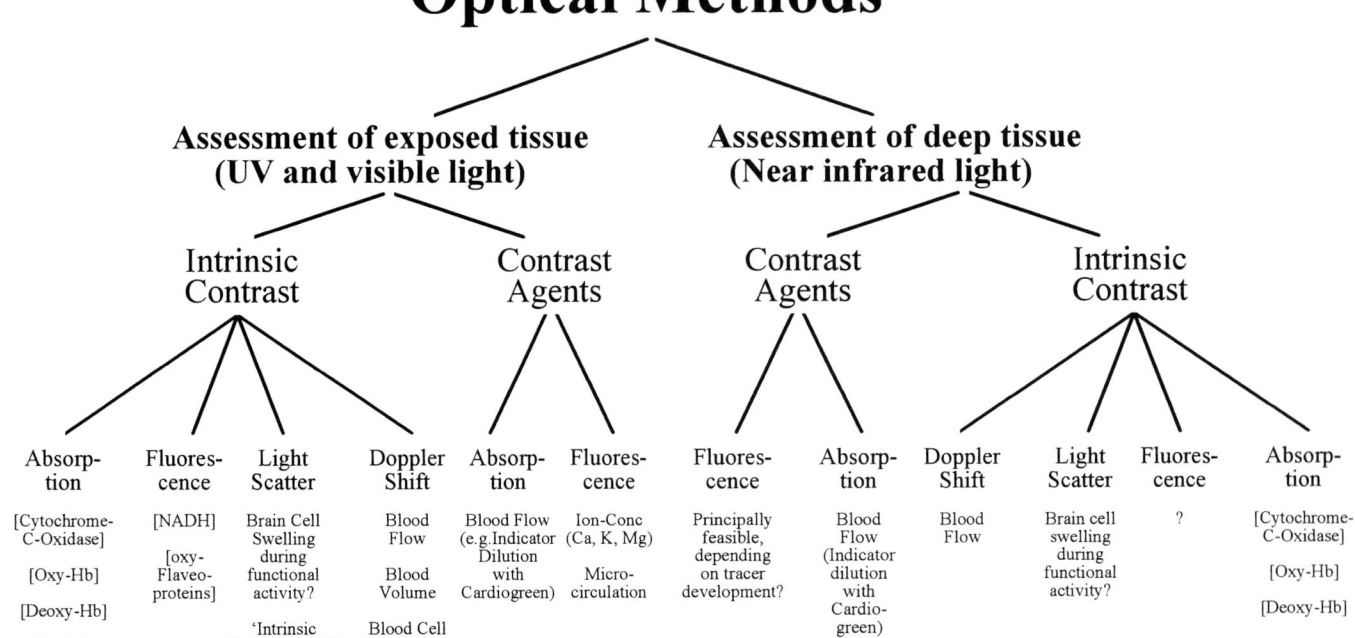

Figure 3. Classification of optical methods.

Even better penetration is achieved by light in the adjacent near-infrared range of approximately 700 to 1000 nm, permitting investigations of the brain even through the intact skull (77). At higher wavelength penetration into tissue is again poor due to the high water absorption of light.

Depending on the penetration properties of the light involved, different optical methods may be divided into those which require the direct exposure of the tissue to the illuminating light and those which assess noninvasively deeper tissues or organs below the surface (Fig. 3).

Optical Measurements on Exposed Tissues

Methods that require exposure of tissue usually employ a light source that emits light in the visible or UV light range. Penetration of this light into tissue is limited to 1 mm or less. These approaches in turn can be divided into those attempting to measure endogenous optical tissue properties and those (see below) employing the administration of a contrast agent.

Measurements of endogenous tissue properties are often referred to as *intrinsic signals,* and measurements that take advantage of contrast agents are referred to as *extrinsic signals.* A particularly well-known example consists of intrinsic and extrinsic signals from brain tissue that can be recorded during functional activation of exposed brain tissue (56).

Optical Measurements of Intrinsic Optical Tissue Properties

Endogenous optical tissue properties include light absorption due to the presence of absorbing substances, the measurement of autofluorescence that allows the measurement of fluorescent tissue components such as NADH and oxidized flavoproteins, the assessment of light scattering changes, and the assessment of Doppler shifts due to the interaction of light with moving blood cells.

Assessment of Endogenous Molecules by Measurement of Light Absorption. As illustrated in Fig. 1, oxygenated hemoglobin, deoxygenated hemoglobin, and cytochrome-C-oxidase have characteristic light absorption patterns. When visible light is used, penetration depth is limited to the outer 200 to 1000 μm of the tissue; hence relatively small tissue volumes are investigated. From the reflection spectra, concentration changes in oxy- and deoxy-Hb, total Hb, oxygen saturation, and cytochrome-oxidase oxygenation may be determined (46, 133).

Measurement of Endogenous Substances by Measurement of Autofluorescence. In vivo fluorimetry, the fluorescence measurement of endogenous substances, was pioneered in Chance's laboratory (14). *NADH fluorimetry* takes advantage of the fluorescence of NADH and permits the assessment of the NADH/NAD redox state. Excitation wavelengths are usually in the ultraviolet range, 337 nm and 366 nm (106, 131). In order to cancel out signal changes due to local blood volume changes, the method is usually combined with reflectometry (106, 131). *Fluorimetry of oxidized flavoproteins* is performed at a somewhat higher wavelength, e.g., at 460 (165) or 441.5 nm (excitation), and the maximum of fluorescence lies around 540 nm. Frequently, fluorimetry of NADH and of oxidized flavoproteins is performed simultaneously (13).

Assessment of Light Scattering of Tissue. The assessment of changes in light scattering has been performed indirectly. It has been shown that brain slices change their transmittance for light in the wavelength range between 450 and 800 nm considerably during induced synaptic activity (95). It is believed that this finding reflects reduced light scattering on functional activation, and there is evidence that this change in the optical property of tissue may be induced by transient changes in cellular volume (3, 95). Technically, a better way to assess these changes in light scattering may be the measurement of path length changes, e.g., using a phase-modulation or time-resolved optical system. From a physiologic point of view, these measurements are interesting because they may indicate the possibility of measuring functional brain activity that is not dependent on neuronal-vascular coupling.

Assessment of Doppler Shift, Laser-Doppler Flowmetry (10, 119, 156). As the name implies, this approach relies on the measurement of a Doppler phase shift of photons. The method has been suggested by Stern (156), and it has been applied to several tissues in the meantime. In order to make the measurements insensitive to hemoglobin oxygenation, the wavelengths used are usually close to the isosbestic points of oxy-Hb and deoxy-Hb. Usually, the tissue is directly exposed, light from the laser diode is guided through a fiberoptic device on the surface of the tissue, and the backscattered light is detected by the same fiberoptic. Newer devices include a scanning procedure of the incident light that allows the blood flow measurement to cover a larger area (176).

Optical Assessment Using Contrast Agents

There are several ways to use contrast agents in optical studies. One can measure changes in light absorbance due to the presence of an agent, or the contrast agents can be fluorescent or phosphorescent dyes.

Absorbent Contrast Agents. Changes in absorbance of tissue may be induced by contrast agents that have different light-absorbing properties than the tissue of investigation. After intraarterial or intravenous injection of a nondiffusible contrast agent (an agent that stays in the blood and does not enter tissue), light absorption in the tissue changes transiently, and flow of the agent through the investigated tissue may be monitored by continuously measuring absorption of light. Under certain assumptions, the area of the indicator dilution curve obtained is proportional to local blood volume (*BV*). By assessing mean transit time *(MTT)* of the tracer, blood flow *(BF)* may be calculated from $BF = BV/MTT$ (33). For principal problems associated with the indicator dilution approach, the reader is referred to Weisskoff et al. (177).

Fluorescent Dyes. There are several ways that fluorescent dyes may be employed to assess tissue function. If, for example, a fluorescent agent such as fluorescein is injected into the bloodstream, it is bound to plasma proteins and therefore remains within the plasma compartment of the blood. Blood cells are not labeled and are therefore identified as nonlabeled particles within the blood. Using this approach, combined with a microscopic imaging device, dynamics of the microcirculation can be monitored under different physiologic conditions (172).

Another interesting group of fluorescent dyes changes its fluorescent properties in reaction to different physiologic conditions. Dyes change their fluorescence behavior, for example, depending on the local pH (125), Ca concentration (8), Mg concentration (12), cAMP concentration (1), and a number of other substances. When these dyes are loaded into the cellular and/or the intracellular space, measurements of the respective physiologic condition/concentration can be performed by measuring fluorescence within the tissue sample.

Phosphorescent Dyes. Phosphorescent dyes can be quenched by oxygen; in other words, increasing oxygen pressure causes an increase in the rate of decay of phosphorescence. This is associated with a shorter lifetime and thus a decrease in total phosphorescence intensity. Therefore, phosphorescence lifetime measurements may be used to measure oxygen pressure. When phosphorescent oxygen probes such as Pd-coproporphyrin and Pd-mesoporphyrin are loaded into tissue, the oxygen pressure of tissue can be measured. The light detector is a photomultiplier or a photointensified CCD camera. Several applications of this technique in biologic systems have been reported (135, 167).

Near-Infrared Techniques

Taking advantage of the excellent tissue-penetration properties of near-infrared light allows the assessment of biologic tissues located deep within the body. Most prominently, the adult human brain can be examined noninvasively through the intact skull using near-infrared devices.

Absorption Measurements Using Near-Infrared Techniques

Commercially Available Approaches. Several commercially available near-infrared devices have been built to assess concentration changes of substances such as oxy-Hb, deoxy-Hb, or cytochrome-C-oxidase according to a modified Lambert-Beer law (20), as described above. Usually, a multiwavelength approach is employed with several laser diodes as light sources (e.g., the pioneering dual-wavelength system used by Chance's group [15], an NIRS instrument by Shimadzu as used by Hoshi and Tamura [73], and systems by Hamamatsu) (20, 171). The light detector usually is a photomultiplier. These techniques do not measure path length of the light directly. In order to quantitate changes in concentration, a certain value for the differential path length factor (DPF) is assumed based on measurements performed in similar experimental conditions. Thus a value of 6.26% ($\pm$14.1%) has been given for the adult human head, a value of 4.16% ($\pm$18.8%) for the adult arm, and 5.51% ($\pm$18%) for the adult leg (31). The standard deviations of these figures indicate a considerable potential error in individual subjects. This error will become considerably larger when examinations are performed on subjects with brain diseases. Therefore, it is mandatory for the next generation of near-infrared systems to implement strategies for path length determination simultaneously with each measurement.

Approaches to Determine Optical Path Length for Better Quantitation of Concentration Changes. Using a white continuous-wavelight source (e.g., halogen) covering the whole wavelength range from 700 to 1000 nm, an entire spectrum may be measured (21, 104). The reflected light is passed through a grating, and the spectrally dispersed light is then projected on the light-detecting CCD camera, where the horizontal axis becomes the spectral axis. This approach evidently has a higher spectral resolution and may therefore permit better separation of the contribution of the different absorbers in tissue. In addition, it allows the assessment of water absorption peaks at 820 and 970 nm. Assuming a constant water concentration in tissue, changes in the water absorption of light are a measure of changes in path length. By determining the relative concentration of deoxy-Hb to the (known) total water concentration, an absolute concentration of deoxy-Hb can be calculated (104).

Another way to assess path length or path length changes is the time-resolved approach. Employing extremely short (on the order of picoseconds) laser pulses and measuring the reflected light at a high temporal resolution (44, 143, 182) the distribution of time of flights of photons can be measured.

Another approach uses intensity-modulated light as light source and determines the phase shift of the frequency modulation after passage to the tissue. From the phase shift, path length also can be determined (31, 87).

Measurement of Scattering Using Near-Infrared Techniques

NIRS systems that measure changes in path length of light may be used to detect events in tissue that mainly or solely produce changes in light scattering. The same approaches that were discussed in the preceding chapter are employed for such studies: (a) assessment of the water absorption peak by acquiring a whole spectrum in the near-infrared range (21, 104), (b) measurement of the time of flight of photons using ultrashort laser pulses and a time-resolved detector (44, 143, 182), and (c) the phase-modulation approach (31, 87). Using a phase-modulation approach, Gratton et al. have reported rapid signal changes in the human brain that may correspond to electrophysiologic events (52).

Measurements of Fluorescence and Phosphorescence Using Near-Infrared Techniques

So far such measurements that are principally feasible have not been reported. However, since dyes in the red and near-infrared light range are currently being developed, such measurements seem to be on the horizon. The wide range of possible measurement parameters (see above) makes this a very promising approach for the future.

Assessment of Doppler Shifts Using Near-Infrared Techniques

This is another interesting approach that seems principally feasible. Recently, a prototype of such a device has been developed by Chance's group. Further developments may bring an analogy to the widely used laser-Doppler approach into the arena of noninvasive studies in human subjects.

Near-Infrared Developments Toward Functional Imaging

The near-infrared techniques mentioned above are single-site measurements. The first multisite applications have been reported by Hirth (68) and Maki et al. (96). Multisite measurements also will be easily implemented in the CCD camera approach, where input from several fibers may be displayed vertically displaced on the CCD camera; hence the vertical axis becomes a spatial dimension (104).

The next step involves attempts toward near-infrared imaging. The first approaches have employed the above-mentioned time-resolved approach, and for image reconstruction, only ballistic photons, i.e., photons that are not or little scattered, were used. For image generation, backprojection algorithms similar to those used in x-ray computed tomography were used (144). The disadvantage of these methods is that in tissues thicker than a few centimeters there are extremely few ballistic photons. It seems clear now that for the majority of applications this approach is not feasible. Therefore, attempts are made to include scattered photons in the measurements. In these studies, light transport is modeled according to known diffusion properties of light in tissue. The first NIRS imaging systems have been presented in animal models (144).

ORGANS OF INVESTIGATION

Optical Measurements on Exposed Tissues

The main limitation of these methods is the necessity of tissue exposure. In animal studies, in order to access the brain, different cranial window methods (for an overview, see Haber [58]) have been developed that allow tissue observation with optical devices such as (confocal) light microscopy (170), devices for the assessment of autofluorescence (107), laser-Doppler flowmetry (26, 59, 60), and the special case of intrinsic brain signals (47, 54). In human subjects, the studies are therefore limited to the skin, tissues that can be accessed by endoscopic measures (57, 93, 141), or other more or less invasive placement of probes, e.g., in the intensive care unit (58) or the intraoperative arena (27, 67, 79, 158, 164).

Optical Measurements of Intrinsic Optical Tissue Properties

Assessment of Endogenous Molecules by Measurement of Light Absorption. Oxygenated hemoglobin, deoxygenated hemoglobin, and cytochrome-C-oxidase are being measured, e.g., using the so-called EMPHO device in brain tissue of the Mongolian gerbil (107), the rabbit lung (71), the rabbit eye vasculature (45), the rat heart (185), muscle, and liver, and the human brain (70).

Measurement of Endogenous Substances by Measurement of Autofluorescence. In vivo fluorimetry (NADH and/or flaveoproteins) has been performed in Mongolian gerbil brain (107), dog brain (115), gerbil brain (65), rat heart (66), rabbit cornea (103, 127), rabbit liver (161), and rat kidney (186).

Assessment of Light Scattering of Tissue. As indicated before, measurements of light scattering on exposed tissue have been done indirectly on brain slices, in which changes in light transmittance have been taken as indication for increased synaptic activity of brain cells (95). These findings represent one example of functional imaging of brain tissue using "intrinsic signals."

Functional Brain Imaging Using Intrinsic Signals. Whereas the above-mentioned approaches have a clear measurement parameter such as concentration of a certain substance, intrinsic signal recordings are defined primarily by their striking agreement with electrophysiologic assessment of brain cell activity (55) and less well defined regarding the actual measurement parameter. Exposed brain tissue is illuminated with light at a certain wavelength in the visible or near-infrared range. A slow-scan CCD camera records pictures from the exposed part of the cortex. Pictures are digitized and divided by a blank trial picture to correct for uneven illumination. The resulting "blank adjusted" pictures represent the activity map of the corresponding stimulus, and such maps correspond surprisingly well with electrophysiologic measurements or activation images obtained after loading of brain tissue with voltage-sensitive dyes. In whole animals, the most important contributions to the signal may stem from changes in oxy-Hb, deoxy-Hb, and total Hb concentration. In addition, changes in light scattering and cytochrome oxygenation also may contribute to the observed signals. The latter contribution is probably of particular importance in analogous experiments performed on blood-free brain slice preparations (95). By definition, these experiments are all performed on brain tissue. Examples of successful applications include the assessment of seizure propagation in isolated whole-brain prepartions of the guinea pig (43), the analysis of the layout of iso-orientation domains in the cat visual cortex (9), the analysis of ocular dominance columns in the primate striatae cortex (5), the analysis of shape and motion processing in area MT of the owl monkey (97), imaging cell volume changes and neuronal excitation in the hippocampal slice (3), assessing the somatosensory whisker barrel cortex in the rat (113), and numerous others.

Laser-Doppler Flowmetry (LDF). In principle, the method can be applied to any tissue that is blood perfused. Due to the limited depth penetration of current LDF devices, applications are limited to organs or tissues that can be exposed directly. This limits clinical applications to the skin and to procedures that involve the invasive exposure of tissues (61, 78). Studies have been presented, for example, on skin (36, 119, 138), muscle (62, 92), lung, parathyroid gland (78), intestinal mucosa (137), kidney (119, 128), liver (17), testis (23), and brain (26, 59, 147). Measurements have been validated by comparisons with other blood flow techniques. For the brain, for example, those validation studies were performed by Haberl et al. (59) and Skarpedinsson (147) using the hydrogen clearance method and by Dirnagl et al. (26) using the [^{14}C]iodoantipyrine method.

Optical Assessment Using Contrast Agents

Absorbent Contrast Agents. Most studies in which optical properties of tissues are measured during administration of a contrast agent have been performed on the brain (22, 33). In order to measure cerebral blood flow, tracers that induce transient changes in light absorbance of the tissue are administered into the intravascular space. The blood-brain barrier prevents these contrast agents from entering the extravascular space.

Fluorescent Dyes. Fluorescent dyes have been loaded in various types of cell cultures in order to measure intracellular calcium concentration (16, 53, 132, 184), pH (145), cAMP concentration (139), and other ion concentrations. Such studies are principally also feasible in more complex systems such as brain slices and intact brain (89, 163). Functional studies using voltage-sensitive dyes have been performed on cultured rat heart cells (41, 42). Most studies, however, have been performed on brain tissue (2, 114, 142).

Phosphorescent Dyes. Oxygenation measurements with phosphorescent dyes have been performed in several tissues such as human tumors (157), the brain of newborn piglets (124, 154), the heart of newborn piglets (134), the cat brain cortex (179), and the rat costal diaphragm (129).

Near-Infrared Spectroscopy (NIRS)

Most functional NIRS studies have been performed on brain and muscle tissue (attempts to image structural alterations of breast tissue are not covered in this review) (37, 130). There are a few reports on investigation of the liver. Studies were performed on rat liver after transplantation (120), rabbit liver during hemorrhage and hypoxia (83, 84), and the liver of human children after transplantation (162). The main problem with studies on liver in adult human subjects is the pronounced movement of the liver with respiration.

One study has been reported on rat kidney (168) assessing the effect of ischemia-reperfusion.

Studies on Muscle

A number of studies have been performed on dog muscle (30), on human muscle (98) under normal conditions and during and after exercise (6, 99, 110, 111, 155, 159) and ischemia (24), in peripheral vascular disease (18, 86, 110), in patients with heart failure (100, 180), and in metabolic myopathies (4).

Studies on Neonatal Brain

Due to the smaller head size and thinner bone, but also due to the practical difficulty of performing other imaging procedures such as CT or MRI, the neonate's brain has been examined frequently with NIRS (7, 11, 19, 25, 32, 38, 40, 150). Studies are principally possible in transmission mode; however, many studies also have been performed in reflection mode. Cerebral oxygenation changes have been assessed in preterm infants with low-dose versus high-dose surfactant therapy (28, 39, 148), within 24 hours after birth asphyxia (166), during hypothermic circulatory arrest (88), and during endotracheal suctioning (151), to measure the effect of hypoxemia and bradycardia (94), during in-

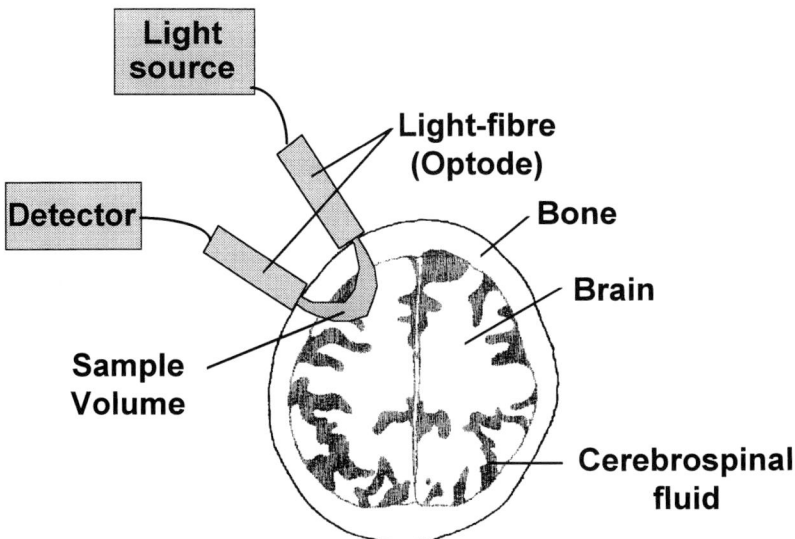

Figure 4. Volume of investigation in near-infrared spectroscopy (NIRS) performed in reflection mode of the adult human brain.

duction of extracorporeal membrane oxygenation (91), and after the administration of indomethacin (108). Some studies on the neonatal brain have been performed in utero and during labor (29, 126). Results have been favorably compared with an ^{133}Xe clearance (149) blood flow measurement.

Studies on the Adult Human Brain

Increasingly, NIRS studies are performed on the adult human brain. The crucial issue and prerequisite for these studies is the definition of the volume under investigation. This volume depends on the distance of the optodes (light fiber endings attached to the head), the geometry of the head, and other individual factors such as presence of hair, hair and skin pigmentation, etc. Usually, the sample volume is assumed to be a banana-shape structure beneath the optodes (Fig. 4). Increasingly sophisticated model calculations that take into account the multilayer composition of the head are currently modifying this picture. There might by tunneling of light at interfaces of compartments with different optical properties such as cerebrospinal fluid with gray matter and gray matter with white matter. Therefore, significant amounts of light might be confined to just the gray matter beneath the optodes. It may be possible to differentiate between contributions of different depths beneath the brain surface by time-resolved studies, and such studies may allow one to get information also about tissue deeper than the gray matter.

A number of NIRS studies of the adult human brain (34, 35, 152) focused on more or less global changes in cerebral oxygenation, e.g., during mild hypoxia (63), during cardiopulmonary bypass (160), during + Gz-acceleration in order to simulate conditions in rockets or airplanes (49, 50), during cardioverter defibrillation testing (146), after stellate ganglion blockade (123), during carotid endarterectomy (82, 101, 140, 178, 183), during ventricular fibrillation (90), during cardiac surgery (116), in patients with head injury (81), during hypercapnia and hypocapnia (153), and during cerebral hypoxia (109). It must be mentioned that the ability to assess brain tissue oxygenation as opposed to extracerebral oxygenation with the particular device used by the latter group has been questioned by others (48, 64). A study by Chance's group has shown that after head trauma it was possible to detect the development of intracranial hematoma using a near-infrared device (51).

Studies on Functional Brain Activation

Recently, a number of studies have demonstrated the ability to assess changes in NIR parameters occurring during localized brain activity in adult human subjects (15, 69, 72,

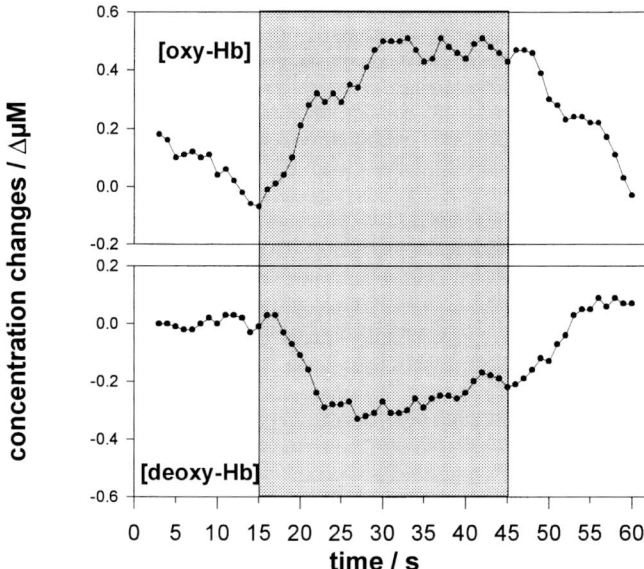

Figure 5. Response of near-infrared parameters oxygenated and deoxygenated hemoglobin (oxy-Hb, deoxy-Hb) to functional brain activation. Measurement was performed over the occipital cortex during rest (30-second observation of blank computer screen) and during observation of a moving colored object (30-second shaded period). The stimulation was repeated 10 times and averaged, time locked to stimulus onset subsequently.

73, 75, 76, 80, 120, 121, 171, 172). Responses have been measured to cognitive activation (69, 72, 73, 171), a mirror drawing task (121), visual stimulation (80, 112, 171), and motor activation (85, 96, 117). The typical NIRS response to a localized increase in brain activity is an increase in the concentration of oxy-Hb and a decrease in the concentration of deoxy-Hb. An example is given in Fig. 5. For an overview, see Obrig and Villringer (118). The results of functional NIRS assessment of brain activation have been compared with PET (72, 174). It has been shown that changes in total Hb concentration and CBF as measured by PET correlate positively (174). In addition, it has been shown that changes in deoxyhemoglobin concentration, as measured by near-infrared spectroscopy, correlate positively with changes in the BOLD contrast of MRI during performance of a motor activation task (85).

Pathologic brain activation has been studied in rats during epileptic seizures (74), during spreading depression (181), and during epileptic seizures in adult human patients (173).

REFERENCES

1. Adams SR, Harootunian AT, Buechler YJ et al. Fluorescence ratio imaging of cyclic AMP in single cells. *Nature,* 349, 694–697 (1991).
2. Albowitz B, Kuhnt U. Epileptiform activity in the guinea pig neocortical slice spreads preferentially along supragranular layers: Recordings with voltage sensitive dyes. *Eur J Neurosci,* 7, 1273–1284 (1995).
3. Andrew RD, MacVicar BA. Imaging cell volume changes and neuronal excitation in the hippocampal-slice. *Neuroscience,* 62, 371–383 (1994).
4. Bank W, Chance B. An oxidative defect in metabolic myopathies: Diagnosis by noninvasive tissue oximetry [Comments]. *Ann Neurol,* 36, 830–837 (1994).
5. Bartfeld E, Grinvald A. Relationships between orientation-preference pinwheels, cytochrome oxidase blobs, and ocular-dominance columns in primate striate cortex. *Proc Natl Acad Sci USA,* 89, 11905–11909 (1992).
6. Belardinelli R, Barstow TJ, Porszasz J, Wasserman K. Changes in skeletal muscle oxygenation during incremental exercise measured with near-infrared spectroscopy. *Eur J Appl Physiol,* 70, 487–492 (1995).
7. Benaron DA, Benitz WE, Ariagno RL, Stevenson DK. Noninvasive methods for estimating in vivo oxygenation. *Clin Pediatr Phila,* 31, 258–273 (1992).
8. Bird GS, Rossier MF, Hughes AR et al. Activation of Ca^{2+} entry into acinar cells by a non-phosphorylatable inositol trisphosphate [Comments]. *Nature,* 352, 162–165 (1991).
9. Bonhoeffer T, Grinvald A. The layout of iso-orientation domains in area 18 of cat visual cortex: Optical imaging reveals a pinwheel-like organization. *J Neurosci,* 13, 4157–4180 (1993).

10. Bonner R, Nossal R. A model for laser Doppler measurements of blood flow in tissue. *Applied Optics,* 20, 2097–2107 (1981).
11. Brazy JE. Cerebral oxygen monitoring with near-infrared spectroscopy: Clinical application to neonates. *J Clin Monit,* 7, 325–334 (1991).
12. Brocard JB, Rajdev S, Reynolds IJ. Glutamate-induced increases in intracellular free Mg^{2+} in cultured cortical neurons. *Neuron,* 11, 751–757 (1993).
13. Chance B. Optical method. *Annu Rev Biophys Biophys Chem,* 20, 1–28 (1991).
14. Chance B, Cohen P, Jobsis F, Schoener B. Intracellular oxidation-reduction states in vivo. *Science,* 137, 499–508 (1962).
15. Chance B, Zhuang Z, Unah C et al. Cognition-activated low-frequency modulation of light absorption in human brain. *Proc Natl Acad Sci USA,* 90, 3770–3774 (1993).
16. Chandra S, Morrison GH. Imaging elemental distribution and ion transport in cultured cells with ion microscopy. *Science,* 228, 1543–1544 (1985).
17. Chavez Cartaya RE, Ramirez Romero P, Calne RY et al. Laser-Doppler flowmetry in the study of in vivo liver ischemia and reperfusion in the rat. *J Surg Res,* 56, 473–477 (1994).
18. Cheatle TR, Potter LA, Cope M et al. Near-infrared spectroscopy in peripheral vascular disease. *Br J Surg,* 78, 405–408 (1991).
19. Cooper CE, Elwell CE, Meek JH et al. The noninvasive measurement of absolute cerebral deoxyhemoglobin concentration and mean optical path length in the neonatal brain by second derivative near-infrared spectroscopy. *Pediatr Res,* 39, 32–38 (1996).
20. Cope M, Delpy DT. System for long-term measurement of cerebral blood and tissue oxygenation on newborn infants by near infra-red transillumination. *Med Biol Eng Comput,* 26, 289–294 (1988).
21. Cope M, Delpy DT, Wray S et al. A CCD spectrophotometer to quantitate the concentration of chromophores in living tissue utilising the absorption peak of water at 975 nm. *Adv Exp Med Biol,* 248, 33–40 (1989).
22. Crumrine RC, Lamanna JC. Regional cerebral metabolites, blood flow, plasma volume, and mean transit time in total cerebral ischemia in the rat. *J Cereb Blood Flow Metab,* 11, 272–282 (1991).
23. Damber JE, Bergh A, Fagrell B et al. Testicular microcirculation in the rat studied by videophotometric capillaroscopy, fluorescence microscopy and laser Doppler flowmetry. *Acta Physiol Scand,* 126, 371–376 (1986).
24. De Blasi RA, Quaglia E, Gasparetto A, Ferrari M. Muscle oxygenation by fast near-infrared spectrophotometry (NIRS) in an ischemic forearm. *Adv Exp Med Biol,* 316, 163–172 (1992).
25. Delpy DT, Cope MC, Cady EB et al. Cerebral monitoring in newborn infants by magnetic resonance and near-infrared spectroscopy. *Scand J Clin Lab Invest Suppl,* 188, 9–17 (1987).
26. Dirnagl U, Kaplan B, Jacewicz M, Pulsinelli W. Continuous measurement of cerebral cortical blood flow by laser-Doppler flowmetry in a rat stroke model. *J Cereb Blood Flow Metab,* 9, 589–596 (1989).
27. Dodson TB, Neuenschwander MC, Bays RA. Intraoperative assessment of maxillary perfusion during Le Fort iosteotomy. *J Oral Maxillofac Surg,* 52, 827–831 (1994).
28. Dorrepaal CA, Benders MJ, Steendijk P et al. Cerebral hemodynamics and oxygenation in preterm infants after low- versus high-dose surfactant replacement therapy. *Biol Neonate,* 64, 193–200 (1993).
29. Doyle PM, O'Brien S, Wickramasinghe YA et al. Near-infrared spectroscopy used to observe changes in fetal cerebral haemodynamics during labour. *J Perinat Med,* 22, 265–268 (1994).
30. Duhaylongsod FG, Griebel JA, Bacon DS et al. Effects of muscle contraction on cytochrome a, a3 redox state. *J Appl Physiol,* 75, 790–797 (1993).
31. Duncan A, Meek JH, Clemence M et al. Optical pathlength measurements on adult head, calf and forearm and the head of the newborn infant using phase resolved optical spectroscopy. *Phys Med Biol,* 40, 295–304 (1995).
32. Edwards AD, Brown GC, Cope M et al. Quantification of concentration changes in neonatal human cerebral oxidized cytochrome oxidase. *J Appl Physiol,* 71, 1907–1913 (1991).
33. Eke A. Reflectometric mapping of microregional blood flow and blood volume in the brain cortex. *J Cereb Blood Flow Metab,* 2, 41–53 (1982).
34. Elwell CE, Cope M, Edwards AD et al. Quantification of adult cerebral hemodynamics by near-infrared spectroscopy. *J Appl Physiol,* 77, 2753–2760 (1994).
35. Elwell CE, Owen Reece H, Cope M et al. Measurement of adult cerebral haemodynamics using near-infrared spectroscopy. *Acta Neurochir Suppl (Wien),* 59, 74–80 (1993).
36. Engelhart M, Kristensen JK. Evaluation of cutaneous blood flow responses by 133Xenon washout and a laser-Doppler flowmeter. *J Invest Dermatol,* 80, 12–15 (1983).
37. Ertefai S, Profio AE. Spectral transmittance and contrast in breast diaphanography. *Med Phys,* 12, 393–400 (1985).
38. Fahnenstich H, Schmidt S, Krebs D, Kowalewski S. Intracranial hemodynamics in phenobarbital administration. *Z Geburtshilfe Perinatol,* 196, 74–77 (1992).
39. Fahnenstich H, Schmidt S, Spaniol S, Kowalewski S. Relative changes in oxyhemoglobin, deoxyhemoglobin and intracranial blood volume during surfactant replacement therapy in infants with respiratory distress syndrome. *Dev Pharmacol Ther,* 17, 150–153 (1991).
40. Faris F, Thorniley M, Wickramasinghe Y et al. Noninvasive in vivo near-infrared optical measurement of the penetration depth in the neonatal head. *Clin Phys Physiol Meas,* 12, 353–358 (1991).
41. Fast VG, Kleber AG. Anisotropic conduction in monolayers of neonatal rat heart cells cultured on collagen substrate. *Circ Res,* 75, 591–595 (1994).
42. Fast VG, Kleber AG. Cardiac tissue geometry as a determinant of unidirectional conduction block: Assessment of microscopic excitation spread by optical mapping in patterned cell cultures and in a computer model. *Cardiovasc Res,* 29, 697–707 (1995).
43. Federico P, Borg SG, Salkauskus AG, MacVicar BA. Mapping patterns of neuronal activity and seizure propagation by imaging intrinsic optical signals in the isolated whole brain of the guinea pig. *Neuroscience,* 58, 461–480 (1994).

44. Ferrari M, Wei Q, Carraresi L et al. Time-resolved spectroscopy of the human forearm. *J Photochem Photobiol B*, 16, 141–153 (1992).
45. Frank K, Funk R, Kessler M, Rohen JW. Spectrometric measurements in the anterior eye vasculature of the albino rabbit: A study with the EMPHO I. *Exp Eye Res*, 52, 301–309 (1991).
46. Frank KH, Kessler M, Appelbaum K, Dummler W. The Erlangen micro-lightguide spectrophotometer EMPHO I. *Phys Med Biol*, 34, 1883–1900 (1989).
47. Frostig RD, Lieke EE, Ts'o DY, Grinvald A. Cortical functional architecture and local coupling between neuronal activity and the microcirculation revealed by in vivo high-resolution optical imaging of intrinsic signals. *Proc Natl Acad Sci USA*, 87, 6082–6086 (1990).
48. Germon TJ, Young AE, Manara AR, Nelson RJ. Extracerebral absorption of near-infrared light influences the detection of increased cerebral oxygenation monitored by near-infrared spectroscopy. *J Neurol Neurosurg Psychiatry*, 58, 477–479 (1995).
49. Glaister DH, Jobsis Vandervliet FF. A near-infrared spectrophotometric method for studying brain O_2 sufficiency in man during $+ Gz$ acceleration. *Aviat Space Environ Med*, 59, 199–207 (1988).
50. Glaister DH, Miller NL. Cerebral tissue oxygen status and psychomotor performance during lower body negative pressure (LBNP). *Aviat Space Environ Med*, 61, 99–105 (1990).
51. Gopinath SP, Robertson CS, Grossman RG, Chance B. Near-infrared spectroscopic localization of intracranial hematomas. *J Neurosurg*, 79, 43–47 (1993).
52. Gratton G, Fabiani M, Friedman D et al. Rapid changes of optical parameters in the human brain during a tapping task. *J Cogn Neurosci*, 7, 446–456 (1995).
53. Grega DS, Werz MA, MacDonald RL. Forskolin and phorbol esters reduce the same potassium conductance of mouse neurons in culture. *Science*, 235, 345–348 (1987).
54. Grinvald A, Frostig RD, Siegel RM, Bartfeld E. High-resolution optical imaging of functional brain architecture in the awake monkey. *Proc Natl Acad Sci USA*, 88, 11559–11563 (1991).
55. Grinvald A, Lieke E, Frostig RD et al. Functional architecture of cortex revealed by optical imaging of intrinsic signals. *Nature*, 324, 361–364 (1986).
56. Grinvald A, Lieke EE, Frostig RD, Hildesheim R. Cortical point-spread function and long-range lateral interactions revealed by real-time optical imaging of macaque monkey primary visual cortex. *J Neurosci*, 14, 2545–2568 (1994).
57. Guslandi M, Polli D, Sorghi M, Tittobello A. Rectal blood flow in ulcerative colitis. *Am J Gastroenterol*, 90, 579–580 (1995).
58. Haberl RL. Optical access to the brain: How artificial are cranial window techniques? *Adv Exp Med Biol*, 333, 177–181 (1993).
59. Haberl RL, Heizer ML, Ellis EF. Laser-Doppler assessment of brain microcirculation: Effect of local alterations. *Am J Physiol*, 256, H1255–H1260 (1989).
60. Haberl RL, Heizer ML, Marmarou A, Ellis EF. Laser-Doppler assessment of brain microcirculation: Effect of systemic alterations. *Am J Physiol*, 256, H1247–H1254 (1989).
61. Haberl RL, Villringer A, Dirnagl U. Applicability of laser-Doppler flowmetry for cerebral blood flow monitoring in neurological intensive care. *Acta Neurochir Suppl (Wien)*, 59, 64–68 (1993).
62. Hakim TS. Is flow in subpleural region typical of the rest of the lung? A study using laser-Doppler flowmetry. *J Appl Physiol*, 72, 1860–1867 (1992).
63. Hampson NB, Camporesi EM, Stolp BW et al. General oxygen availability by NIR spectroscopy during transient hypoxia in humans. *J Appl Physiol*, 69, 907–913 (1990).
64. Harris DN, Bailey SM. Near-infrared spectroscopy in adults. Does the Invos 3100 really measure intracerebral oxygenation? *Anaesthesia*, 48, 694–696 (1993).
65. Haselgrove JC, Bashford CL, Barlow CH et al. Time resolved 3-dimensional recording of redox ratio during spreading depression in gerbil brain. *Brain Res*, 506, 109–114 (1990).
66. Hassinen I, Ito K, Nioka S, Chance B. Mechanism of fatty acid effect on myocardial oxygen consumption: A phosphorus NMR study. *Biochim Biophys Acta*, 1019, 73–80 (1990).
67. Hemingway DM, Angerson WJ, Anderson JH et al. Monitoring blood flow to colorectal liver metastases using laser-Doppler flowmetry: The effect of angiotensin II. *Br J Cancer*, 66, 958–960 (1992).
68. Hirth C, Obrig H, Villringer K et al. Mapping of the human motor cortex using near-infrared spectroscopy. *NeuroReport*, in press (1996).
69. Hock C, Mullerspahn F, Schuh-Hofer S et al. Age dependency of changes in cerebral hemoglobin oxygenation during brain activation: A near-infrared spectroscopy study. *J Cereb Blood Flow Metab*, 15, 1103–1108 (1995).
70. Hoper J, Gaab MR. Effect of arterial PCO_2 on local HbO_2 and relative Hb concentration in the human brain: A study with the Erlangen micro-lightguide spectrophotometer (EMPHO). *Physiol Meas*, 15, 107–113 (1994).
71. Hoper J, Plasswilm L. Micro-lightguide spectrophotometric measurement of changes in local haemoglobin oxygenation and concentration in the rabbit lung induced by hypoxia and hyperoxia. *Int J Microcirc Clin Exp*, 14, 282–288 (1994).
72. Hoshi Y, Onoe H, Watanabe Y et al. Nonsynchronous behavior of neuronal activity, oxidative metabolism and blood supply during mental tasks in man. *Neurosci Lett*, 172, 129–133 (1994).
73. Hoshi Y, Tamura M. Dynamic multichannel near-infrared optical imaging of human brain activity. *J Appl Physiol*, 75, 1842–1846 (1993a).
74. Hoshi Y, Tamura M. Dynamic changes in cerebral oxygenation in chemically induced seizures in rats: Study by near-infrared spectrophotometry. *Brain Res*, 603, 215–221 (1993b).
75. Hoshi Y, Tamura M. Detection of dynamic changes in cerebral oxygenation coupled to neuronal function during mental work in man. *Neurosci Lett*, 150, 5–8 (1993c).
76. Hoshi Y, Tamura M. Multichannel near-infrared optical imaging of brain activity. *Neuroscience Protocols*, Module 4, 155–169 (1994).
77. Jobsis FE. Noninvasive, infrared monitoring of cerebral and myocardial oxygen sufficiency and circulatory parameters. *Science*, 198, 1264–1267 (1977).

78. Johansson K, Ander S, Lennquist S, Smeds S. Human parathyroid blood supply determined by laser-Doppler flowmetry. *World J Surg,* 18, 417–420 (1994).

79. Jones NF. Intraoperative and postoperative monitoring of microsurgical free tissue transfers. *Clin Plast Surg,* 19, 783–797 (1992).

80. Kato T, Kamei A, Takashima S, Ozaki T. Human visual cortical function during photic stimulation monitoring by means of near-infrared spectroscopy. *J Cereb Blood Flow Metab,* 13, 516–520 (1993).

81. Kirkpatrick PJ, Smielewski P, Czosnyka M et al. Near-infrared spectroscopy use in patients with head injury. *J Neurosurg,* 83, 963–970 (1995).

82. Kirkpatrick PJ, Smielewski P, Whitfield PC et al. An observational study of near-infrared spectroscopy during carotid endarterectomy. *J Neurosurg,* 82, 756–763 (1995).

83. Kitai T, Tanaka A, Tokuka A et al. Quantitative detection of hemoglobin saturation in the liver with near-infrared spectroscopy. *Hepatology,* 18, 926–936 (1993a).

84. Kitai T, Tanaka A, Tokuka A et al. Changes in the hepatic oxygenation state during hemorrhage and following epinephrine or dextran infusion as assessed by near-infrared spectroscopy. *Circ Shock,* 41, 197–205 (1993b).

85. Kleinschmidt A, Obrig H, Requardt M et al. Simultaneous recording of cerebral blood oxygenation changes during human brain activation by MRI and near-infrared spectroscopy. *J Cereb Blood Flow Metab,* in press (1996).

86. Komiyama T, Shigematsu H, Yasuhara H, Muto T. An objective assessment of intermittent claudication by near-infrared spectroscopy. *Eur J Vasc Surg,* 8, 294–296 (1994).

87. Kurth CD, Steven JM, Benaron D, Chance B. Near-infrared monitoring of the cerebral circulation. *J Clin Monit,* 9, 163–170 (1993).

88. Kurth CD, Steven JM, Nicolson SC et al. Kinetics of cerebral deoxygenation during deep hypothermic circulatory arrest in neonates. *Anesthesiology,* 77, 656–661 (1992).

89. Lamanna JC, Griffith JK, Cordisco BR et al. Intracellular pH in rat brain in vivo and in brain slices. *Can J Physiol Pharmacol,* 70 (Suppl), S269–S277 (1992).

90. Levy WJ, Levin S, Chance B. Near-infrared measurement of cerebral oxygenation. Correlation with electroencephalographic ischemia during ventricular fibrillation. *Anesthesiology,* 83, 738–746 (1995).

91. Liem KD, Hopman JC, Oeseburg B et al. Cerebral oxygenation and hemodynamics during induction of extracorporeal membrane oxygenation as investigated by near-infrared spectrophotometry. *Pediatrics,* 95, 555–561 (1995).

92. Linderoth B, Herregodts P, Meyerson BA. Sympathetic mediation of peripheral vasodilation induced by spinal cord stimulation: Animal studies of the role of cholinergic and adrenergic receptor subtypes. *Neurosurgery,* 35, 711–719 (1994).

93. Lindsberg PJ, Siren AL, Feuerstein GZ, Hallenbeck JM. Antagonism of neutrophil adherence in the deteriorating stroke model in rabbits. *J Neurosurg,* 82, 269–277 (1995).

94. Livera LN, Spencer SA, Thorniley MS et al. Effects of hypoxaemia and bradycardia on neonatal cerebral haemodynamics. *Arch Dis Child,* 66, 376–380 (1991).

95. MacVicar BA, Hochman D. Imaging of synaptically evoked intrinsic optical signals in hippocampal slices. *J Neurosci,* 11, 1458–1469 (1991).

96. Maki A, Yamashita Y, Ito Y et al. Spatial and temporal analysis of human motor activity using noninvasive NIR topography. *Med Phys,* 22, 1997–2005 (1995).

97. Malonek D, Tootell RB, Grinvald A. Optical imaging reveals the functional architecture of neurons processing shape and motion in owl monkey area MT. *Proc R Soc Lond [Biol],* 258, 109–119 (1994).

98. Mancini DM, Bolinger L, Li H et al. Validation of near-infrared spectroscopy in humans. *J Appl Physiol,* 77, 2740–2747 (1994).

99. Mancini DM, Ferraro N, Nazzaro D et al. Respiratory muscle deoxygenation during exercise in patients with heart failure demonstrated with near-infrared spectroscopy. *J Am Coll Cardiol,* 18, 492–498 (1991).

100. Mancini DM, Henson D, Lamanca J, Levine S. Respiratory muscle function and dyspnea in patients with chronic congestive heart failure. *Circulation,* 86, 909–918 (1992).

101. Mason PF, Dyson EH, Sellars V, Beard JD. The assessment of cerebral oxygenation during carotid endarterectomy utilising near-infrared spectroscopy. *Eur J Vasc Surg,* 8, 590–594 (1994).

102. Masters BR, Falk S, Chance B. In vivo flavoprotein redox measurements of rabbit corneal normoxic-anoxic transitions. *Curr Eye Res,* 1, 623–627 (1981).

103. Masters BR, Riley MV, Fischbarg J, Chance B. Pyridine nucleotides of rabbit cornea with histotoxic anoxia: Chemical analysis, noninvasive fluorometry and physiological correlates. *Exp Eye Res,* 37, 1–9 (1983).

104. Matcher SJ, Cooper CE. Absolute quantification of deoxyhaemoglobin concentration in tissue near-infrared spectroscopy. *Phys Med Biol,* 39, 1295–1312 (1994).

105. Matcher SJ, Cope M, Delpy DT. Use of the water absorption spectrum to quantify tissue chromophore concentration changes in near-infrared spectroscopy. *Phys Med Biol,* 39, 177–196 (1994).

106. Mayevsky A, Chance B. Intracellular oxidation-reduction state measured in situ by a multichannel fiber-optic surface fluorometer. *Science,* 217, 537–540 (1982).

107. Mayevsky A, Frank K, Muck M et al. Multiparametric evaluation of brain functions in the Mongolian gerbil in vivo. *J Basic Clin Physiol Pharmacol,* 3, 323–342 (1992).

108. McCormick DC, Edwards AD, Brown GC et al. Effect of indomethacin on cerebral oxidized cytochrome oxidase in preterm infants. *Pediatr Res,* 33, 603–608 (1993).

109. McCormick PW, Stewart M, Goetting MG, Balakrishnan G. Regional cerebrovascular oxygen saturation measured by optical spectroscopy in humans. *Stroke,* 22, 596–602 (1991).

110. McCully KK, Halber C, Posner JD. Exercise-induced changes in oxygen saturation in the calf muscles of elderly subjects with peripheral vascular disease. *J Gerontol,* 49, B128–B134 (1994).

111. McCully KK, Iotti S, Kendrick K et al. Simultaneous in vivo measurements of HbO_2 saturation and PCr kinetics after exercise in normal humans. *J Appl Physiol,* 77, 5–10 (1994).

112. Meek JH, Elwell CE, Khan MJ et al. Regional changes in cerebral haemodynamics as a result of a visual stimulus measured by near-infrared spectroscopy. *Proc R Soc Lond [Biol],* 261, 351–356 (1995).

113. Narayan SM, Santori EM, Toga AW. Mapping functional activity in rodent cortex using optical intrinsic signals. *Cereb Cortex,* 4, 195–204 (1994).

114. Nelson DA, Katz LC. Emergence of functional circuits in ferret visual cortex visualized by optical imaging. *Neuron,* 15, 23–34 (1995).

115. Nioka S, Smith DS, Chance B et al. Oxidative phosphorylation system during steady-state hypoxia in the dog brain [Comments]. *J Appl Physiol,* 68, 2527–2535 (1990).

116. Nollert G, Mohnle P, Tassaniprell P, Reichart B. Determinants of cerebral oxygenation during cardiac surgery. *Circulation,* 92, 327–333 (1995).

117. Obrig H, Hirth C, Junge-Huelsing JG et al. Length of resting period between stimulation cycles modulates hemodynamic response to a motor stimulation. *Adv Exp Med Biol,* in press (1996).

118. Obrig H, Villringer A. What is the typical NIRS-response to functional brain activation? *Adv Exp Med Biol,* in press (1996).

119. Oeberg PA, Tenland T, Nilsson GE. Laser Doppler flowmetry: A noninvasive and continuous method for blood flow evaluation in microvascular studies. *Acta Med Scand,* 687 (Suppl), 17–24 (1984).

120. Ohdan H, Fukuda Y, Suzuki S et al. Simultaneous evaluation of nitric oxide synthesis and tissue oxygenation in rat liver allograft rejection using near-infrared spectroscopy. *Transplantation,* 60, 530–535 (1995).

121. Okada F, Tokumitsu Y, Hoshi Y, Tamura M. Gender- and handedness-related differences of forebrain oxygenation and hemodynamics. *Brain Res,* 601, 337–342 (1993).

122. Okada F, Tokumitsu Y, Takahashi N et al. Region-dependent asymmetrical or symmetrical variations in the oxygenation and hemodynamics of the brain due to different mental stimuli. *Cognitive Brain Res,* 2, 215–219 (1995).

123. Okubo Y, Ogata H. Brain blood volume measured with near-infrared spectroscopy increased after stellate ganglion block. *Masui,* 44, 423–427 (1995).

124. Olano M, Song D, Murphy S et al. Relationships of dopamine, cortical oxygen pressure, and hydroxyl radicals in brain of newborn piglets during hypoxia and posthypoxic recovery. *J Neurochem,* 65, 1205–1212 (1995).

125. Paradiso AM, Tsien RY, Machen TE. Digital image processing of intracellular pH in gastric oxyntic and chief cells. *Nature,* 325, 447–450 (1987).

126. Peebles DM, Spencer JAD, Edwards AD et al. Relation between frequency of uterine contractions and human fetal cerebral oxygen saturation studied during labour by near-infrared spectroscopy. *Br J Obstet Gynaecol,* 101, 44–48 (1994).

127. Piston DW, Masters BR, Webb WW. Three-dimensionally resolved NAD(P)H cellular metabolic redox imaging of the in situ cornea with two-photon excitation laser scanning microscopy. *J Microsc,* 178, 20–27 (1995).

128. Pollock DM, Arendshorst WJ. Tubuloglomerular feedback and blood flow autoregulation during DA1-induced renal vasodilation. *Am J Physiol,* 258, F627–F635 (1990).

129. Poole DC, Wagner PD, Wilson DF. Diaphragm microvascular plasma PO_2 measured in vivo. *J Appl Physiol,* 79, 2050–2057 (1995).

130. Profio AE, Navarro GA, Sartorius OW. Scientific basis of breast diaphanography. *Med Phys,* 16, 60–65 (1989).

131. Renault G, Raynal E, Sinet M et al. In situ double-beam NADH laser fluorimetry: Choice of a reference wavelength. *Am J Physiol,* 246, H491–H499 (1984).

132. Rich KM, Hollowell JP. Flunarizine protects neurons from death after axotomy or NGF deprivation. *Science,* 248, 1419–1421 (1990).

133. Rosenthal M, Feng ZC, Raffin CN et al. Mitochondrial hyperoxidation signals residual intracellular dysfunction after global ischemia in rat neocortex. *J Cereb Blood Flow Metab,* 15, 655–665 (1995).

134. Rumsey WL, Pawlowski M, Lejavardi N, Wilson DF. Oxygen pressure distribution in the heart in vivo and evaluation of the ischemic "border zone." *Am J Physiol,* 266, H1676–H1680 (1994).

135. Rumsey WL, Vanderkooi JM, Wilson DF. Imaging of phosphorescence: A novel method for measuring oxygen distribution in perfused tissue. *Science,* 241, 1649–1651 (1988).

136. Sahlin K. Noninvasive measurements of O_2 availability in human skeletal muscle with near-infrared spectroscopy. *Int J Sports Med,* 13 (Suppl 1) S157–S160 (1992).

137. Sakaguchi M, Hosie KB, Gourevitch D et al. Laser Doppler assessment of human colonic blood flow. *J Med Eng Technol,* 14, 188–189 (1990).

138. Salerud EG, Tenland T, Nilsson GE, Oberg PA. Rhythmical variations in human skin blood flow. *Int J Microcirc Clin Exp,* 2, 91–102 (1983).

139. Sammak PJ, Adams SR, Harootunian AT et al. Intracellular cyclic AMP, not calcium, determines the direction of vesicle movement in melanophores: Direct measurement by fluorescence ratio imaging. *J Cell Biol,* 117, 57–72 (1992).

140. Samra SK, Dorje P, Zelenock GB, Stanley JC. Cerebral oximetry in patients undergoing carotid endarterectomy under regional anesthesia. *Stroke,* 27, 49–55 (1996).

141. Sawant P, Bhatia R, Kulhalli PM et al. Comparison of gastric mucosal blood flow in normal subjects and in patients with portal hypertension using endoscopic laser-Doppler velocimetry [Comments]. *Indian J Gastroenterol,* 14, 87–90 (1995).

142. Senseman DM. High speed optical imaging of afferent flow through rat olfactory bulb slices: Voltage sensitive dye signals reveal periglomerular cell activity. *J Neurosci,* 16, 313–324 (1996).

143. Sevick EM, Chance B, Leigh J et al. Quantitation of time- and frequency-resolved optical spectra for the determination of tissue oxygenation. *Anal Biochem,* 195, 330–351 (1991).

144. Shinohara Y, Takagi S, Shinohara N et al. Optical CT imaging of hemoglobin oxygen-saturation using dual-wavelength time gate technique. *Adv Exp Med Biol,* 333, 43–46 (1993).

145. Siczkowski M, Ng LL. Culture density and the activity, abundance and phosphorylation of the Na+/H+ exchanger isoform 1 in human fibroblasts. *Biochem Biophys Res Commun,* 209, 191–197 (1995).

146. Singer I, Edmonds HJ. Changes in cerebral perfusion during third-generation implantable cardioverter defibrillator testing. *Am Heart J,* 127, 1052–1057 (1994).

147. Skarphedinsson JO, Harding H, Thoren P. Repeated measurements of cerebral blood flow in rats. Comparisons between the hydrogen clearance method and laser Doppler flowmetry. *Acta Physiol Scand,* 134, 133–142 (1988).

148. Skov L, Hellstrom Westas L, Jacobsen T et al. Acute changes in cerebral oxygenation and cerebral blood volume in preterm infants during surfactant treatment. *Neuropediatrics,* 23, 126–130 (1992).

149. Skov L, Pryds O, Greisen G. Estimating cerebral blood flow in newborn infants: Comparison of near-infrared spectroscopy and 133Xe clearance. *Pediatr Res,* 30, 570–573 (1991).

150. Skov L, Pryds O, Greisen G, Lou H. Estimation of cerebral venous saturation in newborn infants by near-infrared spectroscopy. *Pediatr Res,* 33, 52–55 (1993).

151. Skov L, Ryding J, Pryds O, Greisen G. Changes in cerebral oxygenation and cerebral blood volume during endotracheal suctioning in ventilated neonates. *Acta Paediatr,* 81, 389–393 (1992).

152. Slavin KV, Dujovny M, Ausman JI et al. Clinical experience with transcranial cerebral oximetry. *Surg Neurol,* 42, 531–539 (1994).

153. Smielewski P, Kirkpatrick P, Minhas P et al. Can cerebrovascular reactivity be measured with near-infrared spectroscopy? *Stroke,* 26, 2285–2292 (1995).

154. Song D, Olano M, Wilson DF et al. Comparison of the efficacy of blood and polyethylene glycol-hemoglobin in recovery of newborn piglets from hemorrhagic hypotension: Effect on blood pressure, cortical oxygen, and extracellular dopamine in the brain. *Transfusion,* 35, 552–558 (1995).

155. Stainsby WN, Brechue WF, O'Drobinak DM, Barclay JK. Oxidation/reduction state of cytochrome oxidase during repetitive contractions. *J Appl Physiol,* 67, 2158–2162 (1989).

156. Stern MD. In vivo evaluation of microcirculation by coherent light scattering. *Nature,* 254, 56–58 (1975).

157. Stone HB, Brown JM, Phillips TL, Sutherland RM. Oxygen in human tumors: Correlations between methods of measurement and response to therapy. [Summary of a workshop held November 19–20, 1992, at the National Cancer Institute, Bethesda, Maryland.] *Radiat Res,* 136, 422–434 (1993).

158. Tamaki N, Ehara K, Fujita K et al. Cerebral hyperperfusion during surgical resection of high-flow arteriovenous malformations. *Surg Neurol,* 40, 10–15 (1993).

159. Tamaki T, Uchiyama S, Tamura T, Nakano S. Changes in muscle oxygenation during weight-lifting exercise. *Eur J Appl Physiol,* 68, 465–469 (1994).

160. Tamura M. Noninvasive monitoring of brain oxygen metabolism during cardiopulmonary bypass by near-infrared spectrophotometry. *Jpn Circ J,* 55, 330–335 (1991).

161. Tanaka A, Kitai T, Tokuka A et al. Increased span of oxido-reduction states between pyridine nucleotide and cytochrome c oxidase in the regenerating rabbit liver as measured by arterial ketone body ratio and near-infrared spectroscopy. *Res Exp Med (Berl),* 193, 353–359 (1993).

162. Tanaka A, Tanaka K, Kitai T et al. Living related liver transplantation across ABO blood groups: Evaluation of hemodynamics with tissue near-infrared spectroscopy. *Transplantation,* 58, 548–553 (1994).

163. Them A. Intracellular ion concentrations in the brain: Approaches towards in situ confocal imaging. *Adv Exp Med Biol,* 333, 145–175 (1993).

164. Tracy CA, Pool R, Gellis M, Vasileff W. Blood flow of the areola and breast skin flaps during reduction mammaplasty as measured by laser Doppler flowmetry. *Ann Plast Surg,* 28, 160–166 (1992).

165. Tsubota K, Laing RA, Kenyon KR. Noninvasive measurements of pyridine nucleotide and flavoprotein in the lens. *Invest Ophthalmol Vis Sci,* 28, 785–789 (1987).

166. Van Bel F, Dorrepaal CA, Benders MJ et al. Changes in cerebral hemodynamics and oxygenation in the first 24 hours after birth asphyxia. *Pediatrics,* 92, 365–372 (1993).

167. Vanderkooi JM, Maniara G, Green TJ, Wilson DF. An optical method for measurement of dioxygen concentration based upon quenching of phosphorescence. *J Biol Chem,* 262, 5476–5482 (1987).

168. Vaughan DL, Wickramasinghe YA, Russell GI et al. Is allopurinol beneficial in the prevention of renal ischaemia-reperfusion injury in the rat?: Evaluation by near-infrared spectroscopy. *Clin Sci (Colch),* 88, 359–364 (1995).

169. Villringer A, Dirnagl U. Coupling of brain activity and cerebral blood flow: Basis of functional neuroimaging. *Cerebrovasc Brain Metab Rev,* 7, 240–276 (1995).

170. Villringer A, Haberl RL, Dirnagl U et al. Confocal laser microscopy to study microcirculation on the rat brain surface in vivo. *Brain Res,* 504, 159–160 (1989).

171. Villringer A, Planck J, Hock C et al. Near infrared spectroscopy (NIRS): A new tool to study hemodynamic changes during activation of brain function in human adults. *Neurosci Lett,* 154, 101–104 (1993).

172. Villringer A, Planck J, Stodieck S et al. Noninvasive assessment of cerebral hemodynamics and tissue oxygenation during activation of brain cell function in human adults using near-infrared spectroscopy. *Adv Exp Med Biol,* 345, 559–565 (1994).

173. Villringer A, Them A, Lindauer U et al. Capillary perfusion of the rat brain cortex. An in vivo confocal microscopy study. *Circ Res,* 75, 55–62 (1994).

174. Villringer K, Minoshima S, Hock C et al. Assessment of local brain activation: A simultaneous PET and near-infrared spectroscopy study. *Adv Exp Med Biol,* in press (1996).

175. von Siebenthal K, Bernert G, Casaer P. Near-infrared spectroscopy in newborn infants. *Brain Dev,* 14, 135–143 (1992).

176. Wardell K, Jakobsson A, Nilsson GE. Laser Doppler perfusion imaging by dynamic light scattering. *IEEE Trans Biomed Eng,* 40, 309–316 (1993).

177. Weisskoff RM, Chesler D, Boxerman JL, Rosen BR. Pitfalls in MR measurement of tissue blood flow with intravascular tracers: Which mean transit time? *Magn Reson Med,* 29, 553–558 (1993).

178. Williams IM, Mead G, Picton AJ et al. The influence of contralateral carotid stenosis and occlusion on cerebral oxygen saturation during carotid artery surgery. *Eur J Vasc Endovasc Surg,* 10, 198–206 (1995).

179. Wilson DF, Gomi S, Pastuszko A, Greenberg JH. Microvascular damage in the cortex of cat brain from middle cerebral artery occlusion and reperfusion. *J Appl Physiol,* 74, 580–589 (1993).
180. Wilson JR, Mancini DM, McCully K et al. Noninvasive detection of skeletal muscle underperfusion with near-infrared spectroscopy in patients with heart failure. *Circulation,* 80, 1668–1674 (1989).
181. Wolf T, Obrig H, Villringer A, Dirnagl U. Extra- and intracellular oxygen supply during cortical spreading depression in the rat. *J Cereb Blood Flow Metab,* in press (1996).
182. Wyatt JS, Cope M, Delpy DT et al. Measurement of optical path length for cerebral near-infrared spectroscopy in newborn infants. *Dev Neurosci,* 12, 140–144 (1990).
183. Yamane K, Shima T, Okada Y et al. Near-infrared spectrophotometric monitoring for cerebral ischemia during the occlusion of the internal carotid artery at CEA. *No Shinkei Geka,* 22, 947–953 (1994).
184. Zheng JQ, Felder M, Connor JA, Poo MM. Turning of nerve growth cones induced by neurotransmitters [Comments]. *Nature,* 368, 140–144 (1994).
185. Zundorf J, Tauschek D, Frank K et al. Monitoring of redox-state of respiratory enzymes and myoglobin oxygenation in the working rat heart in normoxia and oxygen deficiency. *Adv Exp Med Biol,* 317, 583–592 (1992).
186. Zurovsky Y, Sonn J. Fiber-optic surface fluorometry-reflectometry technique in the renal physiology of rats. *J Basic Clin Physiol Pharmacol,* 3, 343–358 (1992).

Functional Imaging, edited by
Gustav von Schulthess and Jürgen Hennig.
Lippincott–Raven Publishers, Philadelphia, © 1998.

8

Radio Waves:
Magnetic Resonance

Jürgen Hennig

SOME BASICS

This chapter gives an overview on the basics of functional in vivo magnetic resonance imaging (MRI). The topics are presented in a way that is as self-consistent as possible, with cross-references to other chapters wherever possible. It is thus not required to read this chapter from the beginning to the end in order to get an understanding of every particular topic. Readers who take image formation for granted can thus, for example, skip to the later sections.

The topic of this chapter is magnetic resonance imaging (MRI), which is based on the interaction of electromagnetic radiation with atomic nuclei. It is therefore worthwhile to recollect some facts about atoms in order to understand this interaction.

Atomic nuclei are sitting at the heart of matter. Molecules are built from positively charged nuclei surrounded by negatively charged electrons. The attractive and repellent electromagnetic forces between these particles tie the molecules together: Attractive forces hinder the particles from tearing apart; repulsive forces prohibit them from collapsing into nothingness. The size of this force is tremendous, and the only reason we do not feel it is that positive and negative charges are exactly balanced in our bodies. If we had only a 1% surplus of negative charge and we were to meet somebody suffering from the same excess, the repellent force would be enough to lift the entire earth!

Mass is very unevenly distributed between the positive and negative charges: 99.946% of our mass rests in the (positively charged) nuclei, only 0.054% can be attributed to the electrons. This difference in mass between the two moieties leads to our picture of molecules, where the nuclei constitute the rigid structural parts and the electrons serve as a glue that binds the molecule together.

J Hennig: Department of Radiology, University Hospital, Freiburg, Germany.

With mass and electric charge, we have already noted two of three important properties of nuclei. The last one is spin, and it is this one that is responsible for the magnetic resonance phenomenon. The spin of an atomic nucleus is much harder to imagine than its mass and electric charge. This is because we can accept mass and electric charge as properties with an intrinsic value of their own. We do not need to have an image of an object in order to accept that it has mass and electric charge. Spin, however, at least in its common use, relates to a motional property of an object and therefore requires some image of the spinning object.

Atomic nuclei are much too small to be visible. Their diameter is on the order of 10^{-15} m, which is several orders of magnitude smaller than the wavelengths of light. According to the principle of wave propagation set forth in Chap. 1, it is thus impossible to form an image of a nucleus even with the most fanciful microscope. Visible light interacts with a nucleus as little as a 10-m ocean wave is refracted by some pollen on its surface.

In order to form an image of a nucleus by optical principles, radiation with a wavelength on the same scale or preferably shorter would be required. Such waves would, however, have energies in the gigaelectronvolt range (see Chap. 1) and thus would drastically interfere with the atoms; they would kick them miles away rather than being absorbed, reflected, or refracted and thus form an image. One is therefore forced to say that atoms do not look like anything at all.

This is, of course, a rather awkward fact, especially from a didactic point of view: For explaining the spin of a nucleus and its interaction with radiation, we would like to use some visual help such as diagrams and graphs. How should we visualize something that doesn't look like anything at all?

When forming an image by any imaging process that doesn't work, we can build a somewhat abstract image by looking at the spatial distribution of some property that we perceive as relevant. The distribution of mass would be a likely candidate. At time scales relevant for our perception (and for an MR experiment), the mass appears to be spherically and homogeneously distributed inside a nucleus. In this sense, a perfect sphere is a quite sensible image of a nucleus and much less artificial than it appears from the diagrams in this chapter.

It is still difficult to imagine a perfect sphere rotating around itself. In order to perceive rotation of a body, we need some surface feature (like the clouds on Jupiter or the craters on the moon) as a landmark. How can we distinguish a rotating perfect sphere without any such landmark from a nonrotating one? This is actually a very good question and one that brings us close to the actual MR experiment. In order to make such a distinction, we can make use of the fact that a rotating body reacts in a totally different way to an outside force than a nonrotating one. The easiest such demonstration is to use a spinning top. If we do not spin it and place it on a table at a skew angle, it will just fall down. If we start spinning it and then place it on the table, it will start circling on a cone defined by the skew angle between the axes of rotation and the table (Fig. 1). This strange motion

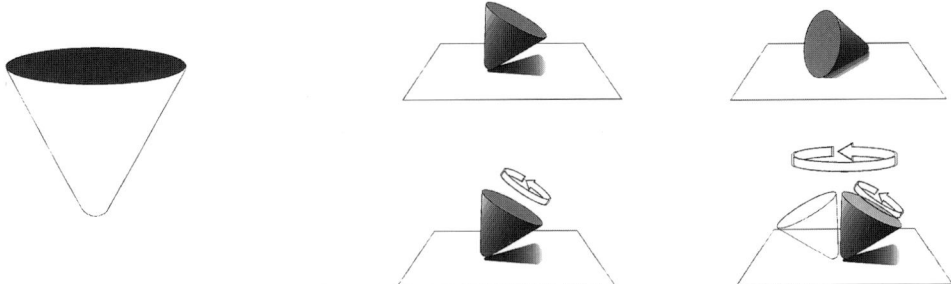

Figure 1. How to distinguish a rotating from a nonrotating body. A nonrotating body will fall down when it is placed at a tilted angle on a plane (*top*). A rotating body will start to precess around a vertical axis (*bottom*).

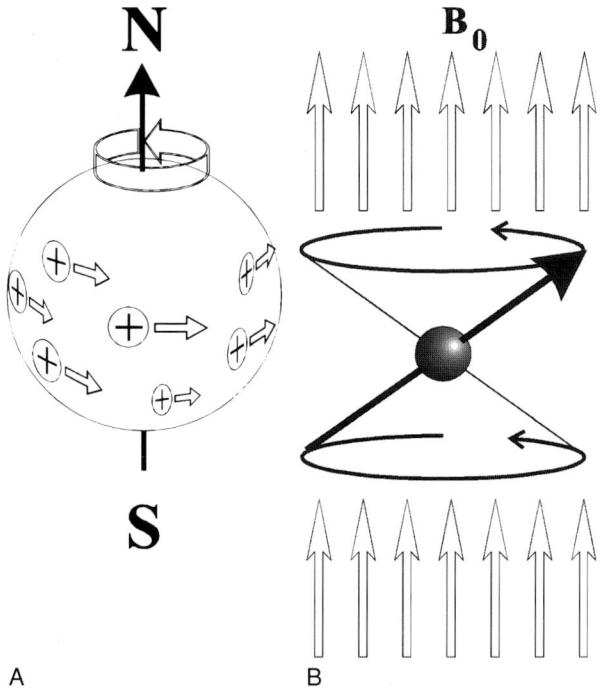

A

B

Figure 2. Classic picture of nuclear spin and precession. Protons can be thought of as small spheres carrying a positive electric charge. The current loop generated by its rotation ("spin") generates a magnetic moment (**A**). When placed into an outer magnetic field, quantum mechanics allows only two angles of orientation with respect to the direction of the outer field. Protons thus precess on a cone with an opening angle of ±54°44′ (**B**).

is called *precession.* The force that is used for this demonstration is, of course, gravitation.

Gravitation is a much too weak force to lead to any measurable effects at the scale of the nucleus. Fortunately, nuclei are sensitive to other forces as well. Nuclei have electric charges. If an electric charge runs in a circle, it will produce a circular current, which in turn produces a magnetic field. This is the principle of any electromagnet. If a spinning nucleus is placed into a magnetic field, it will therefore feel a force due to the interaction with the magnetic field and thus will precess with a precession frequency that is proportional to the magnetic force between the nucleus and the field (Fig. 2). The proportionality constant is called the *gyromagnetic ratio,* which is a constant for every type of nucleus. The simple equation that connects the precession frequency with the strength of the magnetic field (called the *magnetic flux density*) is called the *Larmor equation:*

$$\omega = \gamma B \tag{1}$$

The gyromagnetic ratio is determined by the combined magnetic moments of the nucleons (protons or neutrons) contained in the atomic nucleus, both of which are magnetic. Just like bar magnets thrown together into a box, the magnetic moments have a tendency to cancel each other pairwise.

Nuclei that are made of an odd number of nucleons will thus possess a spin. For even-numbered nuclei, the spins of the individual nucleons might cancel, but they may not necessarily do so. For a deuterium nucleus, for example, which is composed from 1 proton and 1 neutron, the spins add up to yield spin 1, whereas in oxygen, with 8 protons and 8 neutrons, all spins cancel to give spin 0. A very remarkable distinction between the macroscopic world of our experience and the microscopic world of elementary particles is the fact that at the level of atoms and electrons, things do happen not in a continuous fashion but as stepwise transitions between discrete states. In the most simple case of the excess of one elementary magnetic moment, two such states exist, which can be labeled *parallel* and *antiparallel* to an outer field.

The precession cone of the nucleus can thus only take on discrete angles (see Fig. 2). For a two-state nucleus, this angle is 54°44′. In a practical experiment a single spin is never observed but always an ensemble consisting of a huge number of spins. There is

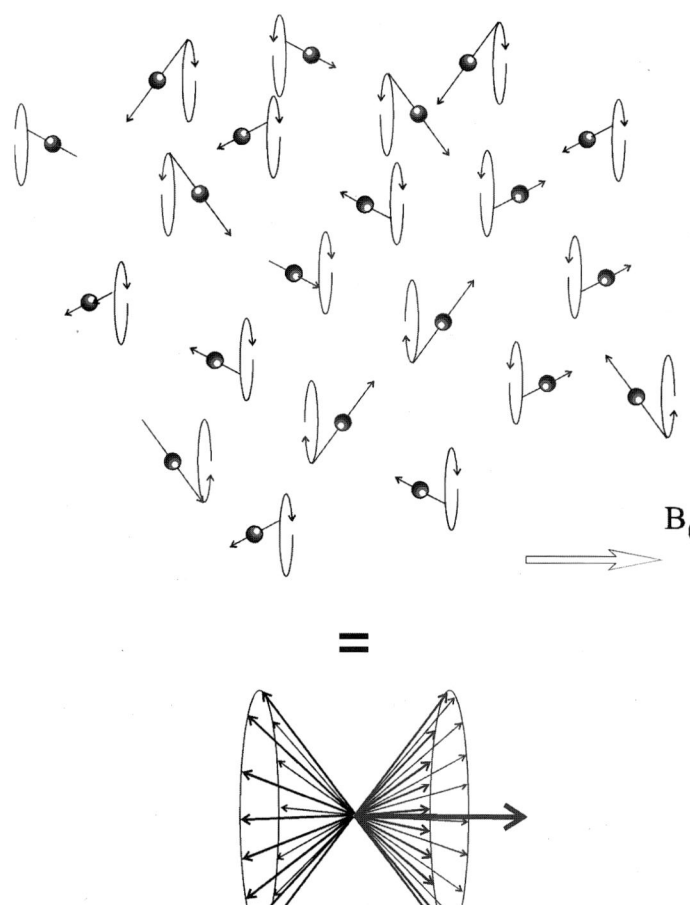

Figure 3. The total magnetization is the sum of all spin vectors that precess either parallel (*red*) or antiparallel (*black*) to the outer field. After vector addition, all contributions orthogonal to B_0 will cancel out due to the random orientation of the vectors. The resulting macroscopic magnetization vector will thus be aligned parallel to B_0, reflecting the slight excess of protons with parallel orientation in thermal equilibrium. See also Color Plate 17.

no preferred location for the spin vectors around the precession cone. They will therefore be distributed randomly, and the observable macroscopic magnetization will be a vector aligned along the outer field (Fig. 3 and Color Plate 17).

The chemical behavior of each element is defined by the number of protons it carries. For all elements, isotopes exist that are distinguished by the number of neutrons. The number of neutrons does not affect the chemical behavior of an atom; it does, however, change its spin. Most elements therefore possess at least one isotope with a magnetic moment.

In the first experiments measuring the Larmor frequency of protons bound in molecules, the surprising observation was made that for some substances various resonance signals were observed, although the gyromagnetic ratio is a fundamental constant and does not allow any modifications. From the Larmor equation it therefore had concluded that the magnetic field varies slightly at the location of the various observed protons. This variation can be attributed to the interaction of the electronic structure of a molecule with the outer magnetic field. The width and location of the resonance lines are thus a very sensitive probe for the molecular structure of the substance under study. This experiment therefore formed the basis of nuclear magnetic resonance (NMR) spectroscopy as an extremely successful tool for analytical chemistry. The structure-dependent frequency differences are called the *chemical shift* σ, which is given as a proportionality constant to the applied field. The modified Larmor equation thus reads

$$\omega = \gamma B(1 - \sigma) \tag{2}$$

Since the electronic environment of different elements varies considerably, the chemical shift ranges from several hundred parts per million (ppm) for atoms with strong interactions of electrons and nuclei to only a few parts per million for nuclei like hydrogen.

Quantum theory requires spins to occur only in discrete states s. These are related to the spin quantum number S according to

$$s = S, S - 1, S - 2, \ldots, -S$$

For $S = \frac{1}{2}$, this gives $s = \frac{1}{2}$ and $-\frac{1}{2}$. The total number of states s is thus given by $2S + 1$.

The opening angle α of the precession cone to the magnetic field B_0 can be calculated from s and S via

$$\cos \alpha = \frac{s}{\sqrt{S(S + 1)}}$$

For protons with $s = \frac{1}{2}$ and $S = \frac{1}{2}$, this yields $\cos \alpha = 1/\sqrt{3}$ and $\alpha = 54°44'137''$.

The magnetic moment of a proton is given by $m = 1.41 \times 10^{-26}$ J T^{-1}. The force acting on m in a magnetic field gradient G of 1 T/m, which is in the range of the gradients at the opening of a superconducting magnet used in MRI, is given by

$$F = mG = 1.41 \times 10^{-26} \text{ J T}^{-1} \cdot 1 \text{ T/m} = 1.41 \times 10^{-26} \text{ N}$$

One mole ($= 18$ g) of water contains $2 \times 6.023 \times 10^{23}$ protons. In the macroscopic world of daily experience, objects always chose the energetically favorable position. If this also would apply to protons in the magnetic field gradient, the total force would be

$$F = 1.41 \times 10^{-26} \times 2 \times 6.023 \times 10^{23} = 16.98 \text{ mN}$$

This is still small but would be measurable. The energy difference between the two spin states is, however, so small that an appreciable number of spins will go to the energetically unfavorable $s = -\frac{1}{2}$ state. For the distribution in thermal equilibrium, the ratio between the occupation of both levels is given by the Boltzmann law:

$$n_1/n_2 = \exp(-\Delta E/kT)$$

where n_1 and n_2 are the number of spins in the two states, ΔE is the energy difference, k is the Boltzmann constant, and T is the absolute temperature.

The energy difference can be calculated from the resonance frequency by

$$\Delta E = h\nu = hw = h\gamma B$$

according to the Larmor equation.

For $B = 1$ T, this yields $\Delta E = 1.055 \times 10^{-34}$ Js $\times 2.675 \times 10^8$ s^{-1}T$^{-1} \times 1$ T $= 2.82 \times 10^{-26}$ J. With $k = 1.38 \times 10^{-23}$ J/K, the Boltzmann distribution can be calculated as

$$n_1/n_2 = \exp[-2.82 \times 10^{-26} \text{ J}/(1.38 \times 10^{-23} \text{ J/K} \times 293 \text{ K})]$$

$$= 1 - 6.97 \times 10^{-6}$$

This means that the excess of protons in the energetically favorable state is only about 1 in 150,000 protons. The attractive force acting on 1 mol of water is thus only 1.18×10^{-7} N, which is only about 1 part per million (ppm) of its weight.

The fact that only a small fraction of the spins goes into the more favorable $+\frac{1}{2}$ state seems to counteract our intuition. A ball will always go downhill and a compass needle will always point due north. This could lead to the notion that for elementary particles a different kind of physics applies compared with our ''real'' world. This is, however, not the case. The difference lies merely in amplitude. Whenever the term in the numerator of the exponential term of the Boltzmann law takes on some macroscopically observable value, the population distribution goes to zero, which means that all macroscopic systems go to the lowest energy level in thermal equilibrium. A waiter with some basic idea about the numbers involved will thus immediately bend down and pick up a fork that has fallen down from a table, since its probability of getting back onto the table by itself is extremely low.

A further modification of the spectrum can occur if nuclei with different chemical shifts interact with each other. Such an interaction, called *j-coupling,* acts like an elastic string connecting the two nuclei and leads to the generation of signal modulations just like in elastically coupled penduli. The result of such a j-coupling is a splitting of the spectral lines. The amount of this splitting in frequency units depends only on the strength of the coupling but not on the field strength such that spectra from coupled substances do not simply spread out linearly with increasing field. Coupling is an important phenomenon for MR spectroscopy (see below) but also has subtle influences of the appearance of, for example, the signal from fat in MRI.

MEASURING THE MR SIGNAL

The Free Induction Decay

In the first NMR experiment performed by Purrcell (173) and independently by Bloch (14) in 1946, the NMR signals were measured by observing the response of the nuclear spins following continuous irradiation with radio (rf) waves at the resonance frequency. The frequency distribution or spectrum of the probe was then determined by varying either the rf frequency or the magnetic field, which is equivalent according to the Larmor equation.

This measurement technique has been considerably improved using the "pulse and acquire" experiment designed by Ernst in 1966 (57). The earlier continuous-wave experiment is equivalent to determining the color of an object by shining monochromatic light onto it and then varying the color of the lamp and observing the reflected intensity as a function of the incident color. The "pulse and acquire" technique corresponds to exhibiting the object to a bright white light flash, where the response immediately yields the full color spectrum.

The latter approach is much faster and more efficient. Prerequisite are receptors that can filter out the various color components from the light beam. For optical measurements, such receptors (our retina, optical dyes, etc.) can be easily found. For NMR measurements, the technical realization is, however, not so straightforward. Rf receivers that allow one to distinguish frequencies in the very narrow range defined by the chemical shift of the nuclei do not exist.

The ingenious solution to the problem of how to use a receiver that is equally sensitive to all relevant frequencies and still able to filter out a spectrum using a "pulse and acquire" approach follows from the equivalence of a spectrum in the frequency domain to temporal variations of a signal in the time domain. By definition, a spectrum is the representation of a frequency distribution. In the time domain, each frequency can be represented as a sine wave. Any frequency distribution in the spectral domain can thus be represented as a superposition of sine waves in the time domain. The distribution of resonance frequencies in a spectrum can thus be derived from a frequency analysis of the temporal variation of the signal following a short "white" pulse that simultaneously excites all spins irrespective of their resonance frequency (Fig. 4).

The strength of the signal depends on the amplitude of the excitation pulse. The pulse consists of an electromagnetic wave and thus constitutes a time-variable magnetic field B_1. It can be demonstrated that spins will start precessing around the direction of this field when its frequency is exactly equal to the resonance frequency in the main field B_0. Since the pulse acts on all spins in the probe, this precession can be visualized as a rotation of the total magnetization vector around B_1. After the pulse, the magnetization vectors will again precess around B_0. But now the situation is different compared with thermal equilibrium, where all spin vectors are distributed randomly on the precession cone; after the pulse, the net magnetization vector will rotate around B_0. If a loop of wire is placed around the probe, a current induced by electromagnetic induction can be observed just like in an electric generator. This observable signal is called the *free induction decay* (FID) (Fig. 5).

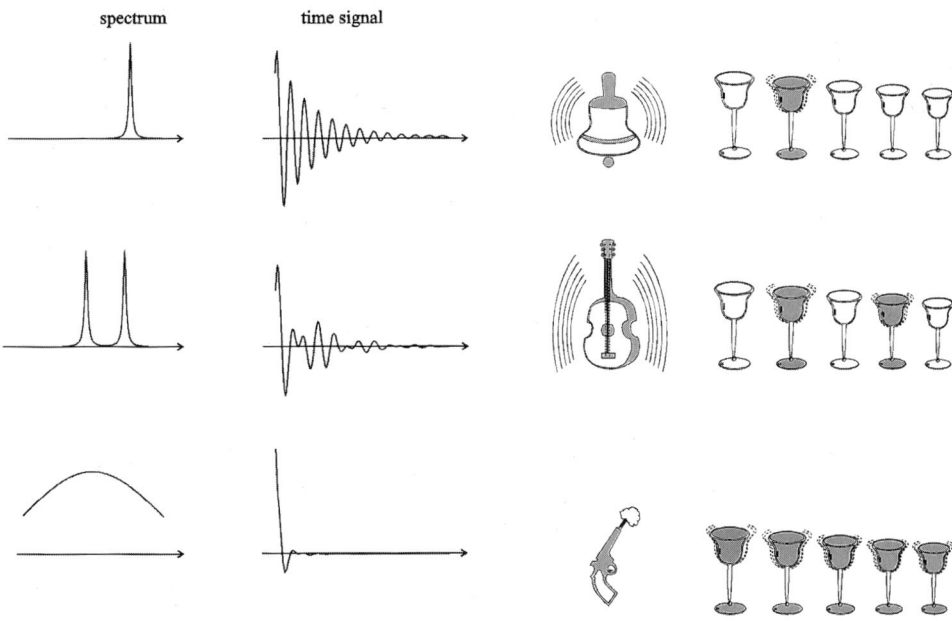

spectrum   time signal

Figure 4. Correspondence of frequency spectrum and time domain and resonance. The spectrum of a pure tone from a bell contains one single frequency. The corresponding temporal pattern of the sound waves is a decaying sinusoid. A pure tone will bring a glass with matching resonance frequency to vibration (*top*). Two tones plucked simultaneously on a guitar contain two frequencies; the time signal then corresponds to a superposition of two sinusoids. Two glasses will start to resonate (*middle*). A pistol shot has a very short time signal; the corresponding frequency spectrum contains a broad range of frequencies. Correspondingly, all glasses will start to resonate (*bottom*).

The motion of the spin system can be classically described by the Bloch equations, which—including the effect of the B_1 field—read

$$\frac{dM_x}{dt} = \gamma(M_y B_z - M_z B_{1y}) - \frac{M_x}{T_2}$$

$$\frac{dM_y}{dt} = \gamma(-M_x B_z + M_z B_{1x}) - \frac{M_y}{T_2}$$

$$\frac{dM_z}{dt} = \gamma(M_x B_{1y} - M_y B_{1x}) - \frac{M_z - M_0}{T_1}$$

where B_{1y} and B_{1x} correspond to the x and y components of the rf field B_1 and M_0 to the equilibrium magnetization. T_2 and T_1 denote the time constants for decay of the transverse magnetization M_x and M_y and the return to equilibrium, respectively.

In the laboratory frame, B_z is equal to B_0, and B_1 will be rotating with the frequency of the rf field. For convenience, the Bloch equations are normally transformed into a coordinate system that rotates with the frequency ω_{rf} of the rf field B_1. The precession frequency γB_0 is then replaced by an effective precession frequency $\Omega = \gamma B_0 - \omega_{rf}$, and B_1 becomes constant.

For some special cases, the Bloch equations can be solved analytically: After a B_1 pulse with B_1 aligned to the y axis of the rotating coordinate system with a flip angle α, a transverse magnetization $M_{tr} = M_x = M_0 \sin \alpha$ will be created. Solution of the Bloch equations for the ensuing free induction decay leads to

$$M_x(t) = M_{tr0} \cos(\Omega t) \exp(-t/T_2)$$

$$M_y(t) = M_{tr0} \sin(\Omega t) \exp(-t/T_2)$$

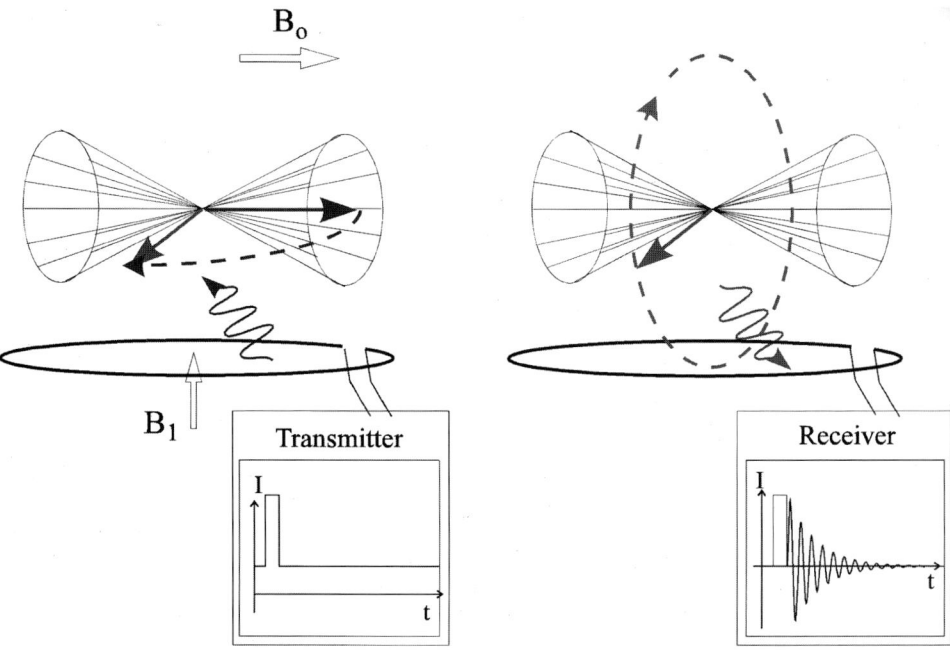

Figure 5. "Pulse and acquire" MRI experiment. The MR equivalent of the "pistol shot" experiment in the preceding figure consists of the application of a brief electromagnetic field B_1 with a frequency at the Larmor frequency of the protons. This will deflect the macroscopic magnetization from its equilibrium position parallel to B_0. After switching off B_1, the macroscopic magnetization vector will then precess around B_0. The precession of the macroscopic magnetization induces an alternating electric current in the receiver coil (which often but not always is identical to the transmitter coil).

The signal will be at a maximum when the net magnetization is orthogonal to B_0. In the jargon of MR, this corresponds to an excitation with a flip angle of 90°. All equilibrium magnetization, which is called *longitudinal* or *z-magnetization,* has then been converted to transverse magnetization. If B_1 gets larger, the transverse magnetization will get smaller again until—for a flip angle of 180°—it vanishes because the net magnetization is now again aligned with B_0 but points in the opposite direction. This is called *inversion.*

The observable magnetization and thus the signal intensity is always equal to the vector component of the net magnetization, which is given by

$$I = I_0 \sin \alpha \tag{3}$$

where α is the so-called flip angle of the pulse.

This signal will persist as long as the total magnetization has some component in the transverse plane. The various parameters affecting the signal decay are discussed in the following section.

It should be noted that there are some significant differences between the "pulse and acquire" experiment used in MR and the observation of an object with visible light. If we shine a light onto an object, the light will be absorbed, and the pigment molecules go to an excited state. When they drop back to equilibrium after a few microseconds, they will reemit light, which can be observed. In terms of an MR experiment, the absorption and transition to the excited state would correspond to the application of an inversion pulse, which also brings the nuclei from their ground state to the only available excited state. A lot of patience is required, however, in order to observe the equivalent of optical fluorescence in MR, since the lifetime of the excited magnetic state is on the order of several thousand years. (The actual lifetime is considerably shorter due to mechanisms discussed in the next section.)

The measurement of the coherent transverse magnetization via induction of an electric current in an appropriate receiver coil does not involve a transition of the nucleus from the excited state to the ground state. It is comparable with the resonance vibration that builds up in a glass placed on a piano that starts to ''sing'' when the appropriate key is hit. The coupling between the nucleus/piano string and the receiver coil/glass is much too weak to involve any appreciable energy transfer from one to the other (although in principle an energy transfer is, of course, involved); the piano tone will not be appreciably shortened by the resonating glass. Only if a more rigid connection between the resonator and the source is made will significant energy transfer with concordant damping of the signal take place. Such conditions, called *radiation damping,* can be created in experiments on small probes. They are, however, of little relevance for in vivo MR experiments.

As a final note, it should be mentioned that the equivalent of an MR experiment can be realized with visible light also. Due to the dramatically reduced lifetime of the excited state for optical transitions, such experiments require pulses with a duration in the picosecond or even femtosecond range, the generation and exact control of which require some extremely sophisticated equipment.

Spin Echoes

Once the possibility of creating coherent transverse magnetization via an rf pulse has been recognized, one can immediately start to play some more tricks with it above the already mentioned spin excitation and inversion, which are performed on z-magnetization. In his seminal paper from 1950, Hahn dealt with the question of what happens if an rf pulse is applied to already existing transverse magnetization (86).

If some time delay between the excitation pulse and a following rf pulse is included, spins will have precessed by some phase angle determined by their Larmor frequency and thus by the magnetic field at the location of the spins. For a large object such as a human body, this field might easily be not absolutely constant across the whole volume of examination. Some actual numbers might yield a feeling of the importance of such inhomogeneities. For a waiting time of 10 ms, the magnetization vectors of two spins will be opposed if the difference in their Larmor frequencies is equal to $1/(2 \times 10$ ms) $= 50$ Hz. In a 1-T magnet, the Larmor frequency is around 42 MHz. The corresponding field inhomogeneity is thus 50 Hz/42 MHz, or 1.2 parts per million! Since the net magnetization is given by the vector sum of all magnetization components, the signal will have vanished due to this field inhomogeneity effect. If there are just two magnetization moieties positioned at points on the field that are 1.2 ppm apart, the vectors will come in phase again after 20 ms and the signal will come back and so forth. For a continuous distribution of spins along a continuous magnetic field profile, the initial coherence will, however, never be restored. The signal will thus be zero, although in each small-volume element transverse magnetization will still be present.

Let us now consider what happens when a 180° pulse is applied at the time of such total incoherence. The magnetization vectors will then be rotated by 180° around B_1 and will thus lie on the opposite side of the transverse plane. This means that the spins that have accumulated the largest phase will lag the furthest behind. After the pulse, spins will continue to precess with their respective Larmor frequencies. It is now easy to see that after a time that is equal to the time between the excitation pulse and the second pulse, all spins will be realigned again (Fig. 6A). They will thus form a so-called spin echo. An even simpler model to describe the formation of echoes is to use a phase graph. In this presentation, the phase of the spins is plotted as a function of time in a cartesian coordinate system. Dephasing of spins due to some difference in Larmor frequency with respect to an arbitrary reference is then represented as a straight line, the slope of which will be proportional to the off-resonance frequency (see Fig. 6B and Color Plate 18). A 180° pulse will invert the phases. The phase graphs of all spins will cross the baseline at the same time, independent of their slopes. As long as all spins remain stationary and

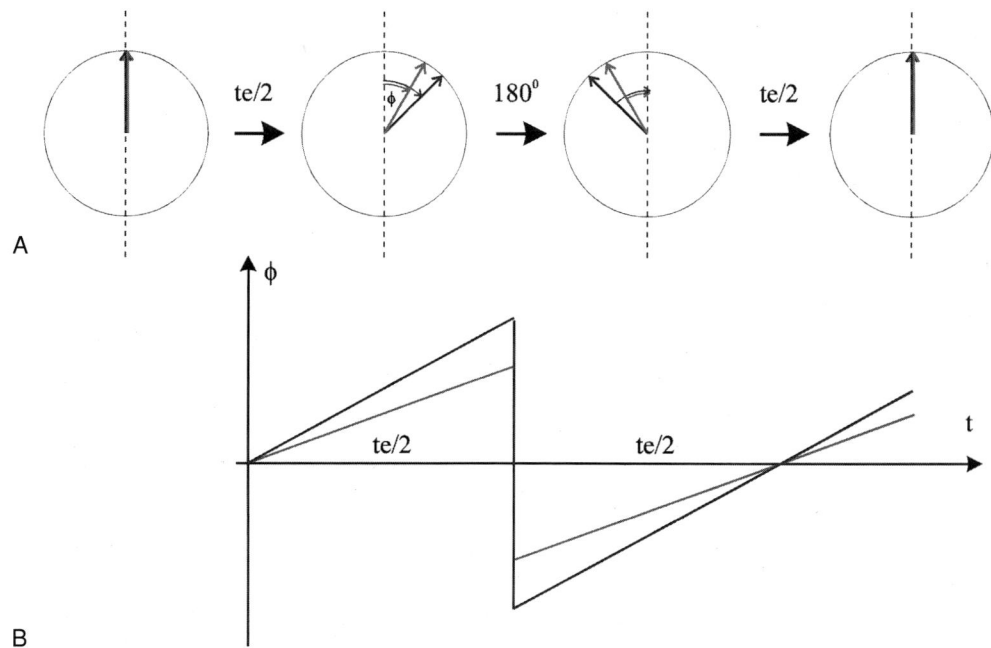

Figure 6. Spin echo with phase diagram. Two spins with slightly different Larmor frequencies will precess by a slightly different angle ϕ during a time $t_e/2$ after excitation. If the vectors are rotated by 180° by an appropriate additional rf pulse, the faster spin (*blue*) will lag behind. After another time interval $t_e/2$, both spins will again be parallel, and an echo is formed **(A)**. The accumulated phase angle of the spins also can be represented in a phase diagram **(B)**. A constant frequency will lead to a tilted phase graph; the tilt angle is proportional to the rotation frequency. Echo formation is then characterized by the intersection of the phase graphs of the spins on the baseline. See also Color Plate 18.

do not suffer from additional effects that might change their phase, it can be taken for granted that echo formation takes place at each baseline crossing, and we can pick one phase graph as representative for the whole spin system in order to get the most comprehensive description of the formation of spin echoes.

The 180° pulse that leads to echo generation is called the *refocusing pulse* in such a spin-echo experiment. It should be emphasized that this distinction between the initial excitation pulse and the following refocusing pulse is merely semantic and does not reflect any difference in the physics of these pulses. The refocusing pulse will thus act as an inversion pulse for any z-magnetization that happens to be present at the time of its formation, and the excitation pulse also will act on any transverse magnetization that might happen to be present due to some previous pulse.

If more than one refocusing pulse is applied, and if the flip angle of the pulse is not equal to 180°, more signals can arise. All these can be understood by tracing the tips of the magnetization vectors according to the Bloch equations, although even for the understanding of the refocusing behavior following a refocusing pulse with 90° flip angle more than two magnetization vectors need to be traced in order to convince oneself that an echo will be formed. In general, magnetization vectors will not be exactly aligned at the time of echo formation but rather will point in roughly the same direction. The signal amplitude of such echoes will then be somewhat reduced compared with a fully coherent 180° echo. An easy way of bookkeeping the occurrence of signals after any arbitrary sequence of pulses is offered by the extended phase graph algorithm, which is demonstrated in Fig. 7 and Color Plate 19. Repetitive application of the splitting of the phase graphs at each rf pulse will produce all possible refocusing pathways, where echo formation will occur at each zero-crossing point. The extended phase graph algorithm for

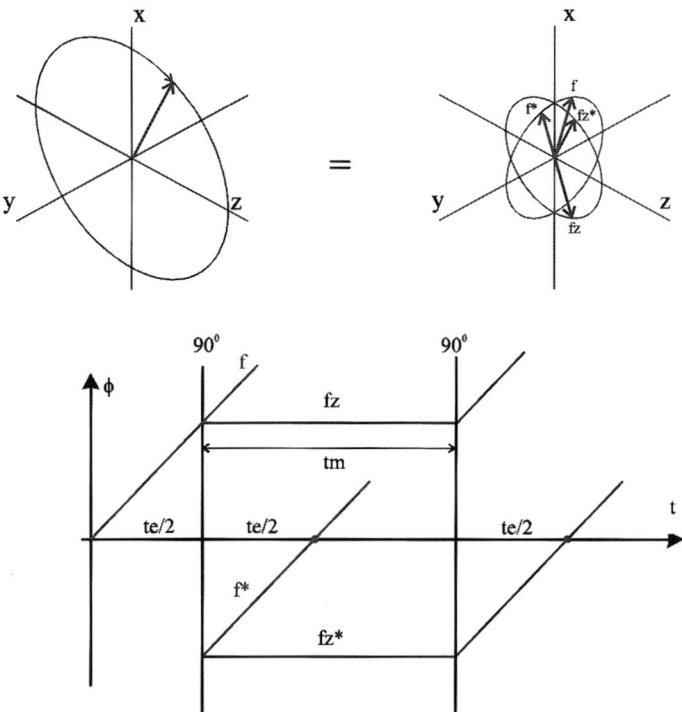

Figure 7. Decomposition of magnetization vectors. The extended phase graph. Any magnetization vector generated by applying a 1-90° pulse to magnetization that has precessed by *f* can be decomposed into four parts: one part *f*, which is parallel to the vector before the pulse; one part *f**, which is symmetrical to *f* around the *x* axis and thus behaves as if a 180° pulse had taken place; and two vectors f_z and f_z^* in the *xz* plane, which represent *z*-magnetization. After this decomposition, the formation of the various echoes easily follows from the extended phase graph. Spin-echo formation follows from the phase graph of *f** after the first refocusing pulse (*red*). The second pulse converts f_z^* into *f**, which then forms the stimulated echo (*blue*) no matter where the (*red*) graphs of the initial *f* and *f** magnetizations have gone to meanwhile. See Color Plate 19.

three pulses shows the development of the various spin echoes and so-called stimulated echoes (Fig. 8).

RELAXATION TIMES

T_1 Relaxation

It has already been mentioned in the preceding section that the fluorescence lifetime, which means the time for which nuclei will stay in their excited state before they spontaneously drop back to equilibrium, is on the order of several thousand years due to the very low energy difference between the two states. Spins consequently can do with some outside help to get back to their ground state (15). Such help is afforded for nuclei in molecules in solution by Brownian motion of molecules in the surrounding ''bath.'' Since molecules will have a more or less inhomogeneous distribution of electric charges, their tumbling motion will invariably lead to the generation of electromagnetic fields.

Due to the random motion of the molecules, these fields will, of course, not have a single fixed frequency like the B_1 field used for rf pulses. The frequency spectrum nevertheless will have some amplitude at the Larmor frequency. The magnetic component of this field at the Larmor frequency will interact with the nuclei and will lead to what is called *T1 relaxation*, which brings the nuclei back to equilibrium. For molecules with

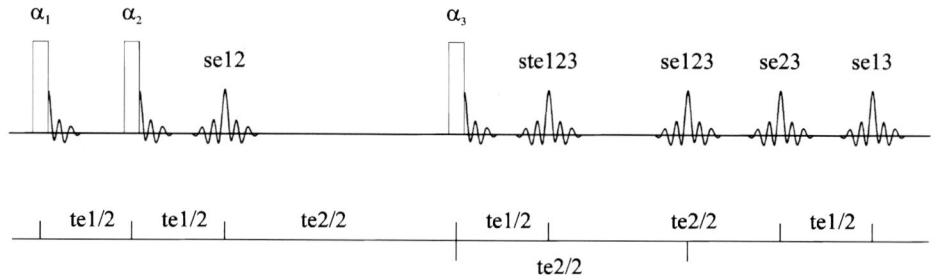

Figure 8. Signal formation in a three-pulse experiment. Three rf pulses will in general form eight signals: one free induction decay from each pulse, three spin echoes se_{12}, se_{13}, and se_{23} from each pair of pulses, one spin echo se_{123}, which has been refocused twice and the stimulated echo ste_{123}.

a weak internal magnetic moment, this interaction, called *dipole-dipole interaction,* is dominated by the interaction with other nuclei in the bath.

Pure radiative interactions between the nuclei are not sufficient to bring the spin system into equilibrium. If this were the case, it would be possible to restore equilibrium by applying an external rf pulse. In "Some Basics" it was mentioned that continuous irradiation with an rf pulse will lead to an equal population of ground and excited states and thus to saturation rather than equilibrium. In order to restore equilibrium, the energy, which comes from the induced transition from excited state to ground state, has to be converted into thermal energy; otherwise, it will lead to a transition from the ground state to the excited state of another spin.

T1 relaxation is thus a quite subtle process by which a molecule in the bath approaches the nucleus, induces a transition by "tickling" it on the right frequency, but then annihilates the emitted energy by putting it into motion. Since the Larmor frequency varies with field strengths, T1 relaxation times also will be field-dependent. For small molecules observable in MRI, the fast-exchange model is valid, and T1 typically will become longer with increasing field strength.

Measuring T1

In analytical applications, the most common T1 measurement is performed using an inversion-recovery sequence. In this experiment, first a 180° pulse is applied, which inverts the equilibrium magnetization. After a waiting time t_i, the signal is read out either as an FID or a spin echo (Fig. 9). $M_z(t_i)$ will then be given by

$$M_z(t_i) = M_0[1 - 2 \exp(-t_i/T1)] \qquad (4)$$

which will then be converted into an observable signal intensity by an excitation pulse.

Given the long relaxation times T1 of organic tissues, which are on the order of several hundreds of milliseconds up to several seconds, this experiment is intrinsically quite slow, especially since it requires a waiting time of 3 to 5 T1 in order to restore thermal equilibrium prior to repetition. This experiment is thus only rarely conducted in MRI imaging, although it yields beautiful T1-weighted images. More frequent is its application in order to nullify signal from some particular tissue that is not desired to be present in the image. Fat suppression in the STIR sequence (26) and suppression of cerebrospinal fluid (CSF) in the FLAIR experiment (87) are two such examples (see "Perfusion and Diffusion," following). Suppression of multiple tissues with different T1 times is also possible by applying more than one inversion pulse with appropriate timing prior to signal readout. The contrast behavior of the visible tissues will then become strongly nonlinear and complex.

A faster and thus for in vivo MRI much more common pulse sequence is given by the progressive saturation sequence. Here the signal acquisition is repeated at a time that

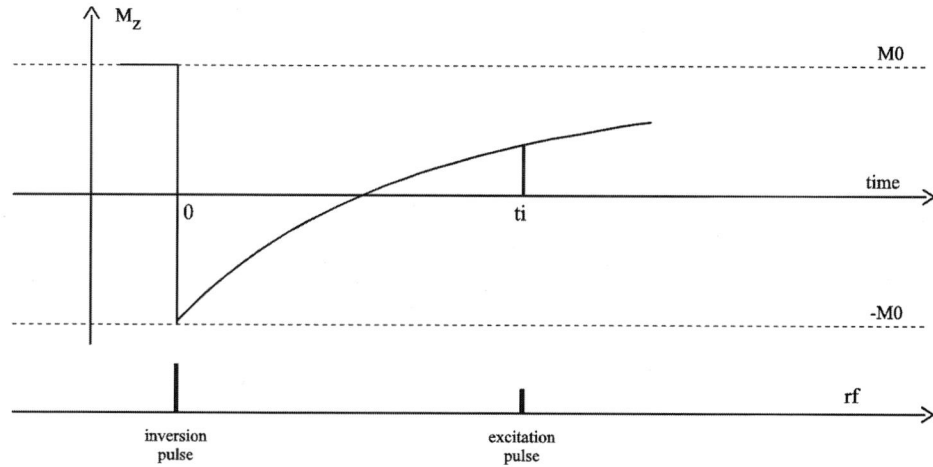

Figure 9. Principle of inversion recovery experiment. An initial 180° pulse inverts z-magnetization, which then recovers with T1 toward equilibrium. After a time t_i, an excitation pulse is applied, which converts the then existing z-magnetization into transverse magnetization and thus a signal.

is shorter than T1 (Fig. 10). Signal will then not be allowed to recover to equilibrium, and M_z will go to a steady-state value M_{ss} given by

$$M_{ss} = M_0 \exp(-t_r/T1) \tag{5}$$

T2 Relaxation and T2* Decay

In addition to the processes leading to T1 relaxation, the fluctuating electromagnetic fields generated by Brownian motion will lead to some interactions that do not require a transition between ground and excited states and thus do not affect the net z-magnetization. One such interaction is small fluctuations of the magnetic field that lead to small variations of the Larmor frequency of the nuclei. After a few such random variations,

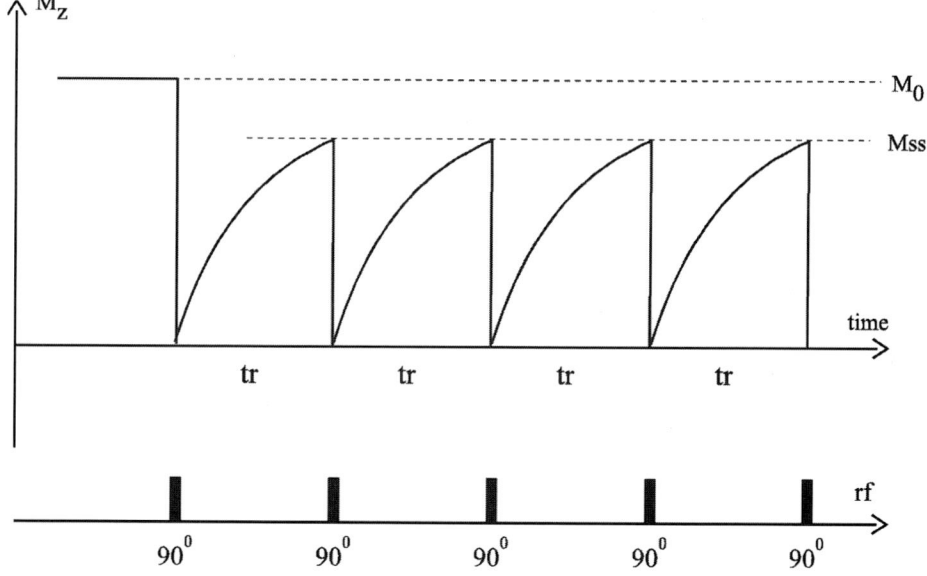

Figure 10. Progressive saturation experiment. Repetitive application of 90° excitation pulses with a time interval t_r leads to the establishment of a steady-state magnetization M_{ss}.

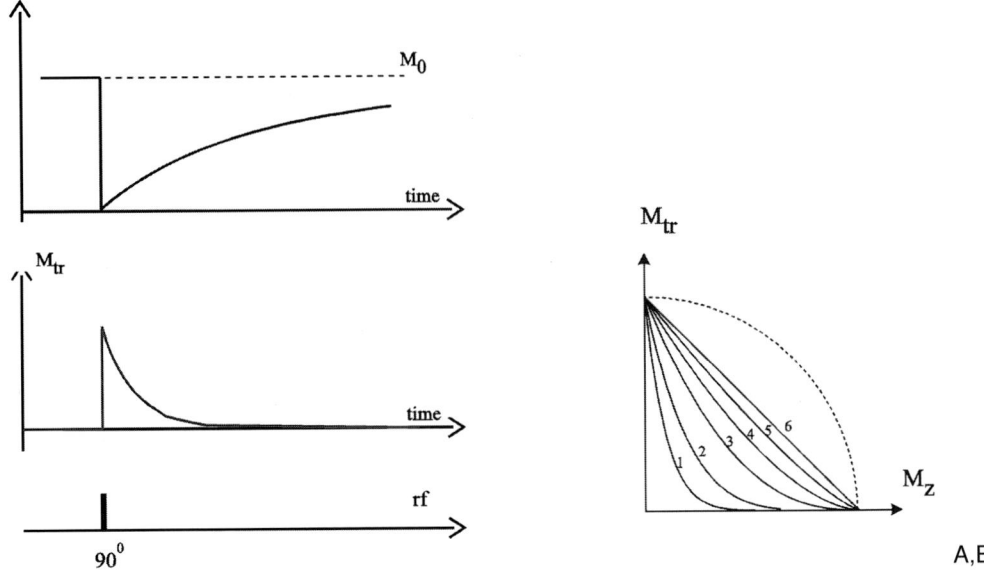

Figure 11. Signal evolution after an excitation pulse including T1 and T2 relaxation. The z-magnetization M_z (**A,** *top*) will return to thermal equilibrium with the relaxation time T1, whereas transverse magnetization M_{tr} decays with T2 (**A,** *bottom*) (**A**). The trajectories of the tips of the magnetization vectors as a function of T2 = nT1 are shown in (**B**) for n = 0.1 (1), 0.2 (2), 0.4 (3), 0.6 (4), 0.8 (5), and 1. For $n > 1$ (T2 > T1), the trajectory would eventually grow out of the dotted circle, which means that magnetization would grow by relaxation in clear contradiction to thermodynamics.

the magnetization vectors will lose coherence, and the net transverse magnetization will decay. Eventually, the signal will be zero, although the number of excited nuclei can still be the same as immediately after excitation.

This signal decay by interactions on the molecular scale is called *transverse* or *T2 relaxation* (1, 9). T1 and T2 relaxations are thus formally treated as two independent phenomena due to the fact that one requires the exchange of energy, whereas the other does not. A full description of a "pulse and acquire" experiment including relaxation is given in Fig. 11.

In spite of their formal separation, T1 and T2 relaxation are closely linked. T1 relaxation brings back magnetization into thermal equilibrium. Since equilibrium magnetization is pure z-magnetization, which does not induce any current in a surrounding coil, the transverse signal will necessarily have vanished. One is therefore forced to say that any process leading to T1 relaxation will invariably lead to T2 decay as well, but not vice versa. In addition, T2 will be shortened by no-energy interactions. T2 thus is always shorter than or at most equal to T1. Since the local modulations responsible for the acceleration of T2 compared with T1 show little or no field dependence, T2 will be less field-dependent than T1 in the range used for MRI. In general, some T2 shortening will be observed in most tissues when going to a higher field.

Since T2 and T1 are dependent on the mobility of the molecules in which the observed protons are bound, both will vary considerably with molecular weight. Especially T2 will be significantly shortened in larger molecules due to a process called *spin diffusion,* which describes the fact that all protons within one such molecule feel the precession of all the others very efficiently due to the rigid geometry of the molecule. T2 of protons in macromolecules is thus so short that MRI observes only protons in small molecules, the most abundant of which is free water. Compared with a pure solution, the observed T2 and T1 times of tissues will nevertheless be shortened. One important and ubiquitous mechanism for this shortening is the exchange of protons between hydrophilic groups on protons and free water (40). During the short time of attachment to the protein, protons will feel the high relaxation rate of the large molecule. The observed T2 and T1 times will thus be a time-averaged value.

There are other processes on a more macroscopic scale that also lead to loss of coherence. Changes of the Larmor frequency due to minute variations of the magnetic field across the probe have already been mentioned in the section describing the spin-echo experiment. Such changes might be caused either by the limited field homogeneity that can be achieved in a whole-body magnet or by interaction of the bulk magnetic properties of the tissue under study with the main magnetic field. The latter effect is called *susceptibility effect*. The homogeneity of superconducting whole-body magnets is 3 to 10 ppm across a 40- to 50-cm homogeneous volume. Susceptibility effects for organic tissue are on the order of a few parts per million up to several tenths of parts per million for deoxygenated blood with its strong magnetic moment.

If the location of spins remains fixed with respect to the magnetic field, the field variations will lead to spin dephasing, which can be refocused in a spin-echo experiment. A different situation occurs when spins move randomly across an inhomogeneous field. In this case, the dephasing will depend on the random path and will thus not be automatically refocused by a spin-echo experiment. The importance of this dynamic susceptibility effect depends, of course, on the scale of the field variations. For steep susceptibility-dependent field gradients occurring, for example, around small blood vessels, this effect can be appreciable. It will be discussed further in the section on diffusion and perfusion.

T2 effects are often cited to represent some intrinsic property of the tissue under study, whereas T2* effects reflect the signal decay due to the experimental conditions. Whereas in general this is true, it also should be noted that a continuous transition exists between T2* and T2 effects when susceptibility effects take place on a smaller and smaller scale. The various mechanisms leading to signal decay are represented schematically in Fig. 12 and Color Plate 20.

Measuring T2

The relaxation time T2 is normally measured using a spin-echo experiment. It can be determined either by repetitive measurements with variable echo time t_e or—more elegantly—by making a multiecho experiment, where signal is read out at—preferably—equidistant echo times (144), and the whole decay curve is thus acquired in a single experiment (Fig. 13 and Color Plate 21). T2* can be measured simply by analyzing the signal decay of the FID. For a homogeneous liquid sample, T2 will normally follow a monoexponential curve. This is not necessarily true for T2*, which depends on the actual distribution of spins with different Larmor frequencies across the probe. Representing T2* as the constant of a monoexponential decay curve is thus only an approximation.

A special case is T2* effects caused by the dynamic susceptibility effect. These also will affect the signal amplitude in a spin-echo effect and therefore contribute to the measured T2. Due to the nature of the random walk, the extent of signal attenuation, however, will depend on the echo time of the measurement. From Fig. 12 it can be deduced that the effect will get smaller for smaller echo spacing. This is similar to going to camp in the forest with a number of kids and trying to keep them together by letting them report back at the camp at regular intervals: If the intervals are short, they will never move far away from the camp; if the intervals get larger, their "dephasing" gets stronger and stronger. Eventually, they will get totally lost—but that's another story.

BASICS OF MRI

The resonance frequency for protons in a 1-T magnet, which is a common field strength in MR tomography, is roughly 42 MHz. According to the conversion table in Chap. 1, this corresponds to a wavelength of several meters. The image resolution for wave optical image formation is connected with the wavelength used by the Rayleigh criterion (see Chap. 1, Fig. 1). If we want to achieve a resolution of 1 mm for a diagnostic imaging device, this immediately leads to an apparatus with a detector size of several hundred meters. On the other hand, an imaging device that can fit into a hospital room

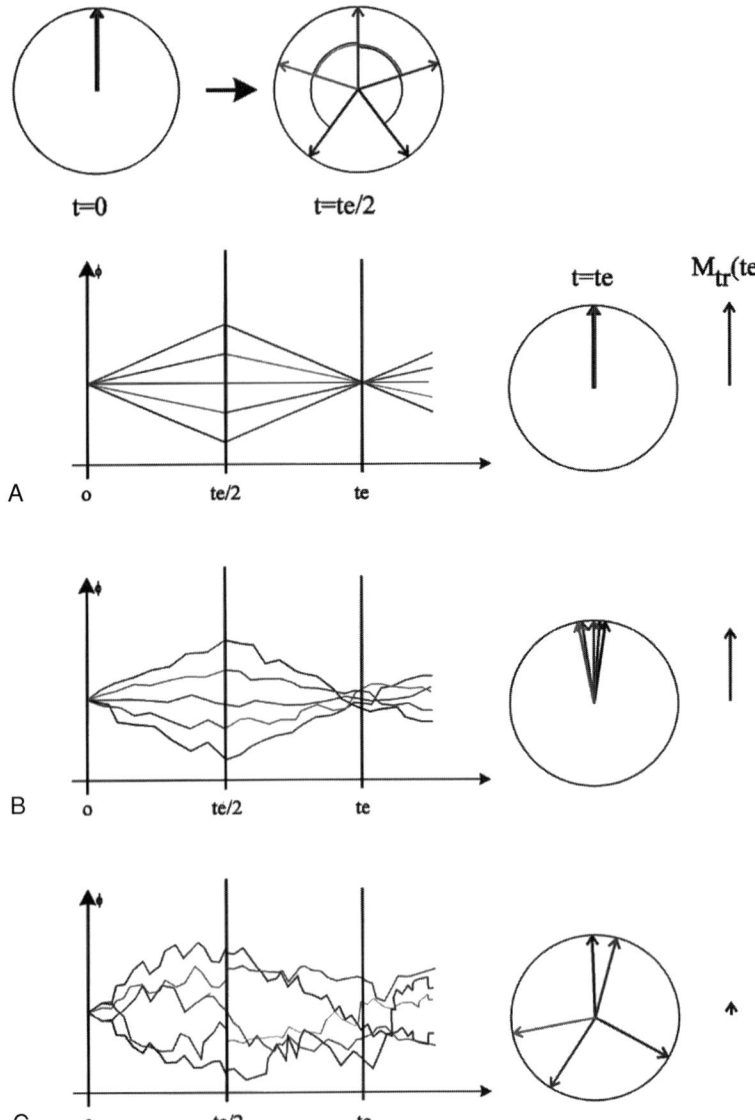

Figure 12. Effect of fluctuations of the precession frequency on the measured T2 relaxation. Three cases are shown that are all categorized by coherence at $t = 0$ and an even distribution of magnetization vectors at the time $t_e/2$ of application of the refocusing pulse but with varying temporal fluctuations of the Larmor frequency of the observed spins as a consequence of, for example, motion in an inhomogeneous field. Static spins **(A)** will be perfectly refocused at $t = t_e$. Spins with some slight fluctuation in their resonance frequencies will be slightly defocused at $t = t_e$ **(B)**. If the fluctuations become large or the time scale of the fluctuations becomes shorter, eventually no spin refocusing can be observed any more (dynamic susceptibility effect) **(C)**. See Color Plate 20.

will have a resolution that at best allows one to determine whether the patient is in the hospital but not be able to make any meaningful diagnostic image of him or her.

This demonstrates that forming an image by MRI cannot be based on the principles of wave propagation, although these principles fully apply to the actual measuring process.

One could in principle increase the magnetic field strength until the wavelength approaches a useful range. Apart from the fact that this is technically unfeasible (a 1-T magnet already has more than 100,000 times the earth's magnetic field, and its construction constitutes a remarkable engineering feat), Fig. 1 in Chap. 1 also demonstrates that at higher frequencies the body very quickly becomes opaque, which violates the most

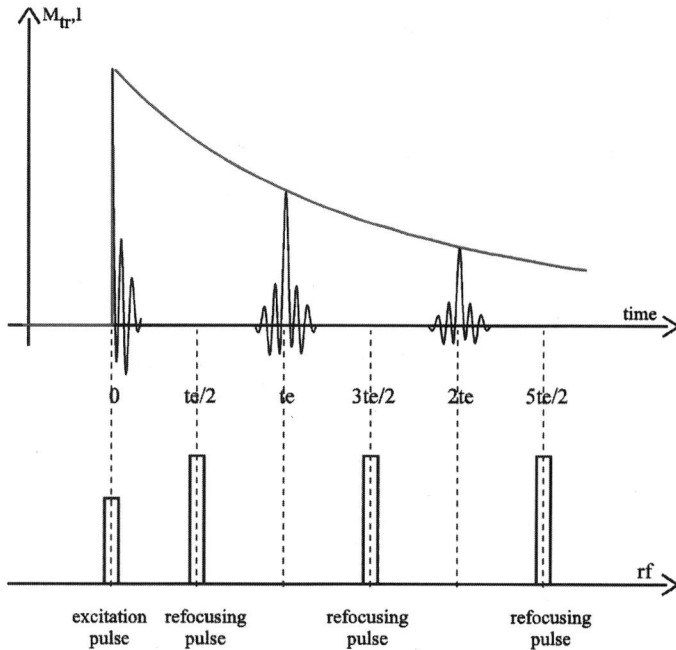

Figure 13. Principle of multiecho T2 measurement. Application of equidistant refocusing pulses leads to the formation of an echo train at times t_e, $2t_e$, $3t_e$, etc. See Color Plate 21.

important precondition for any imaging technique. The ingenious trick that is used to overcome the apparent impossibility of making images with millimeter resolution using waves with wavelengths of several meters is based on the Larmor equation (see "Some Basics"): Since the resonance frequency is directly proportional to the magnetic flux density, the location of spins can be mapped by varying the magnetic field across the probe (Fig. 14 and Color Plate 22). The position of spins along the direction of the gradient will then be identified by their resonance frequency. Unfortunately, this principle works only in one dimension at a time; it is impossible to shape a magnetic field in three dimensions such that each point in space is uniquely identified by its local field and thus Larmor frequency. Making an MRI image thus will be a stepwise process in which the three spatial directions have to be selected consecutively. This requires a combination of rf pulses and switched magnetic field gradients. The first MRI image was produced by Lauterbur in 1973 (128). The backprojection encoding he used for spatial encoding (see Chap. 1) has meanwhile been replaced for most routine imaging applications by the two-dimensional Fourier transform technique (124), which has some important advantages, especially with respect to artefact behavior. The essential steps of image formation according to this approach are described in the next sections.

The Slice-Selection Gradient

The first step in an MRI experiment is selection of the plane of the image. This is done by applying the excitation pulse in the presence of a magnetic field gradient (207), which is then called the *slice-selection gradient* G_s. The excitation profile across the selected slice will depend on the frequency profile of the pulse. A pulse with frequency ω_1 in Fig. 14 will select spins at location x_1; ω_2 will select those at x_2.

A profile that is ideal for MRI imaging should be exactly rectangular; it should excite (or refocus) all spins within the desired slice uniformly and not affect spins outside at all. It can be shown that such a profile cannot be realized by any pulse of finite lengths. If only a limited time is allotted to such a pulse, only more or less good approximations to such an ideal shape can be generated. The number of pulse shapes that will approximate a desired profile within a certain margin of error is infinite. Various sophisticated

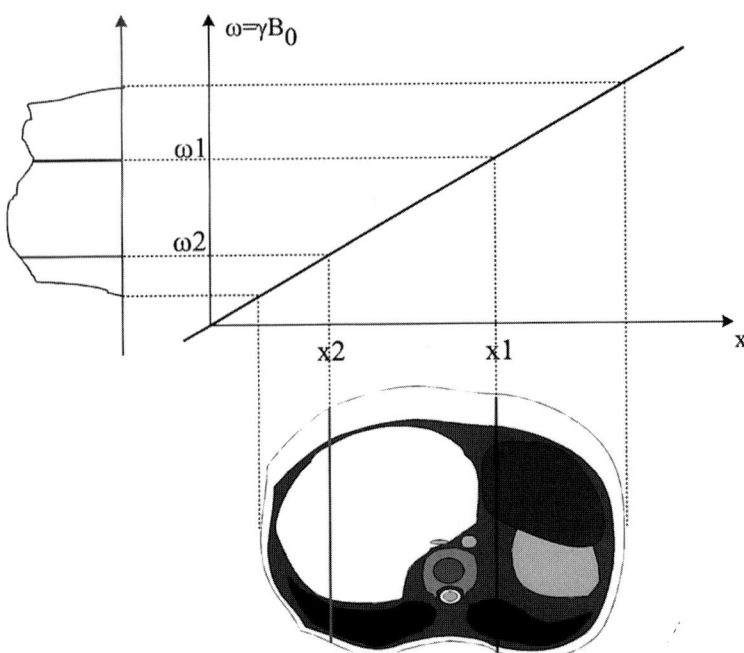

Figure 14. Principle of spatial encoding with constant gradient. If a linearly varying magnetic field (=constant magnetic field gradient) is applied across a body, the Larmor frequency will vary linearly across the body. The signal intensity at the frequencies ω_1 and ω_2 of the acquired frequency spectrum thus corresponds to the measured magnetization from spins at positions x_1 and x_2, respectively. See Color Plate 22.

optimization algorithms exist that can be used to generate such pulses. Depending on their minimization criteria, they will lead to dramatically different pulses that nevertheless generate nearly identical excitation profiles.

Slice profiles are normally defined by a bandwidth, which defines the frequency interval within which the pulse affects the observed spins. There is no clear convention as to how this bandwidth should be defined. Often the frequency width at half height is cited, which means that some spins at the feet of the pulse that lie outside the so-defined slice thickness also will be affected. Another measure would be the width at a 5% level, which leads to slightly larger nominal slice thickness.

Pulses are time invariant as long as the intrinsic time scale of the pulse is long compared with the duration of one Larmor precession and short compared with the relaxation times. Halving the length of a pulse and doubling its amplitude in order to maintain the same flip angle will thus double its bandwidth.

The slice thickness s_{th} for a pulse of a given bandwidth bw can be simply calculated from the slope of the slice selection gradient G_s:

$$s_{\text{th}} = \frac{2\pi bw}{\gamma G_s} \tag{6}$$

For a given gradient strength, the slice thickness will thus be proportional to bw. Short pulses that optimize the timing of a pulse sequence thus require strong gradients if thin slices are to be observed.

A lower limitation to the duration of a pulse and thus an upper limitation to the pulse bandwidth is given by the fact that the pulse power grows with the square of its amplitude. Halving the pulse width thus will lead to a fourfold increase of the rf power for a pulse with the same flip angle. Given current hardware restrictions, a bandwidth of 5 to 10 kHz is the maximum achievable value; a common value is 1 to 2 kHz. Apart from technical limitations, heat absorption from the body limits the applicable power, especially at higher fields.

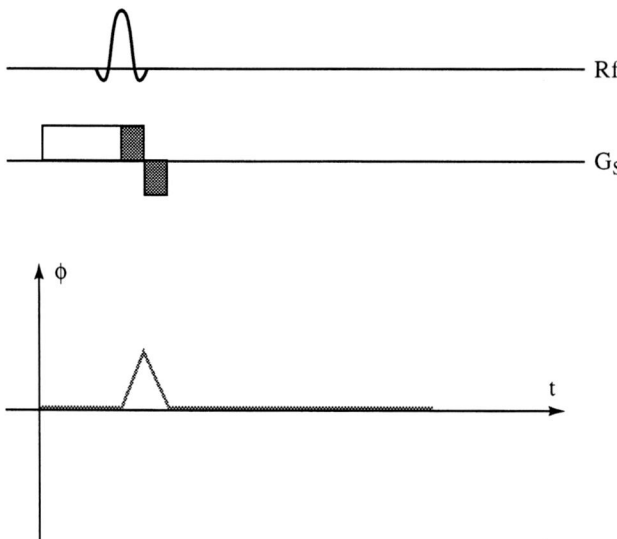

Figure 15. Pulse sequences with slice selection. The first step of an MRI sequence is slice selection. Application of an rf pulse with limited bandwidth under a slice-selection gradient leads to excitation of spins in a small section of the body defined by the Larmor equation. Due to the finite length of the pulse, some dephasing of spins will be observed even directly after the pulse that is undone by an appropriate negative lobe of the slice-selection gradients. For most commonly used pulses, the dephasing can be said to be linear and the (nominal) time of spin coherence can be assumed to be at the center of the pulse. The refocusing gradient lobe thus has to be equal to the area of the gradient between the center and the end of the pulse (*shaded areas*).The de- and refocusing of spins are also shown in the phase graph at the bottom of the diagram.

The first step of an imaging sequence can thus be diagramed as shown in Fig. 15. The negative lobe of the slice-selection gradient is necessary in order to compensate for the dephasing of spins across the slice during the finite time of the pulse during which the slice-selection gradient is on. For most commonly used pulses, the center of the pulse can be taken as the origin of a linear phase evolution. The amplitude of the compensating gradient (often called *trim gradient*) can then be calculated such that the areas under the relevant part of the positive and negative gradient lobes are identical.

More advanced pulse designs deliver the spins more or less in phase at the end of the pulse. This allows for a smaller compensating gradient, which can be important for fast imaging techniques.

The Read Gradient

For a linear magnetic field (constant gradient; see Fig. 14), the frequency distribution of the signals will directly reflect the distribution of spins along the gradient. A generalization of this principle to two dimensions is, however, unfeasible. Any profile of a magnetic field that we might generate can be represented as a contour map. For any continuous field this map will show contour lines that indicate locations of equal field just like the contour map of a mountain range represents places of equal altitude. Spins along each such contour line will thus have identical Larmor frequencies and thus cannot be distinguished by the MR spectrum.

A feasible way to resolve the location of spins in two dimensions is to measure one-dimensional projections along various projection angles. This was in fact the basis for the first MRI experiment published by P. Lauterbur in 1973 (130). Image reconstruction can then be performed by the so-called filtered backprojection algorithm (see Chap. 1). Prerequisite for Lauterbur's technique, as well as any of the schemes described below, is the availability of magnetic field gradients that can be applied in any spatial direction.

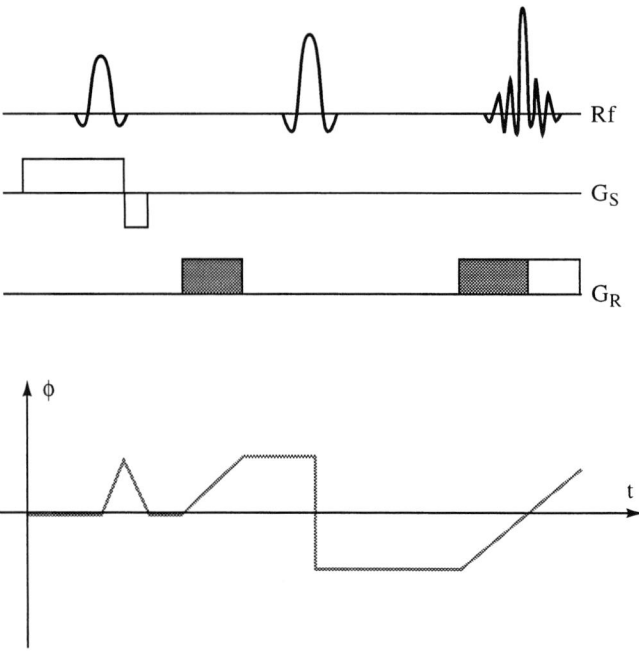

Figure 16. Pulse sequence with readout gradient. For frequency encoding along one of the in-plane directions of the selected slice, signal is read out under a readout gradient. If the readout gradient is just switched on at the time of the echo, spins will dephase very fast, and the signal will be complicated by the switching characteristics of the magnetic field gradients. Thus normally spins are dephased first by a gradient lobe (*gray*) between the excitation and the refocusing pulse. Signal can then be read out continuously as a sping echo if the area of the readout gradient after the refocusing pulse is chosen such that it matches the defocusing lobe exactly at the time t_e for echo formation. This is also shown as a phase graph at the bottom of the figure.

Backprojection is intuitively easy to understand at least in principle (understanding the mathematics of image reconstruction is something different). It is, however, rarely used in MRI due to the more beneficial properties of so-called two-dimensional Fourier transform (2DFT) imaging. 2DFT imaging also uses frequency encoding in one image dimension, called the *readout direction*. A spin-echo version of such a sequence including the slice selection and readout gradients is shown in Fig. 16.

Note that the occurrence of the echo at the proper time necessitates thorough adjustment of the gradient. Contrary to a spin echo under a constant field inhomogeneity, signal formation in time-variant magnetic field gradients does not automatically occur at the proper time: If the defocusing lobe of the readout gradient in Fig. 16 is too large, the echo will be shifted to the front of the proper refocusing time, and inhomogeneity effects will not be properly refocused.

The Phase-Encoding Gradient

Similar to backprojection, 2DFT imaging relies on repetitive acquisitions under a readout gradient that yields spatial resolution along one axis. Contrary to backprojection techniques, the readout gradient is kept constant from one acquisition to the next. Spatial resolution in a direction orthogonal to the readout gradient is achieved using a phase-encoding gradient prior to acquisition. This gradient is switched off during acquisition; its effect, however, will be present in the phase of the observed signals.

In order to understand how phase encoding works, it should first be noted that the dephasing of spins under a given magnetic field gradient of finite duration will be proportional to the distance of the spins along the gradient; spins further out will see a stronger magnetic field and will thus precess faster and accumulate a larger dephasing (Fig. 17A and Color Plate 23). Second, it should be noted that the dephasing is propor-

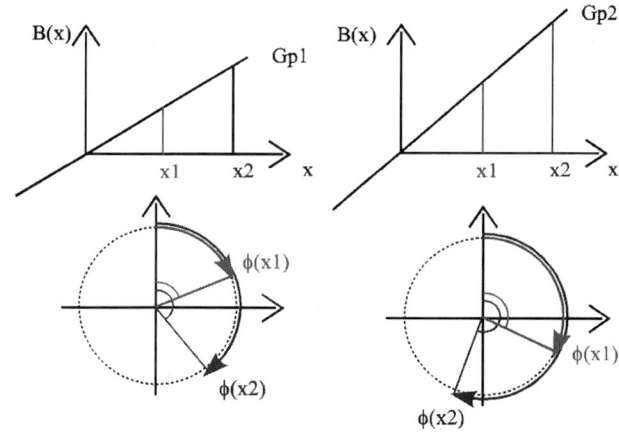

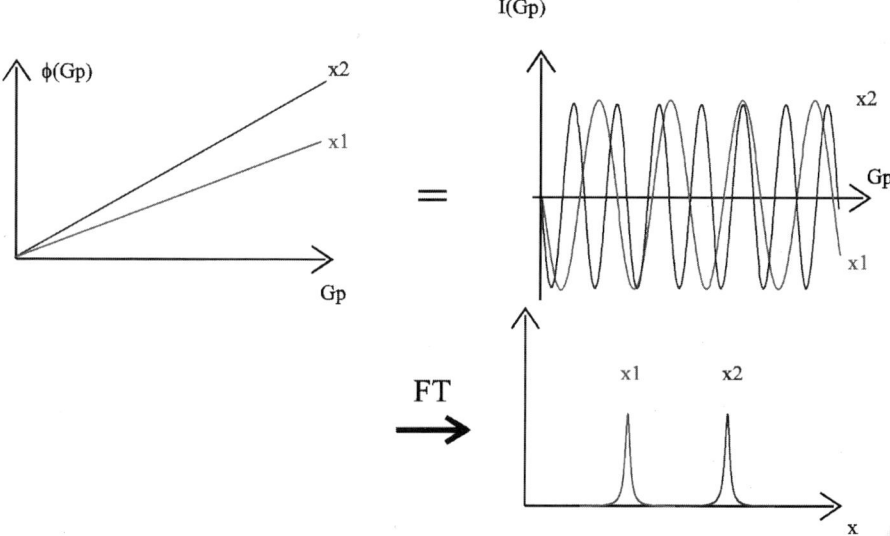

Figure 17. Principle of phase encoding. The dephasing of spins will be proportional to their distance along the phase-encoding gradient (*top left*). It will also be proportional to the strength of the gradient (*top right*). If the amplitude of the gradient is changed from one acquisition to the next, the signal phase will thus increase linearly, where spins closer to the center show a smaller slope than those further out (*bottom left*). A linearly varying phase is equivalent to a constant frequency, whereas a steeper slope corresponds to a higher frequency. Frequency analysis will thus generate signals whose frequencies correspond to the locations of spins (*bottom right*). See Color Plate 23.

tional to the amplitude of the gradient. Taking these two points together, a gradient can be applied before each acquisition step such that the amplitude of this gradient will be stepwise increased from one acquisition to the next. The phase of spins located along this gradient will then increase linearly, where the slope of this increase will be directly proportional to the distance to the center of the gradient. The last step is the recognition that phase is not a linear property but runs in circles. A signal with a linearly increasing phase is nothing but a sinusoidal wave exactly like a free-induction decay (Fig. 17B). The slope of the phase represents the frequency of the wave. The location of spins along the phase-encoding gradient can thus be derived from Fourier transformation of the data along this direction.

The full diagram of a 2DFT imaging sequence is thus shown in Fig. 18. The conventional way to sample all differently phase-encoded projections consists in repeating the

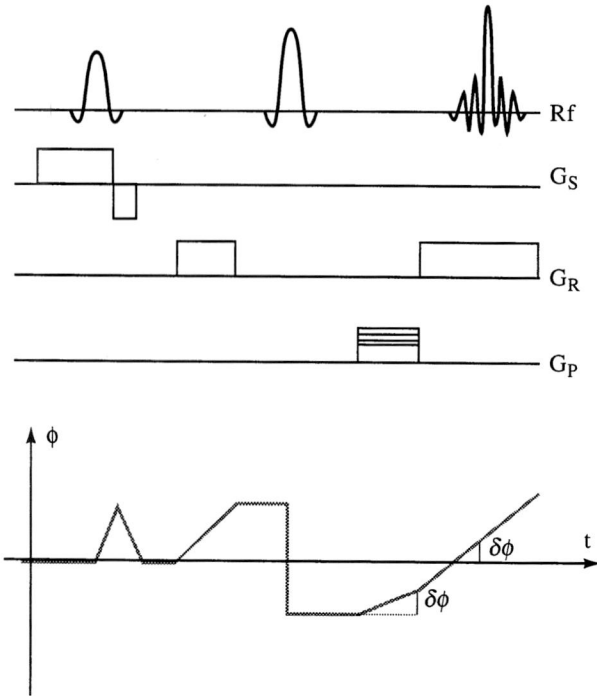

Figure 18. Pulse sequence with phase encoding. The varying phase-encoding gradient is applied immediately before signal acquisition. Note that inclusion of the phase-encoding gradient in the phase graph at the bottom will lead to a residual signal phase *df* at the time of echo formation, which is equivalent to saying that the time of refocusing depends on the position of the spins along the direction of the phase-encoding gradient. A proper echo is thus only formed in the one acquisition step carrying zero (=no) phase encoding.

experiment under variation of the phase-encoding gradient until all data required for two-dimensional (2D) image reconstruction have been acquired.

Three-Dimensional (3D) Data Acquisition

The idea of phase encoding can be carried further to a 3D experiment. Here, an additional phase-encoding gradient is applied in the direction reserved for slice selection in a 2DFT experiment (Fig. 19). Acquisition of a full 3D data set requires the application of all 2D phase-encoding gradients for each 3D phase-encoding step. The total number

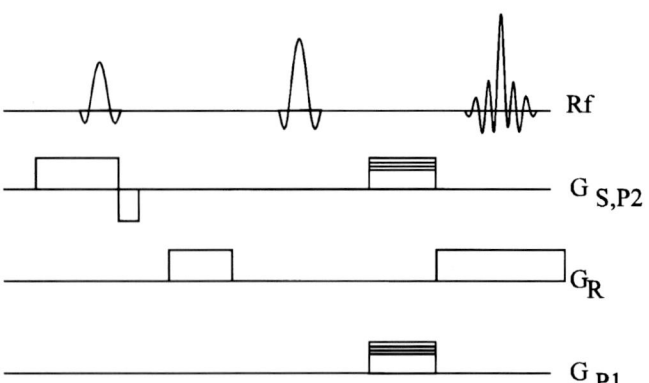

Figure 19. 3D pulse sequence. The concept of phase encoding can be applied in more than one spatial direction. In a 3D (volumetric) acquisition sequence, a second phase-encoding gradient is applied in the direction of the slice-selection gradient (which can be omitted altogether if data acquisition is to be performed for the whole body under study).

of projections to be measured will then be $n_{2D} \times n_{3D}$. The large number of projections restricts the application of 3D imaging to fast imaging sequences in order to stay within reasonable limits for the total acquisition time.

Other techniques such as x-ray computed tomography also allow the reconstruction of 3D image data sets. These are, however, based on stacks of parallel 2D images, whereas 3D MRI uses true 3D data acquisition.

THE FOURIER TRANSFORMATION

Sampling

Frequency analysis is a very common task in everyday life. Our ear (plus the auditory system in the brain) is an extremely sensitive apparatus to analyze periodic pressure waves. Filtering out certain frequencies from a complex signal also can be performed by simple mechanical devices such as the already mentioned resonating glass (see Fig. 4). The mathematical analysis of a complicated function of time seems to be, however, quite tricky. How can the frequency components be filtered out of a complicated curve such as the MR signal acquired under a readout gradient? One would first think of trying to use some kind of a fitting procedure in order to find out whether some particular frequency component is contained in the time function. One might even think of more sophisticated algorithms that match the time function to one frequency after the other until the whole (and in principle infinite) frequency spectrum is covered. To develop an algorithm for performing this task seems to be, however, a gargantuan task.

In view of the apparent complexity of the problem, the algorithm devised by the Comte du Fourier at the time of the French Revolution seems to be staggeringly simple. He used a very simple and nevertheless extremely powerful concept of how to measure the likeness of two functions: Do a point-by-point multiplication, and add up the result. The total sum—or for a continuous function, the integral—will be a measure of the likeness of the two functions. This is, of course, pointless if it is done only once. The resulting number only gets a meaning if it is compared with the result of other such correlations. For the analysis of frequencies, the set of functions with which the time signal is correlated is composed of sinusoids with frequencies covering the whole infinite range (Fig. 20 and Color Plate 24). Mathematically, this yields an extremely compact formula (19):

$$S(\omega) = \int_{-\infty}^{\infty} s(t) \exp(-i\omega t) \, dt \tag{7}$$

Here $s(t)$ represents the signal to be analyzed, and the exponential term is a short-hand notation for a 2D wave that takes into account that the waves to be analyzed are in general not planar waves but functions along two coordinates. In mathematical representation it is quite useful to represent the two orthogonal components by the real and imaginary parts of a complex number rather than in the x and y coordinates of a cartesian coordinate system. The terms *real* and *imaginary* are simply labels to symbolize two orthogonal directions, and no mysticism should be attached to their meaning. For a corkscrew wave like an FID, the real part will be shifted by 90° with respect to the imaginary.

The Fourier transform reads

$$FT[s(t)] = S(\omega) = \int_{-\infty}^{\infty} s(t) \exp(-i\omega t) \, dt$$

Backtransformation then yields

$$IFT[S(\omega)] = \frac{1}{2\pi} \int_{-\infty}^{\infty} S(\omega) \exp(i\omega t) \, d\omega = \frac{1}{2\pi} s(t)$$

For the sake of symmetry, the scaling factor $\frac{1}{2\pi}$ in the backtransformation often is equally attributed as $\sqrt{\frac{1}{2\pi}}$ to both the forward and back Fourier transforms.

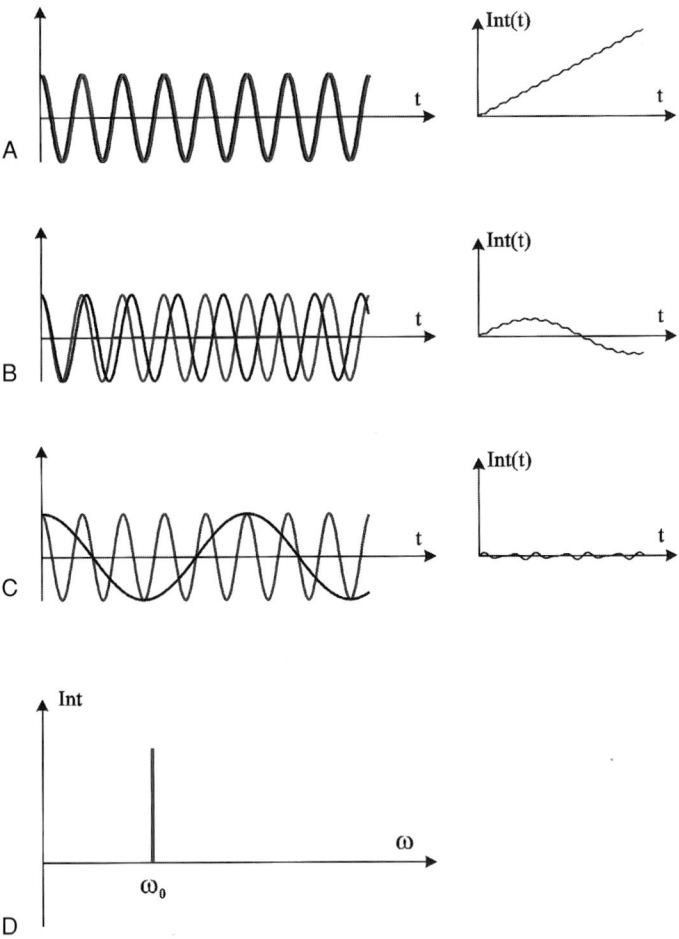

Figure 20. Principle of Fourier transformation. The concept of frequency analysis by Fourier transformation uses the calculation of the running sum of the product of the function to be measured (*red*) with sinusoids with varying frequencies (*blue*). Only when both frequencies match will the two signals stay in phase and their running sum Int(*t*) grow arbitrarily **(A)**. Even for a slight mismatch of the two frequencies, signals eventually will get out of phase, and their running sum oscillates around zero **(B)**. For larger frequency mismatch, the running sum will stay very close to zero. The longer time is left running, the larger will be the ratio of the linearly growing on-resonance value to the off-resonance oscillations **(C)**. Extrapolated to infinite time, the resulting scaled spectrum will show a nonzero value only at $\omega = \omega_0$ **(D)**. See Color Plate 24.

Finite Sampling

In any physical measurements, the time for measuring a time function will be finite. The spectrum of the time function will then be given by the spectrum of the infinite function convoluted with the Fourier transform (FT) of the rectangular sampling window, which can be presented formally by a function that is 1 inside the sampling period and 0 outside.

The Fourier transform of a rectangular function is a so-called sinc function that follows the equation:

$$S(\omega) = \frac{\sin(\omega)}{\omega} \tag{8}$$

The spectrum of any function that is truncated by a finite sampling window will thus show sinc-shaped lines rather than delta functions. The width of the sinc shapes will be inversely proportional to the length of the acquisition period; the longer the sampling window, the sharper will be the lines. The side bands of the sinc function decay very slowly. Figure 20 demonstrates that this results in a very natural process for comparing

SOME IMPORTANT BASIC PROPERTIES AND THEOREMS OF FOURIER TRANSFORMATION

Addition Theorem

The Fourier transform of a sum of two functions is identical to the sum of the Fourier transforms of each function:

$$FT[s_1(t) + s_2(t)] = FT[s_1(t)] + FT[s_2(t)]$$

Shift Theorem

The Fourier transform of a function that is shifted by τ in time is equal to the Fourier transform of the unshifted function multiplied by a frequency-dependent phase shift:

$$FT[s(t - \tau)] = \exp(-i\omega\tau)*S(\omega) \qquad \text{(see Fig. 34)}$$

Convolution Theorem

The convolution integral of two functions $s_1(t)$ and $s_2(t)$ is defined as

$$s_1(t)*s_2(t) = \int_{-\infty}^{\infty} s_1(\tau)s_2(t - \tau)\, d\tau$$

The convolution theorem states that the Fourier transform of the convolution integral is equal to the product of the Fourier transforms of the two functions:

$$FT[s_1(t)*s_2(t)] = FT[s_1(t)]FT[s_2(t)]$$

One important application of these symmetry properties regards the use of magnitude versus phase-sensitive spectra. For an exponential decay, the real part $R[S(\omega)]$ of its Fourier transform represents a nice and narrow Lorentzian line. Its imaginary part $I[S(\omega)]$, however, yields a dispersion line whose wings stretch out to infinity. The magnitude spectrum $M[S(\omega)]$ is defined as

$$M[S(\omega)] = \sqrt{R[S(\omega)]^2 + I[S(\omega)]^2}$$

and will consequently show a much worse resolution compared with the real part $R[S(\omega)]$ (which is the reason why high-resolution MR spectroscopy always uses phase-corrected spectra). This can be considerably improved by using the symmetry conditions of Fourier transform: First, the exponential decay is made symmetrical by adding a time-reversed copy to its front. A time reversal also reverses the real and imaginary parts of the spectrum. By symmetry, the time-reversed dispersion curves in the imaginary part will then cancel out on combination according to the addition theorem. Thus a nice and narrow Lorentzian will remain in the real part and even after taking the magnitude of the spectrum.

by physical necessity finite functions rather than the infinite functions required by the mathematics of Fourier transformation.

In information theory, the sinc function is also called the *point-spread function* of finite sampling (see Chap. 1). It represents the amount by which information is blurred in any finite measurement. When listening to music, this blurring is not perceived due to the fact that the length of the notes is much longer than one wavelength. If the note a′ with a frequency of 880 Hz is played, for example, as a ¹⁄₁₆ note in a 120-beats-per-minute tempo (allegro), its duration will be ¹⁄₃₂ second. The first side lobe of the perceived sinc spectrum will then be 32 Hz away, which is less than one note.

If the frequency of the carrier note is reduced, the blurring will be the same in absolute units. At lower tones, this does, however, correspond to ever-increasing tone intervals

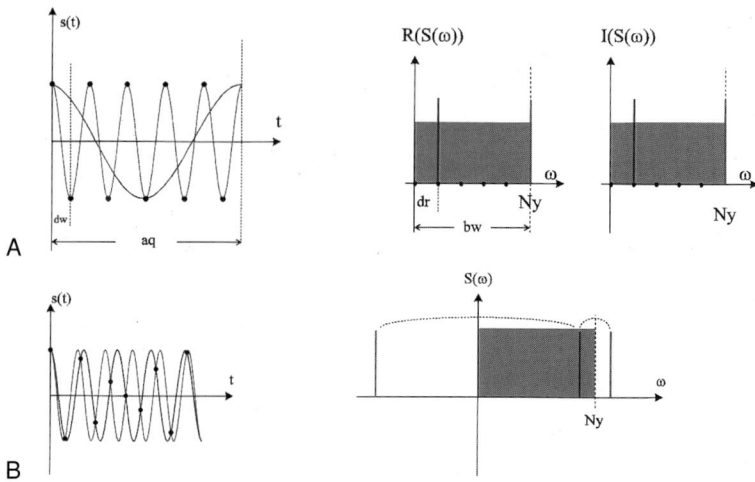

Figure 21. The Nyquist frequency and aliasing. For discrete sampling of the (real) time function with a dwell time *dw*, the highest detectable frequency for discrete sampling requires two sampling points per period. This defines the Nyquist frequency (*red* in **A**). A higher frequency (*red* in **B**) will have identical values at the discrete sampling points than a frequency that is mirrored back at the Nyquist frequency (*blue*) in **B**. By symmetry, folding back also occurs with respect to the zero point of the spectrum. The first nonzero frequency in the discrete frequency domain defines the spectral resolution *dr*. Its time function contains one frequency period over the acquisition window *aq* (*blue* in **A**). See Color Plate 25.

due to the proportional scale in music. Fast runs will therefore appear "dirtier," the lower they are placed on the tone scale. Playing $1/16$ notes in the bass range will produce nothing but a deep rumble, whereas for a soprano the tones can be clearly distinguished.

Discrete Sampling

In a physical measurement, the sampled signals have to be converted to digital data prior to Fourier transformation. Sampling will take place at discrete intervals and is normally performed at equidistant time intervals called the *dwell time dw*. This representation of a continuous function by a finite number of data points has some important consequences.

It is evident that the highest frequency that can be detected will be determined by the spacing of the sampling points. Above a certain threshold frequency the signal will be "folded back" by the discrete sampling. Figure 21A and Color Plate 25 demonstrates that one period of the maximum sampling frequency corresponds to two dwell times. This is the so-called *Nyquist theorem:*

$$\mathrm{Ny} = 1/(2dw) \tag{9}$$

Frequencies that exceed the Nyquist frequency *Ny* will be folded back into the sampling window (Fig. 21B):

$$S(\mathrm{Ny} + \omega) = S(\mathrm{Ny} - \omega) \tag{10}$$

This is called *aliasing*. Signals from all frequencies will thus be folded back into a sampling window, the bandwith *bw* of which is equal to Ny. Aliasing will fold not only spectral lines back into the acquisition window but also random noise. It is therefore wise to use an appropriate filter prior to Fourier transform in order to nullify all signal components outside the sampling window.

The resolution is solely defined by the acquisition time. Faster sampling will only increase the spread of spectral coverage. If the argument is reversed, it can be stated that the spectral resolution is not affected by the sampling rate. This is often used in so-called

SOME USEFUL RELATIONS FOR DISCRETE FOURIER TRANSFORMATION

The mathematics of the Fourier transformation requires complex data as input. The n sample points of the digitized signal are thus alternatively labeled as the real and imaginary parts of the input function for the Fourier transform; the spectrum after Fourier transform will then contain $n/2$ complex data points. The acquisition time will be given by

$$aq = n\ dw$$

The spectral resolution dr will be given by the bandwidth divided by the number of (complex) data points:

$$dr = \frac{bw}{(n/2)} = \frac{2bw}{n}$$

The Nyquist theorem can be expressed by the relations

$$Ny = \frac{1}{(2\ dw)} = bw = \frac{n}{(2aq)}$$

This yields

$$dr = \frac{1}{(n\ dw)} = \frac{1}{aq} = \frac{2Ny}{n.}$$

The resolution thus depends only on the acquisition time. For a given aq, increasing the number of data points will thus increase bw; the number of data per unit frequency will, however, remain constant.

The Nyquist theorem states that spins with frequency $f = 0$ at the lower edge of the sampling window and those with $f = Ny$ acquire a phase difference of $180°$ per dwell time. The frequency difference between adjacent points in the spectrum is identical to the resolution dr. Thus spins in adjacent voxels will acquire a phase difference of $360°$ over the whole acquisition time.

oversampling, where data are sampled faster than strictly necessary and the relevant part of the spectrum is cut out after Fourier transformation.

Aliasing shows that the Fourier transform does not distinguish between the actual frequencies and their equivalents of the higher harmonics of the Nyquist frequency. Fourier transformation of data within a finite sampling window is thus equivalent to Fourier transform of infinite periodic repetitions of the same functions. This illustrates that a large discrepancy of the data at the end of the acquisition window to the beginning can lead to serious artefacts (Fig. 22).

It also shows how this effect can be expressed in terms of the point-spread function. Any real object is represented by a more or less homogeneous distribution that is forced onto a discrete and equidistant grid by Fourier transformation. It was shown in Chap. 1 that the intrinsic image resolution can be described by the point-spread function (PSF), which represents the image of a discrete data point (180). The point-spread function for a discrete acquisition window will be a sinc function. In discrete Fourier transform, this sinc function will be projected onto the sampling grid. For a sample located at the center of the magnet, the discrete points of the data matrix after Fourier transform will coincide with the zero crossings of the sinc function, and a point really will be represented by a point. If the sample point falls between two grid points, this is not the case any more. The resulting artefact first distributes the signal intensity into two adjacent voxels, but it also leads to slowly decaying signal artefacts further on. High-intensity structures can thus lead to blurring all over the image. This is no serious concern for conventional MRI.

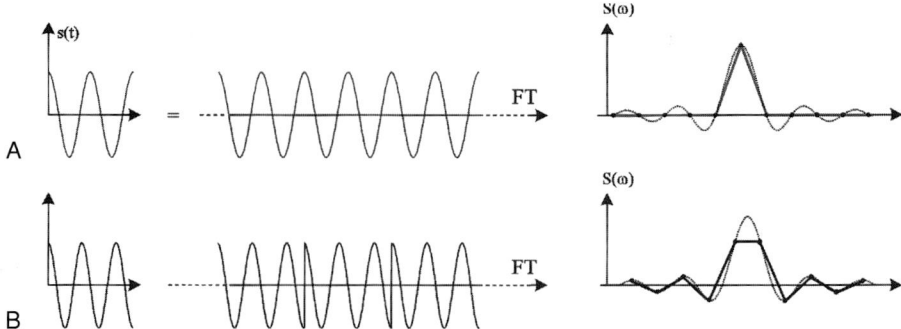

Figure 22. Periodicity of Fourier transformation. The Fourier transformation of any finite time function (*left*) is identical to infinite replications of the same function. This demonstrates why the discrete Fourier transformation of a function that continuously loops back from the end looks rather benign **(A)**, whereas the sudden jump implied by different starting and end points of the time function leads to severe ringing artefacts **(B)**.

It is, however, a serious concern for chemical-shift imaging, where low-intensity metabolite signals are to be observed.

For non-point-like distributions of spins, the dephasing of signals across each voxel also has to be taken into account. This will lead to signal attenuation, which increases with increasing signal dephasing. As a result, this dephasing will act as a weak low-pass filter, which will lead to a slightly modified point-spread function that decays faster than the sinc function of a discrete point.

In conclusion, Fourier transform can be said to be a very benign transformation algorithm at least if the number of data points is sufficiently large that the result of Fourier transform is dominated more by what's happening inside the sampling window and less by the effects occurring at both ends of the acquisition window. Depending on the demands on image quality, 8 to 16 data points can be said to be a lower bound at which Fourier transform can be used with some compromise; 32 data points are already a comfortable number to work with. For a lower number of data points, other algorithms should be used for frequency analysis in order to avoid the rigid constraints of discrete Fourier transform.

Finally it should be noted that discrete Fourier transform in principle does not require equidistant sampling points. The ubiquitous use of an equidistant sampling grid is dictated by practical considerations rather than by any fundamental reason: Fourier transformation of an equidistant sampling grid can be performed very fast and efficiently using the fast Fourier transform algorithm (34), whereas the calculations needed for step-by-step calculation of the Fourier integrals are very time-consuming even on powerful computers.

k-Space

It has been shown that spatial encoding in MRI is done by Fourier transformation in both image dimensions. Rather than being collected in a linear array for one-dimensional Fourier transform, data are being placed into a 2D matrix. Fourier transformation is then performed (at least formally) first row by row; the results of the first Fourier transform are then Fourier transformed again column by column. The 2D domain of the sampled data is called *k-space.*

From the point of view of image formation, the image dimensions are given in spatial units (which are derived from the frequency domain by the Larmor equation). Due to inversion by Fourier transform, *k*-space is consequently mapped out in units of 1/m. These are determined by the integrated amplitude of the gradient between adjacent sampling points (Fig. 23). Note that the time domain has thus vanished; we get from one point in *k*-space to an adjacent point by applying a certain incremental gradient no matter whether this is done in time by sampling under a constant gradient (as in the read domain)

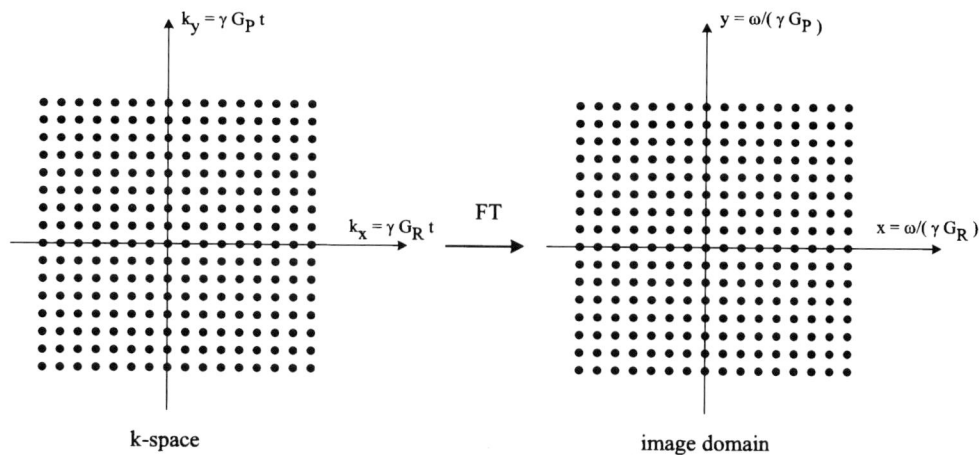

Figure 23. *k*-space and its coordinates. An MR image is mapped out in frequency units; the spatial coordinates are derived by the Larmor equation. The corresponding Fourier domain is called *k-space*, the coordinates of which are mapped out by the area under the respective gradient between adjacent sampling points.

or by applying an incremental gradient prior to acquisition (as in the phase-encoding direction). Since the *k*-space coverage is determined by the integral (or area) of the gradients, data acquisition using strong gradients and short acquisition times will lead to identical images as acquisition with weaker gradients and longer sampling times at least mathematically. Signal-to-noise considerations as well as possible artefacts will, however, narrow down the useful range of acquisition parameters for a given pulse sequence.

It is quite useful to discuss some of the consequences of the basic properties of Fourier transformation for MRI. By looking at the *k*-space data in Fig. 24 it becomes apparent that most of the signal intensity is located in the center of *k*-space. This is a consequence of the inverse relation of the extent of Fourier transformation pairs in their respective domains; since an image has a broad distribution of intensities, its Fourier transformation correlate is expected to have a narrow distribution. It should be emphasized that this focusing of data in *k*-space is no intrinsic property of Fourier transformation but solely determined by the particular intensity distribution encountered in in vivo MRI. If an object containing only discrete points arranged in a regular lattice is imaged, the *k*-space distribution will be much more extensive.

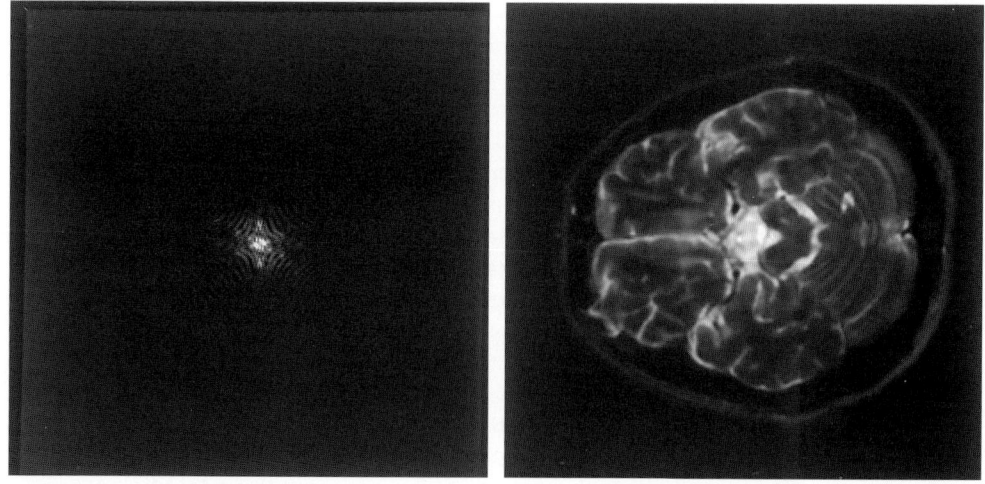

A   B

Figure 24. MRI data *k*-space versus image. The *k*-space data **(A)** demonstrate high signal intensity in the center and appear to be rather featureless further out. The information content of the image **(B)** resulting after 2D Fourier transformation of **(A)** is identical to that of **(B)**.

This inhomogeneous distribution of information can be wrapped up in the following statement:

The center of k-*space represents the image contrast, whereas the outer parts yield the spatial resolution.*

Since acquiring more data does not incur a severe penalty in the read direction, a reduction of the *k*-space data is normally done in the phase-encoding direction alone. After Fourier transform, an image with an identical field of view is generated, but at somewhat reduced resolution.

A further important property of data in *k*-space is their symmetry; due to the echo-formation mechanism, a spin echo will have a symmetric real (cos) part and an antisymmetric (sin) part. From the symmetry relations discussed above, it follows that the image will then contain real-only data. One-half the *k*-space data should therefore yield sufficient information, and the other half can be filled in by symmetry:

$$R[s(k_x, k_y)] = R[s(-k_x, -k_y)], \qquad I[s(k_x, k_y)] = -I[s(-k_x, -k_y)] \qquad (11)$$

In practice, this is used for the so-called half-Fourier technique (60), which—contrary to acquiring the central half of data—maintains the full image resolution. Its penalty is a reduced signal-to-noise ratio due to the sampling of only half the intensity-containing part of the data. The center of *k*-space has, of course, to be known exactly in order for the symmetry conditions to apply. Any slight shift will mix the real and imaginary data according to the shift theorem. Signal-to-noise ratio can be improved and artefacts from improper definition of the symmetry center be avoided if slightly more than half of *k*-space is sampled such that all the important data at its center are actually measured. An important prerequisite for half-Fourier imaging is, of course, that the acquired signals are really symmetric and not disturbed by some nonsymmetric mechanism such as T2* effects in gradient-echo imaging (see below).

The Physics of Image Formation

Signal-to-Noise Considerations

The intrinsic low signal-to-noise ratio is one of the major concerns in MRI. Any discussion of the signal-to-noise ratio has to take both the signal and the noise into account (see Chap. 1).

The signal intensity in a given experiment scales with the size of the voxel. It will consequently go up in proportion to the slice thickness and be inversely proportional to the square of the in-plane resolution. The noise in MRI is mainly caused by the electromagnetic fluctuations caused by Brownian motion of the molecules in the patient's body. Noise caused by electronic noise of the receiver system is relevant only at low field strength (<0.5 T), although an exact break-even point between both noise sources depends on many factors and is difficult to predict.

The amount of noise going into each image is then determined by the total amount of this random noise perceived by the receiver coil; a large coil will see more noise than a smaller coil. Since the noise fluctuations are, of course, not spatially encoded by the imaging gradients, the total noise from the total volume seen by the coil will go into each image, no matter what the dimensions of the image.

A consequence of this consideration is that a smaller coil invariably will produce a better signal-to-noise ratio than a larger one, even if both are built perfectly in the sense that both receive all the incoming signal. It is thus advisable to always use the smallest possible coil to cover the volume of interest.

Random noise is determined by its power per frequency unit. If data are sampled under a strong readout gradient, each image element (pixel) will contain a larger frequency spread and thus contain noise, where the intensity of the noise scales with the square root of the acquisition bandwidth (189). In a practical experiment, images produced with stronger gradients at reduced acquisition times and thus increased bandwidth will therefore be more noisy. The optimal bandwidth (and therefore gradient amplitude) depends on various factors, which will be discussed in more detail below.

Signal-to-noise ratio can always be improved by repeating the experiment and averaging the data. The signal will grow proportionally to the number of replications, whereas random noise grows only with its square root. Signal-to-noise ratio will thus grow as the square root of the number of averaged scans. The number of averaged data is abbreviated most commonly as *nex* in order to avoid confusions due to the fact that one average semantically already implies the existence of at least two data sets for averaging.

This square root dependence yields the most significant improvements for the first few averages; afterwards the gain in signal-to-noise ratio will be painstakingly slow. Consequently, the intrinsic signal-to-noise ratio for a single acquisition should not be too far off the desired mark.

Finally, it should be noted that the repetitive acquisition with increasing phase-encoding gradient already serves as an averaging process for the signal in each and every pixel. This can best be demonstrated by looking at an imaging experiment on a sample that contains spins only in the central voxel located at the zero point of all gradients. These spins will not see the effect of the phase-encoding gradient and thus produce the same signal in each and every acquisition step. Acquiring 256 phase-encoding steps will thus improve their signal-to-noise ratio by a factor of 16 compared with a single acquisition. From the shift theorem it follows that this consideration applies for all other pixels as well. This fact is responsible for the intrinsic advantage of 2D data acquisition compared with 1D (line scan) or even single-point measurements.

The importance of such considerations has already been mentioned for half-Fourier imaging; acquiring only one-half the data leads to a loss in signal-to-noise ratio by a factor of $\sqrt{2}$ if the size of the voxels is maintained. For the acquisition of the central half of k-space, this signal loss, of course, is more than compensated by the fact that the voxel size is effectively doubled by this particular selection of k-space lines.

If the spatial resolution is increased by going from 256 to 512 phase-encoding steps, the same argument applies; the reduction of the voxel size by a factor of 2 is countered by a gain of $\sqrt{2}$ due to the increased number of ''averaging'' steps. The resulting image will thus suffer from a loss in signal-to-noise ratio by only a factor of $\sqrt{2}$, which still is often considered as prohibitive and allows the acquisition of 512 $\times$ 512 or even 1024 $\times$ 1024 only for images with a very high intrinsic S/N ratio.

The effective averaging taking place for each phase-encoding step is especially beneficial for true 3D acquisition compared with consecutive slice-selective imaging. Since data from all spins are acquired in all acquisition steps, $n_{2D} \times n_{3D}$ acquisition steps will lead to an improvement of a factor $\sqrt{n_{3D}}$ compared with consecutive acquisition of parallel 2D images.

Increasing the number of phase-encoding steps while maintaining the spatial resolution is often preferable to averaging, since it leads to an increased field of view in the phase-encoding direction and thus reduces the danger of aliasing artefacts. Especially for 3D acquisitions, where the small voxel size sets a lower limit regarding the number of averages to be used, it is most often advisable to invest the necessary number of repetitions into a large matrix and dispense with averaging altogether.

Signal-to-Noise Ratio and Fast Imaging. Given these very basic arguments, a reference signal-to-noise ratio can be defined using common imaging parameters. A typical data-acquisition time is on the order of 10 ms per projection, corresponding to a bandwidth of 50 kHz. For a typical image matrix of 256 $\times$ 256, this leads to a total net acquisition time of 256 $\times$ 10 ms = 2.56 s. This is the minimum time necessary to acquire all k-space data for that particular bandwidth, omitting all practical limitations given by the gradient and rf system. No matter what exceedingly clever imaging sequence is being used, a shorter acquisition time maintaining the same resolution can only be achieved at the cost of an increased sampling bandwidth with a concordant reduction in signal-to-noise ratio. This loss in signal-to-noise ratio sets the final limitation for the speed of

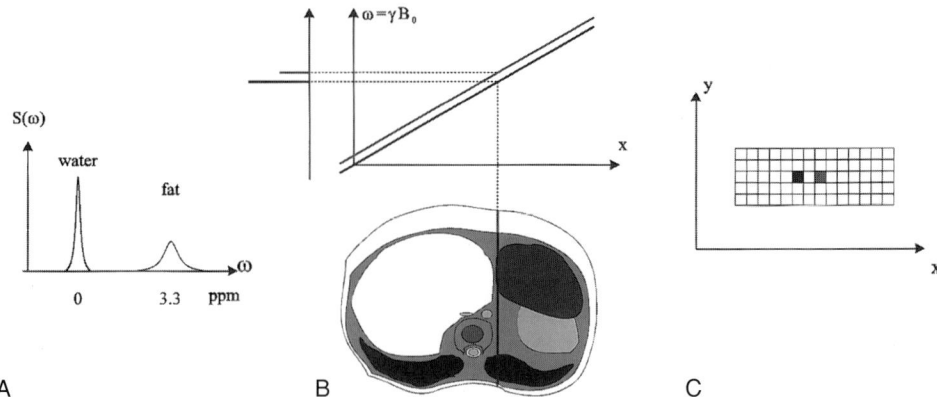

Figure 25. Chemical-shift misregistration. The proton signals from fat and water are separated by about 3.3 ppm **(A)**. This chemical-shift frequency adds to the gradient-dependent Larmor frequency. Fat (*red*) and water (*blue*) spins from the same position will thus be slightly displaced in the spectrum measured under the gradient **(B)** and thus appear shifted in the final image **(C)**. See Color Plate 26.

MRI. Even if space age technology would eventually allow the acquisition of an image in let's say 10 ms, the resulting signal-to-noise ratio would be at least 16 times lower compared with the reference value and thus be practically useless for most purposes. The practical compromise chosen for many of the subsecond acquisition sequences in use today is a reduction in the image resolution, which brings the signal-to-noise ratio back to tolerable levels. It must be emphasized that this limitation is a very fundamental one that does not depend on the actual sequence being used and which can only be alleviated if dramatic improvements in the basic signal-to-noise ratio can be achieved.

Chemical-Shift Misregistration

It has already been pointed out in the introduction that nuclei in different molecular surroundings ''see'' slightly different magnetic fields due to interactions between the outer field and the electrons inside the molecule. This chemical shift effect is extremely useful for MR spectroscopy, which will be discussed elsewhere. For MRI, only two different tissue moieties have to be taken into consideration, which are characterized by different chemical shifts. The signals from free water, which makes up most of the signal observed in MRI, and those from protons in aliphatic groups are separated by a chemical-shift difference of about 3 to 3.5 ppm (Fig. 25A and Color Plate 26).

Fourier transformation does not, of course, distinguish between frequency differences caused by chemical shift and those caused by gradients. A signal from fatty tissue will thus look exactly like one from water protons at a slightly different location. As a consequence, fatty tissue will appear slightly displaced (see Fig. 25C) (190).

For a conventional imaging scheme, where data are acquired line by line by repeating the same projection step with all parameters identical except an increment of the phase-encoding gradient, this displacement takes place only in the read direction, since corresponding data points in the phase-encoding direction are read out at identical acquisition times. (For more sophisticated acquisition schemes, this need not necessarily be true.) As an example, let us take an image acquired on a 1-T magnet using a matrix size of 256 × 256 shift, a field of view of 25 cm, and an acquisition bandwidth of 25 kHz. The pixel size in frequency units will then be given by approximately 3.3 ppm at 1 T, corresponding to a frequency shift of 140 Hz, or 1.4 pixels. Chemical-shift misregistration will be decreased when the size of the pixel in frequency units is increased. For a given field of view, this is achieved by increasing the gradient amplitude and the acquisition bandwidth. The penalty for this is a reduction of signal-to-noise ratio. It should be noted that chemical-shift misregistration goes up with increasing field strength. At 0.2 T, where

3 ppm correspond to roughly 25 Hz, it is more or less negligible, whereas on a 4-T system (which is the strongest field for whole-body systems currently available) it will be more than 500 Hz and requires extremely strong gradients in order to keep it at a tolerable level.

It should be noted that chemical-shift misregistration also occurs in the slice-selection direction; the selected slice for lipids will always be slightly displaced from that of water protons. The extent of the displacement will depend on the ratio of the bandwidth of the excitation pulse to the chemical-shift difference. For a 1-T system, the chemical-shift difference of 130 Hz amounts to something like a 10% chemical-shift displacement if pulses with a typical bandwidth of 1000 to 1500 Hz are being used.

MRI HARDWARE

From the requirements for an imaging sequence, it is apparent that an MRI system must contain a magnet, electronics for generating rf pulses, an rf transmitter, gradients (and their power supplies), rf coils, the analogue and digital components for signal processing, and finally, a powerful computer to handle all image-acquisition steps as well as to provide an intuitive and easy-to-use user interface for the technician who operates the machine and who is not necessarily an expert in MRI methodology nor a computer enthusiast. The requirements for a routine system are reliability, optimal image quality, low downtime, and high reproducibility, all at the lowest cost possible. Naturally, some compromise has to be made in practice, since not all criteria can be met simultaneously. In the following, some essential features of the salient components will be discussed.

Magnet

The magnet is the single most expensive part of most MRI systems. The vast majority of MRI systems built today use superconductive magnets (Fig. 26). Superconductors allow achievement of high magnetic fields up to currently 4 T for a whole-body system. The fact that the magnet has to be charged only on installation and will maintain its

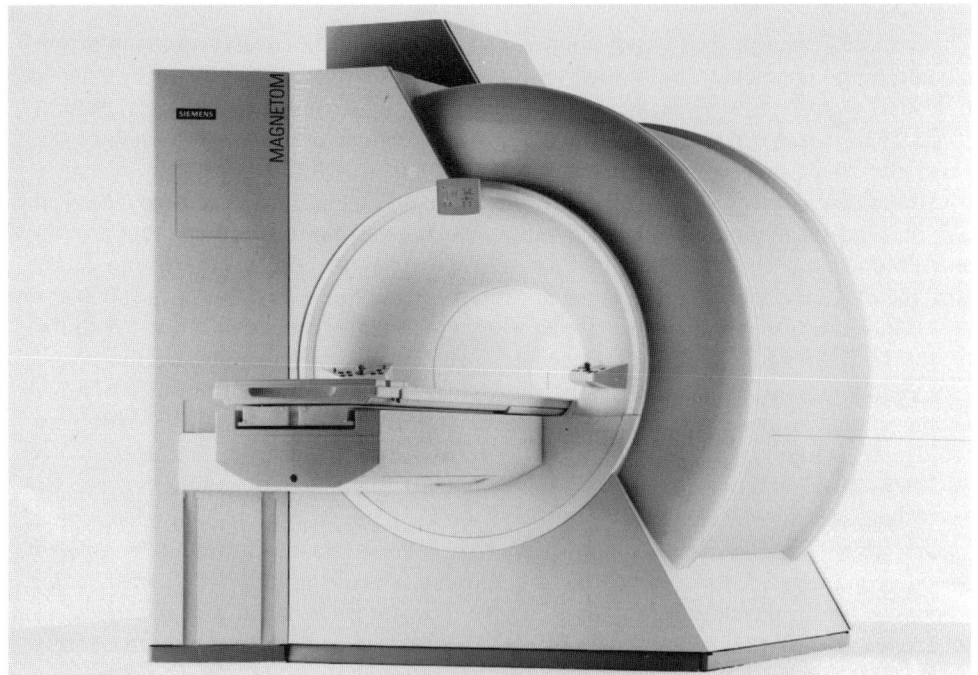

Figure 26. Routine MRI system with superconductive magnet. (Harmony Magnetom Vision, Siemens, Germany.)

magnetic field as long as the very low temperature of $-269°C$ (4 K) is maintained leads to a very high temporal stability of the magnetic field. The very high current density that can be sustained by the superconductive wire allows the construction of very compact magnets with very high homogeneity.

A disadvantage of this technology is the high cost of the superconductive wire (Nb/Ti and Nb/Sn) as well as the complex technology of manufacturing. The requirement of cooling by liquid helium is no problem in industrialized countries but a serious concern in developing nations. A further limitation is the very costly development of new designs caused by the fact that a superconductive coil cannot be unwound after fabrication. A magnet has therefore to work on the first try; later modifications are not possible. This has led to a very reluctant progress in the development of new designs. A further limitation for the magnet design is the need to keep the coil at ultralow temperature, which requires additional space for the insulating dewar.

Most current magnet designs (at least up to field strengths of 2 T) use self-shielded magnets, where the magnet contains two coils with opposite polarity such that the desired magnetic field is achieved inside the magnet, whereas the field outside the magnet drops off very fast. This allows placement of MRI systems inside a hospital room with moderate space requirements, whereas for earlier nonshielded magnets the use of adjacent rooms up to 10 m away from the magnet was severely limited by the magnetic fringe field, which prohibited the use of sensitive electronic equipment like computers, patient monitoring devices, etc. Access to this fringe field area also had to be restricted to persons carrying pacemakers and other electronic supports.

High-temperature superconductors currently offer no solution to any of the problems of superconductive magnets. Apart from the fact that currently no such material exists except for some microscopic laboratory specimen that can sustain the necessary high current and magnetic field, an MRI magnet built from such a still hypothetical material will be extremely expensive due to the very difficult manufacturing process of these very brittle materials. A technically more feasible perspective for dealing with the problem of the use of liquid helium is further advancement in cooling technology. Current helium coolers already allow a reduction of the helium refill interval to several months. In one prototype magnet system, helium has already been totally avoided in favor of direct cooling of the magnet coil via thermal contact with a cooling device (GE MRT, General Electric, Milwaukee, WI).

Conventional magnets built from copper wire are drastically cheaper to manufacture compared with supercons. The limited current density that can be sustained by copper wire leads, however, to very bulky designs with very high current requirements, even at field strength, that are moderate compared with superconductors. A field strength of 0.2 to 0.3 T for whole-body magnets is the current maximum, which can be achieved for a reasonably compact magnet with tolerable current requirements. Even then the electrical power demand for the magnet is considerable, which is not only an ecologic but also an economic concern. The increased bulkiness of a copper magnet also does not allow achievement of magnetic field homogeneities in the same range as those for a superconductor. Since the susceptibility effects caused by the inhomogeneous field scale with the magnetic field strength, the disadvantages of such field inhomogeneities are much less severe than commonly perceived for such low-field systems, especially since a number of techniques exist that allow the production of high-quality images even in extremely inhomogeneous fields.

A further disadvantage of resistive magnets is their low temporal stability caused by the fact that the magnetic field directly depends on the external power supply. Even with stabilized power supplies, the stability of such systems is drastically limited compared with superconductors. This is, of course, an important issue, especially for the installation of such systems in developing countries, where they are often installed rather than superconductors due to helium supply problems. The reduced performance of such systems caused by their lower field is then further compromised by stability issues.

Permanent magnets built from magnetic material alone without any supportive electromagnetic coil have become more or less obsolete. Although they possess the intrinsic

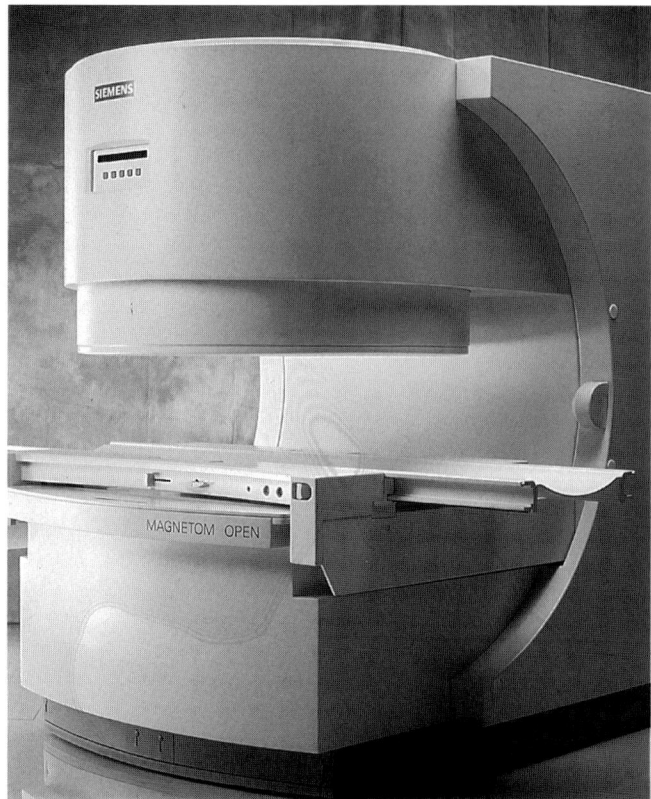

Figure 27. Resistive magnet used in a low-field system operating at 0.2 T. (Magnetom OPEN, Siemens, Germany.)

advantage of no electrical power consumption, their disadvantages of high weight even for low magnetic fields and—even more critical—the extreme temperature stability required for maintaining a tolerable field homogeneity have pushed these systems from the market.

Combinations of resistive magnets with some supporting magnetic yoke are currently proliferating, especially to serve the market in developing countries. They offer field strength on the order of 0.2 to 0.3 T at a reasonable power consumption of 25 to 50 kW and are considerably cheaper to manufacture compared with superconductors (Fig. 27). Whether the attainable image quality is sufficient to proliferate such systems even in developed countries as economic alternatives to more costly conventional systems is open to discussion and requires further developments.

An important current trend is the development of dedicated magnets for a limited range of applications. Such developments are driven by two often conflicting motivations; one is to provide economic systems that are deemed to be adequate for a reduced but still relevant field of applications. An example is a system based on small magnets built for examinations of the extremities. The economic constraints for these systems restrict them to resistive magnets with intrinsically reduced performance compared with state-of-the-art systems even for the desired range of applications. The discussion of the usefulness of such systems is more a political issue than a technical one, especially since these systems open the MRI market to new groups of potential MRI users, which opens up a lot of sensitive issues like self-referral and the responsibility for teaching and education.

The second aim for dedicated MRI is to build optimized systems for a range of applications that are not accessible to conventional scanners. These systems are not necessarily cheaper compared with existing ones; given the prototype character of such new developments, they can in fact be quiet costly. An example is high-end open magnets for MRI intervention (Fig. 28).

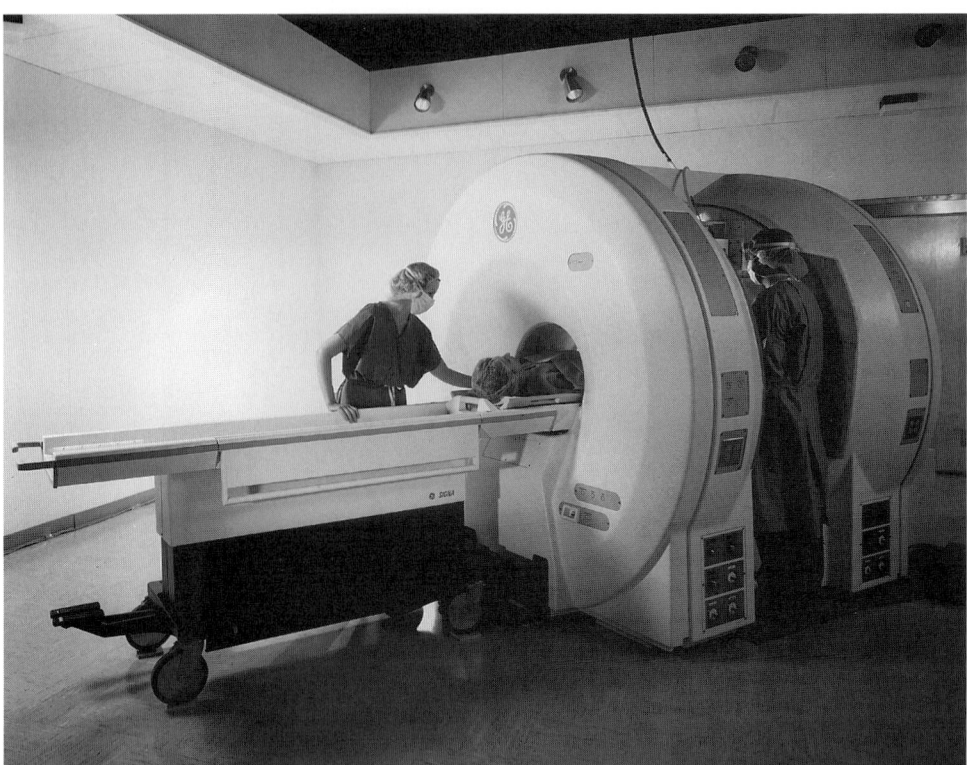

Figure 28. Superconductive 0.5-T magnet system for MRI intervention. (General Electric MRT, Milwaukee, Wisconsin.)

A region of overlap exists between these two groups of novel systems in such that the resistive magnets used for low-end dedicated systems often allow open designs that immediately broaden the range of applications compared with conventional magnets with cylindrical bores. Magnets like the one shown in Fig. 27, which originally were designed as low-end conventional scanners, also allow at least to some degree their use for novel applications such as functional examinations of joints and MRI intervention, especially since the intrinsic demands of these applications with respect to image quality are often considerably reduced compared with those of state-of-the-art MRI diagnosis.

Gradient Coils and Power Supplies

Even preceding the development of actively shielded magnets, active shielding was introduced for gradient systems (140). The motivation was the reduction of eddy currents, which are induced in the metallic and therefore electrically conductive container vessels of superconductive magnets. The structural components of superconductive magnets are commonly built from stainless steel (more recently also from special aluminum alloys). Attempts to replace these metal parts by nonconducting materials have failed due to poor performance under the extreme conditions of ultralow temperature and ultrahigh vacuum required for thermal insulation.

Current loops induced by fast gradient switching can in return cause gradients of opposite polarity that decay only slowly. These gradients interfere with the imaging gradients and can lead to drastic image artefacts, especially for sequences that require highly exact gradient switching.

Conventional whole-body gradient systems were characterized until recently by an amplitude of 10 mT/m and 1 ms switching time. Currently, a generation change has taken place in gradient coil design, as well as in the performance of gradient power supplies. Current state-of-the-art performance parameters are a gradient amplitude of 25 mT/m and a switching time of 0.1 to 0.5 ms. Dedicated gradient systems allow even

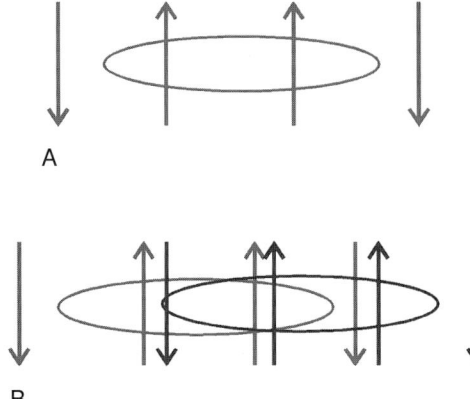

Figure 29. Principle of phased-array coils. A basic axiom of electromagnetism states that the receptive field of a coil is identical to the field generated by a current going through the coil. For a circular single-coil arrangement **(A)** the magnetic fields inside and outside the coil have opposite polarity. In a phased-array coil arrangement **(B)** two coils are intersected such that the field components of each coil inside the other cancel (opposed vectors) such that each coil "sees" only its own receptive field.

faster and stronger gradients. Especially small gradient head coils offer exceedingly high performance with comparatively modest power requirements as a consequence of the fact that the voltage and current demands for a given performance scale with the volume of the gradient coil.

The higher gradient performance allows improvements in imaging speed and quality that open up totally new applications for clinical and especially functional MRI.

rf Coils

A generation change similar in consequence to the leap forward in gradient technology is currently taking place in the design of receiver coils due to the introduction of so-called phased-array coils (115). These coils use an assembly of smaller coils rather than a single large coil in order to maximize the signal-to-noise ratio even for examinations of larger volumes, as in whole-body examinations or examinations of the spine. When conventional surface coils are closely spaced around the volume examined, the signals generated in them will interfere with each other. As a result, such an assembly will not perform better (in fact, normally worse) compared with one single coil. For certain geometric arrangements, the interference can, however, be canceled such that the coils operate truly independent of each other. Each coil will therefore only "see" the limited amount of noise generated in the receptive volume, which is independent of the noise seen by the other coils (Fig. 29). The signal generated in the coils will therefore add up linearly, whereas the noise will grow only as the square root of the number of coils. The total signal-to-noise ratio will therefore be improved drastically compared with a single-coil arrangement.

Originally, phased-array coils were developed for examinations of the spine, where high resolution is desired as well as coverage of a large volume. Meanwhile, such designs have appeared for practically all regions of the body, leading to a significant leap in image quality. The number of segment coils, of course, cannot be increased without limit, since the penetration depth will be determined by the size of one such segment. An array of too many too small coils consequently will deliver high-quality images only from a small volume at the surface of the patient.

rf Transmitter and Receiver Systems

The current trend in the rf transmitter and receiver systems goes to the introduction of more and more digital components, which are easier to produce and maintain compared with analog components. Fully digital signal generation and reception are currently possible up to a few megahertz. Consequently, MRI systems typically use carrier frequencies generated by an analog synthesizer. The signal modulation for generation of the phase- and amplitude-modulated rf pulses as well as the processing of the received signal after downconversion with the carrier frequency is more and more taken over by digital electronics. Tube amplifiers used for the signal transmitters in earlier systems have been more and more replaced by solid-state amplifiers, which offer much better linearity and higher stability and reproducibility.

Computer Platform

A further generation change is taking place regarding the computer platform for modern MRI systems. The previously used midsize mainframe computers are more and more replaced by powerful workstations (SUN, Silicon Graphics). The advantage of such workstations is the availability of a huge amount of processing programs, which are available for such more or less standardized platforms. This includes simple and reliable tools for generating a user-friendly interface as well as sophisticated tools for signal processing. The explosion in postprocessing possibilities afforded by such synergetic effects as compared with the isolated efforts of the previous system software packages has only just begun. Its full potential will only be used when the system software is rewritten to conform to such standards. Current solutions often do not use the full potential of the new platforms due to only half-hearted conversion of the very complex system software to the new platforms. Especially applications in functional examinations tremendously benefit from open software architectures in order to accommodate the various postprocessing routines necessary to derive the functional information from the acquired images.

The high internal flexibility of MRI systems is in marked contrast to the hard-wired solutions common to other modalities. This increasingly flexible design is caused by the still rapid development of MRI methodology, which makes any hard-wired solution obsolete within unreasonably short times. The full flexibility is, however, not accessible to the common user, who works with a still huge number of factory-approved methods. The introduction of new methods very often requires only the downloading of new software, since the system architecture often already allows the realization of new acquisition techniques. Similarly to the developments in the general computer market, the software consequently becomes more and more important compared with hardware developments.

IMAGING SEQUENCES

The literature on MRI techniques contains an abundant variety of different sequences characterized by more or less fancy acronyms. Even when the redundance of such labels, which is caused by the fact that each manufacturer of MRI equipment uses a different name for one and the same sequence, is taken into account, there still remains a quite significant number of different techniques.

Very often imaging sequences are treated in textbooks more or less according to the chronologic order in which they appeared in the literature. Although such an approach does justice to the historical development of the field, it is less appropriate for getting a systematic overview of the various approaches used for generating an image. In the following, historical reminiscences to early imaging schemes that have not found acceptance in current scanners are therefore omitted, and a classification is used according to the different strategies for acquiring k-space data.

In terms of spatial encoding, the task of designing an MRI sequence can be reformulated into finding a means to sample the k-space data necessary for image reconstruction (see the section, "The Fourier Transformation," above). Basically, there are two vehicles that can be used to travel along k-space (Fig. 30). The first is application of a gradient along any of the image dimensions; this will lead to a k-space trajectory in a direction and speed defined by the amplitude of the gradient. The second means of moving around k-space is a refocusing pulse, which inverts the phase and thus brings the spin system to a point located symmetrically across the origin of k-space.

Practically all MRI sequences in routine use today use a rectilinear k-space trajectory. The main reason for this is the fact that a fast computer algorithm called *fast Fourier transform* (FFT) exists for this special case, whereas Fourier transformation of data ac-

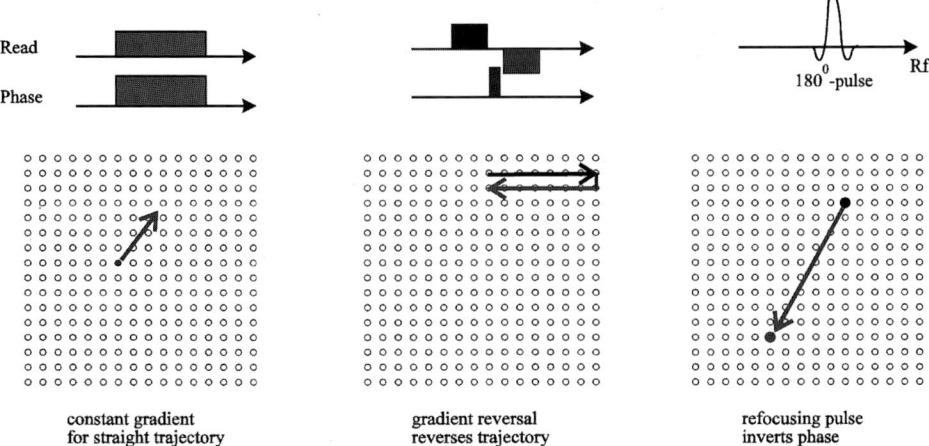

Figure 30. Vehicles in *k*-space. Traveling in *k*-space can be performed basically by two (and just two) different means. Applying a gradient along the direction of the readout gradient and/or the phase-encoding gradient will lead to a trajectory in the direction of the combined gradients (*left*). The figure in the middle shows how three gradient lobes can be used to start a regular line-by-line scan. A refocusing pulse (*right*) will bring the spin system to a point that is mirror symmetric to the origin.

quired along arbitrary trajectories requires significantly longer computation times. Data acquired along nonrectilinear trajectories are in fact normally interpolated onto a rectilinear grid and then transformed by fast Fourier transform in order to avoid the excessive computation times for full Fourier transformation.

Acquisition of one line of *k*-space is very fast and efficient, since it requires data sampling under a constant gradient. For a typical choice of parameters, one such phase-encoding step is typically acquired in about 5 to 20 ms; for fast imaging techniques, acquisition times below 1 ms can be used. The critical step comes after the end of one *k*-space line is reached. There are basically two options on how to continue data acquisition. One is to wait until the spin system has more or less gone back to equilibrium and repeat the acquisition with different phase encoding starting again at the zero point in *k*-space. The sampling speed of such a multiexcitation experiment will be determined mainly by the relaxation behavior between two projection steps. With the commonly long T1 relaxation times of biologic tissue, the waiting time can be appreciably longer than the actual acquisition time in order to maintain a decent signal-to-noise ratio. One possibility to fill this waiting time is to perform a multislice experiment in which the same projection step is applied to parallel slices until the repetition time that leads to the desired T1 contrast is reached (Fig. 31). Since most diagnostic examinations require imaging of a volume that is larger than a single slice, such multislice experiments can be very efficient despite the fact that they often require imaging times of a few minutes.

The second possibility to continue sampling after reaching the end of one *k*-line is to use either gradients or rf pulses or combinations of both in order to trace additional projection lines to fill more than one line of *k*-space per excitation. In the extreme, this approach leads to single excitation techniques that yield one image within very short times around or even below 1 s.

Given the 5- to 20-ms acquisition time per projection, the total pure acquisition time for a 256 × 256 image is on the order of 1.28 to 5.12 s. Most actual imaging sequences require much longer acquisition times. The main reason for the limited sampling efficiency is technical constraints, mainly determined by the limited slew rate of the magnetic field gradients, which need to be switched in order to first select a slice and second to perform proper spatial encoding. Using state-of-the-art gradient systems, the efficiency of data acquisition, which previously was on the order of 10% to 30%, has been increased to 50% or more depending on the actual imaging system used. This does not necessarily mean that all sequences produce one image every 5 s or so. For many multislice tech-

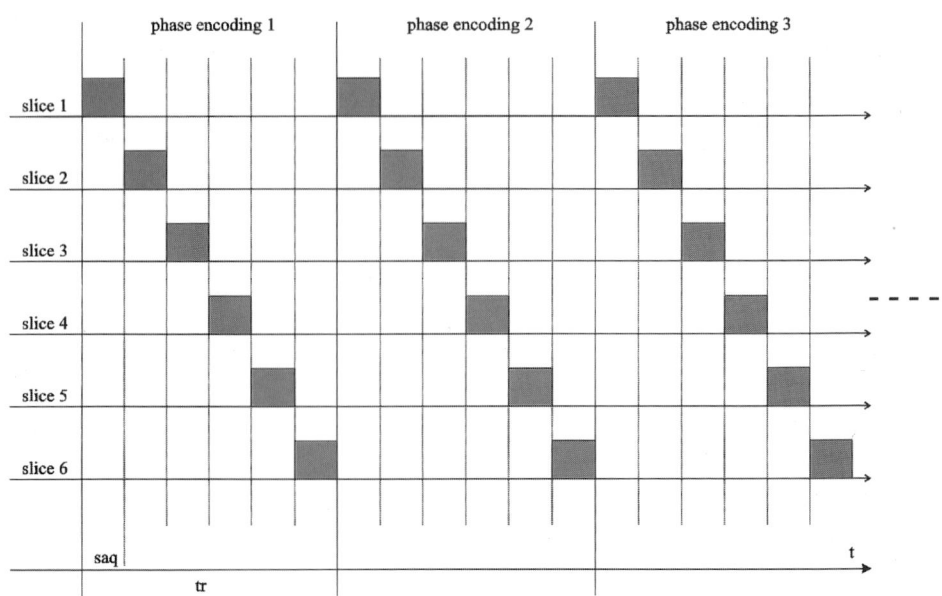

Figure 31. Principle of multislice acquisition. During the waiting time t_r and after finishing data acquisition in one slice (*shaded area*), data are acquired from parallel sections. The number of slices that can be acquired is defined by t_r/s_{aq}, where s_{aq} is the time required for acquisition of a single projection step.

niques, the total acquisition time still lies in the range of a few minutes, during which, however, a considerable number of parallel sections can be imaged.

It should be noted that even with a 100% duty cycle, the image-acquisition time will still be on the order of a few seconds. A reduction of this acquisition time requires shorter acquisition times per line, which—according to the subsection "*k*-Space," above—is invariably accompanied by a reduction in signal-to-noise ratio. Currently, the discussion on fast imaging is focused on the speed and amplitude of the gradient systems, which determine how close to 100% efficiency a given experiment can be performed. The real ultimate limit to imaging speed, however, is signal-to-noise ratio, not gradient performance.

Naturally, the two pure sampling strategies, of course, are only the extremes of a continuum. Methods where more than one *k*-line is acquired per excitation but more than one excitation is used to generate the whole *k*-space data set are often referred to as *hybrid techniques* of the basic single-scan sequence. The term *segmented scan* is used commonly to refer to data-acquisition schemes where the *k*-lines are acquired in several separated groups like the acquisition of a few *k*-lines per ECG cycles for cardiac imaging.

Apart from categorizing imaging techniques into single-excitation or multiexcitation scans, a further distinction can be made according to whether gradient echoes or spin echoes are used for signal generation. Hybrid approaches are also possible, where some of the signals are acquired by gradient reversal and others by spin-echo refocusing.

A very important consideration involves effects caused by the finite sampling time required for data acquisition in any acquisition scheme. In a strict sense, a true image will only be generated by Fourier transformation if all *k*-space points are represented equally. Due to various mechanisms (T1 and T2 relaxation and T2* effects), this condition is not fulfilled in any practical imaging sequence. In addition, phase modulations of the signal will occur due to various mechanisms. Both will lead to typical image artefacts, a general discussion of which was given in the section, "The Fourier Transformation," above. The extent to which any of these mechanisms is relevant for a given sequence will strongly depend on the *k*-space trajectory chosen. In the following, the major sources of artefacts will be discussed for each sequence apart from the intrinsic contrast behavior, since this is one major determining factor in selecting a sequence for a given task.

POCKET DICTIONARY OF COMMONLY USED TERMS IN MRI

Multislice imaging	Imaging scheme in which the same phase-encoding step is acquired consecutively on different (and most often parallel) slices. For n slices and m phase-encoding steps, image acquisition thus follows the sequence (slice selection)$_n$ − (phase encoding)$_m$
Multiexcitation	Imaging scheme in which data are acquired by repeating the same basic imaging sequence and varying the phase-encoding gradient from one acquisition to the next.
Single-shot acquisition	Imaging scheme in which all phase-encoding steps necessary for image reconstruction are acquired after a single excitation pulse.
Hybrid imaging	Formerly used for techniques in which more than one (but not all) phase-encoding steps are acquired per excitation; meanwhile applied in a more general sense for those imaging techniques which are perceived to be conceptionally derived from more generic techniques
Segmented scan	Imaging scheme in which acquisition is performed in segments during each of which a fraction of the total number of phase-encoding steps is acquired

Multiexcitation Sequences

Imaging Properties

In multiexcitation sequences, signal is read out such that each excitation produces one line of k-space. The signal intensity and therefore the image contrast will depend on the evolution of the magnetization prior to data acquisition. Data points along the phase-encoding direction will have (at least in principle) identical weight, since they are required at identical time points during the signal evolution. As long as no variations of the signal amplitude and/or phase exist from one excitation to the next, the image will therefore be a true image in the phase-encoding direction. This condition, however, is not trivial to meet. Especially motion-related effects (pulsatile blood flow and/or breathing) will lead to scan-to-scan nonreproducibility and thus to distinct image artefacts in the phase-encoding direction of the image (94).

The transformation properties in the read direction depend on the signal behavior during data acquisition. The most notable and ubiquitous artefact will be chemical misregistration. It will lead to an apparent displacement of lipid compartments compared with aqueous solutions in the read direction of the image (see the section ''The Physics of Image Formation,'' above and Fig. 25) (190). The effect is minimized if the acquisition bandwidth is large. Since a large bandwidth results in a lower S/N ratio, some sensible compromise has to be found for a given application. Typical values are on the order of 25 to 100 kHz. For lower field systems, smaller bandwidths can be chosen, since the misregistration scales with the field strengths.

Another potential source of artefacts is signal dephasing across the acquisition window. This effect is normally small, since the acquisition time t_{aq} is in general smaller than the T2* of the tissues (t_{aq} = 5 to 20 ms as compared with T2* = 30 to 50 ms). Even for T2* = t_{aq}, the signal amplitude will have dropped only to about 60% at the side of the acquisition window. The resulting signal broadening will be less than the dephasing across each voxel caused by the application of the phase-encoding gradient and will be only appreciable in high-resolution imaging of very thin slices.

The extent and severity of these effects will depend, of course, on the actual pulse sequence used and its relevant parameters.

Spin-Echo Sequence

The spin-echo sequence was the most commonly used imaging sequence during the first decade of clinical MRI (9, 20, 37, 38, 75, 111, 113, 163, 207). Its diagram has already been shown in Fig. 18. The observed signal intensities depend on the parameter's spin density ρ, T1, and T2, which will lead to different image contrast depending on the chosen experimental parameters (echo time t_e, repetition time t_r) (Fig. 32). Although this contrast behavior is more complex compared with the one-dimensional contrast mechanism of x-ray computed tomography, it is nevertheless well behaved enough to deliver images with predictable contrast in a reliable and reproducible fashion. T2* effects—especially effects of the main field inhomogeneity and susceptibility effects that might vary depending on the experimental conditions—are canceled due to spin-echo refocusing. The imaging behavior of spin-echo sequences is therefore extremely benign.

Figure 32 shows the image-contrast dependence on the recovery time t_r and the echo time t_e according to the contrast mechanisms described earlier. For diagnostic imaging, the regimes of spin-density-weighted imaging and T1- and T2-weighted imaging constitute useful imaging modes (Fig. 33). A combination of short t_r with long t_e leads to images with poor signal-to-noise ratios and poor contrast. This is due to the fact that the contrast mechanisms for T1- and T2-weighted scans are running against each other; a T1-weighted scan uses a short recovery time t_r such that signals from tissues with long

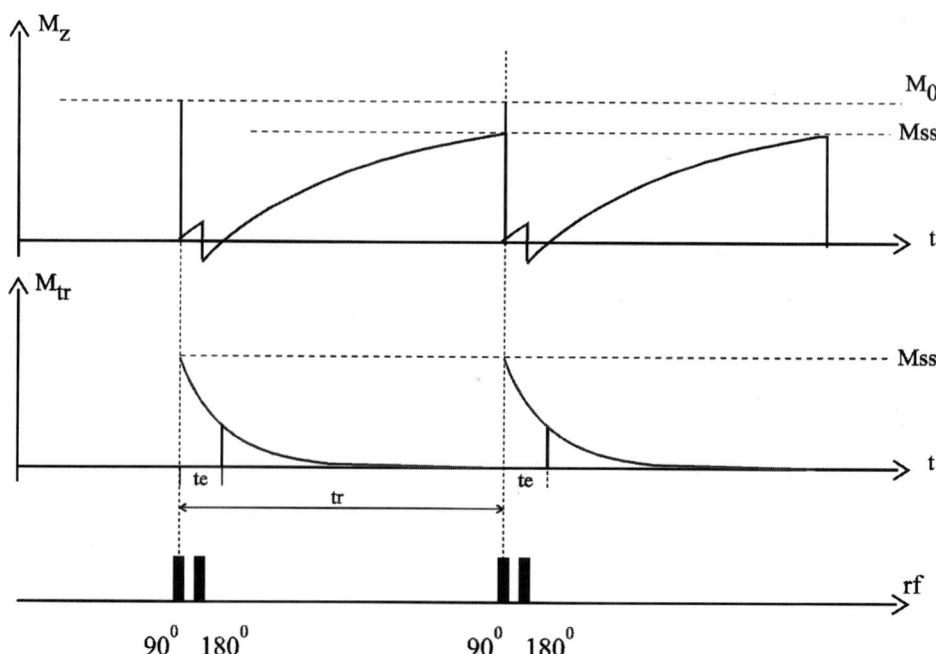

Figure 32. Contrast behavior of spin-echo sequences. The signal intensity in a spin-echo experiment depends on the repetition time t_r, during which T1 relaxation of the z-magnetization M_z into a steady state M_{ss} takes place (*upper diagram*), and the echo time t_e, during which the transverse magnetization M_{tr} decays by T2 relaxation (*lower diagram*). Note the zigzag curve for the T1 relaxation caused by the 180° refocusing pulse, which inverts the already recovered z-magnetization in contrast to the pure progressive saturation experiment shown in Fig. 10.

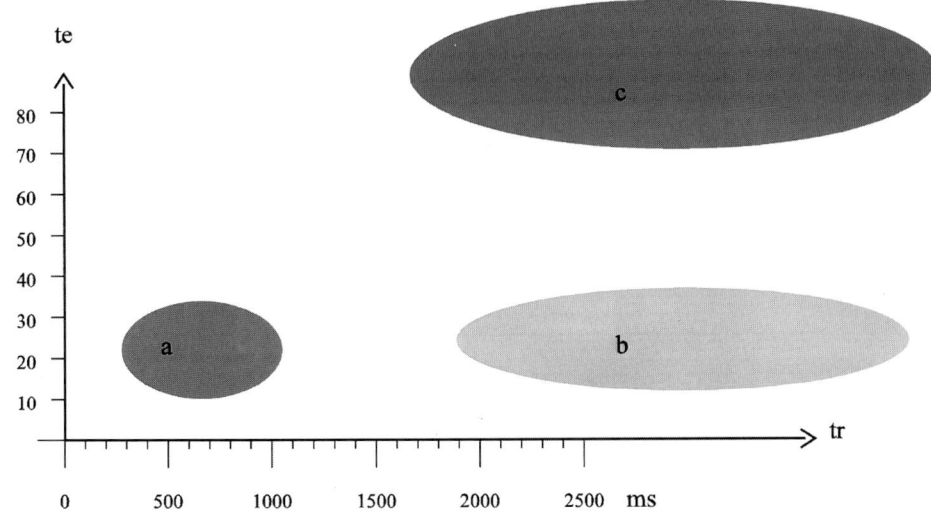

Figure 33. Parameter regimes for spin-echo imaging. Depending on the echo time t_e and the recovery time t_r, images can be roughly categorized as T1-weighted images (*a*), spin-density images (*b*), and T2-weighted images (*c*).

T1 suffer stronger attenuation and therefore yield less signal compared with tissues with short T1 at identical spin density.

For T2 weighting by use of long echo times t_e, tissues with long T2 will give more signal compared with tissues with short T2. In general, the T1 and T2 values of tissues behave in parallel; tissues with long T1 will have longer T2, and vice versa, although the absolute values of T1 and T2 often differ by a factor of 10 or more.

A combination with long t_e with short t_r will thus more or less nullify the contrast between tissues, which is normally undesired in diagnostic applications.

The recovery time t_r is normally used in diagnostic imaging in order to characterize the T1 contrast. Often it is not clear whether the t_r given really signifies the time of recovery, which is the time between the last pulse in a sequence and the next excitation pulse, or the repetition time t_{rep} of the whole sequence. t_r and t_{rep} are connected by

$$t_{rep} = t_r + (n - \tfrac{1}{2})t_e \tag{12}$$

where n is the number of equally spaced echoes. Even if this correction is made, a spin-echo sequence performed with the same t_r compared with a pure progressive saturation sequence will not yield the same contrast due to the T1-dependent differences of the z-magnetization at the start of recovery due to the inversion of z-magnetization by the refocusing pulse (see Fig. 32).

T1-weighted spin-echo sequences, which can be performed within reasonable examination times of 2 to 4 minutes, were the backbone of MRI in the eighties, and they are still in frequent use in many examinations, especially since most diagnostic applications require multislice acquisition. The 20 to 30 projection steps that can be filled into the recovery time of about 500 ms for a T1-weighted scan nicely correlate with the number of slices necessary to get adequate volume coverage for a diagnostic examination. The resulting effective acquisition time of 4 to 6 seconds for one high-resolution image is hard to beat even with sophisticated fast imaging techniques. This sequence—with or without administration of contrast agent—is therefore still a very useful tool in diagnostic imaging despite various faster techniques that have been developed. The intrinsic correction of spin-echo formation for various effects makes it a much more reliable and robust tool compared with more ambitious and sensitive approaches.

T2-weighted imaging using spin-echo sequences with long t_r and long t_e is diagnostically very useful, since many lesions, especially in the central nervous system, appear bright on T2-weighted images. This diagnostic benefit, however, has to be paid for dearly by very long examination times caused by the recovery times on the order of 2 to 4 seconds for such scans. The resulting total acquisition times of 8 to 15 minutes were a major concern regarding patient throughput and consequently the cost-efficiency of diagnostic MRI. The long echo times for T2-weighted scans can be filled by acquiring more than one echo at a late echo time. In the so-called dual-echo sequence, one earlier echo with short t_e is additionally acquired in order to get a spin-density-weighted image. The acquisition of more than one early and one late echo is also possible (63, 74, 76, 79). Due to the vastly increasing number of possible refocusing pathways, however, it becomes more and more difficult to tame all the multiple unwanted signals, which can create severe image artefacts if they occur within the acquisition window (see Fig. 8).

Gradient-Echo Sequence

The gradient-echo sequence omits the formation of a spin echo and directly uses the signal from the free induction decay following the excitation pulse (Fig. 34) (70). From the discussion in the preceding section it is clear that its signal intensity with respect to T1 is considerably higher than that of spin-echo sequences, especially at short repetition times. It therefore has been introduced as one of the first fast imaging techniques useful for routine applications in MRI.

The contrast behavior of gradient-echo sequences is considerably more complex compared with spin-echo sequences (53, 83, 198). The signal generation via inversion of the readout gradient refocuses only the dephasing caused by the preceding negative-gradient lobe. The signal intensity therefore will be identical to that of an FID without any gradient (as long as gradient-dependent effects are ignored). All other mechanisms acting on the FID, such as T2*, chemical shift, susceptibility, etc., will act on the signal phase and/or amplitude. In addition, the short repetition times normally used in gradient-echo imaging lead to the generation of additional signal in the form of spin echoes or stimulated echoes that influence the signal intensity or give rise to artefacts.

T2* Sensitivity and Chemical Shift. The signal of a gradient-echo sequence will be sensitive to various T2* effects, which—contrary to spin-echo acquisition—are not re-

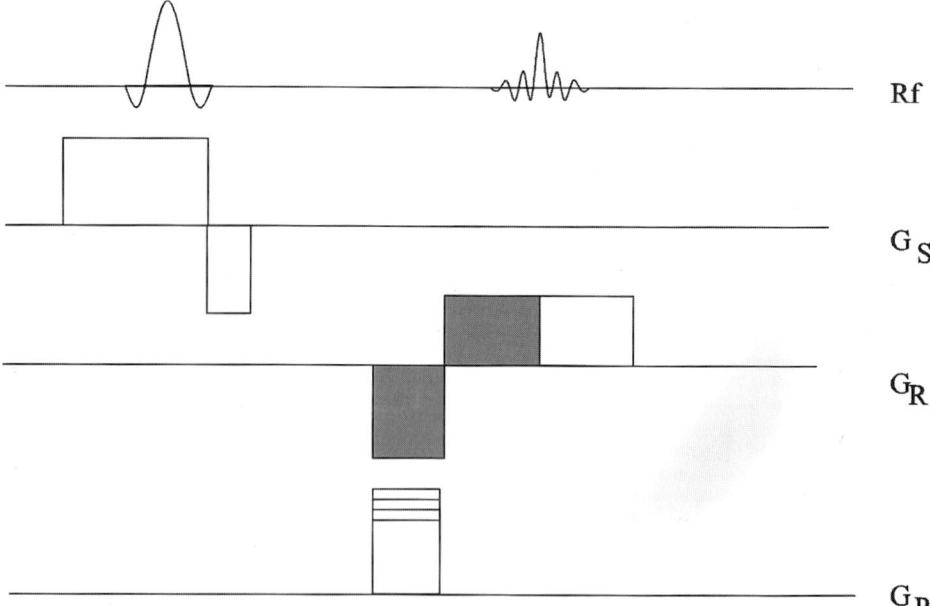

Figure 34. Gradient-echo sequence diagram. *Rf* denotes the rf pulse and signal; G_S, the slice selection gradient; G_R, the readout gradient; and G_P, the phase-encoding gradient. Signal is generated by reversal of the readout gradient and occurs at the time when the area under the positive gradient lobe is equal to the area under the preceding defocusing lobe (*shaded rectangles*).

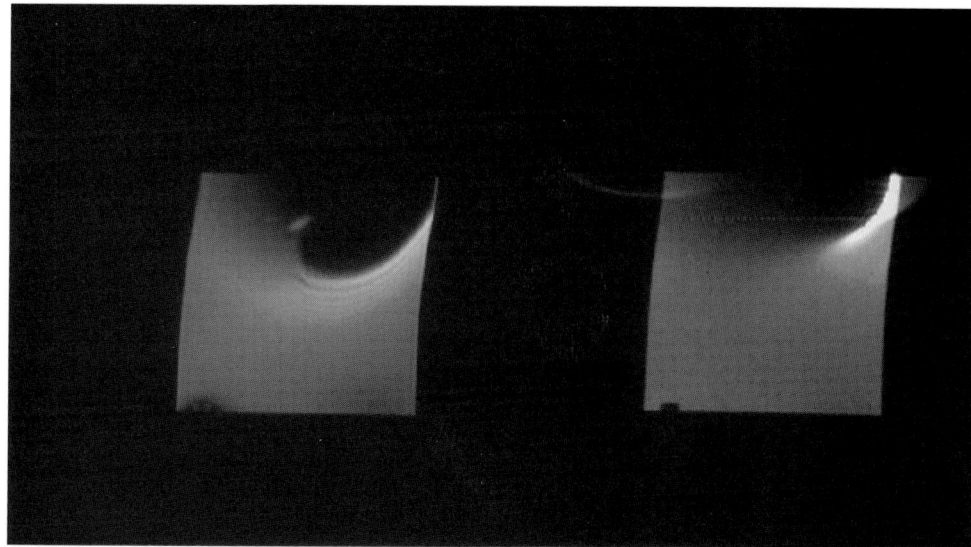

Figure 35. Image acquired with a gradient-echo sequence (*left*) versus a spin-echo image (*right*) in an inhomogeneous field. Both images were acquired with identical parameters, including the receiver bandwidth. The geometric distortions introduced by a paper clip at the top of the square phantom are identical for both methods. The observed amplitude attenuation in the inhomogeneous region is much more pronounced for gradient-echo images.

focused at the time of signal formation (39, 53). These effects will lead to a change in the signal phase and amplitude. Regional variations of the magnetic field along the read-out direction and in the phase-encoding direction will lead primarily to geometric distortions of the image just like in a spin-echo sequence (Fig. 35). In addition, a shift of the echo will occur due to the superposition of the effect of the field inhomogeneity and the gradient. In the readout direction this shift will lead to a shift of the echo time compared with the nominal value determined by the gradient refocusing. A similar shift occurs in the phase-encoding direction for field inhomogeneities along that direction. These shifts are of no practical concern by themselves as long as the amplitude of the readout gradient is large compared with the field inhomogeneity, which is normally (but not always) the case. This susceptibility-dependent shift of the true k-space zero point will increase with increasing echo time. Eventually, the signal in areas with strong local susceptibility effects will get pushed out of the sampled portion of k-space altogether, and the signal from these regions will get lost, which is exactly what has happened in the regions of high field inhomogeneity in Fig. 35.

Magnetic field inhomogeneities in the slice-selection direction will lead to a loss of coherence of spins across the slice and thus to signal attenuation, which is not the case with spin-echo refocusing. Gradient-echo images will thus show the same shape but a different susceptibility-dependent signal attenuation compared with spin-echo images, which is a second factor leading to signal loss in gradient-echo images in Fig. 35. For a linear field inhomogeneity, the dephasing of spins will be proportional to the slice thickness. The gain in signal-to-noise ratio afforded by a thicker slice can then become at least partially compensated by the increased dephasing across the slice. It is thus not always sound advice to try to improve the signal-to-noise ratio in gradient-echo sequences by increasing the slice thickness. Especially in experiments with long echo times, the selection of a thinner slice might be more prudent (Fig. 36).

The second important T2*-related effect acting on the observed signal intensity is chemical shift (see section, "The Physics of Image Formation," above) (5, 171). Since the Larmor frequencies of protons in aqueous and lipid tissues are different (see Fig. 25), their magnetization vectors will show a phase difference that depends on the echo time t_e and the frequency difference $\Delta\sigma$. The observed signal intensity in a gradient-

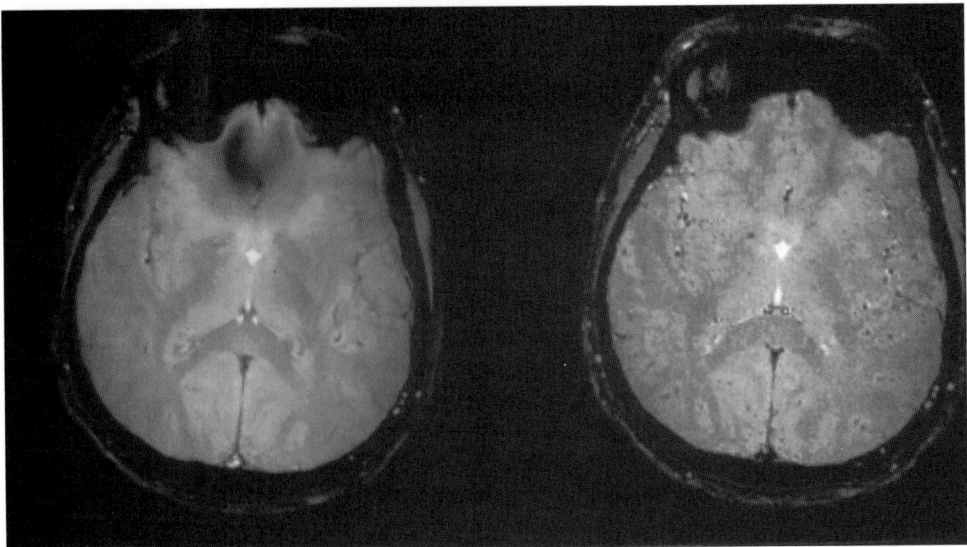

Figure 36. Gradient-echo images of the human head acquired with different slice thicknesses. The signal-to-noise ratio of the image acquired with 8-mm slice thickness (*left*) is much higher compared with a 1-mm image (*right*) in the homogeneous regions at the center of the brain. In the frontal part, however, where strong susceptibility effects occur, the signal in the image with the thicker slice vanishes due to dephasing across the slice, whereas the image on the right shows no significant reduction in signal intensity.

echo experiment will then show an undulating amplitude as a function of t_e. Of special importance are the in-phase and the out-of-phase conditions, which occur at 0, $1/\Delta\sigma$, $2/\Delta\sigma$, . . . (in phase) and $1/(2\Delta\sigma)$, $3/(2\Delta\sigma)$, $5/(2\Delta\sigma)$, . . . (out of phase), respectively, where $\Delta\sigma$ is given in frequency units (Fig. 37 and Color Plate 27). For a 1.5-T magnet, the in-phase echo times are 4.8, 9.6, 14.4, . . . ms, and the out-of-phase echo times are 2.4, 7.2, 12, . . . ms. At lower field strength, the corresponding echo times are proportionally longer.

These numbers are based on $\Delta\sigma$ = 3.3 ppm, which is an approximate mean difference (see Fig. 25). For tissues that contain equal amounts of aqueous and fatty tissue, this

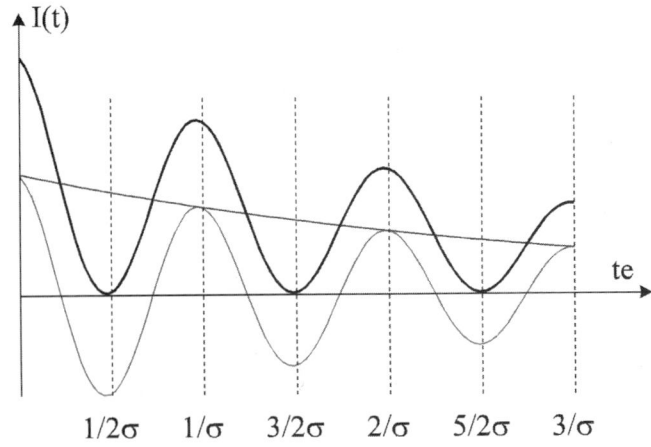

Figure 37. In-phase and out-of-phase effects of chemical shift. The on-resonance signal of water (*blue*) decays with T2* when measured with a gradient-echo sequence. Signal from fat (*red*) in addition shows a chemical-shift-dependent signal modulation. In tissue compartments with equal contributions of fat and water (*black*), this leads to a periodic modulation of the signal amplitude with a period of $1/\sigma$, where σ is the chemical-shift difference between fat and water. See Color Plate 27.

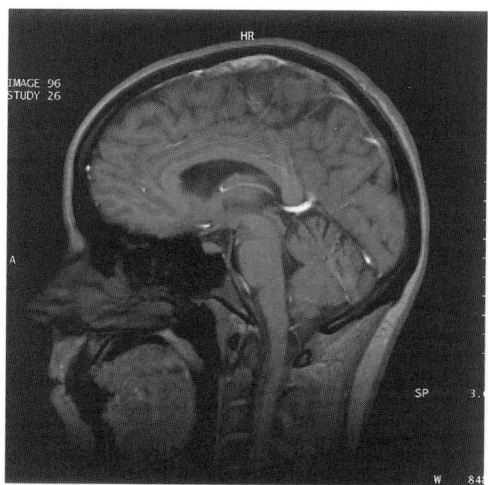 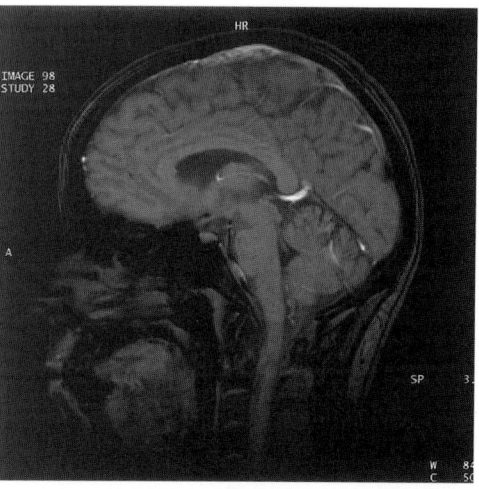

Figure 38. In-phase (*left*) and out-of-phase (*right*) gradient-echo images of a human head (sagittal view). Images were acquired with echo times of 5 and 7.5 ms, respectively, on a 1.5-T system (Siemens Magnetom Vision). Note the artificial darkening at the interface between lipid structures such as subcutaneous fat and tissue. Tissues with mixed content of fatty and aqueous compartments such as bone marrow appear much darker in the out-of-phase image.

effect will lead to periodic cancellations of the signal intensity. This periodic signal behavior can be used to assess the composition of tissue by acquiring images at in-phase and out-of-phase echo times. Care has to be taken, however, in the presence of susceptibility effects. The susceptibility-dependent echo shift might easily lead to a transition from the in-phase to the out-of-phase condition if the susceptibility effect is of the same order as $\Delta \sigma$.

Another consequence of this chemical-shift-dependent dephasing is the occurrence of a dark rim at the interface between fatty and aqueous tissues due to partial volume effects when t_e is chosen to correspond to the out-of-phase condition (Fig. 38). These pronounced dark lines should not be mistaken for true anatomic structures.

The very complex T2*-dependent signal behavior makes it very desirable to perform gradient-echo imaging at the shortest possible echo time, especially in heterogeneous tissue such as the abdomen. The very short echo times at which appreciable effects can occur, however, set severe limitations to the realization of non-T2*-dependent gradient-echo imaging, especially at higher fields. Even at echo times as low as 3 ms, susceptibility effects cannot be neglected at 1.5 T.

T1 Sensitivity. In terms of recovery of longitudinal magnetization, gradient-echo imaging acts as a pure progressive saturation sequence. The considerable literature on this sequence, which has been known in analytical NMR for many decades, is consequently immediately applicable. One important issue is the use of the optimal flip angle to maximize the signal for a given combination of T1 and t_r (Fig. 39). It has been demonstrated that the steady-state transverse magnetization M_{tr} will be reached for a flip angle that is called the *Ernst angle* and is given by

$$M_{tr} = M_0 \frac{1 - \exp(-t_r/T1)}{1 - \cos \alpha \exp(-t_r/T1)} \sin \alpha \qquad (13)$$

This steady state is reached immediately after the first acquisition cycle only if the flip angle is equal to 90°. For smaller flip angles, this initialization period gets progressively longer.

In many imaging applications, optimizing the signal from one tissue is not the major concern. More important is optimizing the contrast between two tissues (such as lesion and healthy tissue). This contrast can be maximized using the difference of the two curves

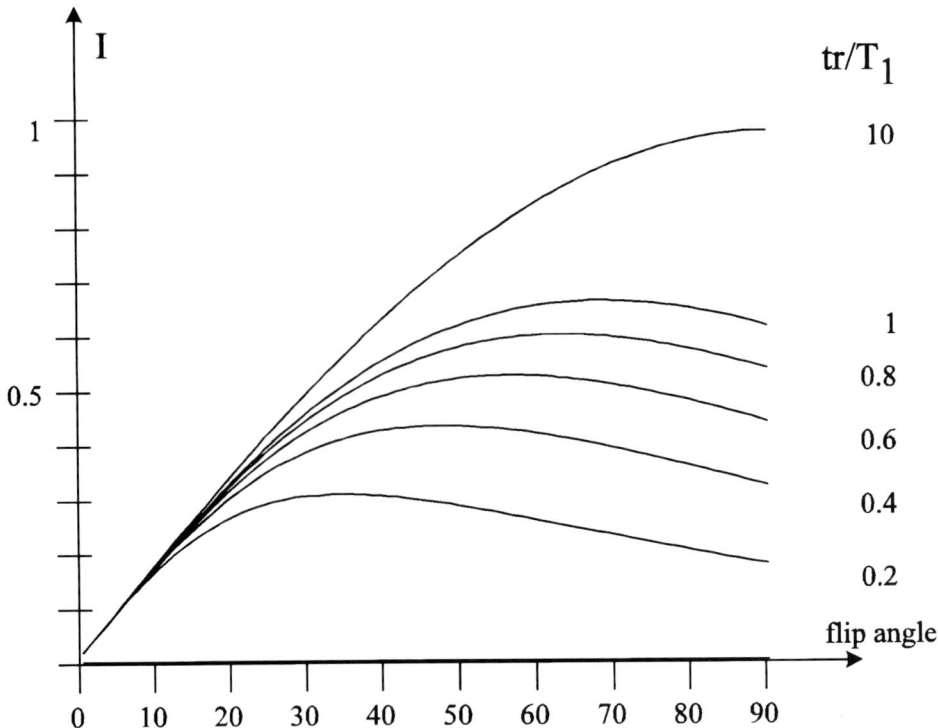

Figure 39. Dependence of the signal intensity on the flip angle for various ratios of $t_r/T1$. It is clearly demonstrated that the optimal flip angle (Ernst angle) decreases with decreasing $t_r/T1$.

representing the $t_r/T1$ of the two tissues. Figure 39 shows, however, that the range of flip angles around the maximum is quite large. Consequently, standardized flip angles are used in most applications.

In slice-selective gradient-echo imaging, a difference in steady-state z-magnetization will occur across the slice due to the imperfect excitation profile. This will considerably attenuate the shape of the slice profile as well as the T1 contrast. T1-weighted gradient-echo images with good rf pulses will show considerably crisper T1 contrast compared with gradient-echo sequences with less well shaped pulses.

T2 Sensitivity: Refocused versus Spoiled Gradient-Echo Imaging. The sensitivity of the FID to T2 is normally overridden by the T2* effects described above. There are, however, other mechanisms by which T2 relaxation can contribute to the signal intensity in gradient-echo imaging.

Earlier, it was demonstrated that any rf pulse will act as a (more or less efficient) refocusing pulse on any transverse magnetization present at the time of its application. For a gradient-echo sequence with short t_r, any subsequent excitation pulse will thus act as a refocusing pulse for previously excited spins. Figure 40 and Color Plate 28 demonstrates the effect of this refocusing behavior. The most notable effect is "even echo refocusing," which will lead to a coincidence of the echo with the FID after two refocusings no matter how strongly signals are defocused within each t_r interval.

Figure 40 also shows the various other signal contributions occurring via various refocusing pathways. Since transverse magnetization decays with T2, all refocused signal contributions will be more or less T2-weighted (53, 80, 83, 90, 96, 198). The combined result of these multiple refocusings is a significant T2 contribution to the observed signal amplitude. The amplitude of these T2-weighted terms strongly depends on the flip angle such that a quantitative assessment of the T2 contrast is not very meaningful in practice, especially for slice-selective pulses with variable effective flip angle across the slice.

The basic amplitude of the direct FID generated by each pulse depends on T1 according to the discussion in the preceding section such that the final image contrast depends on T1 as well as on T2.

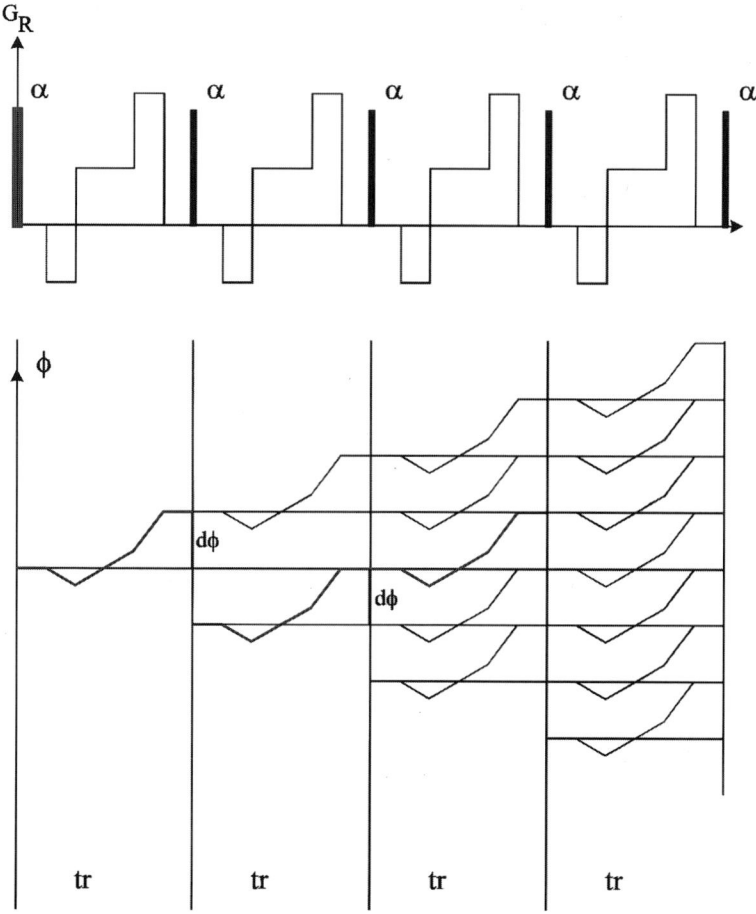

Figure 40. Extended phase graph of unspoiled FLASH. The phase graph shows the fate of transverse magnetization that is generated by the leftmost (*red*) excitation pulse. It is demonstrated that signal contributions (zero crossings in the phase graph) occur whenever the gradients and thus the dephasing $d\phi$ within each t_r interval remain constant. The red graph corresponds to spin-echo formation leading to even-echo refocusing. See Color Plate 28.

It should be noted that the resulting mixed T1/T2 contrast is the normal case for gradient-echo imaging.

As yet phase encoding has been ignored in the discussion. The phase encoding of each signal contribution will be determined by the integral over all phase-encoding gradient loops prior to signal readout. In a naive gradient-echo experiment, where the phase-encoding gradient is applied only once before each acquisition period, the signals, which are refocused via various pathways, will carry different phase encoding. The superposition of these signals will thus lead to images with considerable artefacts. The nature and amount of artefact also will depend on the order of the phase-encoding steps. These artefacts can be avoided if a phase-encoding rewinding gradient is applied after data acquisition such that the total dephasing of the spin system is identical prior to each rf pulse. This sequence is called the *refocused gradient-echo sequence* (Fig. 41).

If a pure T1 contrast is to be maintained, the refocused signals have to be spoiled by appropriate means (53, 70, 83, 96, 198). One possibility is to use additional spoiler gradients between the data acquisition and the next pulse that are varied from one acquisition step to the next. Such gradients are quite inefficient if they are applied along the readout direction, since even a dephasing by 128 $\times$ 180° will keep the refocused signals within the acquisition window of a 256 $\times$ 256 image acquisition according to the Nyquist theorem. A better strategy for gradient spoiling therefore is to apply a linearly

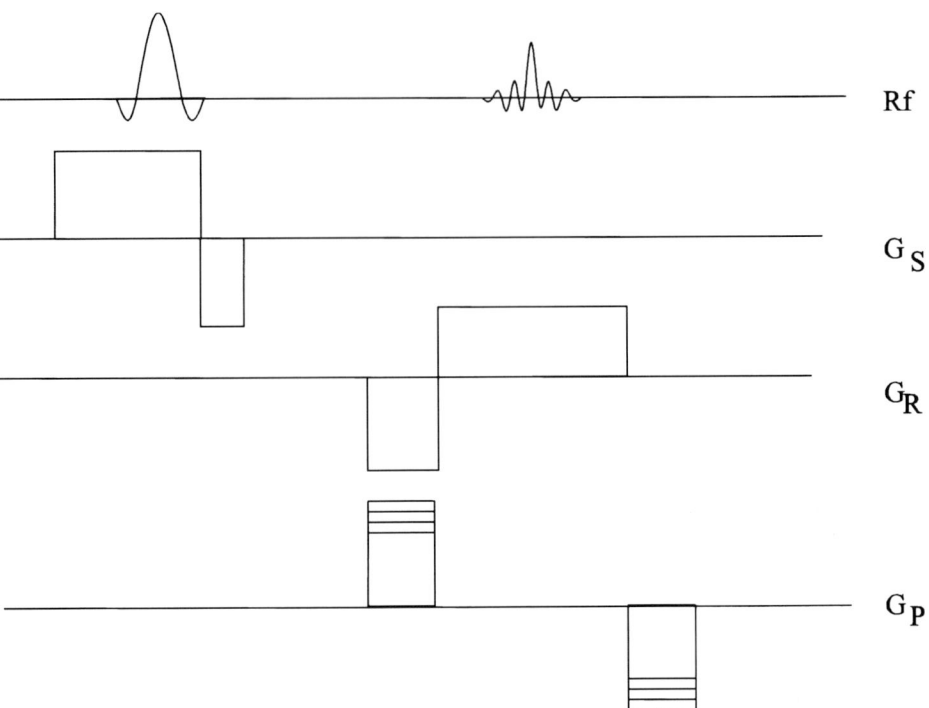

Figure 41. Refocused gradient-echo experiment. Legend as in Fig. 34. In contrast to Fig. 34, the phase-encoding gradient *GP* is rewound after signal acquisition.

increasing spoiler gradient in the slice-selection direction. Even with very strong gradients, spoiling, however, can only be achieved along a few refocusing periods (206).

A significantly better approach at least for limited gradient power is the so-called rf spoiling (35, 213). This uses a progressive change in the phase of the rf pulses. By numerical solution of the Bloch equations, flip angles can be found that lead to more or less near-cancellation of the various refocused signal components as compared with the directly observed gradient echo. Although the exact amplitude of the total refocused signal depends on the T1 and T2 of the observed tissue, some ''magic'' phase increments can be calculated that minimize these signals. Favorable values for this rf spoiling are 117° and 123°, for which gradient-echo images demonstrate predominantly T1 contrast.

Reversed Gradient Echo and FISP. The T2 contrast can be carried to the extreme if the primary FID is suppressed and only refocused components are acquired. A very elegant way to do this is to use a time reversal of the basic gradient-echo experiment (Fig. 42) (80). As shown in Fig. 43, this will lead to observable signals only from components that have experienced at least one refocusing pulse. A disadvantage of this sequence is its intrinsic low signal-to-noise ratio. A large flip angle and short t_r should be used in order to maximize the refocusing efficiency and the number of possible refocusing pathways within the T2 of the tissue. This condition leads, however, to strong signal saturation. Improving the steady-state intensity by going to a lower flip angle and longer t_r will, however, reduce the refocusing efficiency such that a compromise has to be found, which will invariably lead to a low observed S/N ratio. Consequently, this CE-FAST or PSIF technique is used mainly for 3D acquisition, where the reduced S/N ratio is improved by the large number of acquisition steps (see the section, ''*k*-Space,'' above).

An at least theoretically possible approach to maximize the signal from gradient-echo sequences is to refocus the effect of all gradients at the time of the rf pulses (Fig. 44). In the case of perfect refocusing in a perfectly homogeneous magnet, this immediately quenches any echo formation process, for which a total dephasing of all spins is an important prerequisite. The fate of magnetization that has once been excited will, however, crucially depend on the evolution of the phase between two successive rf pulses. As has been discussed for rf spoiling in the preceding section, even a moderate phase

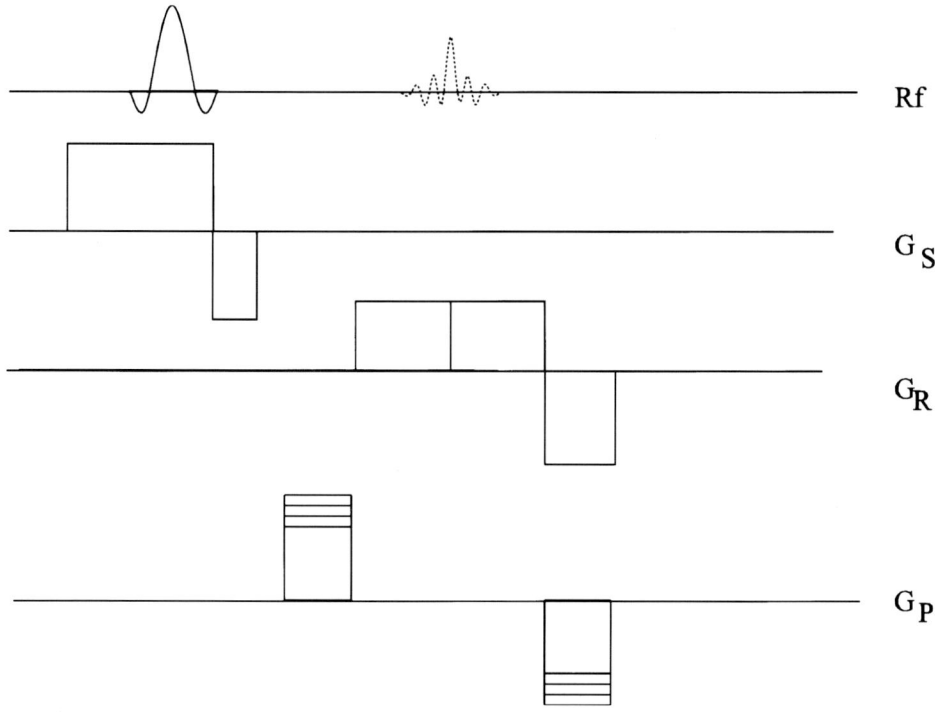

Rf

G_S

G_R

G_P

Figure 42. CE-FAST (PSIF) experiment. The timing diagram shows that this is a time-reversed version of the refocused gradient-echo experiment. Signal is shown as a dotted line, since no signal formation occurs from the immediately preceding rf pulse.

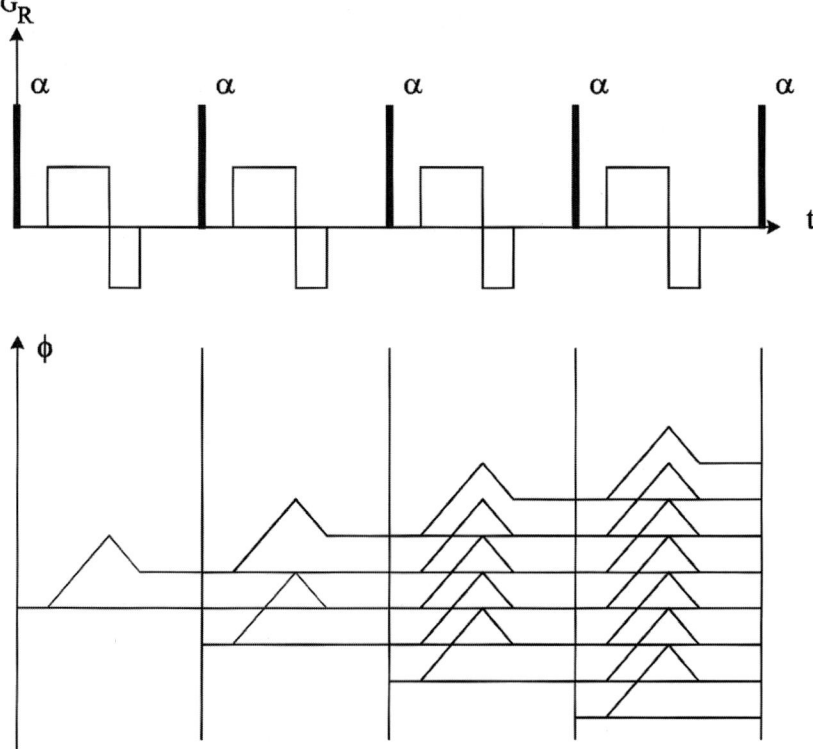

Figure 43. Extended phase graph of CE-FAST. It is demonstrated that the first signal only occurs after refocusing by two successive rf pulses.

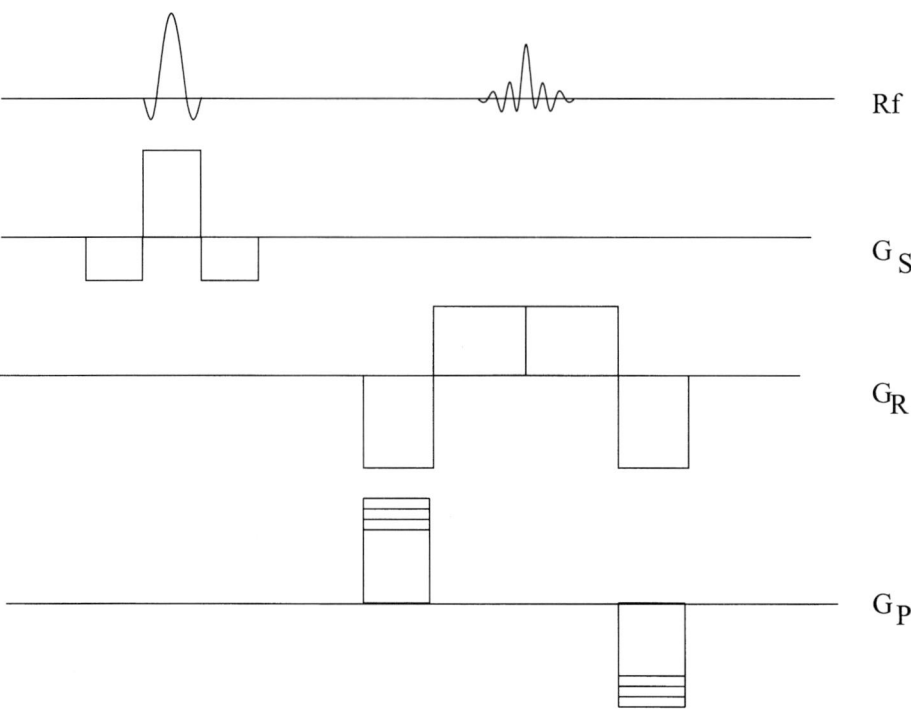

Figure 44. True FISP. Legends as in Fig. 34. All gradients are refocused at the time of the excitation pulse.

shift between successive pulses will lead to a drastically different superposition of the inverted and the directly generated signal components. A phase shift by 180° for a t_r of 10 ms is equivalent to a frequency difference of 50 Hz or approximately 1.2 ppm on a 1-T system, which is below any field inhomogeneity or susceptibility effects. The resulting FISP images therefore will show quite dramatic modulations of the signal amplitude across the images depending on the local field strength. This FISP sequence is consequently not practical for a whole-body system. Following this insight, the so-called FISP sequences implemented in clinical scanners use in reality a simple refocused gradient-echo experiment according to Fig. 41, whose T2 component is insensitive to field inhomogeneities due to the use of true spin and stimulated echoes. Recently, so-called true FISP experiments could be demonstrated using very short echo times such that phase-dependent effects remain at a tolerable level.

Figure 45 shows images with identical timing parameters acquired with spoiled and refocused gradient-echo sequences, CE-FAST (PSIF), and true FISP demonstrating the large differences in contrast behavior due to the different treatment of refocused magnetization in these sequences.

Three-Dimensional Gradient-Echo Imaging. The possibility to perform 3D data acquisition has already been mentioned as a basic option in MRI that can be performed in combination with any arbitrary imaging sequence. Given the fact that Fourier transformation requires at least 16 to 32 data points in order to work well, the minimum number of projection steps for a feasible 3D Fourier transform (3DFT) experiment is 16 (3D projection steps) × 64 (2D projection steps) or 1024 acquisition steps for a data set with very modest matrix size. Consequently, only measurement techniques that allow fast repetition have been used commonly for such 3D acquisitions. It is therefore not surprising that the vast majority of clinical applications of 3D imaging are based on gradient-echo sequences, which allow fast repetition and thus moderate overall acquisition times (71, 82). Even a high-resolution data set with 128 × 128 or even 256 × 256 phase-encoding steps can be acquired in a few minutes using repetition times of 10 to 20 ms.

In addition to their very good and—compared with multislice acquisition—gapless volume coverage, 3D gradient-echo experiments offer the advantage of very pure contrast

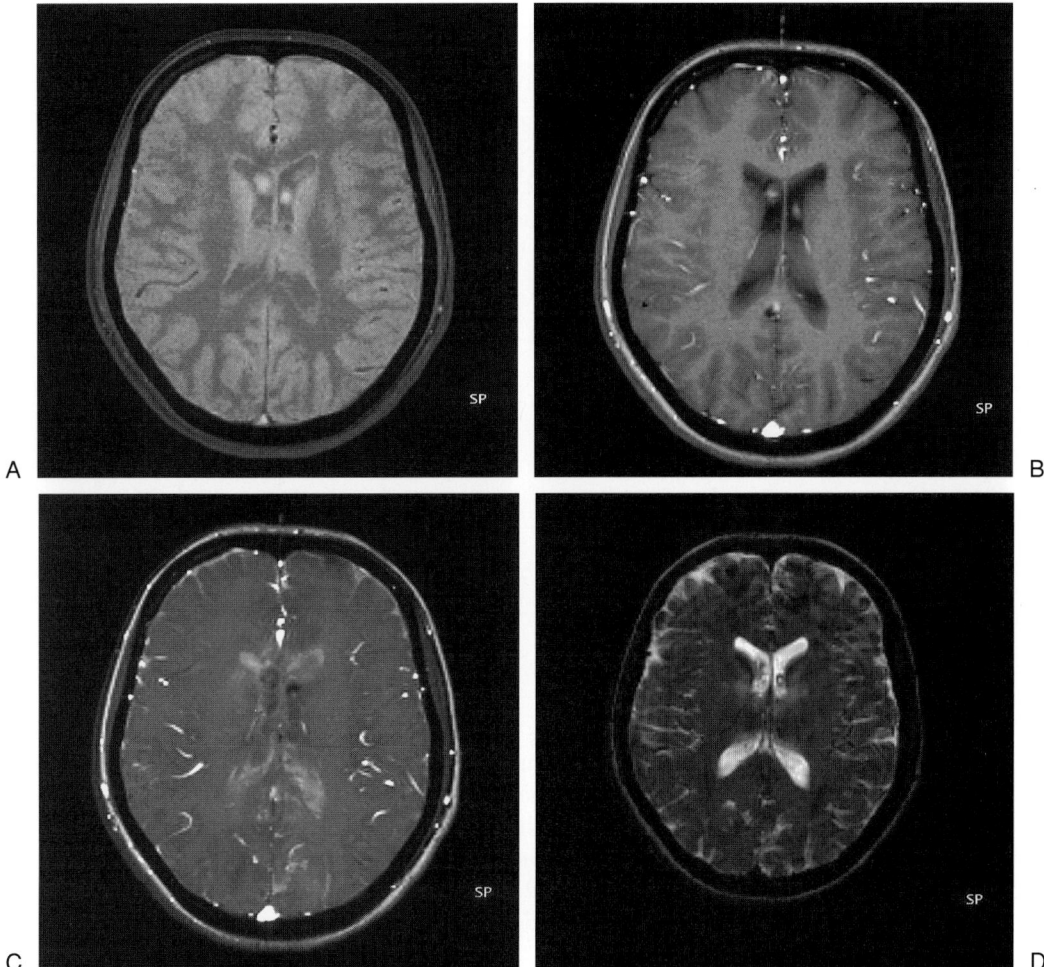

Figure 45. Images of the same transverse slice through the head of a volunteer acquired with gradient-echo sequences with various different experimental parameters. **(A)** Spoiled FLASH with primarily spin density contrast (t_r/t_e = 5 ms/50 ms; flip angle 10°). **(B)** Spoiled FLASH with primarily T1 contrast (t_r/t_e = 5 ms/20 ms; flip angle 60°). **(C)** Refocused FLASH with T1/T2 contrast ($t_r t_e$ = 5 ms/50 ms; flip angle 60°). **(D)** CE-FAST (PSIF) experiment with primarily T2 contrast (t_r/t_e = 5 ms/20 ms; flip angle 60°).

behavior. Using short pulses with a wide bandwidth, it is not difficult to maintain a constant flip angle throughout the volume under examination. This is in marked contrast to slice-selective techniques, where the signal intensity varies across the slice according to imperfections in the slice profile (Fig. 46).

If 3D acquisition is performed with slice selection in order to perform high-resolution imaging of a limited section from the body, each 3D partition will still have a pure contrast described by the actual flip angle at its position. The contrast will, however, vary across the 3D slab, corresponding to a more spin-density-weighted image near the edges of the slice and a more T1-weighted image at the center.

3D Acquisition versus Multislice 2D Acquisition

The advantages of 3D acquisition have already been mentioned as true gapless volume coverage and purer image contrast. For applications demanding 16 to 32 slices out of the body, these advantages are countered by the larger effective volume necessary to deal with the inhomogeneous contrast in slices at the edges of the slab and the suboptimal point-spread function of 3DFT for a low number of partitions. A further practical con-

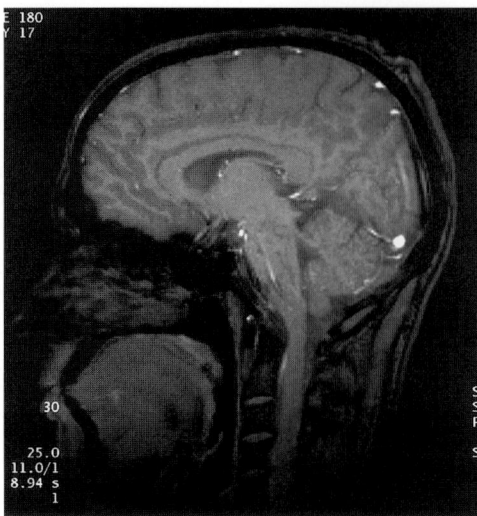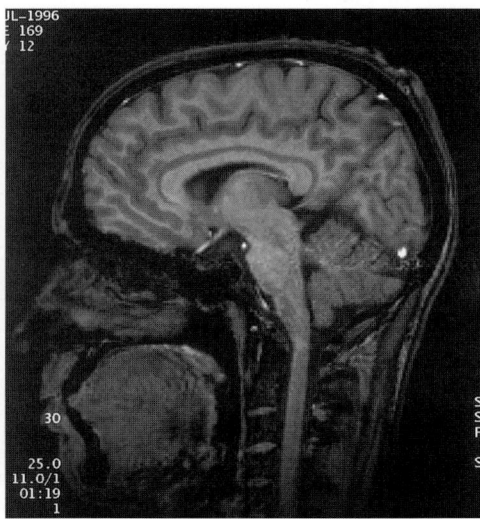

Figure 46. Comparison of a 2D FLASH image (t_e/t_r = 11/25 ms, flip angle 30°, 4-mm slice thickness) (*left*) with a 3D FLASH image (*right*) with identical acquisition parameters. The much crisper contrast of the 3D image (for example, between white matter and gray matter) is demonstrated.

sideration is the longer reconstruction times of 3D data sets. For acquisitions where short repetition times are required in order to achieve a given contrast such that no interleaved multislicing is possible, 3D acquisition is nevertheless clearly superior due to its tremendous gain in S/N ratio, which increases with the square root of the number of partitions n_{3D} compared with consecutive multislice acquisition.

For longer repetition times t_r, the signal intensity will grow with T1. Multislice acquisition might then yield a better S/N ratio (but a totally different contrast) compared with a 3D acquisition.

Single-Excitation Sequences

Single-excitation sequences use only a single excitation pulse in order to generate transverse magnetization, which is then submitted to spatial encoding such that all *k*-space data necessary for image reconstruction are acquired in one single "shot." The time available for signal readout is then determined at maximum by the relaxation time T2 during which the transverse magnetization decays. For signal acquisition as a gradient echo, the even shorter decay constant T2* determines the useful acquisition time. In single-excitation sequences, the various *k*-space data points will be acquired over a much longer time interval after excitation as compared with a multiexcitation experiment, where data points in the phase-encoding direction are acquired at identical times and signal readout occurs within the short 5- to 20-ms interval of the acquisition window. Consequently, changes in signal phase and amplitude across *k*-space will become quite significant, and their effect has to be taken into account when performing such an experiment.

Single-Shot Spin-Echo Sequences (RARE, TSE, FSE)

A conceptionally very simple single-shot experiment based on spin-echo acquisition is the data acquisition in one long echo train, where each echo carries different phase encoding. This possibility has in fact been mentioned in the original paper of P. Mansfield on echo planar imaging, its gradient-echo analogue (141). The reason for the long duration between the first voicing of the concept in 1977 and the first demonstration of its successful implementation on a whole-body system in 1984 followed by another time lag of 7 to 8 years until its widespread introduction to routine imaging lies in the complex behavior of magnetization that is submitted to refocusing pulses with nonideal flip angles.

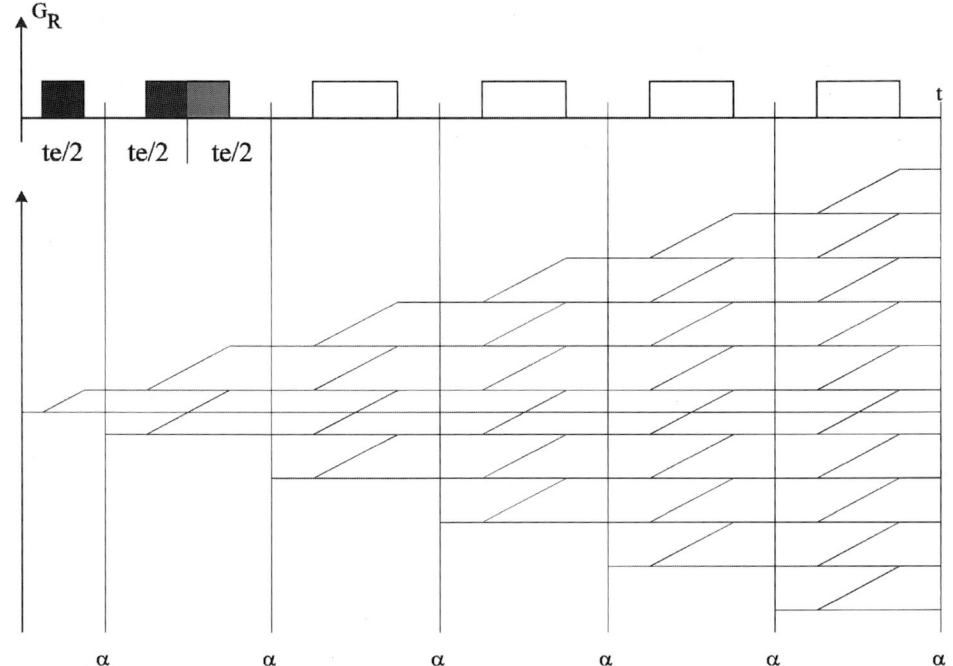

Figure 47. Phase graph for a CPMG sequence (readout gradient only). All signal-generation pathways will coincide if the proper timing is maintained (the time t_e between successive refocusing pulses must be twice the time between the excitation pulse and the first refocusing pulse) and if the gradient is balanced such that refocusing occurs exactly at the center of each refocusing period [the area of the gradient between the excitation pulse and the refocusing pulse must be equal to its area between the refocusing pulse and t_e (*dark gray*) and equal to the area between t_e and the next refocusing pulse (*light gray*)].

A proper single-excitation scheme has to preserve the symmetry of the CPMG multiecho sequence (144). This is achieved by bringing the spin system back to the same state of dephasing prior to each refocusing pulse (Fig. 47). This necessitates first maintaining the proper timing of the sequence and second appropriately adjusting the gradient. An important consideration is that these conditions have to be respected for all gradients, including the phase-encoding gradient.

Only under these conditions will all the 3^{n-1} possible refocusing pathways coincide and thus contribute coherently to the observed signal amplitude. The resulting diagram for the RARE (FSE, TSE) sequence (101, 108) is shown in Fig. 48.

Apart from the avoidance of spurious echoes, this results in surprisingly large echo amplitudes. It can be demonstrated that for an echo train with constant refocusing flip

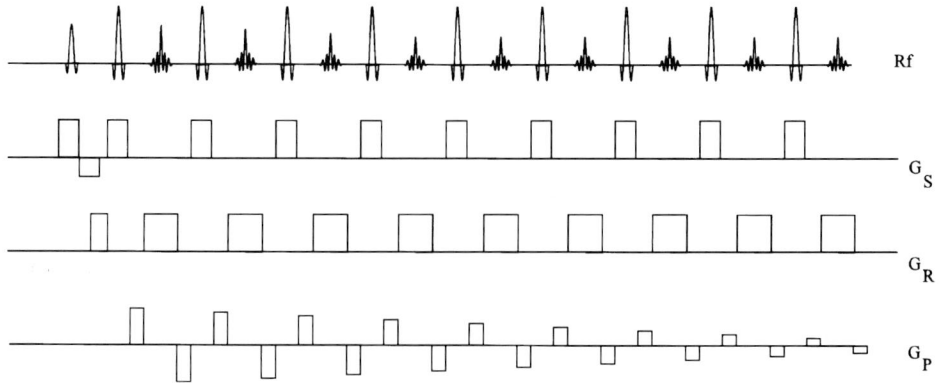

Figure 48. RARE sequence. The phase-encoding gradient *GP* is applied prior to each echo and rewound prior to each refocusing pulse.

angle a, the echo amplitude after several refocusing periods will go to a value given by $\sin(\alpha/2)$ as compared with the multiple refocused value of $\sin^{2n}(\alpha/2)$ for direct formation of the nth spin echo (96, 98). For a refocusing flip angle of 60° corresponding to ⅛th the rf power of a 180° pulse, the signal intensity will thus still be a quite decent 50%.

The ensuing echo train will decay primarily with the relaxation time T2, with additional contributions of T1 via the stimulated echo mechanism as a function of the deviation of the refocusing flip angle from 180°. The phase of the echoes will be constant throughout the echo train as a consequence of spin-echo refocusing. This very stable signal behavior leads to very benign image-transformation properties of the sequence.

Hybrid RARE (TSE, FSE) or Segmented RARE

The signal decay during the echo train will act as a low-pass filter of the image, which leads to broadening along the phase-encoding direction. The extent of the broadening will be given by the echo interval t_e between successive echoes:

$$I_k = I_{k0} \exp(-kt_e/\mathrm{T2}) \tag{14}$$

where I_k is the intensity of the kth echo as measured without phase encoding.

Fast refocusing will produce less blurring than long echo intervals. The minimum echo interval is restricted by the time necessary for the refocusing pulses, as well as by the necessity to apply and rewind the phase-encoding gradient. Even with state-of-the-art gradient systems, the minimum echo time lies on the order of 4 ms; for routine systems, typical values are in the range 9 to 15 ms. Compared with typical soft-tissue T2 relaxation times of 40 to 80 ms, this appears to be quite long for application as a single-shot sequence. Even with $t_e = 4$ ms, the whole echo train for a 256 × 256 image will last 1.024 s, during which signal will long have faded away. The problem can be alleviated by using a segmented (or hybrid) scan with more than one excitation. For an echo train length of n_{ETL}, the efficient signal decay across k-space will then be only

$$I_k = I_{k0} \exp[-kt_e/(n_{\mathrm{ETL}}\mathrm{T2})] \tag{15}$$

The efficient relaxation constant will thus appear to be prolonged by a factor n_{ETL} (Fig. 49). Since the total acquisition time will be reduced by the same factor as compared with a conventional multiexcitation spin-echo experiment, hybrid RARE (TSE, FSE) is an attractive alternative even for quite low echo train lengths in the range of 3 to 8 (108, 145, 146, 159). For a continuous signal attenuation across k-space, the efficient echo

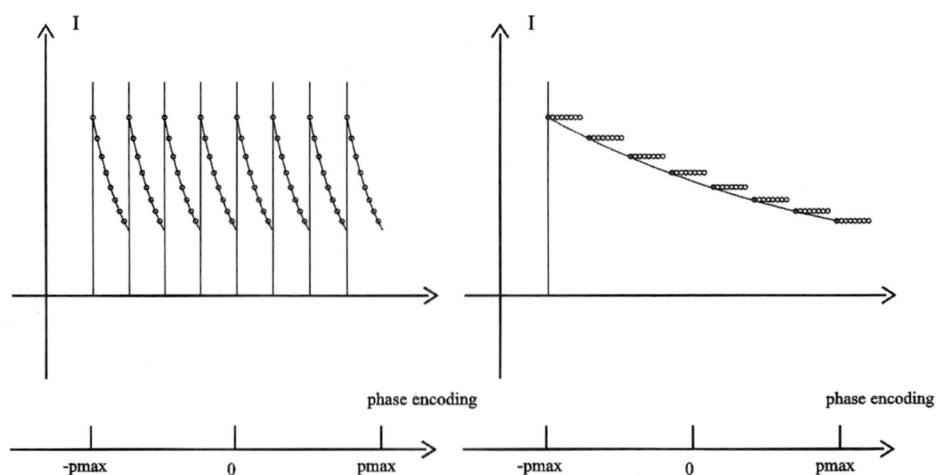

Figure 49. Principle of interleaving for hybrid RARE. Consecutive phase encoding along each echo train (*left*) will lead to a zigzag modulation of the signal intensities, which results in severe image artefacts. If phase encoding is interleaved such that the phase-encoding gradient is incremented n_{ETL} steps between successive echoes, a much smoother intensity profile will ensue (*right*).

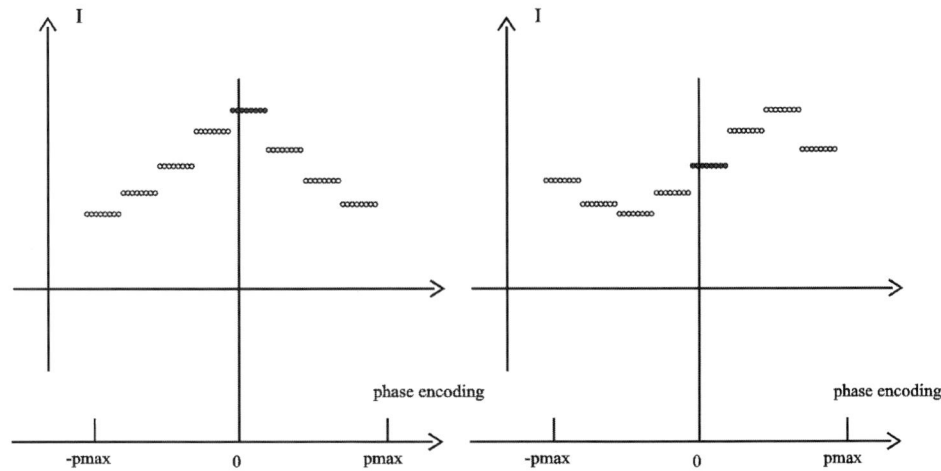

Figure 50. Phase-encoding hybrid RARE. The phase-encoding gradient is varied in an interleaved manner such that echoes acquired at identical echo times in successive excitations carry similar phase encoding. The T2-dependent signal intensities will then vary stepwise along the phase-encoding direction of *k*-space. The phase-encoding zero point can be put into the first (*left*) or any later (*right*) echo.

times should in principle be interleaved, which can be done by various means. In practice, however, the artefacts arising from a more stepwise signal decay are of no consequence.

The contrast of RARE (TSE, FSE) images mainly will be determined by the intensity of the projections carrying low phase encoding according to the discussion in the section "The Fourier Transformation," above. The image contrast can thus be altered significantly from predominantly spin-density-weighted to heavy T2 contrast without any change in the timing of the sequence and thus the underlying signal intensity (Figs. 50 and 51) (108, 145, 146, 158). This allows variation of the image contrast in a very similar manner compared with conventional spin-echo imaging (see Fig. 33). Although the basic contrast of RARE (FSE, TSE) images is identical to that of conventional spin-echo imaging and the vast literature on diagnostic applications can thus be used immediately in planning a considerably faster RARE experiment, there are some notable differences

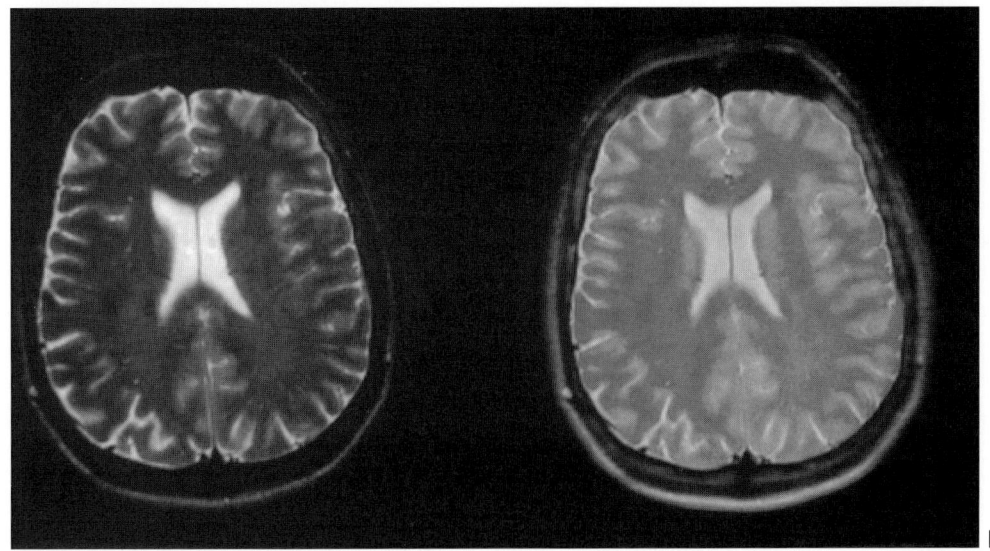

A   B

Figure 51. Images acquired with RARE sequences with identical acquisition parameters except for the order of the phase-encoding steps, which leads to different effective echo times leading to more (**A**, $t_{e,\text{eff}} = 120$ ms) or less (**B**, $t_{e,\text{eff}} = 60$ ms) T2 contrast. (Bruker S 200 Avance 2T.)

in the contrast behavior as a consequence of the much shorter echo spacing that is used in RARE, especially for T2-weighted scans (32, 33).

The first difference arises with respect to the diffusion of particles in local inhomogeneities on a microscopic scale. As was pointed out earlier, the resulting dynamic susceptibility effect will be reduced if several refocusing pulses are used to reach a given echo time in a multiecho experiment compared with a single refocusing (33). Clinically, such microscopic susceptibility differences occur in the very ragged magnetic field profile caused by the accumulation of microscopic particles of magnetic deoxygenated blood. Hemorrhages therefore can appear less conspicuous on RARE images.

A second difference relates to the signal of lipid. As was pointed out earlier, protons in lipid substances are not only heterogeneously bound and thus possess slightly variable chemical shift, they also can show an effect called *j-coupling,* which means that their precession frequencies interact with each other just like two strings that are linked by an elastic band. This interaction leads to an energy transfer with a time constant that is proportional to the strength of the coupling, expressed as the *coupling constant,* which is given in frequency units.

The modulation of the frequency of the coupled spins will lead to a loss of coherence that will not be refocused by a spin-echo experiment. Similar to the diffusion effect, the loss of coherence and thus the signal attenuation will, however, diminish if refocusing times are used that are short compared with the coupling constant. As a result, lipid structures will look somewhat brighter in RARE images compared with their single-echo counterparts (93, 145, 146).

The time savings will in practice only reach the theoretical factor of n_{ETL} if examinations are performed on the limited number of slices that can be squeezed into one repetition interval. Especially for high values of n_{ETL}, the repetition time often has to be increased in order to accommodate the desired number of slices. The time savings will then be somewhat lower then n_{ETL}. This is of no consequence for T2-weighted scans, where the longer t_r leads to improved T2 contrast. It can, however, restrict the application of T1-weighted RARE (TSE, FSE) experiments, where typically 16 to 20 slices have to be acquired with $t_r < 600$ ms in order to ensure proper T1 contrast. Some typical images are shown in Fig. 52.

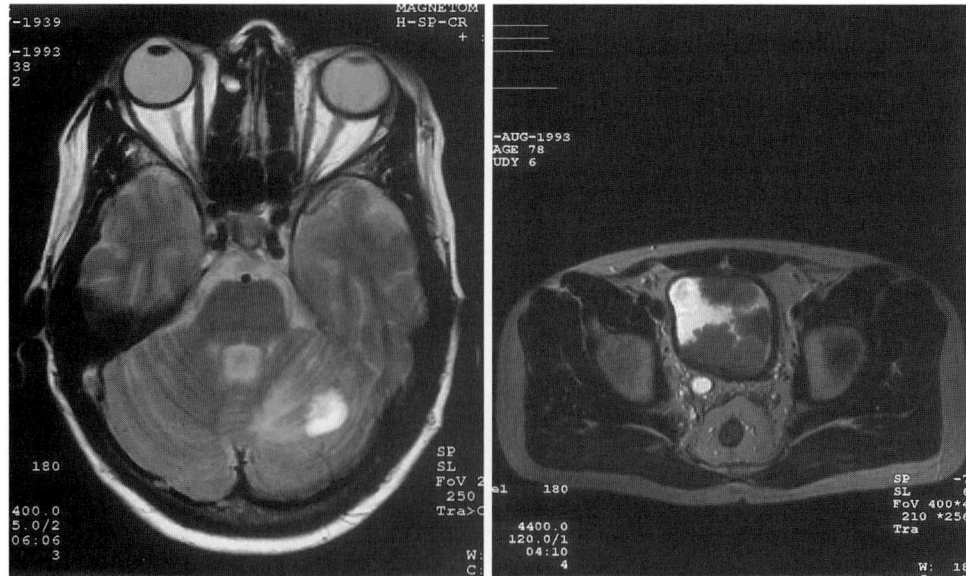

Figure 52. Hybrid RARE images from routine diagnostic examinations. **(A)** Transverse image of the head of a patient with multiple sclerosis. **(B)** Transverse image of a patient with a bladder tumor (both images acquired on Siemens Magnetom Impact Expert at 1 T).

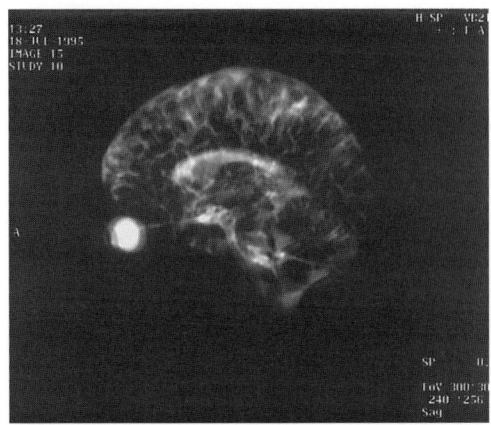 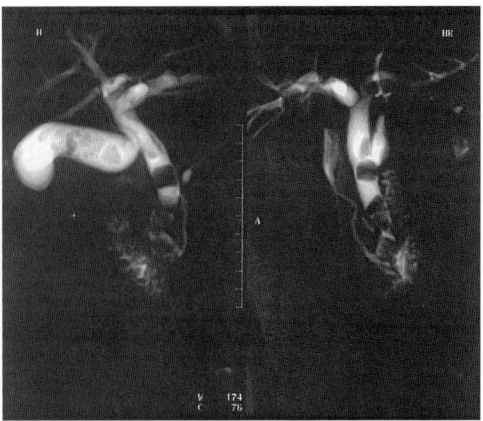

A   B

Figure 53. Two examples for single-shot RARE projection images with fluid-selective contrast. **(A)** A sagittal view of the cerebrospinal fluid-filled spaces of the human head. The bright circles to the left are the eyes, which also appear bright on these heavily T2-weighted images ($t_{e,\text{eff}}$ = 1.2 s; Siemens Magnetom Vision 1.5 T). **(B)** Two views under different projection angles of the gallbladder and the biliary system of a patient with multiple gallstones (*dark shades*) (Siemens Magnetom Impact at 1 T).

Single-Shot RARE (FSE, TSE). The long overall time of the echo train in single-shot RARE will lead to severe attenuation of soft-tissue signals with short T2. For protons in liquids, however, T2 values on the order of several seconds are not uncommon. Single-shot RARE with the phase-encoding zero point shifted to effective echo times on the order of 400 to 600 ms will thus image protons in liquids with extremely high selectivity (101). At t_e = 500 ms, the signal intensity of an aqueous solution with T2 = 1000 ms will be approximately 60% of its initial value, whereas soft-tissue signals with T2 = 50 ms will be reduced to 0.0045%. This technique thus allows highly selective imaging of liquid-filled structures of the body and has found applications as MR-RARE myelography (101), MR-RARE urography (187), MR lymphangiography, and MR-RARE cholangiography (127) (Fig. 53). Due to the scarcity of free liquid in the human body, slice selection can be omitted altogether or thick slices can be used in many clinical applications, which is especially beneficial for the examination of spatially complex structures such as the biliary system or the spinal canal. An additional impact is given to these very fast techniques by the fact that conventional approaches to acquire similar images are quite invasive, requiring the injection of contrast agent and observation by x-ray techniques.

Parenchymal single-shot RARE images (164) have become feasible only recently with the introduction of fast gradient systems, which allow short echo intervals in the range of 4 to 10 ms. For the observation of soft-tissue signals, the phase-encoding zero point should occur not later than 60 to 80 ms. The resulting requirement of asymmetric distribution of the phase-encoding steps over the echo train can be met in two different ways: First, in the so-called HASTE sequence (118), half-Fourier encoding is used, where only one-half the k-space data are actually acquired, whereas the other half is derived by symmetry of the k-space data (60). In order to properly find the symmetry center, some slight overlap is normally used, where the phase-encoding zero point is placed into the 6 to 12 echo and the lower 6 to 12 phase-encoding steps on both sides of k-spaces are acquired (Fig. 54). Second, centric phase encoding can be used, where the phase-encoding zero point is put into the first echo, and phase encoding continues alternatively to the higher positive and negative phase-encoding steps in successive echoes. This, however, will lead to broad background signals from fast-decaying components. It is thus advisable to not use the first 4 to 8 echoes and then commence the phase-encoding scheme.

With new gradient systems, these sequences can be used to produce images with typically 128 phase-encoding steps in 400 to 1000 ms.

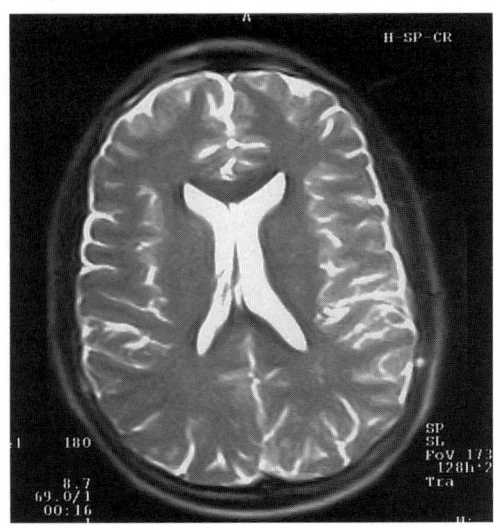

Figure 54. Transversal HASTE image of the head of a volunteer ($t_{e,\text{eff}}$ = 64 ms; t_{aq} = 1.28 s; Siemens Magnetom Vision at 1.5 T).

BURST-Type Sequences

A group of fast imaging methods that also uses spin echoes but with a radically different approach are the BURST techniques (30, 52, 92, 103, 105, 209). The basic concept of these is the somewhat whimsical idea to first make all the rf pulses and then acquire all echoes. This avoids the necessity to apply and rewind phase-encoding gradients between each pair of rf pulses. The generalized phase graph demonstrates that n equidistant pulses under a constant gradient will produce n echoes (Fig. 55). Adding a phase-encoding gradient after the pulse train will produce all data necessary for image reconstruction without the necessity of fast gradient switching. A 64 × 64 image can thus be acquired with very moderate gradient power in 25 to 40 ms.

The optimal S/N ratio of BURST-type sequences can be demonstrated to be given by $\sqrt{n}$, where n is the number of echoes and thus the size of the image matrix in the phase-encoding direction (133, 199). This very severely limits the range of applications of these techniques; for small n, the relative loss increases very sharply compared with conventional spin-echo acquisition. For large n, the dropoff in signal-to-noise ratio is more gradual but eventually reaches a limit where the application of the sequence appears to be unfeasible. 3D applications somewhat make up for the signal loss, especially since saturation between scans is small to start with because of the small flip angles used for the pulses and can be further reduced by echo shifting (52). They also avoid the problem of slice selection, which is possible but somewhat awkward to introduce into 2D BURST.

Nevertheless, BURST appears to be restricted to applications where low spatial resolution and low signal-to-noise ratios can be afforded.

Echo Planar Imaging

Echo planar imaging (EPI) is the oldest fast imaging technique around (139, 141). Although it was developed as early as 1977, it has only recently become widely available due to the development of the fast gradient hardware necessary for its implementation. In its generic form it uses a single-excitation pulse, after which k-space is traversed by reversal of the readout gradient, whereas the phase-encoding gradient is increased in short blips during the switching times of the readout gradient (Fig. 56 and Color Plate 29) (27, 110). Data acquisition therefore uses a spatially encoded free induction decay.

Alternatively, a very weak phase-encoding gradient can be left on during the whole acquisition time. This leads, however, to a zigzag k-space trajectory, which does not allow image reconstruction using the fast Fourier transformation algorithm (Fig. 57). Data have to be interpolated onto a rectangular grid prior to reconstruction, or separate images

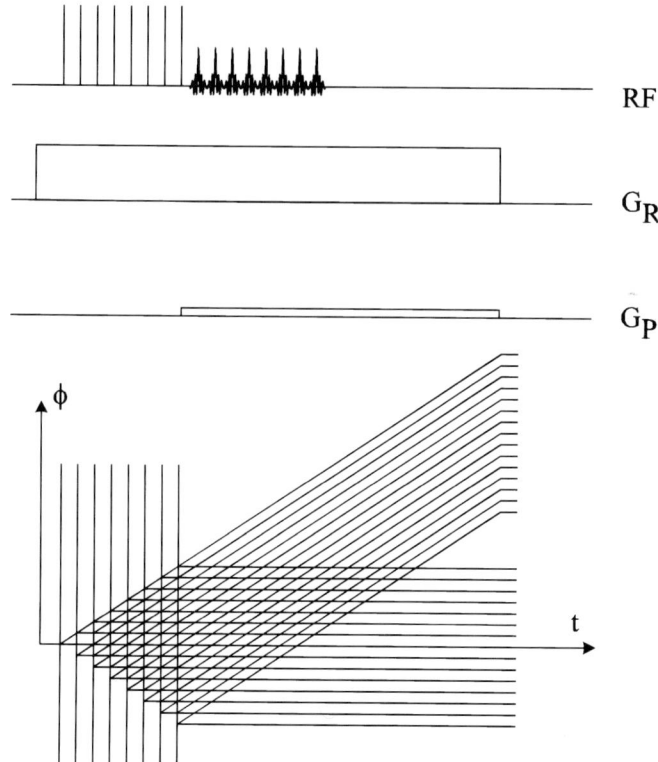

Figure 55. Pulse sequence and *k*-space trajectory BURST. A sequence of eight equidistant hard pulses applied under a constant gradient *GR* will produce a sequence of eight echoes according to the extended phase graph diagram in the lower half of the figure. These signals can be phase-encoded differently by switching on a phase-encoding gradient *GP* immediately after the pulse train.

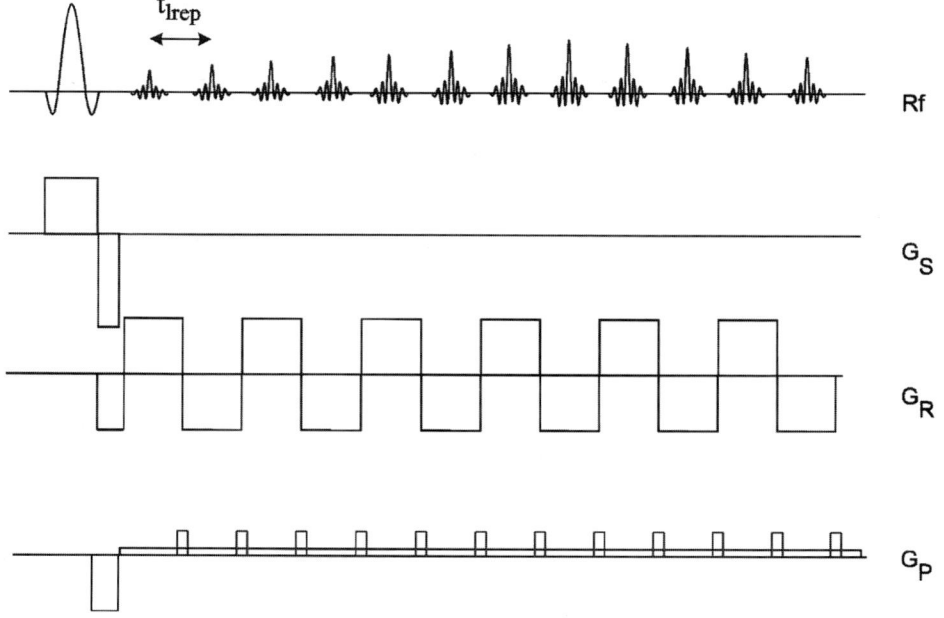

Figure 56. Pulse sequence for echo planar imaging (EPI). A long echo train is generated by repetitive reversal of the readout gradient *GR*, whereas the phase encoding-gradient *GP* is applied either continuously (*blue*) or in short "blips" during the reversal of *GR*. The negative gradient lobe in *GP* directly after the excitation pulse serves as a "prewinder" in order to bring the phase-encoding zero point into a later echo. See Color Plate 29.

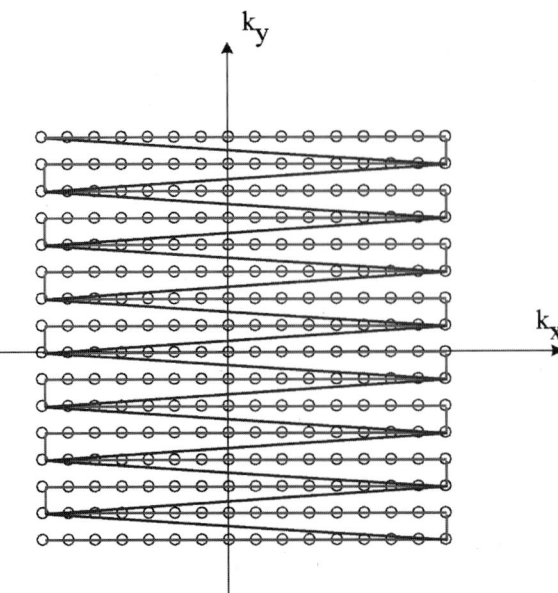

Figure 57. *k*-space trajectory of EPI. Whereas data are sampled line by line in a blipped phase-encoding scheme, continuous phase encoding will lead to a zig-zag trajectory. Data will then not fall onto a rectangular grid necessary for fast Fourier transformation.

have to be reconstructed from the odd and even echoes, respectively; otherwise, severe artefacts will be generated.

Transformation Properties and Artefact Behavior

T2*-Dependent Amplitude Modulation. The signal attenuation in the read direction is very mild, since data acquisition proceeds very fast. Typical acquisition times t_{aq} for one line of *k*-space are 0.25 to 1 ms. For a T2 of 60 ms, the resulting signal decay during 1 ms is only about 2%. Therefore, EPI does not show any appreciable artefacts in the read direction of the image. This is significantly different for the phase-encoding direction, where adjacent points are sampled every t_{lrep}, which is defined by t_{aq} plus the switching time for reversal of the readout gradient. t_{lrep} thus constitutes the effective dwell time for sampling in the phase-encoding direction. The resulting narrow bandwidths make EPI very sensitive to artefacts related to frequency shifts like susceptibility and chemical-shift effects as well as to phase errors, which arise over the total acquisition time.

The T2* decay over the acquisition window constitutes the ultimate barrier for EPI imaging even when T2* = T2 under optimized conditions. For an acquisition time approximately equal to T2, the loss in signal decay due to dephasing across the voxel caused by the phase-encoding gradient is roughly equivalent to the relaxation effect. For longer acquisition times, T2 will act as an additional low-pass filter. The effective image resolution will thus remain the same, even when the acquisition parameters predict a higher nominal resolution.

Structures with long T2 will thus appear sharper than those with shorter T2. This effect can be quite deceptive in EPI images of the head acquired with long acquisition times (150 to 250 ms) and a large image matrix. The long T2 of CSF leads to a sharp image of the ventricular spaces and thus to the impression of high image resolution, which for parenchymal signal is, however, not realized.

Based on a standard 256 × 256 image acquired with a net total acquisition time of 256 × 10 ms = 2.56 s, the 60-ms acquisition time for a parenchymal EPI image already constitutes a reduction by roughly a factor of 40. The required higher acquisition bandwidth will thus lead to a reduction in the S/N ratio by a factor of $\sqrt{40} = 6.5$. This value constitutes a theoretical optimum neglecting all experimental factors that might further decrease S/N ratio. This signal loss is normally compensated by a lower resolution. Even with infinite gradient power, this bandwidth-related S/N ratio loss ultimately limits the achievable resolution of EPI. For imaging of structures with shorter T2, which are typical for applications in the thorax and abdomen, this problem becomes especially severe.

180° ARTEFACTS IN EPI

The *k*-space trajectories for blipped or nonblipped EPI images show that the direction of sampling is reversed in every other line. Any monotonous change in the signal phase or amplitude will thus run in opposite directions. The resulting image therefore can be decomposed into two parts: one that may be called the proper image, which would correspond to an image from data that are acquired by sampling all *k*-space lines in the same direction and a second one that describes the deviation from this regular pattern. For an unblipped phase-encoding scheme, the proper image would be slightly tilted with respect to a blipped EPI image. The artefact, which represents the disturbance by the change in the sampling direction, can vary widely in its appearance. Its basic nature, however, is clear from the earlier discussion. Since the *k*-space data of the artefact are nonzero only in every second line, it will be shifted by half the image matrix, since zeroes in every other line invariably lead to an effective modulation of the signal with the Nyquist frequency. This type of artefact is thus called a *180° artefact*.

Especially for unblipped EPI, this artefact can be so severe that it is prudent to reconstruct images only from data that are acquired in the same sampling direction. With otherwise identical pulse sequence, this requires a two-pass experiment, which then yields two images that are slightly tilted with respect to each other.

Phase Effects. A number of effects occur that will alter the phase of the MR signal over the acquisition time. Due to the change in direction of sampling in every alternate line, the direction of this phase change also will alternate, which in all cases will lead to some 180° artefact for all mechanisms described in the following.

Chemical Shift. The most significant problem in EPI is phase effects, which evolve with the efficient dwell time t_{lrep} (= line repetition time) in the phase-encoding direction. According to the section "Sampling," above, a dwell time of 0.5 ms corresponds to an efficient acquisition bandwidth of 1000 Hz. For a 1.5-T system with a chemical-shift separation of 200 Hz, this means a shift of lipid structures by about 20% of the field of view. EPI consequently has to use fat suppression when applied to parts of the body with significant signals from lipid protons. This is no severe problem for brain imaging, where MRI-visible lipid protons occur only in the scalp and the intrinsic homogeneity is high. For imaging in the thorax and abdomen, the situation is different, since susceptibility effects severely limit shimming of the magnet to a degree that is sufficient for fat suppression. This often can be done only in a limited volume, thus restricting EPI examinations to one or a few slices.

Susceptibility. Even where fat suppression is applicable, EPI is limited by susceptibility effects, which affect the image in various ways: Most significantly, susceptibility effects will lead to appreciable misregistration. EPI delivers thus everything but true images.

For most applications, this does not affect the usefulness of the images, since geometric trueness is seldom an issue in clinical applications. Care has to be taken, however, if the information from an EPI image is to be combined with that from images acquired with some other sequence. Identical loci on images acquired with EPI and some other method with nominally identical spatial parameters easily lie 10 pixels or more apart. This can become especially awkward if some functional information is acquired with an EPI sequence with poor anatomic resolution and the locus of the functional activity is to be derived from a conventional scan.

If the local field inhomogeneity is strong enough, it will shift the phase-encoding zero point for signals from the corresponding voxels. This is of no serious concern as long as the resulting asymmetry of *k*-space acquisition stays within 30% to 40%. If the shift becomes larger, however, additional artefacts will arise from truncation and the stronger and stronger contribution of broad dispersion signals as a consequence of the asymmetry. In the extreme case, the signal can even be pushed over the edge of the acquisition

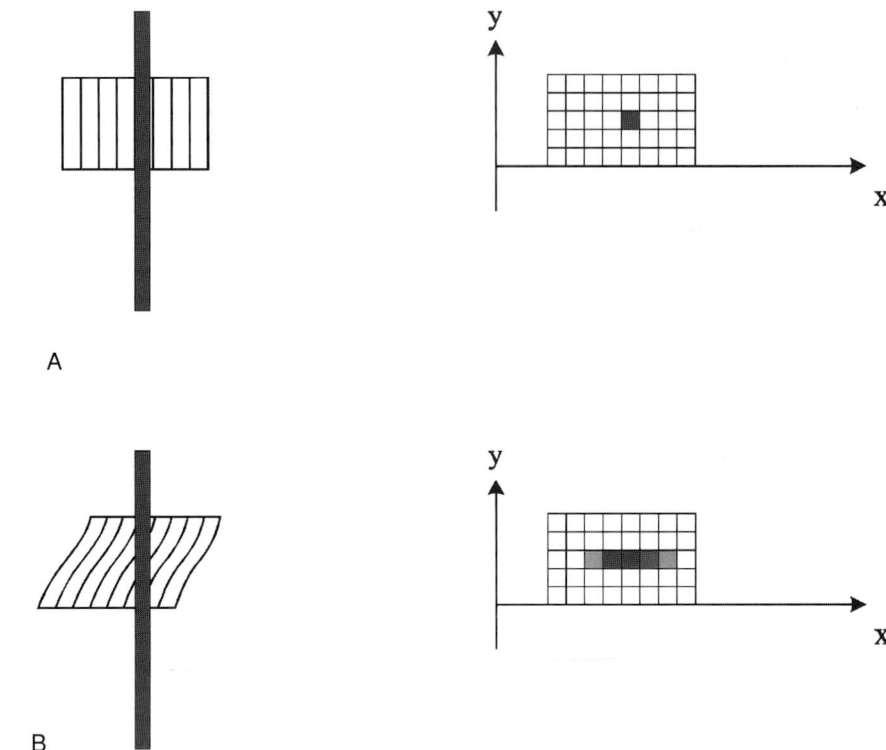

Figure 58. Susceptibility effects in the slice-selection direction. If strong nonlinear susceptibility effects occur across the slice, then the image of a sharp structure **(A)** will appear to be smeared over several pixels **(B)**.

window, and the corresponding structures will vanish from the image altogether (see the section, "T2 Sensitivity: Refocused versus Gradient-Echo Imaging," above, where similar effects are described for gradient-echo sequences with long echo times).

Field inhomogeneities in the slice-selection direction will affect the EPI image in two ways. First, they will lead to image distortions, as discussed previously, that vary across the slice. As a result, images will appear to be smeared (Fig. 58). Second, the field inhomogeneity will spoil the coherence of the spins across the slice and therefore lead to (local) signal attenuation in the images. A comparison of EPI and gradient-echo images of nominally identical geometric parameters shows the significant geometric distortions inherent to EPI (Fig. 59).

Flow and Motion. Flow will lead to gradient-dependent dephasing (25). For flow in the read direction, where the gradients and thus the flow effects are strongest, the flow-dependent phase will evolve in a zigzag fashion as a result of the (partial) compensation in every even refocusing period. As a result, a 180° artefact in the phase-encoding direction of the image will occur. Flow in the phase-encoding direction will show a flow-dependent phase effect that increases quadratically with time. For slow flow (a few pixels over the acquisition time), this will lead to a displacement of, for example, the blood inside a vessel with respect to the vessel wall. For faster flow, appreciable blurring will become visible.

Flow in the slice-selection direction will primarily affect the phase of the signal and go undetected after magnitude calculation. If the vessel is not exactly orthogonal to the image plane, or if the vessel curves downstream from the selected slice, an apparent displacement will occur, since the projection of the spins onto the image plane will have changed at the time of reading out the most significant projections.

It should be noted that most of the flow-related artefacts are quite benign if the flow velocity and direction do not change too abruptly over the acquisition time. Some misregistration and blurring are something one can live with, at least to a certain degree,

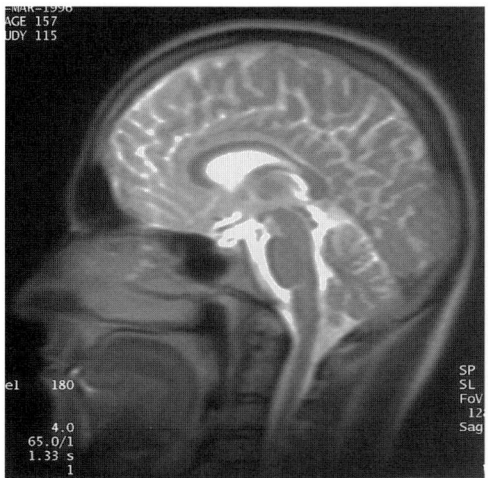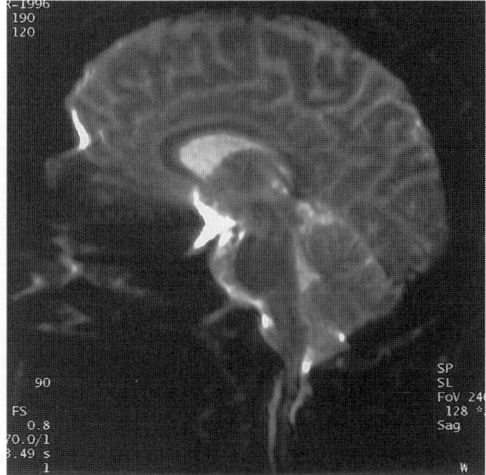

Figure 59. Comparison of a sagittal single-shot RARE image of the head ($t_{e,\text{eff}}$ = 65 ms; 512-ms acquisition time) (*left*) with an EPI image ($t_{e,\text{eff}}$ = 70 ms; acquisition time 140 ms) (*right*) acquired on the same volunteer. Signal from fat is still visible in the RARE image due to spin-echo refocusing. Signal from facial tissue has vanished in the EPI image due to local susceptibility effects, which also lead to strong distortion, especially at the base of the skull and in the brain stem.

and certainly much better than the flow artefacts in multiexcitation sequences, which tend to spread the signal all across the phase-encoding direction of the image. Consequently, one can get away with quite decent EPI images for acquisition parameters (t_e, length of acquisition time) for which one would not even dare to try a multiexcitation scan.

Modifications and Variants

Spin-Echo EPI. A basically very simple but very effective variant of EPI is to use a spin-echo excitation sequence with signal readout by EPI (Fig. 60 and Color Plate 30). If the low-order phase-encoding steps are acquired around the time of spin-echo refocusing, the artefacts for these most important projections will be minimized and the image quality considerably improved (Fig. 61). Small shifts of the phase-encoding order can then be used to introduce selectively some T2* sensitivity if desired. The advantages of spin-echo EPI compared with (FID) EPI are such that this variant is the method of choice for most EPI applications. Restrictions apply when fast repetitions of single-slice scans are needed, where spin echoes show considerably stronger saturation effects compared with FIDs, and for imaging of flow and motion, where outflow or through-the-plane motion between the excitation and refocusing pulse might lead to severe signal loss.

Multiexcitation (Hybrid) EPI. Just like in RARE (TSE, FSE), most of the problems described above can be at least ameliorated by going to hybrid acquisition, which means using more than one excitation in order to cover *k*-space (95, 142). Considerable improvements have been made using hybrid (or segmented) scans for various applications. Hybrid EPI does have some problems, however, that makes it much more difficult to perform than the more robust spin-echo techniques. Progressive saturation will cost in terms of S/N ratio compared with a single-shot scan with its intrinsic infinite t_r. This becomes less and less of a problem for multislice acquisitions.

Since EPI runs with a freely evolving phase of the signal, the requirements for constant phase from excitation after excitation are extremely high. Any phase instability between two excitations will lead immediately to ugly artefacts all over the image. The most ubiquitous sources of such changes are motion between successive excitations. The problem becomes even more notorious because displacing the body also means shifting the susceptibility effects around, which will give rise to additional phase changes. Since the

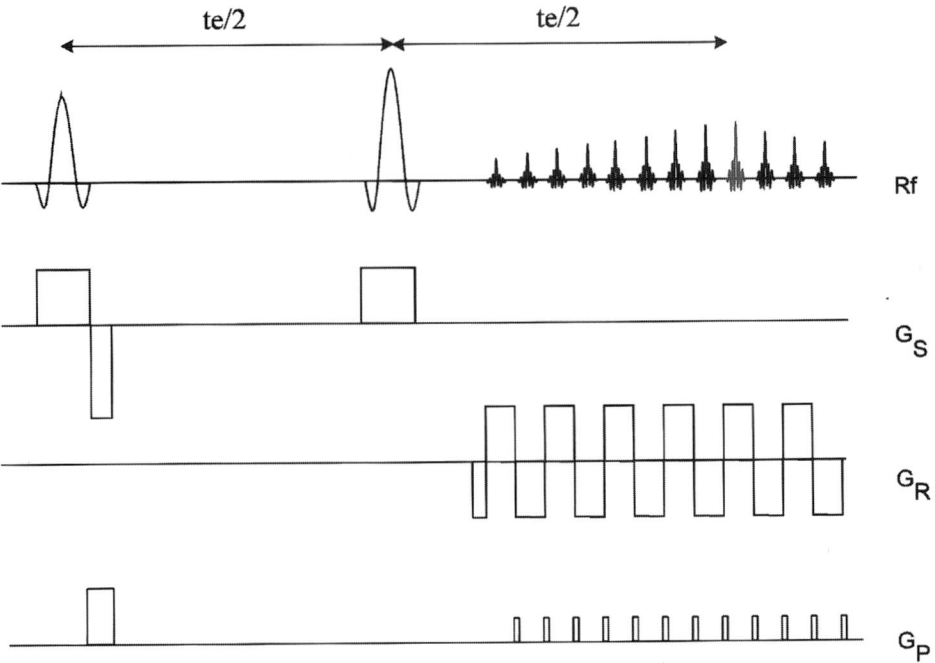

Figure 60. Spin-echo EPI. Signal is generated as a spin echo by applying an excitation pulse followed by a refocusing pulse. The resulting spin echo is then multiplexed by repetitive reversal of the readout gradient G_R. Note that only one signal (*red*) will occur at the proper refocusing time t_e and thus be properly refocused, whereas the others will carry T2* effects depending on their time interval from t_e. See Color Plate 30.

phase of the signal evolves much faster with t_e than with the amplitude, the requirement for maintaining equidistant coverage in terms of the effective t_e is also much more severe than in hybrid RARE, where one can get away with the stepwise effective sampling time shown in Fig. 50. In EPI, time interleave is strictly required in order to avoid severe artefacts.

Finally, flow artefacts, which are quite benign in single-shot EPI, start to become serious in multiexcitation scans.

Nonrectilinear Sampling. The rectilinear sampling scheme used in all techniques discussed so far is mainly chosen by the availability of the fast Fourier transform algorithm.

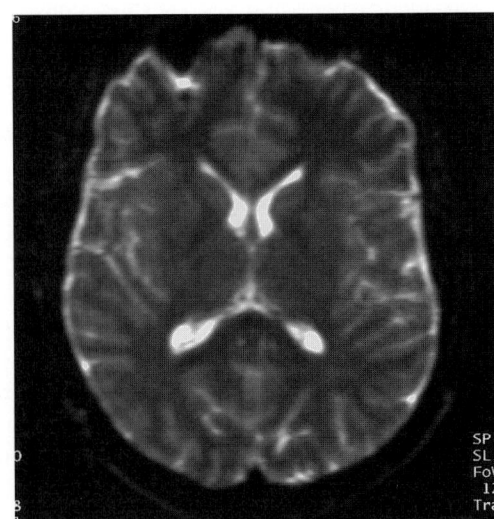

Figure 61. Spin-echo EPI image (transverse section of the head, $t_{e,eff}$ = 70 ms, 128 phase-encoding steps) acquired using a standard gradient system (25 mT/m, 0.6-ms risetime).

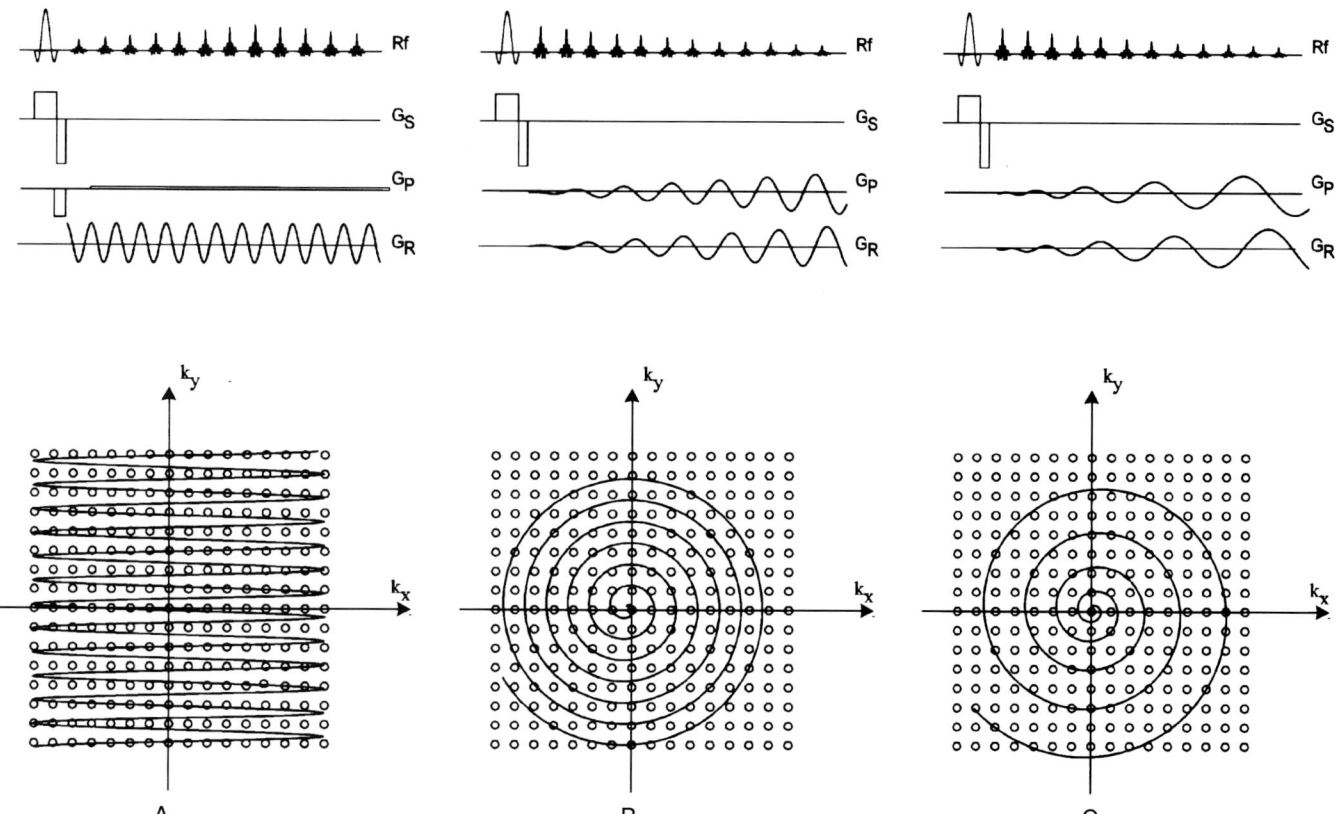

Figure 62. *k*-space trajectories for different approaches to nonrectilinear sampling in EPI. **(A)** A sinusoidal trajectory produced by a sinusoidal readout gradient in connection with a constant phase-encoding gradient. **(B)** A spiral trajectory produced by two sinusoidal gradients with increasing amplitude. **(C)** A hardware-optimized spiral where the switching time decreases with increasing gradient amplitude.

For most conventional sequences it is also a natural approach in terms of sequence performance. Not so for EPI. Rectilinear EPI requires a strong and constant gradient during acquisition and extremely fast switching in between successive *k*-lines. Both requirements are extremely hard to combine in a single-gradient system.

As a consequence, other *k*-space trajectories have been proposed that distribute the current and voltage requirements more homogeneously over the total acquisition. Especially economic in terms of hardware requirements are so-called resonant-gradient designs, by which the gradient coil is part of a resonant circuit that can be driven to a high-amplitude sinusoid with very moderate power requirements. The comparative ease of this design is the reason why the first commercial EPI scanner used this approach.

If such a sinusoidal gradient is combined with a constant phase-encoding gradient, nonrectilinear *k*-space trajectories will occur (Fig. 62A). With a blipped gradient and an appropriately variable dwell time, a rectilinear trajectory can be restored. An even more radical approach is to use two sinusoids in both image dimensions (Fig. 62B). These will produce spiral scans, where the distance between windings is given by the envelope of the sinusoids (2, 149).

A disadvantage of resonant-gradient designs is their inability to perform any of the other MRI sequences described above. Resonant systems are strictly EPI-only systems. Since even slice selection is difficult to realize with a resonant-gradient design, such systems normally restrict their fast gradient to one image dimension only, which is one of the reasons why so few sagittal EPI images have been shown as yet.

In the last few months, gradient systems have been introduced that allow EPI with non-resonant-gradient systems. These offer not only the advantage of being able to combine EPI with a more conventional imaging examination, they also give additional leeway in terms of optimizing k-space trajectories.

Depending on the current and voltage performance of the power supplies, optimized k-space trajectories can be designed at which the system is always running at maximum performance (121). In general, this means sharper edges close to the center of k-space, where the gradient amplitude is low and rounder curves are seen in the outer regions (Fig. 62C). For a spiral scan, the spiral will be steep at the onset, and the height of each winding will decrease gradually when going to the outer high-amplitude regions. Non-spiral approaches like rosettes also have been proposed as efficient trajectories.

A common problem of nonrectilinear scans is the fact that the sampling points do not coincide with a rectilinear sampling grid required by image reconstruction with the fast Fourier transform algorithm. Data have therefore to be interpolated onto a grid prior to fast Fourier transformation. Interpolation is time-consuming at best and might even introduce additional artefacts.

Artefacts. Each k-space trajectory will have its own specific transformation characteristic and thus will display its own characteristic type of artefact. The trajectories, which are optimized in terms of hardware requirements, are not necessarily optimized with respect to their transformation properties.

The basic mechanisms acting on the signal amplitude and phase are, of course, the same for all trajectories. The actual way of k-space coverage will, however, define the type of artefacts that will occur.

For rectilinear EPI, the artefacts could be clearly distinguished according to their effect in the readout or phase-encoding direction. For more isotropic k-space trajectories, no such distinction can be made. Consequently, artefacts will have a different appearance. The advantage of this is that they might be less conspicuous compared with rectilinear EPI. The disadvantage is that they might appear at unexpected locations in the image and thus might not be recognized as such.

A simple demonstration of the vastly different artefact behavior of rectilinear EPI and a spiral scan is chemical shift. In rectilinear EPI, this has been shown to produce misregistration mainly in the phase-encoding direction. For spiral EPI, chemical shift will produce an increasing phase shift of the signal that is more or less tangential. This will lead to a rotational artefact, where in general the outer components of k-space are rotated by a different angle compared with the more central ones. The result will be a blurred-ring artefact.

This leads to a very fast deterioration of the image of structures whose spins are not exactly on resonance. This k-space trajectory–dependent blurring of off-resonance spins can be used to acquire purely on-resonance images by use of a stochastic k-space trajectory (184). This will lead to a near-isotropic distribution of signal intensity from spins that are only slightly off-resonance (or show phase effects due to flow or motion) all over the image, where it will melt into the background noise. These stochastic trajectories, of course, are not optimal in terms of the hardware performance and thus lead to longer acquisition times per image compared with spirals or even rectilinear scans.

Mixed Spin-Echo and Gradient-Echo Excitation: GRASE

After the discussion of what in the previous schematic overview can be called the four generic sequences (spin and gradient echo in single or multiexcitation mode), a few sequences are worthwhile discussing that use a mixed approach with respect to signal generation (hybrids between single- and multiexcitation mode with homogeneous excitation have already been discussed as hybrids of the respective single-excitation sequences). It should be emphasized that the use of the term *hybrid* does not imply any preference of the generic sequences but is simply a label for bookkeeping of the multitude of sequences with no reflection on the originality or creativity of the various sequences. Other categories also could be used, leading to other bookkeeping schemes. Historically, one could find some justification for a system by which a single-echo spin echo and EPI serve as generic sequences and all the others could be labeled as hybrids of these two.

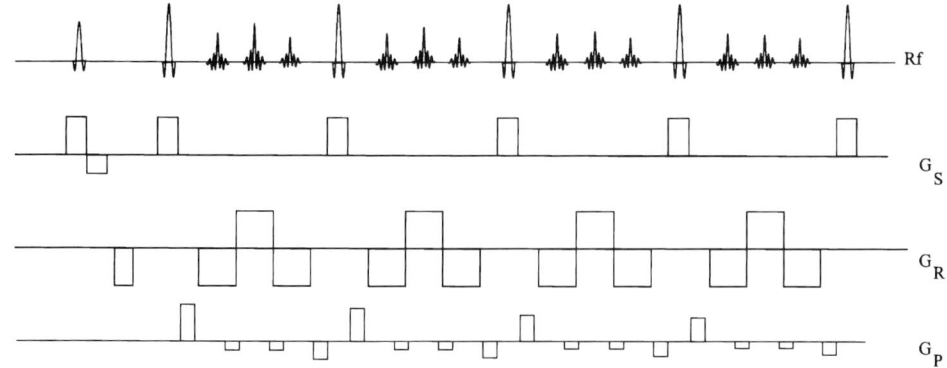

Figure 63. Scheme of the GRASE sequence. GRASE uses a CPMG echo train; thus the conditions for proper refocusing stated for the RARE sequence have to be maintained. By additional reversal of the readout gradient, additional gradient echoes are produced within each refocusing interval.

Depending on which is used as the basic sequence, a mixture of spin echoes and gradient echoes is used in the GRASE technique (Fig. 63) (169). GRASE can be conceived either as a means to ameliorate the dephasing problem of EPI by using rf refocusing on parts of the k-space data or as a significantly faster variant of RARE (TSE, FSE) that allows the acquisition of more than one echo per refocusing interval (61).

Artefacts

The basic properties of spin-echo formation do not change when the signal is read out as several gradient echoes. Therefore, the discussion in the section, "Single-Shot Spin-Echo Sequences (RARE, TSE, FSE)," fully applies to these mixed excitation sequences. This means that the CPMG conditions as described for RARE have to be maintained. The resulting GRASE sequence has been demonstrated to produce single-shot images within acquisition times well under 1 s.

The artefact behavior of GRASE will be considerably better than that of EPI. From the discussion in the section, "Single Excitation Sequences," it should be clear that the improvement comes not so much from the somewhat improved signal amplitude arising from introducing some T2 component into the T2* decay. The main benefit of GRASE compared with EPI lies in the refocusing of some of the phase effects, which have been demonstrated to be the main culprit in EPI. The same argument makes it equally clear, however, that the artefact behavior of GRASE is quite significantly worse than that of RARE (TSE, FSE), which avoids phase deterioration altogether. With respect to chemical-shift effects, for example, even the restriction to two additional gradient echoes at both sides of the proper spin echo will introduce a phase shift by 180° if the gradient echoes occur as little as 1 ms apart from the spin echo on a high-field system. This phase change will translate into more or less drastic image artefacts. This illustrates that even a low gradient-echo admixture practically always necessitates chemical-shift suppression. Similar arguments also apply to other causes of artefacts, such as susceptibility or flow, where GRASE is significantly less robust compared with pure spin-echo techniques.

A second point of concern is the mixed contrast of data acquired with GRASE. This raises the question of how to distribute the acquired data in k-space. Since phase effects are much worse compared with amplitude effects, it is rather advisable to group data together according to their T2*-dependent dephasing. Even then a monotonous weighing function cannot be obtained, and artefacts have to be expected. By optimizing the experimental conditions and using appropriate filter functions, which can be derived by measuring a non-phase-encoded echo train prior to image acquisition, such artefacts can be reduced to a certain degree. Whether the improvements can be made stable and reliable enough to allow image acquisition under routine conditions has as yet to be demonstrated.

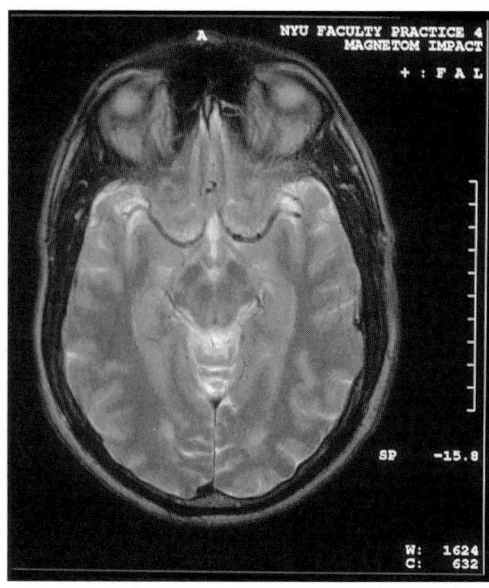

Figure 64. GRASE image of a human head (courtesy of D. Feinberg, New York University, New York, NY).

Currently, GRASE seems to be restricted to imaging of the brain, where exceptionally good images have been demonstrated under optimized conditions (Fig. 64).

APPROACHES TO FAST IMAGING

Optimizing Examination Protocols

Any cheap direct imaging device such as a photographic camera can make an image in a small fraction of a second. The reason why a million dollar system such as an MRI system has so many difficulties in reaching acquisition times in the range of 100 to 1000 ms lies in the fact that in MRI a 2D entity (the image) has to be created from an intrinsically 1D signal. The various techniques described in Chap. 1 for acquiring the data necessary for image reconstruction have their own intrinsic limitation with respect to imaging speed. Table 1 gives an overview of the relevant parameters for a 128×128 image.

It is clear that EPI will be the method of choice if—and only if—one can live with its intrinsic problems (low spatial resolution and chemical shift and susceptibility problems).

For a physicist, the relevant parameter describing imaging speed is very often equal to the imaging time for one single image. In many, if not most, applications this is a

Table 1. *Parameters for a 128 × 128 image*

Imaging sequence	Minimum no. of rf pulses	Minimum no. of gradient-switching steps	Remarks
Spin echo	256	128×6	For fast single slice, low S/N, low contrast
Gradient echo	128	128×4	Low flip angle required
RARE (FSE, TSE)	129	$128 \times 5 + 3$	Rf problems for $t_e < 4$ ms
EPI	1	130	Best S/N ratio per unit time, but intrinsically low resolution
BURST	128	3	Low S/N ratio
GRASE	$128/n_{ge} + 1$	$(128/n_{ge}) \times (2n_{ge} + 4) + 3$	Optimal for single-slice imaging in 100–500 ms

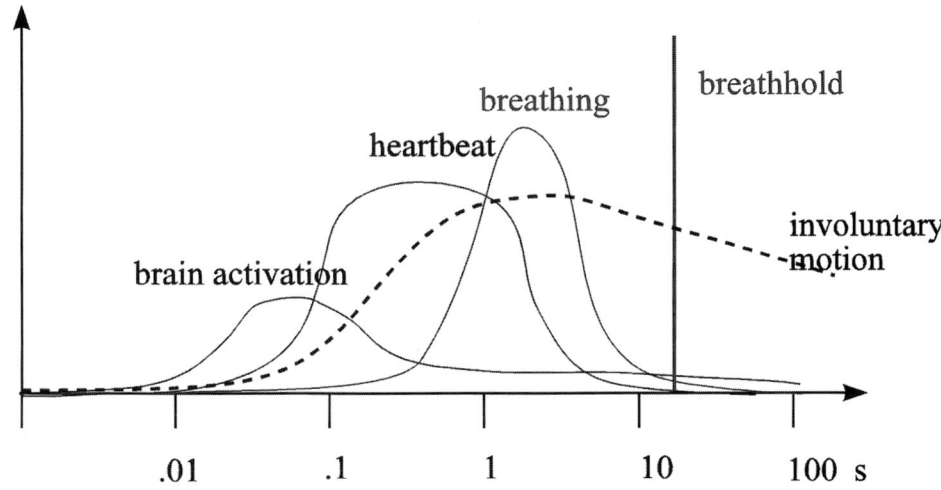

Figure 65. Ranges of relevant physiologic motion. The various physiologic motion regimes are strictly nonlinear. Involuntary motion can occur at all time scales from a few tens of milliseconds up to several minutes. An important threshold is the time a patient (and not a pearl diver) can hold his or her breath, which is in the range of 15 to 20 s. Breathing motion occurs on time scales between 0.1 and 10 s. The heartbeat is more periodic, with a periodicity around 1 s and fast systolic motion components in the region below 100 ms. The electrical response following cortical stimulation as a highly relevant goal for brain activation studies occurs in a range of 10 to 400 ms.

quite meaningless number, however. If a larger-volume coverage is desired, multislice methods or even 3D techniques can easily become the method of choice.

Finally, there exist a quite significant number of applications where fast imaging is desired but not with any compromise to the robustness of the imaging sequence against chemical shift, susceptibility, etc. This applies to many MRI examinations of the abdomen. For these, the intrinsically slower but very robust and reliable spin-echo techniques might be the method of choice for some time to come.

It should be noted that the benefits of fast imaging increase very nonlinearly with the imaging speed (Fig. 65). In the slow range of many minutes, the resulting cost of the examination and the increasing failure rate due to involuntary patient motion are the main problems. These become more or less insignificant for imaging times between 1 and 4 minutes. The next and extremely important threshold is given by the time a patient can hold his or her breath, which should not exceed 15 to 20 s. It thus is of no significant concern if the imaging time can be reduced from 3 to 1 minute; a change by the same factor of 3 from 45 to 15 s, however, can mean a whole new world of applications.

The next lower threshold is image acquisition under natural breathing, which requires acquisition times on the order of 1 to 4 seconds. Below this, imaging the beating heart constitutes a major challenge due to the fact that the systolic motion is extremely fast.

An important consideration for such acquisitions during physiologic motion is the fact that the total data-acquisition time is no good measure for the temporal resolution of most MRI sequences. As demonstrated in the section, "The Fourier Transformation," above, the most significant information in a typical MRI image is concentrated in the center of k-space. The time of acquiring these important k-lines is therefore the relevant factor in assessing the temporal resolution of a given sequence. As a consequence, it has been demonstrated that, for example, snapshot FLASH images of the heart acquired with a total acquisition time of 250 to 300 ms are surprisingly sharp, although the motion of the heart over this period is considerable. Recently, similar effects have been demonstrated using spin-echo-based sequences such as HASTE or RARE myelography, where even ECG-gated images over the heart cycle demonstrated pulsatile motion with a temporal resolution in a range of about 50 ms, although the total acquisition time is on the order of approximately one ECG cycle.

At an even shorter time scale, the spatial-temporal evolution of cortical activation has recently come to the attention of MRI due to the vast success of functional brain imaging (fMRI). The typical time scale of the electrical activity is on the order of 2 to 40 ms, which is not directly accessible to MRI techniques. According to the section, "*k*-Space," above, the limiting factor in this time regime is signal-to-noise ratio rather than any speed-related performance parameters. Therefore, major improvements in signal-to-noise ratio are required in order to get down to the lower end of this range. With current technology, such short acquisition times can only be achieved at the cost of smaller image matrices. This does not necessarily mean low spatial resolution, which, however, helps in terms of signal-to-noise ratio. For sufficiently high signal intensity, high resolution can be maintained using inner volume imaging techniques on small matrices within preselected smaller volumes.

The ultimate limit to MRI is, of course, reached for single-voxel methods, where the temporal evolution of signal from a single voxel is followed. The temporal limit here is given by the time for selecting a single voxel, which can be done easily in 5 to 15 ms.

Given the huge range of available methods and the number of compromises that can be made in terms of spatial resolution, volume coverage, signal-to-noise ratio, etc., it is not always easy to select the proper method for a given fast imaging application. With the strongly nonlinear time resolution of physiologic processes, it is very important to very accurately define the time-resolution requirements as well as the desired volume coverage in order to select the best approach to a given problem. As already mentioned, even a very conventional spin-echo scan can be an extremely efficient tool to cover a large volume using a multislice approach with high spatial resolution.

A special consideration applies to types of examinations with somewhat reduced demands on spatial resolutions, where EPI is a likely candidate as being the method of choice. The dichotomy of the MRI world into those who possess one such EPI scanner, which could not perform anything else, and those who use non-resonant-gradient systems but cannot perform EPI has as yet not allowed us to make a rational assessment of the efficacy of different scan methods for a given purpose. The discussion of the advantages or drawbacks of various techniques consequently very often was based more on myths than on facts. With the advance of fast gradient systems that can perform EPI as well as other scans, this situation currently is changing very rapidly.

Beyond Conventional 2DFT Imaging

Even when the intrinsic temporal resolution of the MRI sequences discussed in the preceding section seems to be insufficiently slow for a given task, there is not yet any need to despair. One very common type of examination where very high temporal resolution is desirable is to monitor changes inside a given volume. These changes might be motional but also might be changes in signal intensity such as contrast changes in first-pass examinations of perfusion or activity-related changes in functional MRI. A great number of methods have been developed to cover such applications, and they are all based on the idea that any such change will affect only a small fraction of the total image data. If the nature of the change can be defined in a way that can be transferred into an imaging experiment, many fewer data points need to be acquired in order to define the current status of the observed volume from a slow high-resolution image acquired prior to the time-resolved study and a much faster experiment, where only the change is measured.

Determination of Main Motional Components

One such example is monitoring of the translational component of motion of a body during an examination. By measuring 1D projections, the main components of motion can be measured very fast (48, 134). Rigid motion components in all three dimensions can thus be measured in three steps.

The resulting signal can be used, for example, in order to measure 1D ventricular motion in so-called line-scan techniques, which are equivalent to M-mode ultrasound

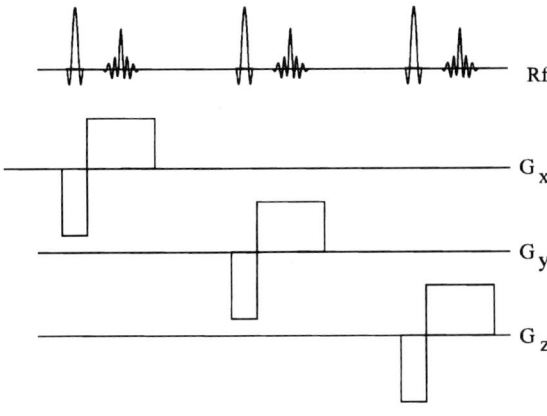

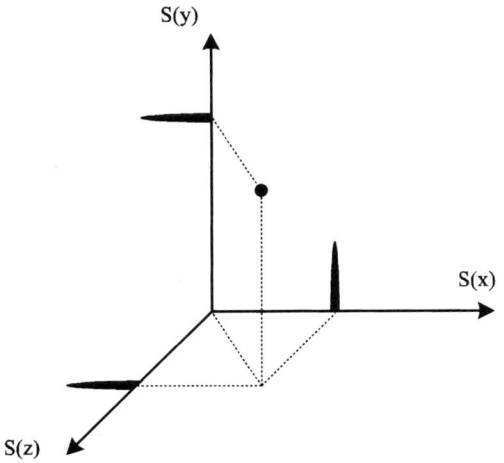

Figure 66. Tip tracking. The locus of a single point can be determined by successive measurement of its three spatial coordinates by a sequence of three gradient echoes under mutually orthogonal gradients.

techniques (see Chap. 11). Such measurements can even be interleaved with a conventional scan and be used for intrascan motion correction using so-called navigator echo techniques (64). Using nonlinear k-line trajectories, motion components in two dimensions have been measured using a single 1D scan (211).

Localization versus Imaging

A more general area of application where 1D projections can be used much more efficiently than pixel-by-pixel imaging techniques consists of examinations where the problem involves locating a comparatively small number of discrete objects within the body. A practical application where a few 1D projections are sufficient to measure is in tip-tracking for interventional MRI (48, 134), where various approaches have been demonstrated to follow the tip of a catheter needle with extremely high temporal resolution. Three 1D projections under appropriate projection angles are sufficient to define the locus and extent of a single point (Fig. 66). Even when more than one signal source is to be located, it has been demonstrated that a very limited number of 1D projections is sufficient to localize several such discrete entities (99). Not only can this principle be used to find and locate discrete structures, but it is also applicable in combination with pre-selection techniques, where a discrete pattern is generated by an appropriate excitation sequence.

Keyhole Imaging and MR Fluoroscopy

The 1D approaches described in the preceding section are restricted to problems where changes in the location or signal intensity are to be monitored that affect either the object

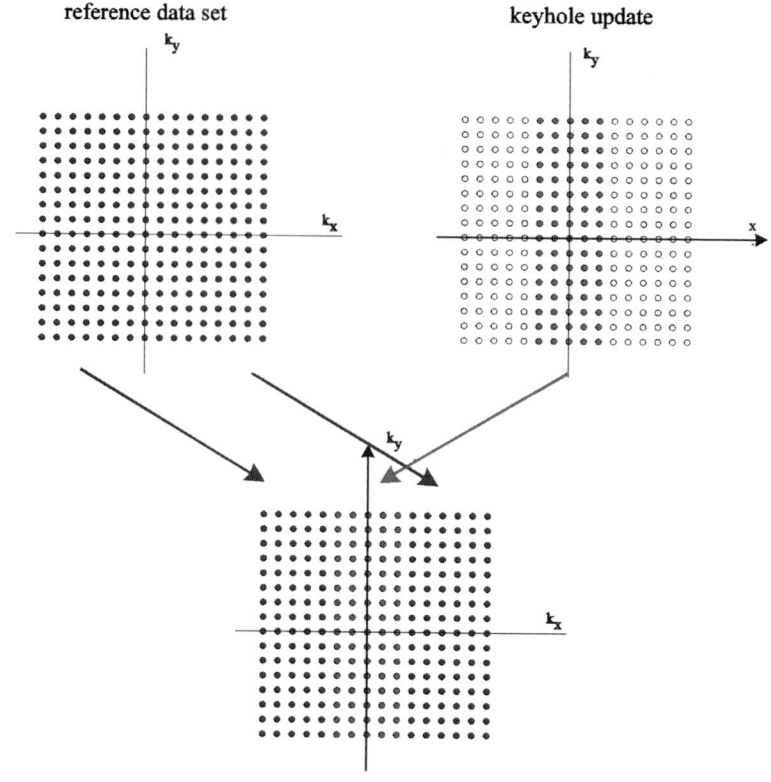

reference data set

keyhole update

combined k-space data of update

Figure 67. Principle of keyhole imaging. First, a fully resolved reference data set is acquired (*blue, top left*). The update images are then acquired with considerably reduced (typically 32) phase-encoding steps normally sampled at the center of *k*-space (*red, top right*). Images are then reconstructed after supplementing the missing *k*-lines in the updated data sets from the reference data (*bottom*). See Color Plate 31.

as a whole or a small subset of sufficiently discrete structures. If changes of a more general nature are to be monitored, where no such a priori confines can be postulated, more spatial information needs to be acquired in order to make a decent assessment of the location and nature of the change. Keyhole imaging has been proposed as a possibility to generate updates of an initial high-resolution scan with much higher imaging speed (200). It follows from the already mentioned property of *k*-space data of medical images that the relevant information of a typical MRI image is restricted to the center of *k*-space. In keyhole imaging, updates are acquired only from a limited subset of *k*-lines around the center of *k*-space. The missing lines are then supplemented from the original high-resolution scan (Fig. 67 and Color Plate 31). As long as the change is small compared with the reference image, the supplemented data will fit very well into the updates, and the resulting combined image will display nearly the same high resolution compared with the reference scan but at an acquisition speed that is typically 8 times faster.

From the addition theorem it follows that the effect image, i.e., the difference of the updated and supplemented images to the reference image, will show the same low resolution defined by the number of updates. Since the change is the relevant information to be monitored, pure keyholing is somewhat cosmetic.

More recently, quite a number of approaches have been published where prior knowledge about the nature of the change is used to refine the keyholing approach. One possibility is to acquire two reference images, one at the beginning and one at the end of the time evolution. If the nature of the temporal evolution is such that changes can be said to occur only at locations that show changes between the two reference images, exceedingly good keyhole images can be reconstructed from very few updates (13). These conditions are typical for bolus tracking of contrast agents, where such an approach has been demonstrated very successfully. Other algorithms using prior knowledge that are

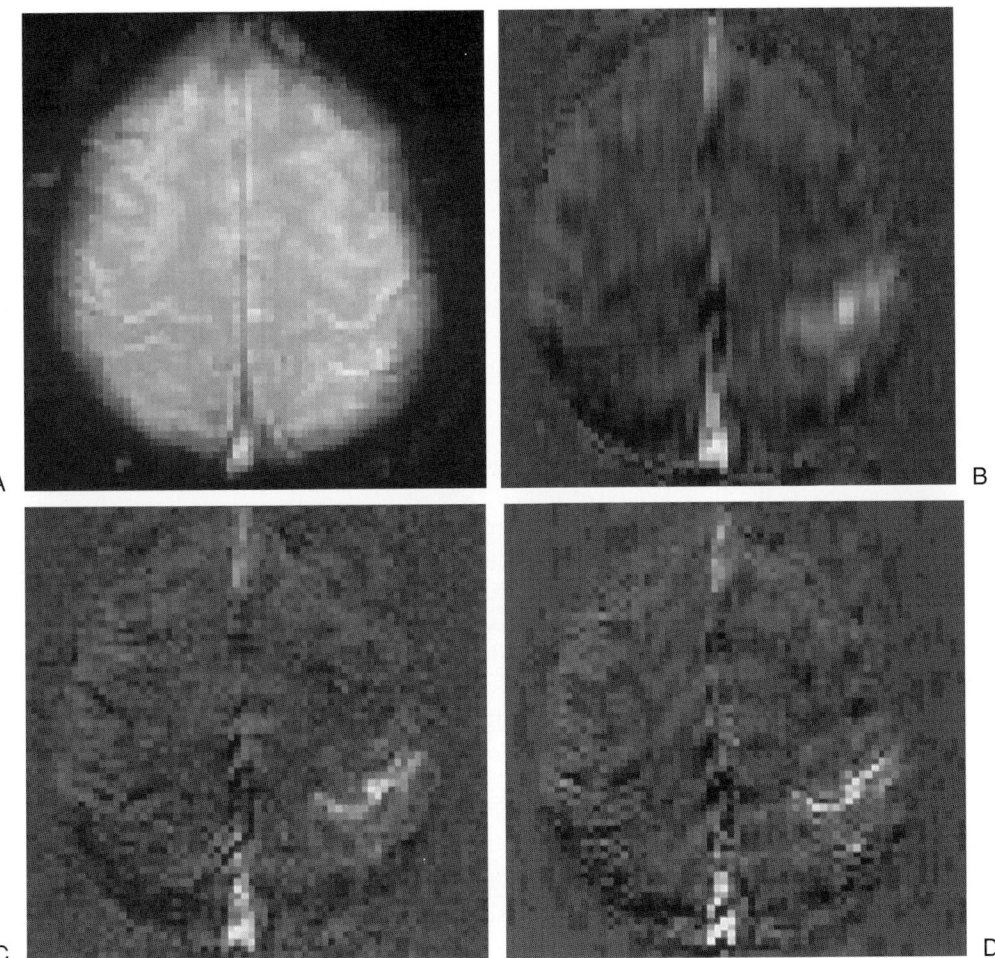

Figure 68. Keyhole images acquired during a brain activation experiment. **(A)** The reference image. **(B)** The low-resolution stimulation image generated by subtraction of the keyhole image based on 32 updates from the reference image. **(C)** The full resolution activation image with signal enhancement in the activated primary motor cortex. **(D)** Keyhole effect image based on 32 updates as in **B** but with improved postprocessing.

based on the fact that the structure of the image remains constant also can be used to improve both the sampling strategy and the reconstruction of keyhole images (Fig. 68) (165).

It should be noted that keyhole imaging is just a special implementation of MR fluoroscopic methods (176) that were described much earlier and which use an adaptive strategy of k-line updates in order to generate a frame rate for observation that is much faster than the actual acquisition rate for one image.

Non-Fourier Approaches: Singular Value Decomposition and Wavelets

It was stressed in Chap. 1 that the number of measures to be acquired for forming an image is given by the number of independent image elements to be observed, which can be much lower than the 65,536 pixels that have to be measured in a conventional 256 × 256 imaging experiment. Defining the relevant image elements is a very active area of research for digital image compression. MRI offers the rather unique possibility to implement some of these compression schemes into a physical measurement process.

One such possibility is wavelet encoding, which can be shown to quite efficiently compress the number of relevant data points. Wavelet-based acquisition techniques have been used in MRI (91). They suffer, however, from intrinsic limitations in signal-to-noise ratio given by the fact that wavelet-encoding measures put only parts of the total information in each scan. The intrinsic averaging that takes place in Fourier imaging thus takes place only partially.

An even more radical approach is singular value decomposition, which is a basic tool in mathematics to create an arbitrary matrix from a hierarchical order of so-called Eigenmatrices that have only diagonal elements. Since such Eigenimages for an $n \times n$ matrix contain only n elements, they can be measured in one single acquisition, at least in principle, if their structure is known beforehand. Although mathematically the number of Eigenimages necessary to fully define a given image is equal to the number of lines, it can be shown that the sum of the Eigenimages converges very fast. With only 16 or even 8 Eigenimages, high-resolution images, which are virtually indistinguishable from the 256×256 reference image, can be reconstructed.

This requires, of course, that the Eigenvalues of the image to be acquired are known beforehand. Just like keyhole imaging, SVD encoding thus requires an initial reference scan as a starting point. The observed changes are then used continually to update the reference image on the fly (''adaptive imaging'').

The problem of implementing this mathematically very simple approach into an MRI sequence is, however, considerable. It requires the use of rf pulses whose profile is defined by the elements of the Eigenmatrices. Data are thus not acquired by leaving transverse magnetization to evolve in k-space under the effect of spatially encoding gradients. Spatial encoding is rather performed by specially shaped pulses, an approach called *frequency encoding.*

Despite the considerable technical problems inherent in such an approach, promising results have already been produced (170).

CONTRAST MANIPULATION

The imaging sequences discussed above already have some built-in sensitivity to a considerable variety of parameters characterizing the tissue under observation. Further contrast manipulation can be carried out either by the application of some extrinsic contrast agent or by manipulation of the MRI signal itself. The first possibility will be covered in the next subsection, whereas the rest of this chapter will be dedicated to the various possibilities to influence the MRI signal directly in order to achieve some sensitivity for some intrinsically MRI-visible parameter.

Contrast Agents

Relaxivity-Based Agents

Contrast agents are used in nearly all imaging techniques (see Chap. 2). Their idea is to apply some extrinsic agent that yields very high contrast and to follow its distribution after oral or intravenous injection. The problem in applying this concept to MRI imaging is the fact that MRI already is based on high concentrations of the most visible compound, namely, protons, for acquiring images without contrast agents. For water protons the effective proton concentration is more than 50 mol/kg. Performing a contrast agent examination based on the visibility of the agent itself thus would require very high concentrations of the agents (1 mol/kg of body weight or more) in order to override the high signal from native tissue. Since the application of high-dose materials is impracticable, MRI contrast agents very early were based not on the visibility of the agent itself but on their effects on their molecular surroundings (Fig. 69).

A typical MRI contrast agent is based on the use of a paramagnetic ion with a high magnetic moment. Rare earth metals, especially gadolinium (Gd), are especially suited (due to their high magnetic moment). Since heavy metal ions, which have strong magnetic moments, are quite toxic in ionic form, the metals are bound in chelates with very strong binding constants. The strong local magnetic moment affects protons in the surroundings of the agent in various ways; if the ion has a high intrinsic mobility, its motion in the outer magnetic field will generate a strong electromagnetic field that will act as

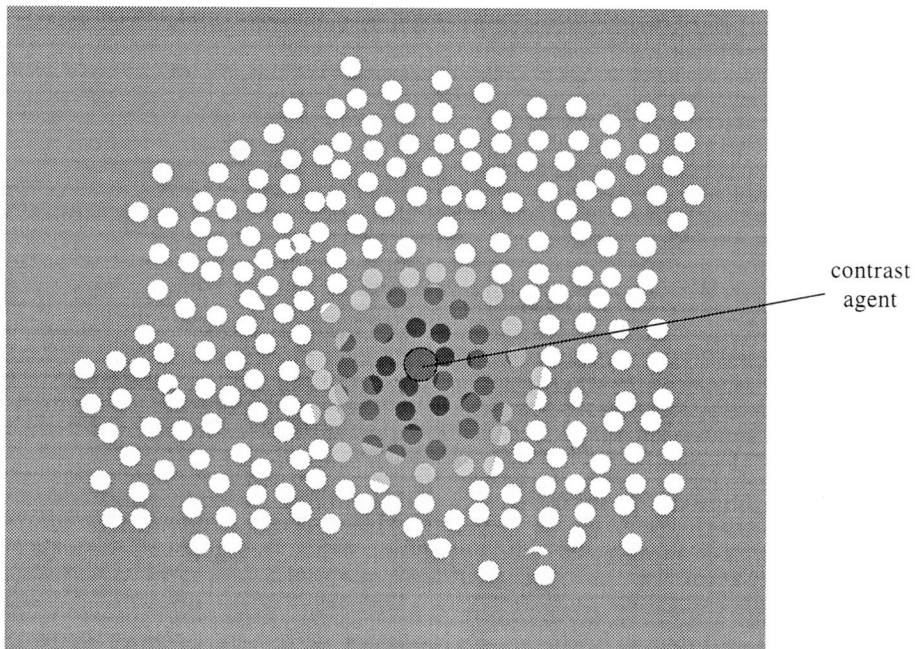

contrast
agent

Figure 69. Indirect effect of MRI contrast agents. The contrast agent molecule itself remains invisible to the MRI experiment. It does affect, however, the visibility of a great number of protons in its surroundings by changing their relaxation behavior. Thus a very low concentration of contrast agent can change the signal in an appreciable number of protons.

an additional source for relaxation. The effect of this dipole-dipole interaction is in principle identical for T1 and T2 and will increase the relaxation rate $1/T1,2_1$ of the surrounding protons:

$$1/T1,2_{\mathrm{eff}} = 1/T1,2_1 + cR_{1,2} \tag{16}$$

where c is the concentration of the agent and $R_{1,2}$ is the T1 or T2 relaxivity of the agent.

Since T1 for normal tissue is much longer than T2, the relative effect for a given cR will affect T1 relaxation much more than T2 relaxation. Consequently, these agents are normally treated as T1 agents. Just like T1 relaxation from the molecular surroundings, the relaxivity of an agent will show some more or less pronounced field strength effect that is directly related to the mobility. In general, relaxivity will increase at lower field strength. Since T1 itself also gets shorter, this does not automatically lead to stronger enhancement at lower field strengths. In fact, for most agents, the reduction in T1 will overcompensate the stronger relaxivity for many relevant tissue types. With the additional lower S/N ratio at lower field strengths, contrast agent examinations can in general be said to be more problematic the lower the field. The search for efficient agents, particularly for low-field magnets, is thus a very active and relevant field of current research.

The effect of the agent, of course, will strongly depend on the imaging sequence used. Some T2 effect will always crawl into any T1-weighted imaging sequence due to the finite time between excitation and signal acquisition. Shortening of T1 will lead to a signal increase in a common partial saturation experiment used for T1 weighting, whereas shortening of T2 will lead to signal loss. Therefore, at some concentration a reversal of the enhancement will occur, when the T2 loss overcompensates the signal gain by shortening T1. The exact shape of the intensity versus concentration curve, of course, will strongly depend on the actual imaging sequence used (Fig. 70). In general, it is prudent to work in a concentration regime where the contrast can be safely assumed to vary (nearly) linearly with concentration.

High concentrations leading to signal obliteration are a serious concern for first-pass studies, where transient local concentrations easily can be several times higher than the steady-state concentration.

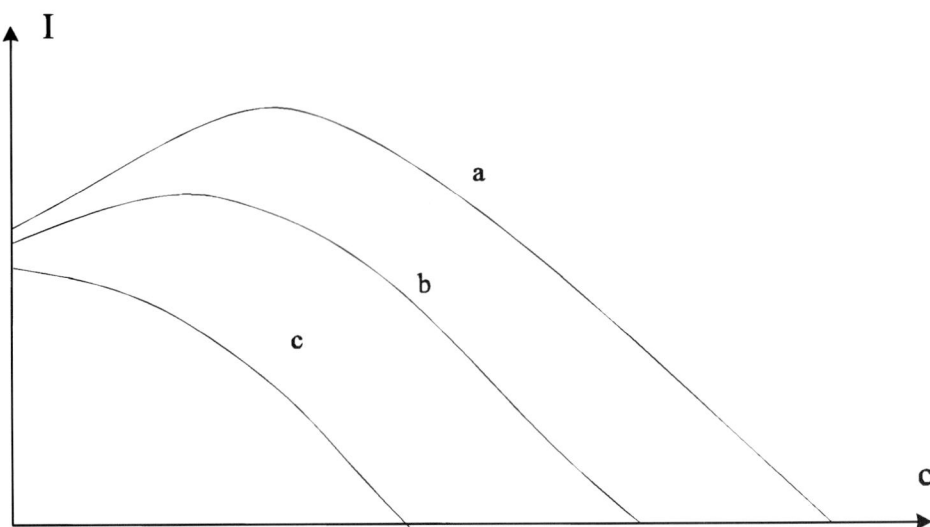

Figure 70. Signal intensity versus concentration of the contrast agent. Most contrast agents lead to a shortening of T1 as well as T2(T2*). The shortening of T1 will lead to an increase in the signal intensity with increasing concentration of the agent (*a*) until a critical concentration is reached at which the T2(T2*)-dependent signal loss compensates the T1-dependent signal gain. At even higher concentrations, the intensity will drop. For stronger T2(T2*)-weighted scans, this signal drop will be reached at lower concentrations (*b*). For purely T2(T2*)-weighted measuring techniques, only the T2(T2*)-dependent signal loss will be observed (*c*).

A second class of paramagnetic compounds does not show a mobility that leads to dipole-dipole relaxation. Such agents will act mainly by the strong local susceptibility field and will be visible by their static or dynamic susceptibility effects. Such agents also can consist of chelate complexes of metal ions. Alternatively, superparamagnetic iron oxide particles (SPIOs) can be used, which create very strong local magnetic fields.

Gradient-echo sequences with long echo times are the most sensitive experiments that can be used to observe T2* agents. Due to the intrinsic sensitivity of such sequences to macroscopic susceptibility effects and chemical shift, their application in the abdomen is restricted. Spin-echo-based sequences are not sensitive to static susceptibility effects; they do, however, show dynamic T2* changes. Consequently, they might be the methods of choice for applications where macroscopic susceptibility effects make the application of gradient-echo-based techniques problematic. Since the dynamic T2* effect is only one aspect of the total relaxivity effect, such spin-echo-based examinations require higher concentrations of the agents in order to generate the same signal attenuation. This disadvantage can be balanced, however, by the often higher S/N ratio of spin-echo techniques, leading to an improved effect-to-noise ratio. It should be emphasized that the balance between static and dynamic susceptibility effect strongly depends on the distribution of the agent. For capillary distribution it has been shown that for capillary sizes below 5 to 10 μm, the dynamic T2* effect will be the dominating factor leading to equal attenuation in spin-echo- and gradient-echo-based experiments, whereas more lumpy distribution of the agents will prefer the static T2* effect.

From the discussion in the section, "Relaxation Times," above, it is not unexpected that SPIOs will start showing T1 relaxivity effects when their size becomes small enough. With diminishing size, the molecular tumbling motion will become faster and faster and finally contain appreciable frequency components at the Larmor frequency.

Distribution-Based Agents

The direct observation of an appropriate contrast agent suffers from two problems: the low intrinsic sensitivity of the MRI experiment, which requires a considerable amount of agent, and the comparatively high signal from the protons observed by MRI. Distribution-based agents try to avoid the latter problem either by using the observation of

ON THE EFFICACY OF CONTRAST AGENTS

The effect of contrast agents with a given relaxivity $R_{1,2}$ depends on the T1,2 of the tissue under study. For a typical example of a tissue with T1 = 1 s and T2 = 100 ms, a relaxivity $R_1 = R_2 = 10$/s will change the relaxation rates to

$$1/T1 = (1 + 10)/s = 11/s \qquad T1 = 99 \text{ ms}$$

$$1/T2 = (10 + 10)/s = 20/s \qquad T2 = 50 \text{ ms}$$

For the same relaxivity, the change in T1 is thus more than 90%, whereas T2 changes by only 50%.

Paramagnetic relaxation agents thus act best if the intrinsic relaxation time is long. Their effect on T1 is thus larger than the T2 effect. For T1 measurements, they will act better at higher fields, where T1 is long.

nuclei other than protons or by using proton-containing compounds with a chemical shift that is sufficiently far away from the resonance frequency of fat or water protons.

The first approach has been used with some limited success by observing compounds containing fluorine. Although fluorine is nearly as MR sensitive as protons, the resulting images suffer from severe S/N ratio problems due to the low concentrations of the agents even under favorable circumstances. Consequently, the spatial resolution of such images cannot be expected to be as high as that of proton images. This especially applies to the observation of pharmacologically active substances, the distribution of which can only be measured with very limited spatial resolution.

Hyperpolarization. An exception to the low sensitivity of distribution-based agents can be hyperpolarized noble gases. It has been known for several decades that the equilibrium distribution of noble gas nuclei in the upper and lower energy states can be altered by optical pumping (1). The total magnetization thus can be increased by a factor of up to 100,000. A tiny concentration of hyperpolarized noble gas (He and Xe both have been used) can thus lead to a signal intensity comparable with that of water protons.

This possibility has been demonstrated only recently to be applicable in MRI (4, 150). Quite a number of problems have to be solved before an assessment can be made about the feasibility and relevance of such an approach for imaging on humans. The problem of preparing an adequate amount of hyperpolarized noble gas has to be solved, as well as that of removing the highly toxic Rb from the preparation mixture. Specially designed imaging sequences have to be used for observation of the hyperpolarized state. After a single 90° pulse, *z*-magnetization will return to zero and from there to its equilibrium value; therefore, everything that can be done in terms of making an MRI image has to be done with a single rf pulse. Even after solving all the technical problems of preparation and administration of the hyperpolarized gas and making an image, it remains to be demonstrated that the then possible clinical applications (lung filling, perfusion measurements?) are of sufficient clinical relevance and the images acquired with this approach sufficiently superior to other, more mundane methods to warrant the high technical effort involved.

Intrinsic Contrast Mechanisms: Basic Concepts—Amplitude or Phase Modulation

As if the large variety of accessible image contrast parameters of the basic imaging experiments with or without contrast agents would not be enough, MRI offers the opportunity to introduce further sensitivity to a number of parameters. In the next two subsections, first the basic approaches to manipulate the image contrast are introduced, and then some examples are shown of how these concepts can be used in various basic approaches to functional MRI. Basically, additional sensitization can be achieved by affecting either the amplitude or the phase of the MRI signal. In the following, first some basic tools for contrast manipulation will be described, followed by some application to

vary morphologic contrast; then MRI methods specially designed for functional examinations will be discussed. Some of the manipulation schemes are conceived to be so
general in nature that they are labeled according to their contrast effect. Examples of this
are inversion recovery, chemical-shift imaging, magnetization transfer, and flow compensation. Other such schemes are more closely related to some particular imaging sequence with which they are used. Magnetization-prepared rapid-gradient-echo imaging
(snapshot FLASH (84), MP-RAGE) (157) and ultrafast low-flip-angle acquisition with
relaxation enhancement (U-FLARE) (164) are examples.

Amplitude-Modulation Schemes

The basic idea used for amplitude modulation is to introduce additional rf pulses into
any of the basic MRI sequences in order to achieve some new contrast or to enhance
some intrinsic contrast sensitivity. It should be noted that the additional contrast parameter works in addition to the intrinsic contrast of the imaging sequence. The resulting
mixed-contrast images consequently often require the acquisition of a reference image
for comparison. The various contrast parameters that are accessible to be introduced via
prepulse schemes are discussed in the following subsection. An important consideration
in implementing such a sequence is the fact that the intrinsic contrast of the imaging
sequence should not overwhelm the additional contrast parameter.

Snapshot FLASH and MP-RAGE. The term *magnetization-prepared rapid-gradient-
echo imaging* (MP-RAGE) is very often restricted to a fast-gradient-echo imaging sequence that is preceded by an inversion (157) that influences the T1 contrast of the
ensuing experiment (Fig. 71). In its broader sense, other contrast parameters can be
introduced into such an experiment as well (84). Important to note is the fact that the
additional contrast fades away over the data acquisition, especially when larger flip angles
are used, which tend to destroy the previous spin memory. It is thus advisable to acquire
the important phase-encoding steps right next to the initial contrast manipulation period.
The usual practice to dismiss the initial repetition steps until the system has reached a
steady state can thus not be applied. In order to minimize artefacts arising from the fact
that the sequence is performed neither near equilibrium nor at a steady state, flip angle
variations along the data acquisition have been proposed that lead to a continuous modulation of the signal envelope and thus minimize image artefacts.

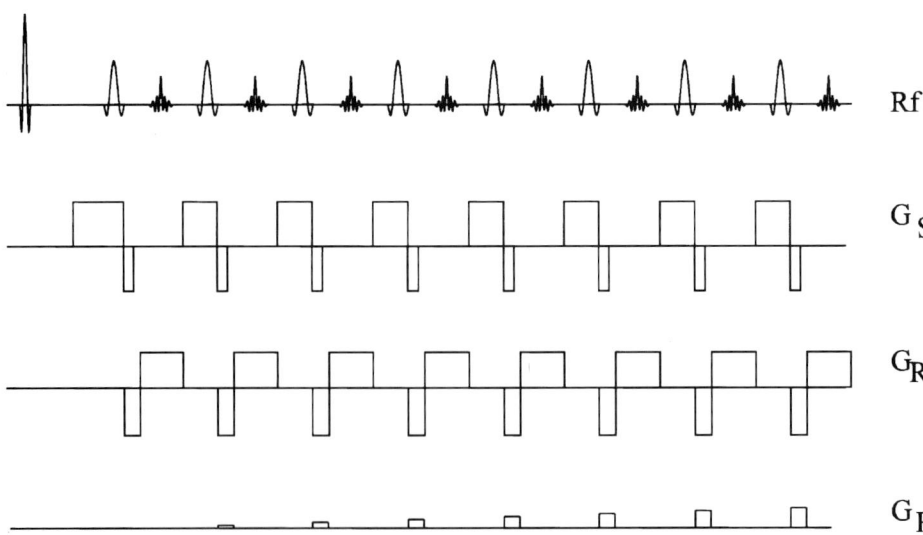

Figure 71. Pulse sequence MP-RAGE. The gradient-echo acquisition is preceded by an
inversion pulse that will affect the *z*-magnetization and thus the signal intensity of the
ensuing gradient echoes.

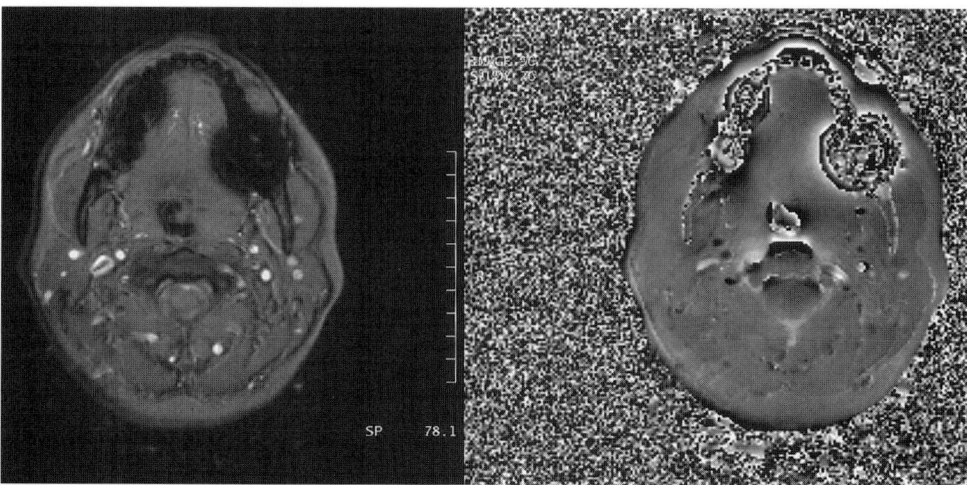

Figure 72. Transverse FLASH image through the human head (*left*) and an image representing the signal phase (*right*). Note phase changes due to susceptibility effects (especially around metal implants in the teeth) as well as phase modulations in vessels due to flow.

Phase Modulation

Phase-modulation schemes have to take place after the initial excitation pulse, since transverse magnetization has to be there before its phase can be modulated. They are thus integrated into the basic imaging sequence.

It has already been mentioned that a number of mechanisms exist that can modify the phase of the MRI signal (susceptibility, motion, chemical shift, etc.). Depending on the nature and exactness of the desired information, these phase effects can be measured with various degrees of refinement.

Phase Images. The simplest approach to measure phase-related signal changes uses a phase image for image display rather than the usual magnitude image. The phase image is calculated on a pixel-by-pixel basis from the complex data set resulting from Fourier transformation instead of or in addition to the usual magnitude calculation. Phase images (and ensuing gradient echoes; Fig. 72) can be used to qualitatively assess severe phase effects like those occurring in vascular flow. They are, however, of limited use for more quantitative measurements, since the signal phase can be influenced by a number of technical parameters and also by more than one physical mechanism.

Phase-Contrast Images. An improvement over the direct phase imaging display is the use of phase-contrast methods, where two data sets are acquired successively such that they differ in the signal phase with respect to the desired parameter only. Flow can be measured in this way (49, 201, 203) as well as a distinction having been made according to the chemical composition of the tissue under study. A problem with phase-contrast techniques is their dependence on the reproducibility of the measurement. They are thus preferably realized by interleaving the acquisition of the two sets in order to minimize the time delay between acquisition of corresponding data.

Preferable implementation of phase-difference techniques uses either a combination of a phase-sensitized scan with a nonsensitized acquisition or two scans with opposite phase sensitization. In principle, however, any two acquisitions can be used so long as they differ in their parameter-dependent signal phase.

MR Interferometry. A different approach to measure some parameter by its phase sensitivity is offered by interferographic techniques (97). The principle of measurement by interference can be derived simply from the basics of wave propagation and is described in Chap. 1. Mathematically, it follows from the shift theorem of Fourier transformation: If two signals are superimposed that are identical but reach the detector by a different route or at a different time, they will form an interference pattern. Any phase change in one of the signals will be converted into a shift of the interference pattern.

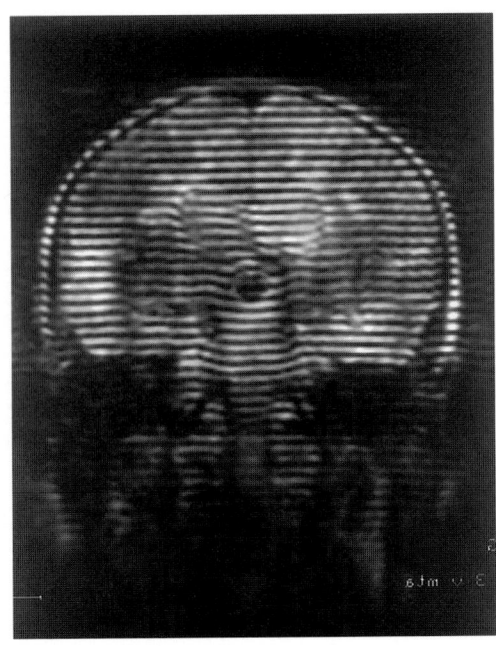

Figure 73. ECG-gated MR interferographic image demonstrating pulsatile brain motion (coronal view). Dislocation of the horizontal interferographic stripes indicates local motion. Note the downward motion of the brain stem at the time of arrival of the arterial pulse wave.

In terms of an MRI experiment, interferometry requires the generation of two signals such that they appear within the same acquisition window. There exists a great variety of excitation schemes that can be used for an interferographic experiment and which can be sensitized for various parameters. The advantage of such an approach compared with phase-contrast methods is the very short time delay between the two signals, which makes this approach very robust against reproducibility artefacts. In addition, the result is immediately available for visual inspection and does not require any postprocessing (Fig. 73). Deriving quantitative data from an interferogram necessitates, however, additional effort in order to regain the initial phase information from the interferograms.

The interferographic display intrinsically has lower spatial resolution than the underlying image. An alternative pattern over at least 2 pixels is the minimum requirement. In order to avoid moiré effects between the interferogram and the pixel matrix of the image, typically a modulation period of 4 pixels is chosen. The interferographic display is thus not very well suited to look at changes that occur on a very small scale like flow in a vessel. It should be emphasized, however, that by reconverting the interferogram into its basic constituent signals, parametric maps can be constructed with the same spatial resolution as the underlying images.

Fourier Techniques. The ultimate method to make use of phase changes is to convert them to a Fourier experiment in which a data set is generated where the phase change caused by the parameter to be measured is varied linearly from one acquisition step to the next. This is exactly identical to the procedure used for spatial encoding of an image. The resulting parameter image will then, however, not contain a spatial coordinate as in a 2DFT image but will display directly the phase sensitivity of the observed signals as an offset of the coordinate of that signal in the parametric image. Fourier techniques, of course, are most suitable for the measurement of phase-sensitive parameters, which can take on a variety of different values inside each measured volume. Fourier techniques thus can be used to measure chemical shift and susceptibility. Their most prominent application in functional MRI is for quantitative exact flow measurements (see next section).

Basic Parameters

Inversion Recovery Imaging

Inversion recovery (IR) imaging does not produce a new type of contrast; it rather can be used to emphasize T1 contrast. The basic concept of inversion recovery was introduced

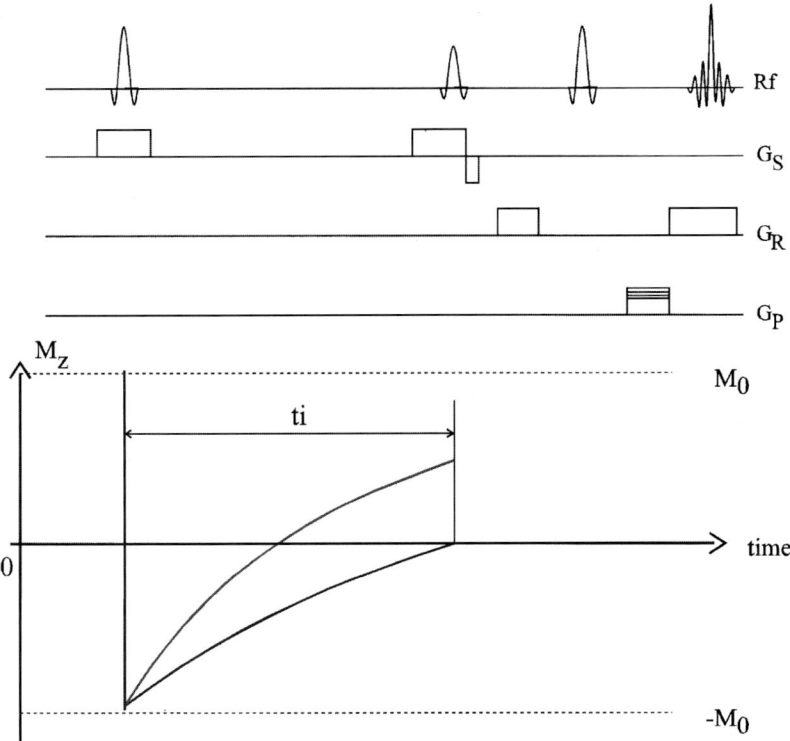

Figure 74. Inversion recovery nulling of signal. If the inversion time t_i is chosen such that the longitudinal relaxation of spins with an appropriate value of T1 is just at its zero crossing (*blue*), then no signal will be generated from those spins. See Color Plate 32.

earlier. By inverting the signal, the effective span of T1-dependent signal amplitudes is effectively doubled compared with progressive saturation sequences. A practical difficulty for IR imaging is the fact that positive and negative signal amplitudes are not distinguished on magnitude images, and thus some ambiguity arises. This can be avoided by using combinations of t_i and t_r such that the signals from the major tissues occur on one side of the zero point (short t_i or long t_i IR).

IR combined with multiexcitation spin echo leads to very long examination times due to the large recovery times required in order to establish good T1 contrast. When combined with RARE (FSE, TSE) or other fast imaging techniques, IR imaging, however, can become a practical and attractive sequence that can be used to resolve, for example, the very subtle T1 difference between gray and white matter of the brain. A very useful feature of IR imaging is its possibility to null the signal from some unwanted compound with a particular relaxation time T1. By putting the excitation pulse at a time where the *z*-magnetization is just at its zero crossing, no signal from that compound will be generated (Fig. 74 and Color Plate 32). This has been used in the STIR sequence for fat suppression (26) (Fig. 75), which will be discussed in the next section and also in the FLAIR experiment, which selectively nulls signal from cerebrospinal fluid (87) (Fig. 76). Multi-inversion experiments that null more than one signal also have been tried with variable success to suppress signals with a broader range of T1 values. A drawback of such an approach can be that the signal intensity of the nonsuppressed entities also will be somewhat affected and occur more or less far from their optimized value without inversion.

Chemical-Shift Selective Imaging (CSI)

The possibility to selectively suppress or enhance the signals from certain chemical entities was a direct legacy of NMR spectroscopy to MRI. Such techniques have been used in analytical NMR for decades and thus were introduced into MRI at a very early

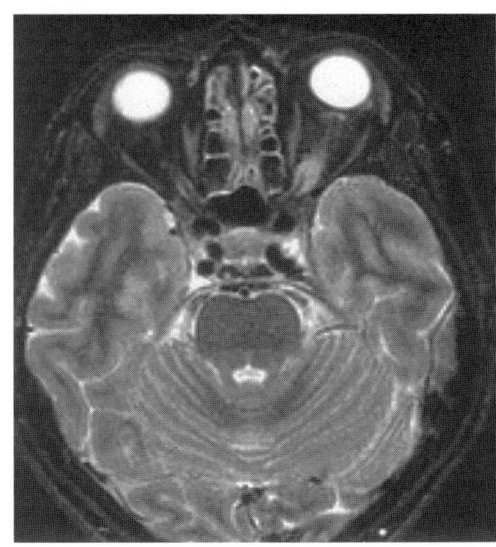

Figure 75. Transverse STIR-RARE image of the human head with an inflammation of the optic nerve. Fat signal is suppressed by adjusting the inversion time. This allows a clear delineation of the bright lesion from orbital fat.

stage. The high-intensity proton signals used for MRI fall into the two chemically different categories of aqueous or lipid tissues that are separated by a chemical-shift difference of about 3.3 ppm. At 1.5 T, 3.3 ppm corresponds to about 200 Hz. This is very small and lies in the order of the magnetic field inhomogeneity or susceptibility effects even at 1.5 T. For field strength below 1 T, chemical-shift selection is restricted to a limited volume in homogeneous tissues, although CSI has been demonstrated on systems as low as 0.23 T.

Even for perfectly homogeneous magnets, CSI becomes unfeasible at low field strengths due to the fact that the selective pulses used for amplitude modulation or the encoding times necessary for phase modulation become prohibitively long.

CSI by Amplitude Modulation. Basically, amplitude modulation or phase modulation can be used to separate fat and water. Amplitude modulation can be achieved by either chemical-shift selective suppression (CHESS), selective excitation, or selective inversion (18, 46, 85, 178) (Fig. 77). The first approach is used most commonly. It includes the application of a selective pulse prior to the imaging sequence that converts all z-mag-

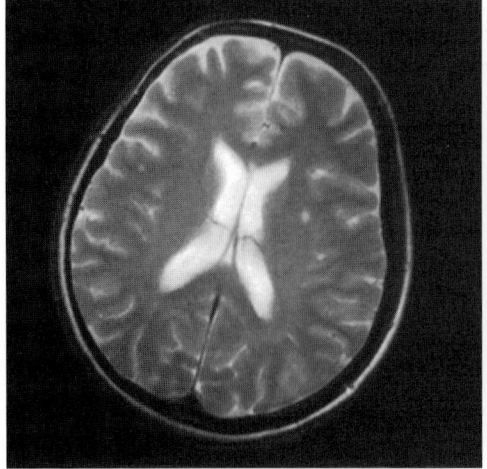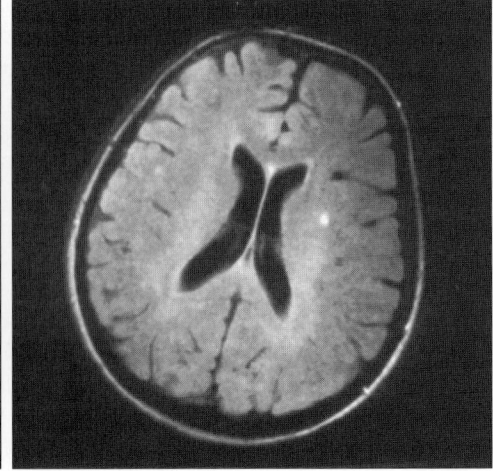

Figure 76. Transversal T2-weighted RARE image (*left*) of a patient with multiple sclerosis compared with an image acquired with a FLAIR-RARE sequence (*right*), where the signal from cerebrospinal fluid (CSF) is nulled by appropriate choice of the inversion time. The demyelination lesions remain bright in the FLAIR image, thus allowing their distinction from CSF.

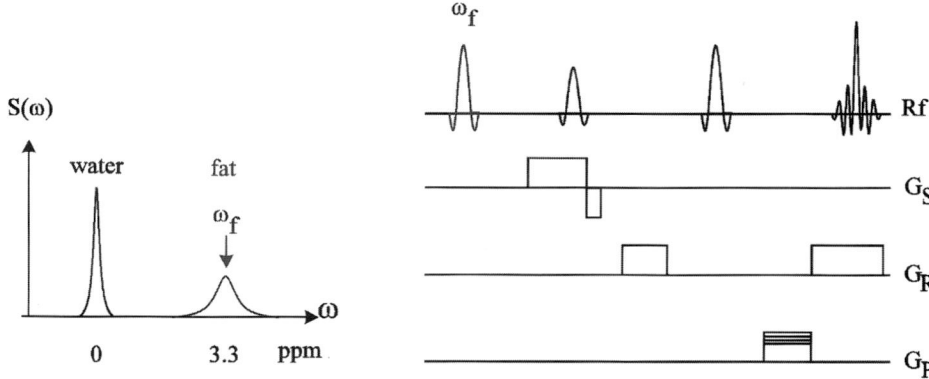

Figure 77. Principle of chemical-shift suppression (CHESS). The image-acquisition sequence (in this case, a spin-echo experiment) is preceded by a saturation pulse with a frequency w_f that is chosen such that the signal of one time between the shift-selective pulse and the excitation pulse is close to zero, then the flip angle of the suppression pulse will be 90°. In practice this is not the case, and the flip angle will be adjusted such that the signal from the unwanted species is minimized.

netization from the unwanted compartment into transverse magnetization, which is then dephased using an appropriate spoiler gradient.

At the time of the excitation pulse of the imaging sequence, no z-magnetization from the presaturated compound will then be available for imaging. If selective images are required for both tissue types, the acquisition has to be repeated using saturation on the second compound.

CSI by Phase Modulation. The different phase evolution of fat and water spins also can be used for CSI. The principle of in-phase and out-of-phase signals was already introduced. Linear combinations of in-phase and out-of-phase images can be used to generate pure fat or pure water images (44). Such experiments can be based not only on gradient-echo sequences but also on spin-echo sequences, where the necessary T2* sensitivity is introduced using some slight time shift of the spin echo.

CSI by T1 Contrast (STIR). A final and very universal method for shift-selective imaging uses the rather homogeneous T1 relaxation times of lipid protons to nullify their signal by a short-term inversion recovery experiment (26). Since this method does not rely on resolving the small chemical-shift difference between fat and water, it can be applied at all field strengths, where the t_i and t_r parameters have, of course, to be adapted according to the field dependence of T1.

A disadvantage of STIR is the fact that the signal intensity of normal aqueous tissues also will be significantly reduced. STIR thus does not deliver very pretty pictures. Since it does show many pathologies quite well, it is nevertheless an attractive diagnostic tool, especially when speeded up by combination with fast acquisition sequences (see Fig. 75).

Magnetization Transfer

The IR and CSI sequences discussed so far do not introduce some new contrast parameter but rather emphasize some already existing signal mechanism. Magnetization transfer makes use of the effect of the relaxation rate of large molecules on the observed water protons by proton exchange (10, 45, 56, 116, 168, 205). If the z-magnetization of protons of proteins is saturated by a sequence as shown in Fig. 78, this saturation will be transferred partially to the water signal by proton exchange between free water and hydrophilic groups at the surface of the protein. The exchange will be more efficient, of course, if more exchangeable protons stay on the macromolecule per unit time. Due to their very short T2, macromolecules show very broad spectral lines. The frequency for the saturation pulse can thus be shifted a significant distance of a few kilohertz away

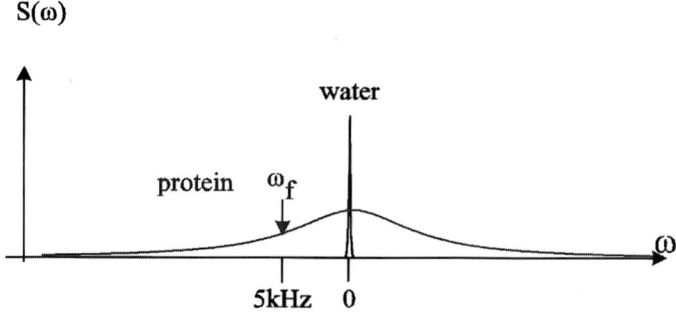

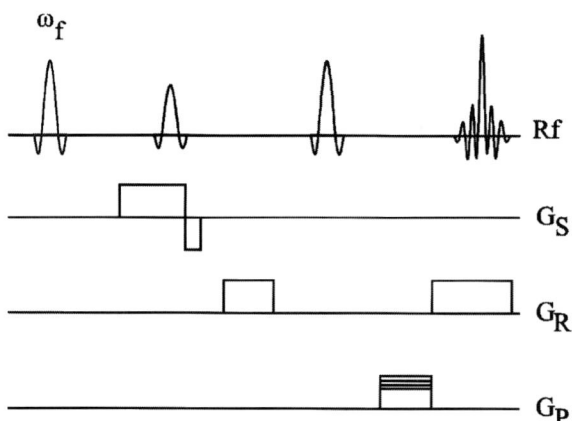

Figure 78. Principle of magnetization transfer sequence. The proton spectrum of proteins is very broad, with a line width of several kilohertz due to the short relaxation time T_2 (*top*). If a chemical-shift selective saturation pulse with a frequency w_f is applied prior to the imaging experiment such that its frequency is far outside the water (and fat) resonances of the spins used for imaging but still within the broad protein peak, the protein signal will be (at least partially) saturated just like in a CHESS experiment (see Fig. 77). This saturation will be transferred to the observed water signal via protons that are exchanged with hydrophilic groups at the surface of the macromolecule.

from the resonance frequency and still hit the protein resonance without directly affecting the signals from water protons. The transferred saturation will then reduce the signal intensity of tissues containing high concentrations of macromolecules with exchangeable protons.

TOWARD FUNCTIONAL MRI

Rigid-Body Motion

The measurement of various types of motion is a central topic for functional MRI. Motion measurements by MRI can be performed on a great variety of types of motion ranging from examinations of the overall motion of the heart or the joints to vascular flow and flow of other body fluids to perfusion and diffusion.

Cine Imaging

The most simple experimental designs use a sequence of images acquired at an appropriate speed in order to make the motion observable on a frame-to-frame basis. For

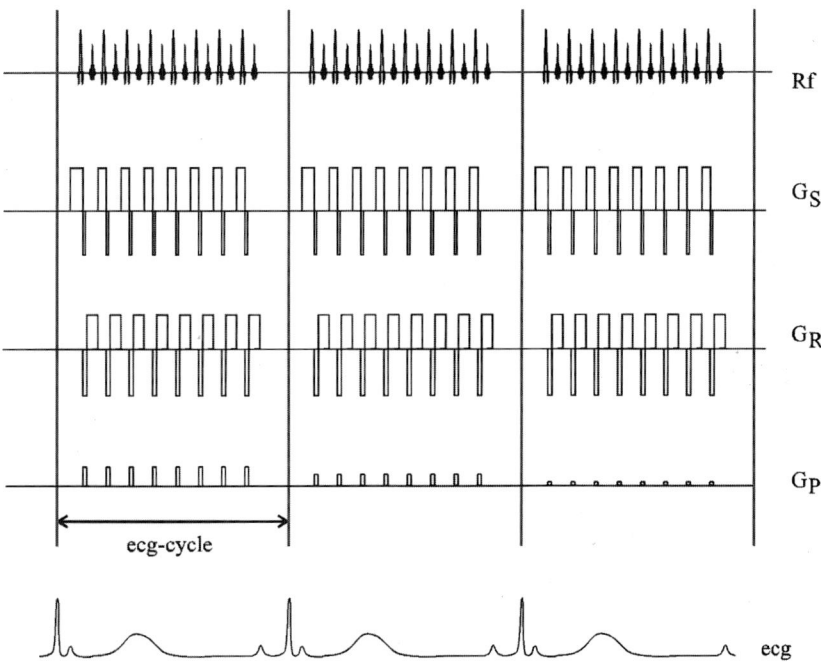

Figure 79. Principle of cine MRI. The acquisition sequence (here a gradient-echo experiment) is gated to the ECG cycle such that a predefined number of projection steps with identical phase encoding is acquired in each ECG cycle. After completion of the scan, one image can then be reconstructed for each time point during the ECG cycle.

examinations of the heart, ECG-gated cine images normally acquired using gradient-echo techniques can be used to study the overall motion of the heart in excellent spatial and temporal resolution (Fig. 79) (68, 185, 202). For cine imaging, a gating signal derived from the ECG of the patient is used to start acquisition of multiple projections on the same slice with identical phase encoding. The phase-encoding gradient is then incremented for the next acquisition cycle following the next gating pulse. After acquiring all phase-encoding steps, images can then be reconstructed for each time increment over the ECG cycle (Fig. 80). Such cine images can be used to derive at least qualitative measures of the cardiac blood flow as well and can help to detect severe functional deficits such as jet flow through septal openings. Widespread application of purely anatomic cine images is restricted by competition by the much cheaper ultrasound. In combination with functional techniques that supply information that cannot be derived by other modalities, MR cine imaging, however, is an extremely useful approach.

Tagging

A step further toward the measurement of velocities of tissues themselves rather than their contours is offered by tagging (6, 16, 22, 143, 156, 208). Tagging belongs to the group of techniques using appropriate prepulses in order to encode information on the signal amplitude of the measured images. Normally, two 90° pulses are used under orthogonal gradients in the image plane to generate a spatial modulation pattern that appears to be superimposed on the image (Fig. 81 and Color Plate 33). If images are acquired at various time intervals after the tagging interval, the local motion of the tagged tissues can be followed by following the displacement of the tagging pattern (Fig. 82 and Color Plate 34). The first experiments demonstrated the possibility of such techniques to monitor myocardial motion. Tagging can be performed in connection with either spin-echo techniques or cine gradient-echo techniques. Although the latter approach is considerably faster, since it allows the acquisition of more than one projection per ECG cycle, it

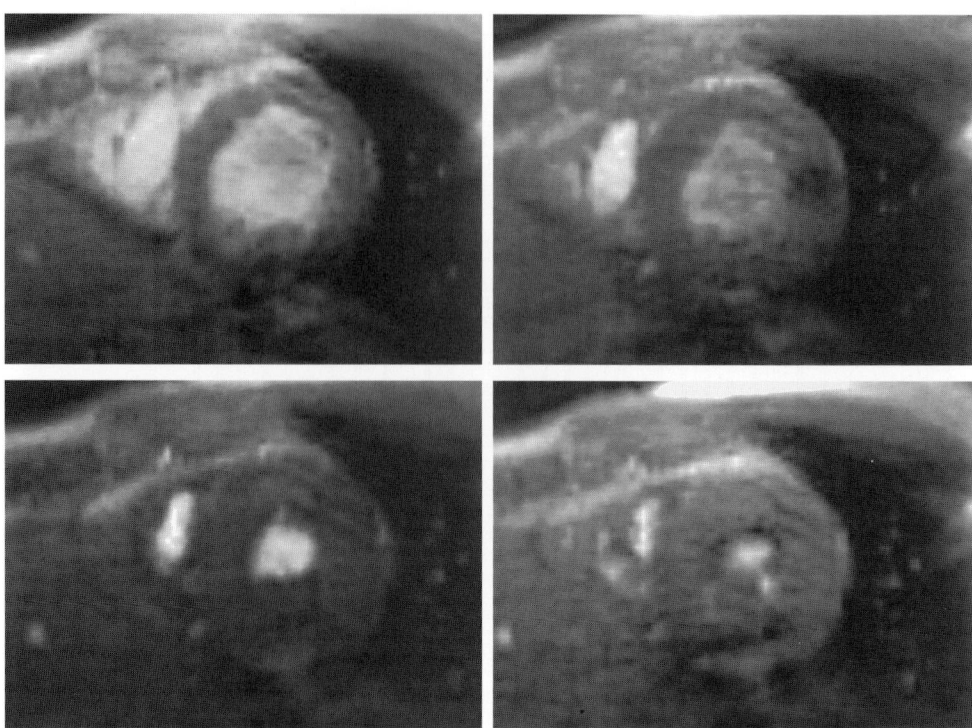

Figure 80. Cine images giving a short-axis view of the heart during systole. Images were acquired within a single breathhold using a segmented gradient-echo sequence.

suffers from fading of the tagging pattern due to the successively longer time delay and the increasing number of rf pulses at later readout times in the ECG cycle.

Tagging versus Interferography. Tagging images look very similar to interferographic images. It should thus be emphasized that they measure quite different parameters. An interferogram is basically a rather abstract image that presents some intrinsic phase information in image format. The displacement of interferographic stripes in a velocity interferogram is by no means connected to any displacement of the tissue under study. The sensitivity and thus the extension of the interferographic stripes can be varied freely by adjusting the motion sensitivity of the experiment. Tagging, on the other hand, shows the locus of the initially tagged spins and thus represents the actual displacement.

For tagging methods, velocity data can be derived from the displacement measurements, at least in principle. A more natural interpretation of tagging images, however, uses stress and strain analysis based on the deformation of the initial tagging pattern. Despite their apparent similarities, both groups of techniques therefore yield very different types of information.

In terms of image properties, there are also some significant differences between both techniques. For interferograms, the spatial resolution is identical to the resolution of the underlying image if the phase information is recalculated from the measured data. The resolution of tagging is limited by the spacing of the tagging pattern, which is considerably lower. An advantage of tagging techniques is their higher signal-to-noise ratio, since for the production of an interferogram the available magnetization always has to be distributed into two different signals.

Flow Measurements

Most MRI sequences demonstrate more or less significant sensitivity to flow. In many applications, this is an annoyance that leads to artefacts and needs to be removed. The sensitivity to flow, however, also can be used to more or less selectively image flow-filled structures such as the vessels (MR angiography) and also to quantitatively measure flow not only of blood but also of cerebrospinal fluid. Basically, for all the types of

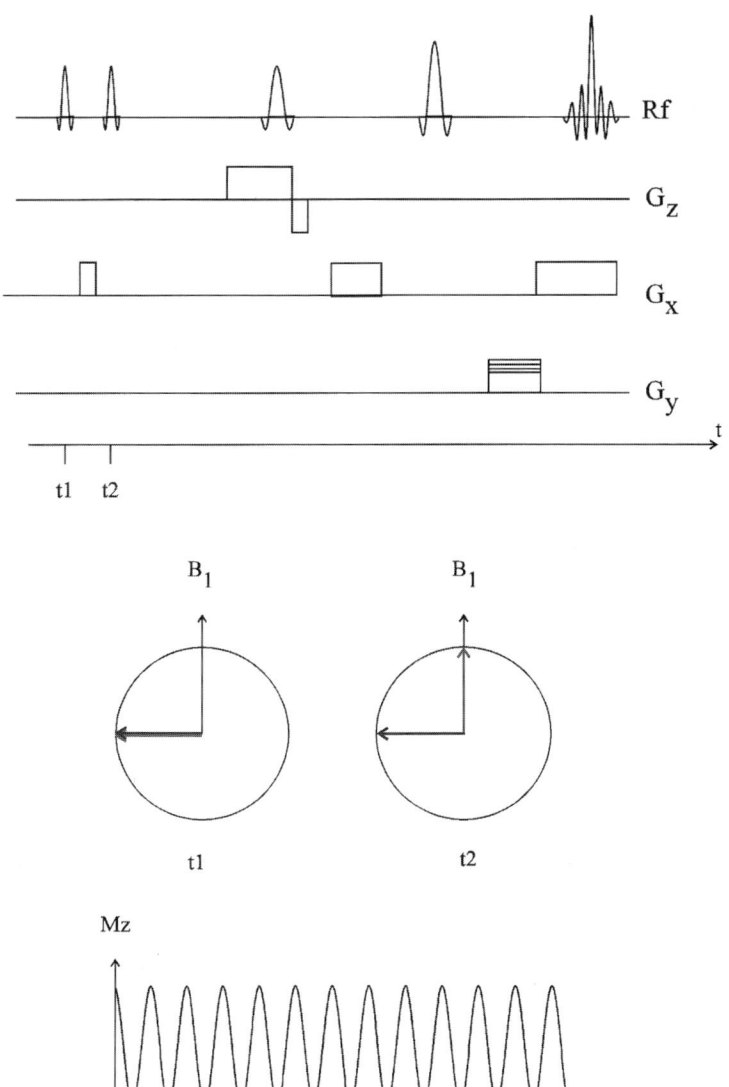

Figure 81. Principle of tagging sequence. The image-acquisition sequence (here a spin-echo experiment) is preceded by two rf pulses with flip anges of 90°. In the time $t_2 - t_1$ between these pulses a gradient in the readout direction is applied such that spins that are in phase at the time t_1 after the first pulse acquire a position-dependent phase along this gradient at time t_2 of the second pulse. The second pulse will then generate a sinusoidal variation of the z-magnetization along G_x that will show up as an intensity variation across the images. This basic recipe can be modified to tag spins in both image directions as well as to improve the sinusoidal signal variation in order to yield a better defined tagging grid. See Color Plate 33.

methods presented in the section, "Intrinsic Contrast Mechanisms," above, implementations exist that are used to demonstrate or measure flow. Generally, flow-sensitive methods are used in conjunction with gradient-echo signal acquisition (including EPI), since the time between the excitation pulse and the refocusing pulse in a spin-echo experiment will invariably lead to signal loss from flowing spins due to outflow between the excitation and the refocusing pulse.

MR-Angiography

Amplitude Methods: Time-of-Flight Angiography. MR angiograms based on amplitude methods make use of the fact that blood flowing into a slice will be unsaturated and thus

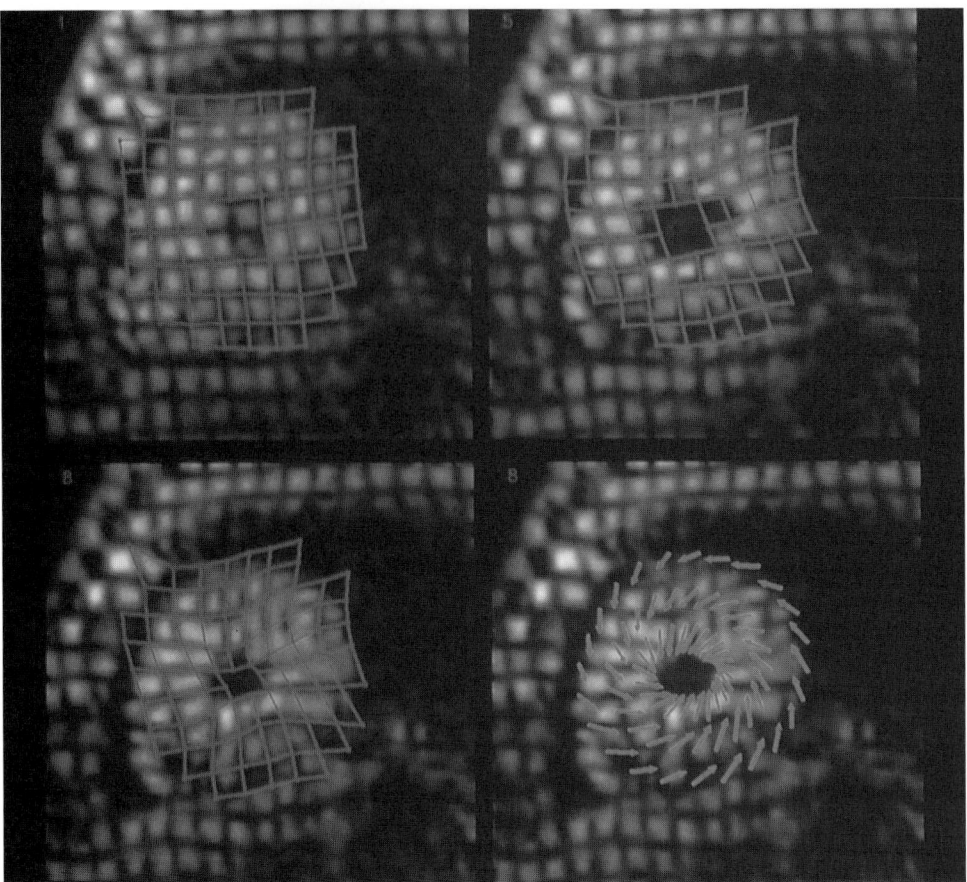

Figure 82. Tagging images of the heart acquired with a modified (C-SPAMM) tagging sequence. The gridlines that are superimposed on the heart are identified (*green*). From the motion of the intersection points on the grid, local velocity vectors (*red lines*, *bottom right*) can be reconstructed. (Courtesy of K. Boesiger, Institute for Biomedicine, Zurich, Philips 1.5 T.) See Color Plate 34.

show comparatively high signal to that from stationary spins, especially if sequences are used that induce strong saturation (Fig. 84 and Color Plate 36).

T1-weighted gradient-echo sequences with short t_r and high flip angles are typical basic experiments for such time-of-flight (TOF) methods (31, 47, 126, 132, 204). For higher field strengths, the longer T1 values of stationary tissue allow sufficient stationary signal suppression without any further means (Fig. 85). At lower field strengths, additional saturation pulses are indicated, which also can be used to distinguish different vessels according to the direction of flow. Further improvements in stationary tissue suppression can be achieved by magnetization transfer, which further reduces most soft-tissue signals but does not affect the water signal from blood.

A typical TOF experiment produces a stack of consecutively acquired 2D images. MR angiograms can then be reconstructed from the resulting 3D data set. The most common algorithm used is maximum intensity projection (MIP), which simply finds the brightest point along a given observation ray. Various approaches exist to improve the reconstruction of the vessel tree ranging from nonlinear MIP variants, which take the local surroundings of each pixel into account, to vessel tracking types of postprocessing routines.

The slice thickness d and the recovery time t_r define the minimum velocity of spins that is necessary to avoid saturation effects. For $d = 2$ mm and $t_r = 10$ ms, only spins that are faster than 20 cm/s will pass through the slice in one projection step. Slower spins typically occurring in smaller vessels will experience some saturation effect and thus appear to be less bright. This saturation of smaller vessels can be avoided by reducing the flip angle. This will, however, lead to an increased background signal from stationary tissue and thus make angiographic reconstruction more difficult.

FLOW AND FLOW COMPENSATION

For the case of a magnetic field that varies linearly in space (constant gradient) and arbitrarily in time and for spins that move along the direction of this gradient, the Larmor equation can be generalized to read

$$\phi(t) = \gamma \int_{t_1}^{t_2} x(t) G_x(t) \, dt$$

For a constant gradient amplitude and a constant velocity v with $x = vt$, this yields

$$\phi(t) = \phi_0 + \tfrac{1}{2} \gamma G_x v (t_2^2 - t_1^2)$$

Higher-order motion (acceleration a with $x = at^2$ or jerk j with $x = jt^3$) produces higher-order motion components. Any arbitrary motion can thus be expressed in terms of components of increasing order in t. The dephasing $\phi(t)$ thus can be expressed as a sum of these motional moments.

$$\phi(t) = \phi_0 + \sum_{1}^{n} \frac{1}{n} \gamma G_x v (t_2^n - t_1^n)$$

Nulling of the nth order motion term requires a minimum of $(n + 1)$ gradient steps (55, 66, 161, 179). Velocity compensation ($n = 2$) thus requires at least three gradients (Fig. 83 and Color Plate 35). For the compensation of higher-order moments, it should be noted that for compensation of the nth moment the increasing exponent invariably will lead to an increase of the sensitivity to the $(n + 1)$th motion moment. For motion with a dominant acceleration term, flow compensation can thus lead to an increase in $\phi(t)$ compared with a noncompensated gradient scheme. Thus, care has to be taken not to overcompensate motional terms. In practical applications, compensation of terms with $n > 2$ have been demonstrated to be favorable only in a limited number of applications.

Additional background suppression can be achieved by magnetization transfer, which will affect most tissue signals but not signal from blood. The highest resolution and sensitivity are achieved using very thin slices. The resulting overall acquisition times, however, can be quite considerable.

An alternative to 2D TOF methods is the acquisition of stacks of 3D data sets where TOF imaging is applied successively to rather thick slabs using 3D Fourier imaging. The increasing saturation will lead to a diminishing signal amplitude of spins flowing deeper into the examined slab. This necessitates 3D TOF techniques to use lower flip angles compared with 2D TOF. In addition, TONE pulses can be used that show an increasing flip angle across the image volume such that saturation at the entering side of the slab is avoided. The resulting signal intensities are then more homogeneous compared with non-TONE methods. The signal intensity will then, however, depend in a rather complex manner on the direction and velocity of flow and can no longer be used in the direct interpretation of the angiograms.

All TOF methods suffer from signal loss at the vessel walls, where the velocities are low and saturation effects strong. TOF angiograms will thus often underestimate the size of a vessel and overestimate the extent of a stenosis, especially when turbulent flow leads to additional signal loss.

Flow compensation as well as rephasing of acceleration and higher-order motion components can be used to reduce signal loss by velocity-dependent dephasing. The additional gradient switching points do lead, however, to longer echo times and therefore stronger T2* effects. Since velocity compensation invariably leads to higher sensitivity to acceleration, care has to be taken about when to apply such a measure. Especially for highly turbulent flow, minimizing t_e might be superior to any compensation scheme.

The large number of parameters (2D versus 3D TOF, magnetization transfer, TONE, slice thickness, t_r, and flip angle) makes it something of an art to define which sequence

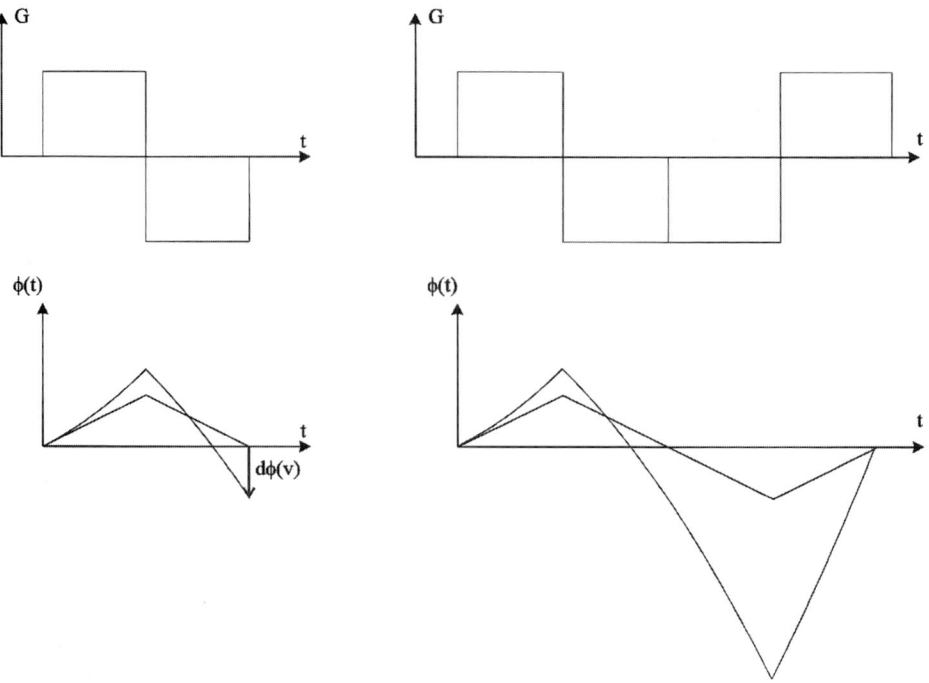

Figure 83. Principle of flow compensation. A bipolar gradient that generates no dephasing of stationary spins (*blue*) will show a quadratic phase graph (*red*) for flowing spins leading to a velocity-dependent phase shift $d\phi(v)$. By symmetry, this phase shift can be compensated by adding a time-reversed copy of the bipolar gradient to the sequence (*right*). See Color Plate 35.

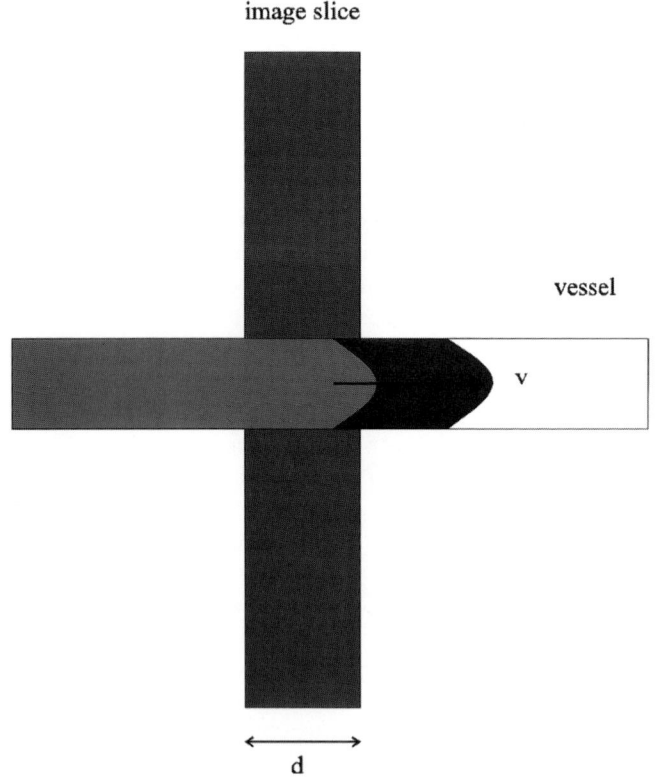

Figure 84. Principle of TOF angiography. Unsaturated spins flow into the slice under examination and thus produce high signal intensity (*red*), whereas stationary spins will give low signal with a heavily T1-weighted gradient-echo sequence. See Color Plate 36.

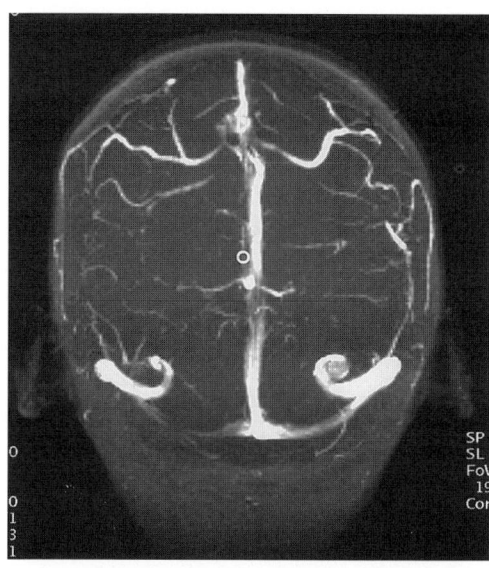

Figure 85. Coronal MIP projection showing a time-of-flight angiogram of a patient with a stenosis of the sagittal sinus (Siemens Magnetom Vision 1.5 T).

to use for a given application. Care therefore has to be taken not to overinterpret MR angiograms. There are, however, many more mechanisms to produce false-positive findings than false-negative findings. A decent and continuous MR angiographic representation of a vessel on an MR angiogram is thus a good sign that there is no pathologic problem with the vessels. A notable exception is fresh thrombi, which might appear quite bright on a TOF angiogram due to the short T1 of spins in a fresh thrombus.

Phase Methods: Phase-Contrast MRA. The flow-dependent phase effect also can be used to produce an MR angiogram by measuring two data sets with different velocity-dependent phases at otherwise identical acquisition parameters (49). This can be achieved by using appropriate velocity-encoding gradients. Since velocity sensitization can only be achieved in one direction per experiment, at least four measurements (one totally flow compensated, one sensitized in each direction) are necessary to produce an angiogram with isotropic flow sensitivity. This leads to quite significant acquisition times, especially since the spatial volume under study normally requires 3D data acquisition. The resulting phase-contrast angiograms pay for all the trouble one has to go to in producing them by at least theoretically a total cancellation of background noise from stationary tissues (Fig. 86). In addition, phase-contrast methods allow at least semiquantitative measures of blood velocities, since the observed signal phase difference can be correlated directly with velocity.

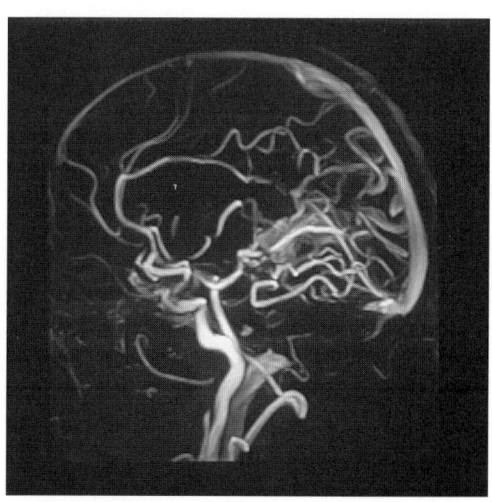

Figure 86. Phase-contrast angiogram of the head of a patient with an AV malformation. (Courtesy of New York University, Siemens Magnetom Vision 1.5 T.)

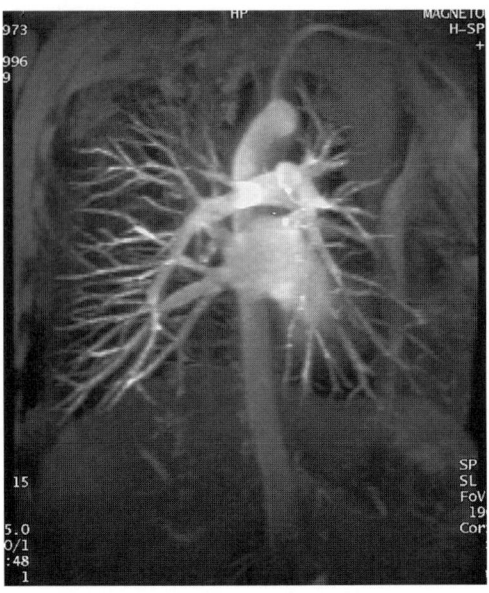

Figure 87. Contrast-enhanced MR angiogram acquired during the bolus passage of contrast agent. The image displays an MIP projection through a 3D data set acquired within one breathhold (20 to 40 s). (Courtesy of H. Bongartz, University Hospital, Basel, Siemens Magnetom Vision 1.5 T.)

Phase-contrast MRA also requires some expertise in its application. For too high velocities, the velocity-dependent phase shift can exceed ±180°, and aliasing occurs. Consequently, the highest velocity that is expected has to be used to define the velocity-encoding (V_{enc} factor) in order to avoid unintentional signal cancellation.

Contrast-Agent-Based MR Angiography

A comparatively recent approach to MR angiography is to use signal changes in blood on introduction of a (preferably) intravascular contrast agent. This yields images of the blood-filled lumen of the vessel comparable with CT angiography (see Chap. 6). The fact that in these techniques no flow information is being used for vessel delineation makes these techniques much more stable against possible flow artefacts. Especially for MR angiography in the abdomen, these techniques have led to significant improvements compared with flow-based methods. In a typical experiment, a fast 3D acquisition using a heavily T1-weighted gradient-echo sequence is performed during the first-pass passage of a contrast agent bolus. The image acquisition, which lasts from 20 to 40 s, is timed such that the bolus passage lasting about 5 to 20 s coincides with the acquisition of the most significant phase-encoding projections (Fig. 87). Even faster angiograms can be produced by projection techniques that allow the image acquisition with a time resolution of better than 1 s (Fig. 88).

Quantitative Flow Measurements

Flow quantitation also can be performed by amplitude (time-of-flight) and phase methods.

Amplitude Methods. Amplitude-based quantitative flow measurements use some variant of a tagging technique, as discussed for soft-tissue motion in the section, ''Multivoxel Techniques,'' below. In-plane tagging can be very useful by suppressing blood signal at a certain position using appropriate saturation pulses and to observe the motion of the saturated spins (7, 107, 204). This is a very useful and practical method to follow the flow patterns in complex vascular situations. Its application does not require special software; it can be applied on any standard scanner that allows the placement of local suppression pulses. Quantitation of flow is possible in principle if the exact time between the application of the saturation pulse and the signal acquisition is known.

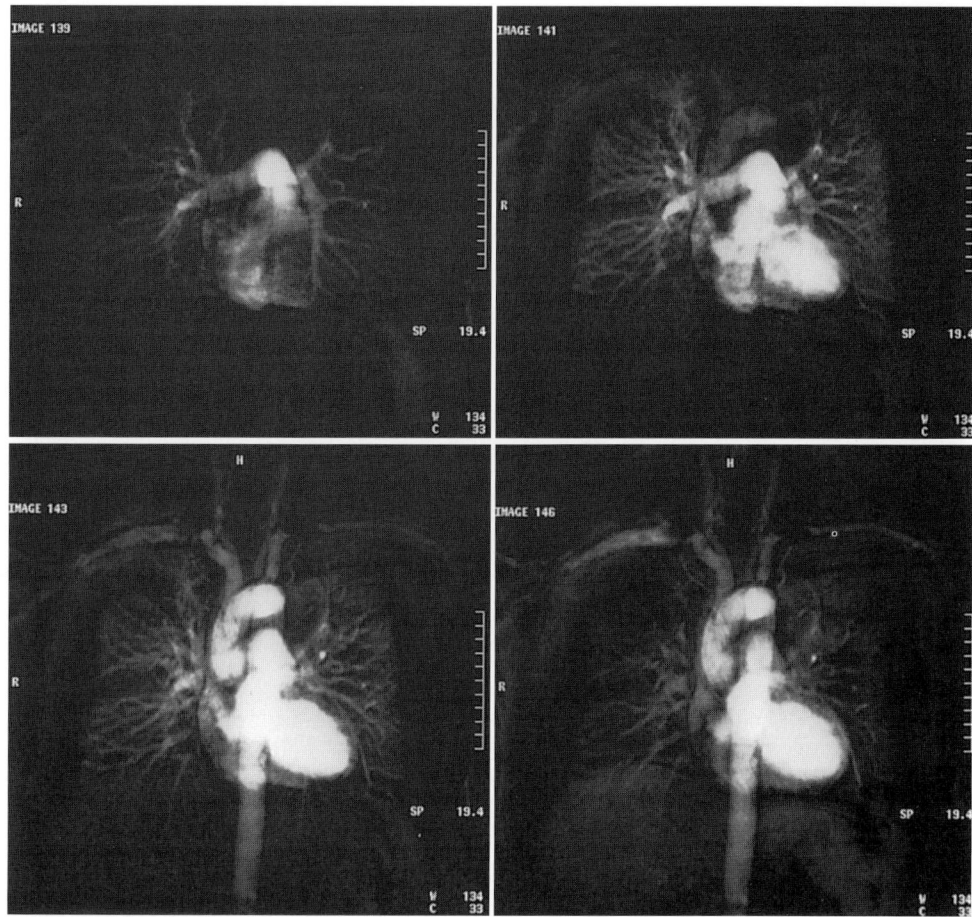

Figure 88. Sequential projection angiogram with contrast enhancement (SPACE) of the human lung acquired during the bolus passage at a rate of one image per second (Siemens Magnetom Vision 1.5 T).

A second approach uses saturation of blood signal in a volume that lies outside the observed slice. By measuring the signal amplitudes in blood vessels as a function of the time and/or distance of the saturation volume to the observed voxels, blood flow can be measured quantitatively. Such techniques have been published already quite early. Their widespread application was, however, hindered by the quite long acquisition times of the required repetitive measurements.

A more recent technique based on the same concept but with a different and much faster implementation is the EPI STAR technique (54). It uses an inversion pulse applied at the tagging region (like the neck of the patient). Signal is then read out using an EPI experiment. Two data sets are acquired, one with and one without the inversion pulse. After subtraction, an image (or 3D data set) is recovered that shows the distribution of the tagged spins from blood. The no-inversion scan is normally acquired by placing an inversion slab symmetrically above the head in order to ensure the symmetry of the two acquisitions.

Phase Methods. The direct interpretation of the signal phase in terms of flow velocities has already been mentioned as a possibility to acquire quantitative flow data (65, 152, 201). Since this essentially constitutes a two-point measurement, the resulting quantitative data are necessarily not very exact and liable to a number of stochastic and systematic errors. The degree of exactness is, however, sufficient for a variety of applications. For more exact and robust quantitation, more than two measurements with different velocity phase encoding have to be performed. In the extreme case, an image of velocity can be

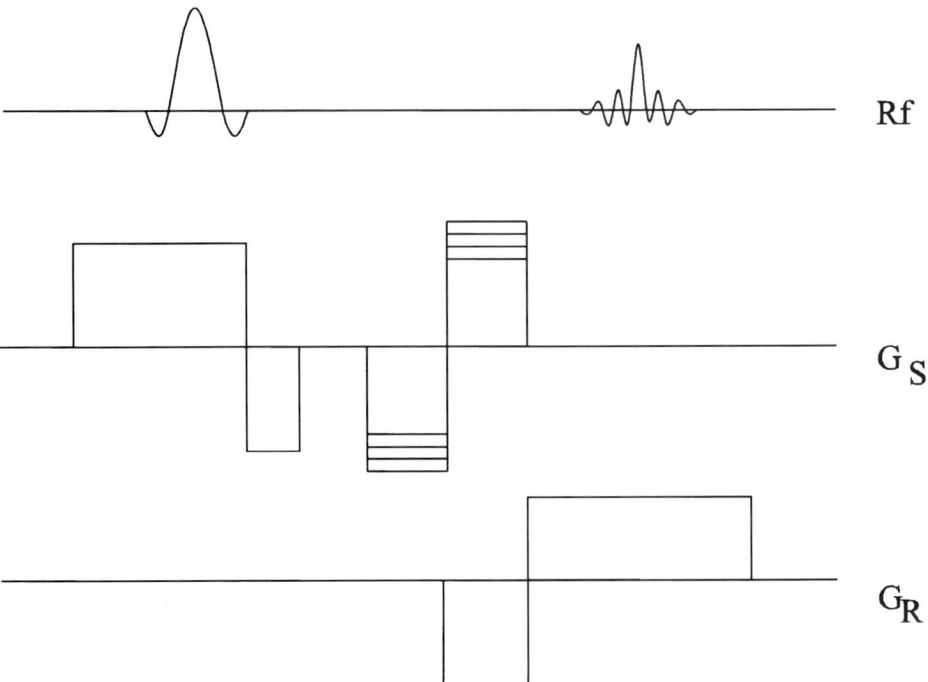

Figure 89. Fast Fourier flow sequence. The experiment uses a gradient-echo approach for signal generation. Phase encoding is then performed not with a unipolar gradient as used in an imaging experiment but with a bipolar gradient, which does not lead to any phase encoding of stationary spins but will lead to a velocity-dependent phase encoding of flowing spins. The resulting image after 2DFT will then show spatial resolution along the read direction only, whereas the phase-encoding direction will encode for velocity.

acquired by using a stepwise incremented bipolar gradient that leaves the phase of stationary spins intact but leads to a velocity-dependent phase change of flowing spins (62, 106, 152). In combination with a gradient-echo technique, this leads to the fast Fourier flow experiment, which allows extremely exact quantitative flow measurements (Fig. 89). The phase-encoding gradient is bipolar in this experiment and thus does not lead to any phase encoding of stationary spins. Moving spins, however, will experience a velocity-dependent phase change that is proportional to the amplitude of the gradient. After Fourier transformation, the location of spins in the phase-encoding direction will thus be determined by their velocity (Fig. 90 and Color Plate 37). Compared with simple phase-contrast methods, Fourier flow techniques have a much higher dynamic range and thus do not require any prior information about the maximum velocity to be expected. If combined with ECG gating, fast Fourier flow can be used to study flow profiles across a vessel in high temporal (10 ms or better) and spatial resolution.

Following the observation that the measured velocity projection images across a slice leave a lot of unused space on the image, modifications have been developed that allow the measurement of flow through more than one cross section in a single acquisition. The resulting multislice Fourier flow experiment not only increases the efficiency of the velocity measurement, but by simultaneous observation of flow in several sections along a vessel, it also allows determination of the propagation velocity of the arterial blood pulse as a potentially useful indicator for the vessel elasticity, which is of interest in studying the development of atherosclerosis.

Although the basic Fourier flow experiment can be performed very fast, the requirement of ECG gating plus the additional Fourier dimension for the velocity domain limits the spatial coverage of the experiment. Full spatial resolution across the slice is normally not required, since vessels normally can be attributed easily by acquiring projections along two or three projection angles. A problem for all quantitative flow measurements,

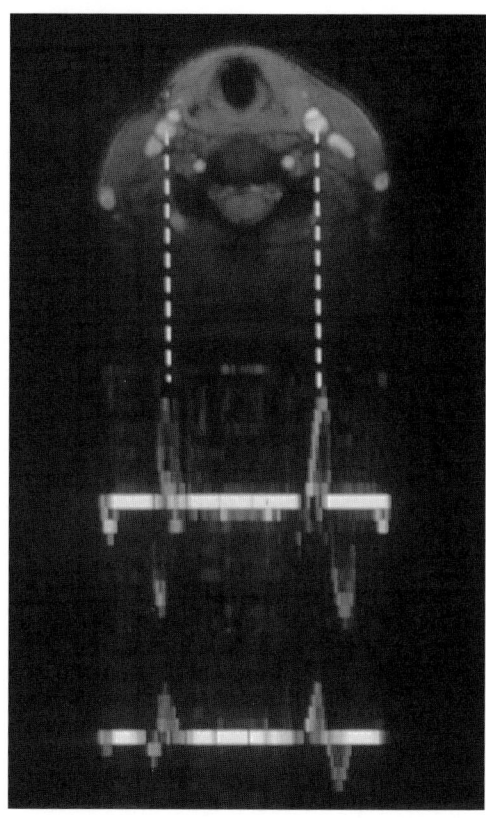

Figure 90. ECG-gated fast Fourier flow images during diastole (*bottom*) and on arrival of the systolic pulse wave (*middle*) displaying flow velocities orthogonal to the transverse section through the neck of a volunteer shown at the top. The flow profiles in veins (*downward*) and arteries are demonstrated. Vessel profiles can be attributed by projection onto the anatomic image (*yellow lines*). See Color Plate 37.

however, is breath-dependent velocity changes that affect flow in most vessels. Segmented acquisition in order to allow flow measurements during breathhold are therefore an important new possibility offered by the strong and fast gradient systems that have been introduced recently.

It should be emphasized that Fourier flow techniques and phase-contrast measurements are not two totally different approaches to flow quantitation but rather the extremes of a continuum. The exactness and dynamic range of the velocity measurements of Fourier flow techniques can be traded for more spatial resolution by reducing the number of flow-encoding steps and increasing the spatial encodes. From the discussion of the Fourier transformation (see above) it should be clear that for less than 8 to 16 encodes in any direction, Fourier transformation might not be the algorithm of choice to derive the phase (and thus velocity) information from the data. Using a reasonable number of flow encodes (4 to 8), data can be acquired that maintain the good quantitation of Fourier flow while still allowing high spatial resolution within reasonable acquisition times.

Perfusion and Diffusion

Techniques Based on Direct Motion Effects

In terms of the MRI experiment, perfusion and diffusion can be treated just like flow or motion experiments, the difference lying in the velocity and topology of flow. Bulk motion as well as regular flow can be characterized by velocity vectors whose direction and amplitude are constant across a reasonable distance. The scale of what constitutes a reasonable distance is defined by the size of the voxel under observation. If changes in the direction and/or velocity of motion occur across a voxel, the observed signal will be the vector sum of the various observed components. If the voxel gets large compared with velocity changes, or if the changes occur over a smaller volume, coherence of the signals will be lost, and the signal will eventually vanish (Fig. 91 and Color Plate 38).

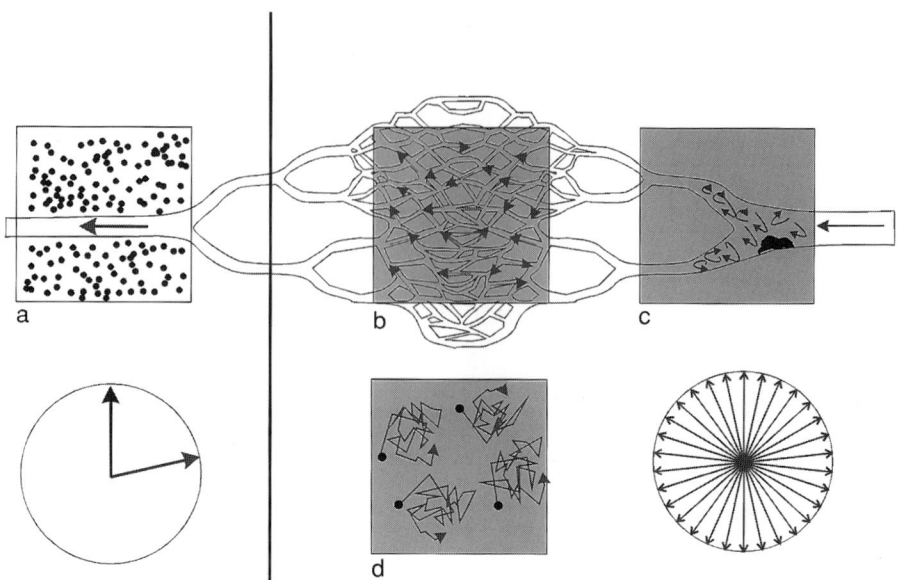

Figure 91. Different effects of flow and motion within a voxel (square box in a–d). Constant flow will lead to an observable phase difference of flowing spins (*red*) as compared with stationary signal **(A)**. Intravoxel flow in capillaries **(b)** as well as turbulent flow around an obstacle **(c)** as well as molecular diffusion **(d)** will all lead to incoherent phase effects and thus to amplitude reduction of the observed signal **(B)**. In terms of an MR experiment, these types of motion are thus equivalent in principle and can only be distinguished by their different inherent velocities. Dephasing around a turbulence is much faster compared with capillary perfusion, which again is faster than molecular motion. See Color Plate 38.

The maximum phase change of a signal will be determined by the motion sensitivity of the sequence used. Full signal cancellation will only occur if the motion-induced phase change across the voxel exceeds 360°. It is thus important to note that motion-sensitive MRI measurements do not a priori distinguish physiologically highly different processes such as turbulent flow, perfusion, and diffusion. A distinction can be made, however, based on the different velocity scales involved.

Perfusion in its strict sense describes the supply of tissue with some substrate (oxygen). Although in principle this includes transport of the substrate across the cell membrane, perfusion in a lesser sense is often used to describe capillary blood flow. Following the intravoxel incoherent motion (IVIM) model of LeBihan (129, 131), capillaries can be assumed to be randomly oriented in the tissue. Flow-sensitive methods applied to capillary flow will thus produce perfusion-related changes in signal amplitude but not phase.

The actual amount of the amplitude change can be calculated by integrating over the signals of the randomly moving spins. The motion velocity will be transformed by integration into an apparent diffusion constant that describes the mean displacement of spins per unit time.

Diffusion of freely mobile spins in a liquid can be described using exactly the same mathematical model that now describes the "random walk" of Brownian motion. A difference between diffusion and perfusion will thus be observed only by the size of the observed amplitude change: The perfusion-related apparent diffusion coefficient is roughly one order of magnitude higher than proper Brownian diffusion. In order to distinguish both mechanisms, a number of experiments have to be performed with an appropriate range of sensitivity to cover both processes.

The basic experiment is based on the method of Stejskal and Tanner (191) and applies two gradient lobes placed symmetrically around the refocusing pulse of a spin-echo experiment (Fig. 92). The diffusion sensitivity can then be calculated from the duration

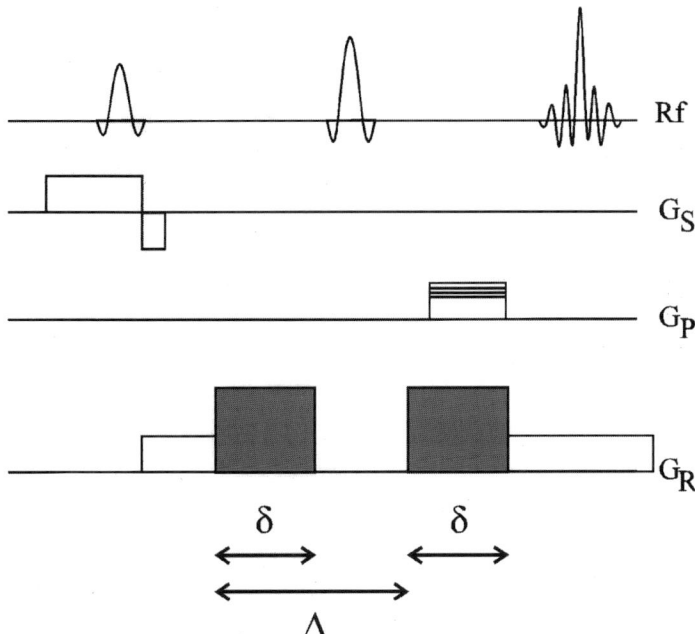

Figure 92. Basic principle of MRI sequence based on a Stejskal-Tanner experiment. Signal is generated as a spin echo. Diffusion sensitivity is achieved by adding the two shaded gradients symmetrically around the refocusing pulse.

and temporal displacement of the gradients. Mathematically, it is expressed by the *b* factor, which corresponds to the integral over the gradient effect.

For gradient strengths in a conventional range of 10 mT/m, quite long diffusion encoding times are required in order to reach sufficiently high *b* factors to achieve appreciable signal attenuation for diffusive protons. Since T2 relaxation is, of course, acting on the signal intensity as well as diffusion dephasing, the signal amplitude might already be considerably reduced at the time of data acquisition by T2 alone.

Conventionally, diffusion-weighted imaging was performed by combining diffusion-weighted acquisition with imaging gradients in a diffusion-weighted spin-echo (or stimulated-echo) multiexcitation experiment (3, 129, 130). Although very nice results could be produced using such an approach, routine application of these techniques suffered severely from motion artefacts due to the extremely high sensitivity of these sequences to motion. Although motion-compensated diffusion weighting is possible, the resulting gradient schemes invariably also will lead to *b* factors that are considerably reduced compared with straightforward approaches.

With the recently available fast and strong gradient sequences, diffusion weighting can be combined with a fast imaging experiment (28, 151, 154) that not only allows considerably faster data acquisition but also leads to tremendous improvements in motion artefacts that—as described in the section, ''Chemical-Shift Misregistration,'' above—are negligible as long as motion is monotonous during the acquisition time. Diffusion-weighted snapshot FLASH (Fig. 93) thus has been demonstrated successfully as well as diffusion-weighted variants of EPI and U-FLARE.

Diffusion and perfusion in structured tissue can be anisotropic if some preferred direction(s) exist. Such anisotropy effects have been observed in white matter of the brain as well as in muscle, including the heart.

Transport-Based Approaches: Bolus Tracking

A second approach to measure perfusion (and to a limited extent also diffusion) is to observe the transport of an appropriate label to the target region. EPI STAR (54) and

DIFFUSION AND PERFUSION

The diffusion coefficient D characterizes the mean square displacement of the molecules:

$$\bar{x} = \sqrt{\langle x^2 \rangle} = (2Dt)^{1/2}$$

This means that for 68% of molecules $-\bar{x} \leq x \leq \bar{x}$

$$\text{in water, } D = 2.2 \times 10^{-3} \text{ mm}^2/\text{s} \quad (\text{at } 20°\text{C})$$

so for $t = 100$ ms

$$(\bar{x} = \sqrt{(2 \times 2.2 \times 10^{-3} \text{ mm}^2/\text{s} \times 0.1 \text{ s})} = 0.02 \text{ mm})$$

$$1 \text{ ms-} \quad 0.002 \text{ mm}$$
$$10 \text{ s-} \quad 0.2 \text{ mm}$$

Typical diffusion coefficient values in vivo

Tissue	D_{tissue}/D_{water}
Muscle	0.61 (parallel to fibers)
Muscle	0.44 (perpendicular to fibers)
Liver	0.25–0.30
Brain	0.45 ($\Delta = 20$ ms), 0.10 ($\Delta = 60$ ms)
Heart	0.34–0.37

Source: From D. Le Bihan, R. Turner, Diffusion and perfusion, in D. D. Stark, W. G. Bradley, *Magnetic Resonance Imaging*. St. Louis: Mosby-Yearbook, 1992.

In biologic tissues, diffusion is often anisotropic and restricted. D depends on temperature. In pure liquid, $D = D_0 \exp(-E_a/kT)$, where E_a is activation energy (in water, $E_a = 0.18$ eV).

In order to quantify the phase effect caused by random motion, the Larmor equation for time-varying magnetic fields (which has already been used for the calculation of the flow-dependent phase) has to be solved for random motion:

$$\phi(t) = \gamma \int_{t_1}^{t_2} x(t)G_x(t) \, dt$$

For a pair of rectangular gradients, this integral yields the Stejskal-Tanner formula:

$$R = \exp\{-\gamma^2 G^2 \delta^2 (\Delta - \delta/3)D^*\} = \exp(-bD^*)$$

where R represents the signal attenuation due to random motion, D^* corresponds to the apparent diffusion coefficient, which represents all random motion effects, and δ and Δ are the duration and separation of the diffusion-encoding gradients according to Fig. 92.

The diffusion sensitivity parameter b depends on the square of the gradient amplitude; stronger gradients thus lead to a dramatic increase in the diffusion sensitivity; b is normally given in units of seconds per square millimeter.

For a spin-echo sequence under a constant gradient, $\delta = \Delta = t_e/2$, and the equation simplifies to

$$R = \exp\{-\gamma^2 G^2 D^* t_e^3/12\}$$

For a diffusion coefficient of liquid water (2.2×10^{-3} s/mm^2), the b factor must be on the order of 50 to 100 in order to measure an appreciable effect. For $t_e = 100$ ms and a gradient amplitude of 10 mT/m, the b factor is about 580 s/mm^2, which leads to a signal attenuation of free water by about 70%. For $t_e = 50$ ms and the same gradient, the signal attenuation is only 15%. Thus strong gradients are essential for diffusion measurements.

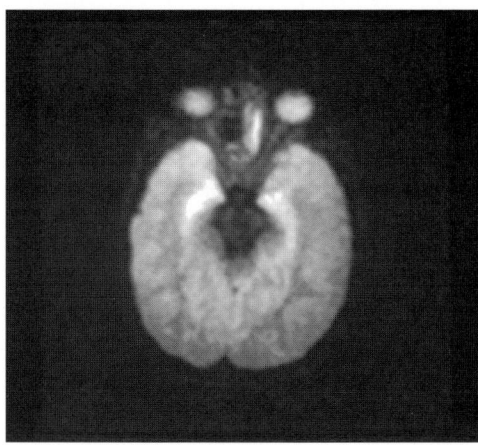

Figure 93. Diffusion image acquired with a diffusion-weighted snapshot FLASH experiment in a 6-year-old child after cardiac arrest and resuscitation. Hippocampus, isthmus of the cingular gyrus, and parts of the occipital lobe appear hyperintense on the diffusion-weighted images. (Courtesy of H. Rumpel, E. Martin, Kinderspital, Zürich, Bruker S 200 2 T.)

other tagging-based techniques have been applied successfully to this purpose (see below). Other transport-based techniques that follow the distribution of some substance that is not normally present in the body also can be used.

A very successful approach is first-pass measurements after bolus application of contrast agents (24, 29, 172, 177). The basics of the kinetics of the distribution of contrast agents in the body are covered in Chap. 2. MR observation of the label distribution follows the changes in signal intensities caused by appropriate contrast agents. At the high local concentrations during bolus passage, induced changes can be either signal increases using T1 agents or signal reduction using T2* agents (see Fig. 70). Both approaches have their advantages and drawbacks.

T1-weighted techniques are normally performed using short echo times and thus suffer only mildly from T2 or T2* effects. The most commonly used imaging techniques with acquisition times on the order of or below 2 s per image required to follow the first-passage effect are based on snapshot FLASH (84). A problem with this approach is the comparatively low enhancement effect in combination with the intrinsically low signal-to-noise ratio of the imaging sequences. Quite low concentrations of the agents have to be used in order to avoid signal attenuation due to T2* effects. Perfusion measurements using this approach are therefore advantageous in the head and problematic outside.

T2*-weighted approaches have the intrinsic advantage of high effect-to-noise ratio due to the fact that signal losses easily reach 100% even with contrast agents that in the steady state are used as T1 agents with positive enhancement. These signal losses are caused by the T2* effects from these agents in the high concentrations observed during the bolus. A disadvantage of T2*-based approaches lies in the fact that the signal attenuation depends not only on the local concentration of the agent but also on its microscopic distribution, since the observed T2* effects are very sensitive to the microscopic environment. The advantage of this sensitivity is the fact that such experiments can be used to study the mechanism of perfusion in considerable detail. The disadvantage is that direct quantitation of perfusion is not possible and can only be performed by elaborate reference measurements in identical tissues.

In order to get relative perfusion maps, T2*-based methods have been demonstrated to be very useful using various types of fast imaging sequences as well as more conventional imaging experiments in connection with keyhole sampling. Since sensitive measurement of static T2* effects using gradient-echo techniques (long t_e gradient-echo imaging or EPI) lead to severe artefacts in body imaging caused by susceptibility and chemical shift; spin-echo-based techniques, which are sensitive to dynamic T2* effects, appear to be advantageous for perfusion measurements outside the head.

Future developments will show whether the use of other fast imaging techniques such as single-shot RARE (HASTE) will improve the effect-to-noise ratio and can be used to reliably and sensitively measure perfusion in organs and pathologies of the abdomen.

A special topic, of course, is perfusion measurements on the moving heart. The tremendous motion effects that appear to be superimposed on the much more subtle perfusion effect make approaches using motion-dependent methods described in the preceding section very problematic, although even anisotropic diffusion imaging has been demonstrated on the heart (175).

Bolus tracking studies of myocardial perfusion have been demonstrated using positive (T1) as well as negative (T2*) contrast with various contrast agents (Fig. 94). Although perfusion deficits could be localized with both methods, quantitation of the observed effects appears to be very problematic in view of the various factors—physiologic effects as well as artefacts—that contribute to the observed signal intensities.

Perfusion measurements based on observation of the distribution of some extrinsic substance were covered earlier in the section on contrast agents.

Deoxygenation Imaging: The BOLD Contrast

Mechanism

MRI experiments can be used for sensitive measurements of the local changes in blood oxygenation. These BOLD (blood oxygenation level–dependent) experiments (166) are based on the observation that deoxygenated hemoglobin has a strong magnetic moment, whereas the paramagnetism is quenched on oxygenation of the iron centers of the molecule. Although this fact has been known for some years (194), it took some time until the first demonstration of an image with contrast based on this effect. Basically, deoxygenated blood acts just like a T2* contrast agent, as described earlier. The main source for the observed signal changes are static and dynamic susceptibility changes, as described earlier.

Since the signal intensity inside a given tissue depends on various factors, absolute deoxygenation imaging appears to be not very practical. An extremely attractive application for BOLD-type examinations, however, is observation of the local change in oxygenation in cortical areas on stimulation.

The typical chain of reasoning for explaining the observed effects runs as follows:

1. Activation of cortical neurons creates a local demand for energy. Since oxygenative glycolysis is the only energy source of neurons in the brain, this results in an increased demand for oxygen and glycogen.
2. This results in increased capillary perfusion in order to supply the neurons with both substrates. The normal assumption is that the increased perfusion more than compensates for the increased oxygen demand.
3. The relative concentration of oxygenated blood is increased despite the increased oxygen consumption.
4. Deoxygenated blood has—in contrast to oxygenated blood—a magnetic moment (Fig. 95B), which leads to a susceptibility effect around vessels with high concentrations of deoxyhemoglobin (Fig. 95C). See also Color Plate 39.
5. The increased relative concentration of oxygenated blood on stimulation thus leads to a decrease in the local susceptibility effect and thus to an increase in the signal intensity as observed in T2*-weighted imaging.

It should be pointed out that this description of the BOLD mechanism is under some discussion. Although experimental data exist that confirm the local increase in oxygen consumption, some experiments performed with PET do not find increased perfusion. Stimulation of different parts of the neuronal processing systems is discussed as a source for the apparent inconsistencies of results from different modalities. Until further light is shed on the mechanism of cortical activation, care has to be taken in the interpretation of results.

In a typical brain activation study, a series of images is acquired with or without stimulation, and the areas of stimulation are identified by postprocessing of the time

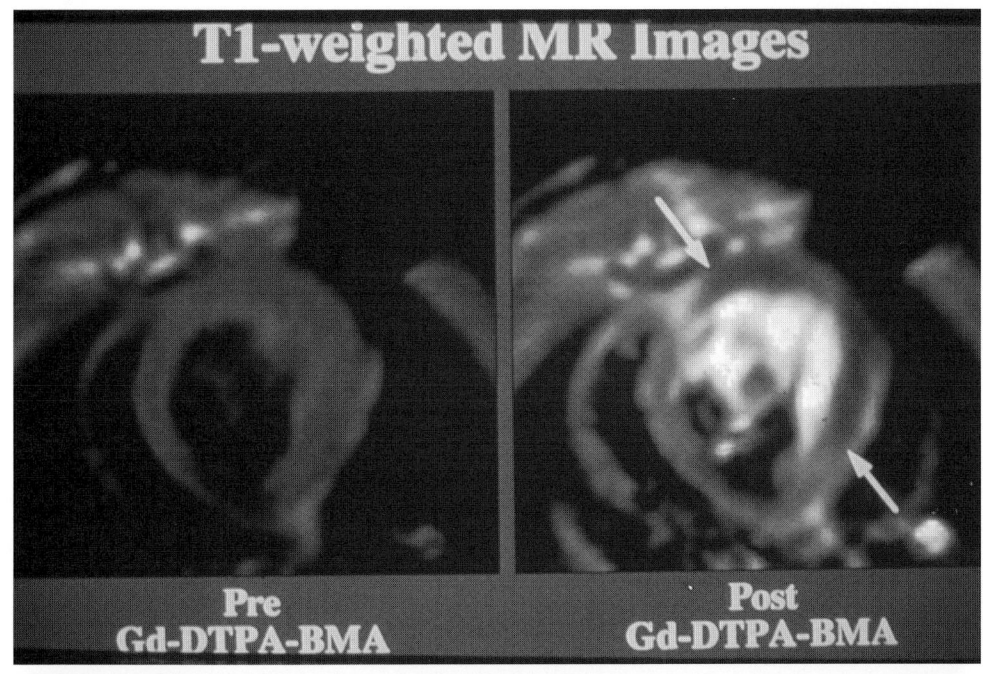

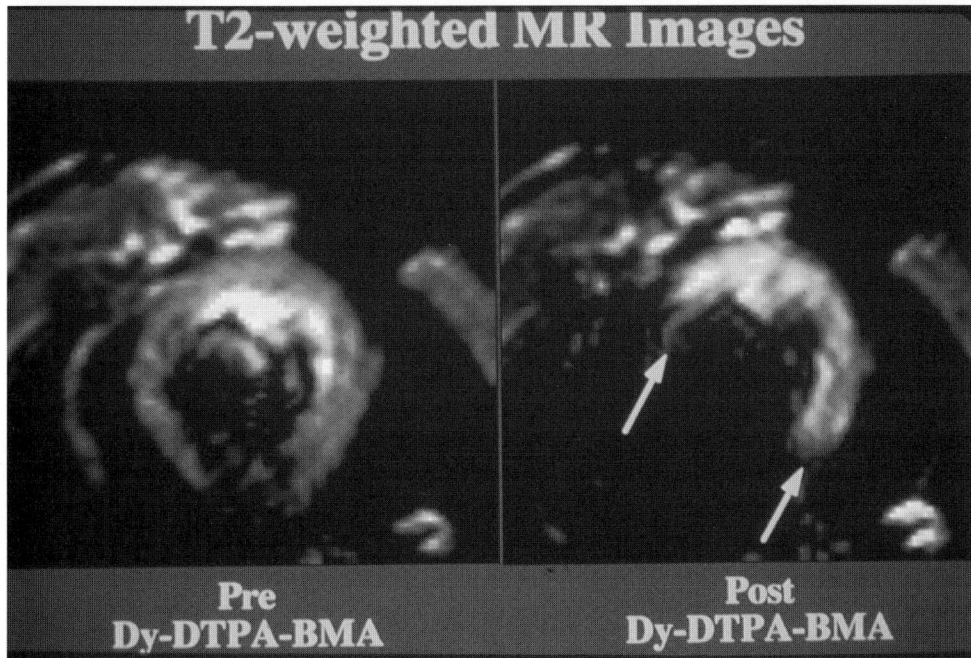

Figure 94. Perfusion images of the heart. The nonperfused area shows up as a dark region in the myocardium after injection of Gd-DTPA-BMA in a T1-weighted scan (*top*). Similary, T2*-weighted imaging can be used to show the infarcted region in bright contrast to normal tissue after injection of a susceptibility agent (Dy-DTPA-BMA). (Courtesy of Ch. Higgins, San Francisco.)

series of data in each pixel element. The number of images per study typically ranges from 16 to several hundred in fast multislice examinations. The possibility to switch the stimulation condition off and on during the examination leads to extremely good robustness of the data against systematic errors compared with a simple before-after examination mode, as normally performed by PET (see Chap. 5).

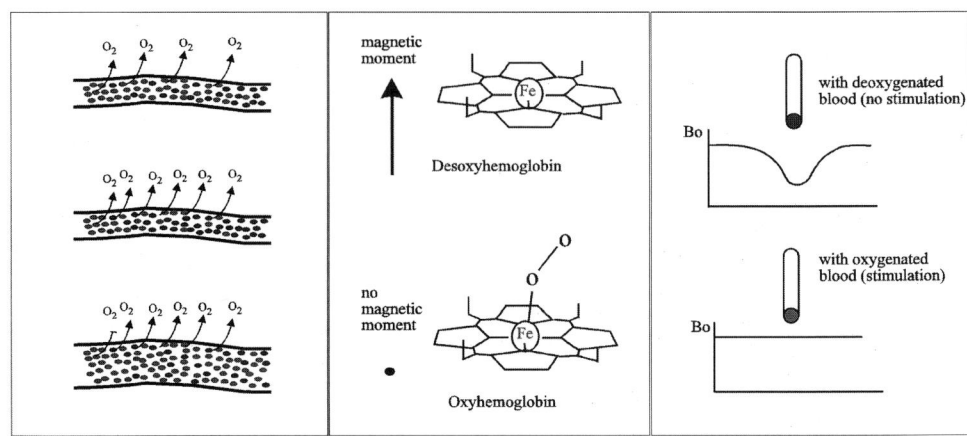

A, B   C

Figure 95. Principle of BOLD mechanism used for brain activation studies. **(A)** The increased energy consumption on stimulation leads to an increased blood supply such that the concentration of oxygenated blood (*red dots* in **A**) is increased compared with deoxygenated blood (*blue dots* in **A**). The increased consumption is thus overcompensated. **(B)** Deoxyhemoglobin has a strong magnetic moment due to free electrons at the iron center. This magnetic moment is quenched by adding an oxygen molecule such that oxyhemoglobin has no magnetic moment. **(C)** The magnetic moment of deoxygenated blood will lead to a strong susceptibility effect in the surroundings of a vessel with a high content of deoxyhemoglobin, whereas no such effect will be observed around vessels filled with oxyhemoglobin. Upon activation, the susceptibility effect around capillary vessels will thus change, which can be observed with appropriate susceptibility-dependent measurement sequences. See Color Plate 39.

Measuring Methods

A great number of different techniques has been proposed for application in functional brain imaging. The proper choice of an experiment depends, of course, on the type of examination to be performed. In general, there exist two types of studies to be performed by functional MRI: finding locations of activation to some kind of stimulation paradigm and physiologic examinations, where the area of activation is known beforehand and some information is desired about the actual mechanism of the observed effects.

Localization of Activated Areas. The search for areas of activation following increasingly complex stimulation paradigms has found an increasingly vast number of applications in neurophysiologic research in the recent past. It normally requires examination of some not too limited volume of interest that can be performed either by multislice examination or by true 3D approaches. Repetitive single-slice scans on a planar section containing the area of interest, which have been the approach normally chosen in the initial stage of functional MRI, have become more or less obsolete except for some limited applications where justified.

The bulk of the existing functional MRI studies has been produced either with EPI (Fig. 96) (125, 196) or with conventional T2*-weighted gradient-echo imaging (Fig. 97) (73, 119). For EPI, asymmetric spin-echo variants commonly have been used, where the zero phase-encoding step is put into a projection with an appropriate time delay to proper spin-echo refocusing in order to get appropriate T2* contrast. Three-dimensional EPI is feasible, but normally, multislice acquisition is preferred. This not only avoids signal saturation but also minimizes phase artefacts from nonreproducibilities between successive acquisition steps.

T2*-weighted gradient echo is considerably slower than EPI and thus has been called the ''poor man's approach'' to functional imaging. The long susceptibility encoding time (typically around 60 ms for a 1.5-T system) indeed sets a lower limit to the image acquisition time. This disadvantage, however, can be at least somewhat reduced by either an interleaved multislice experiment using the MUSIC (multislice interleaved acquisition) sequence (Fig. 98) (136) or by interleaving the excitation pulses of successive projection steps in the PRESTO sequence (Fig. 99) (135). In addition, gradient-echo imaging does

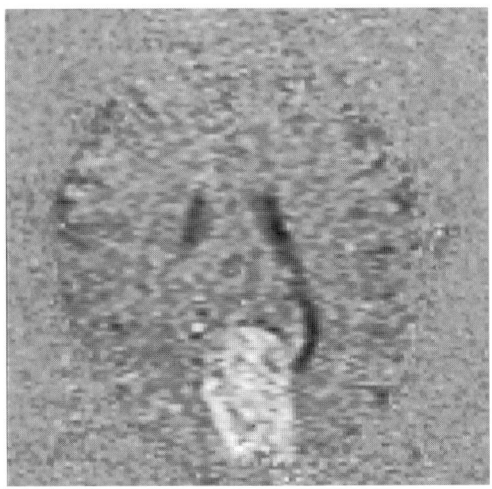

Figure 96. BOLD effect image of the visual cortex as acquired with an EPI sequence. The image is a difference image between images acquired during stimulated and nonstimulated periods in a time series with four stimulation periods (eight images each) interleaved with four resting periods (eight images each). Apart form the bright signal enhancement in the visual cortex, residual signals due to CSF fluctuations are shown (Siemens Magnetom Vision 1.5 T).

allow true 3D acquisition. Since multiexcitation sequences do not have inherent limitations to spatial resolution, they also allow higher resolution compared with EPI scans and have been demonstrated to be successful at looking within the submillimeter structures of the visual processing system (148).

Keyhole techniques also have been applied successfully to speed up the acquisition time of gradient-echo sequences.

Since, on the other hand, segmented EPI acquisitions can be used to overcome the low resolution of single-shot EPI, the two measurement modes are beginning to merge more and more into each other. The current competition between EPI-only and gradient-echo-only scanners caused by technical limitations is expected to make a place for a more rational discussion, when direct comparisons can be made, that allows an optimal choice for a given type of application.

First comparative studies of EPI versus FLASH-type experiments indicate that EPI certainly gives optimal volume coverage, whereas the effect-to-noise ratio per unit of time appears to be higher in gradient-echo experiments. EPI thus seems to be the faster and more elegant experiment if the observed effect is strong enough, whereas gradient-echo experiments yield better results if the examination time can be made sufficiently long. Care should be taken, however, that the intrinsically higher signal-to-noise ratio of gradient-echo images might easily be lost by the higher sensitivity of the experiment to nonreproducibility artefacts (see next section).

In addition to these techniques, other sequences have been applied successfully to functional MRI. Approaches using single-shot RARE (FSE, TSE, HASTE) sequences

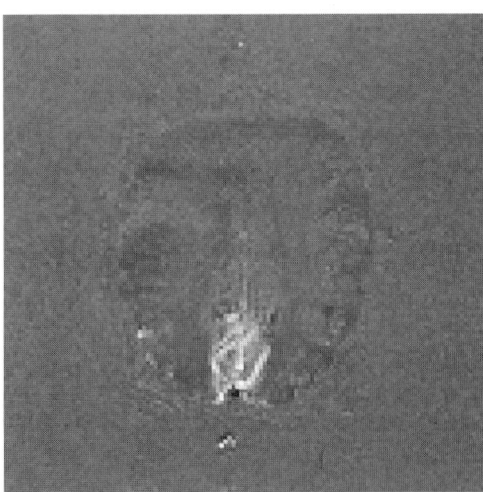

Figure 97. FLASH stimulation images acquired in the same paradigm and during the same session as Fig. 96 with a BOLD-sensitive gradient-echo sequence ($t_e = 60$ ms).

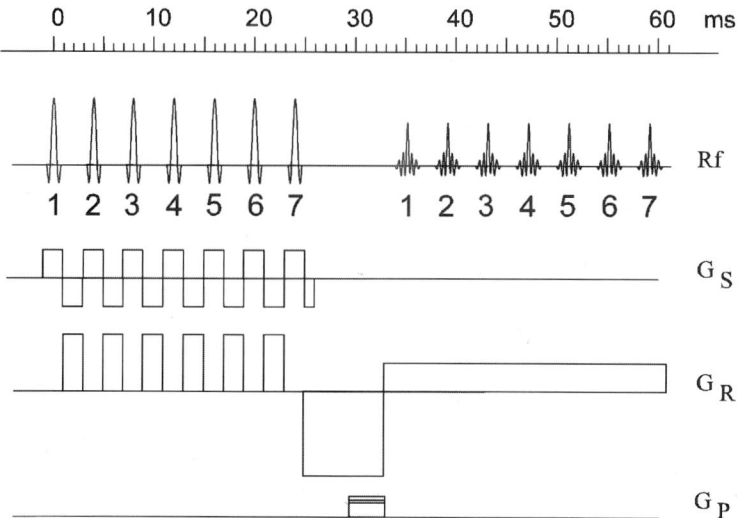

Figure 98. Diagram of the MUSIC sequence. The long echo time necessary for susceptibility encoding is filled with the excitation of multiple parallel slices, whose signals are then read out subsequently.

with or without contrast modification to enhance susceptibility contrast have been demonstrated to be quite advantageous due to their low intrinsic sensitivity to various types of artefacts (102, 114).

Time-Resolved Measurements. The task in time-resolved measurements is not so much to find activated cortical areas but rather to assess what is going on in a predefined region that is known to be activated during a given paradigm. The best way to first localize

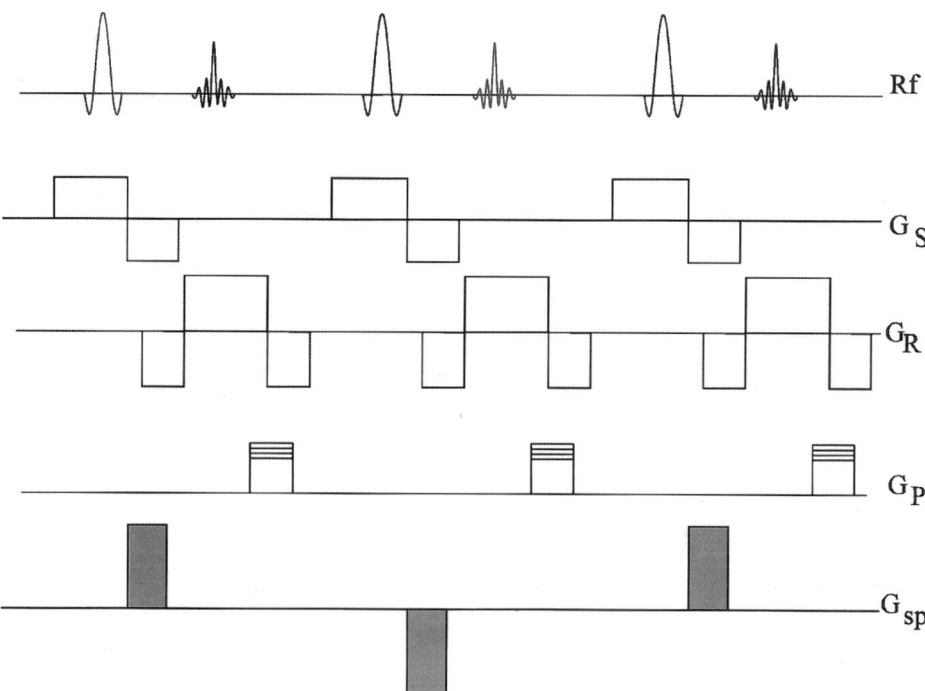

Figure 99. Diagram of the PRESTO sequence. With proper adjustment of the gradients and by adding a spoiling gradient G_{sp} to any of the three gradient directions, a signal is generated not from the excitation pulse preceding each data acquisition but by the pulse in the preceding time interval.

these areas is, of course, to perform one of the experiments described in the preceding section.

There are quite a number of reasons why one could be interested in time-resolved experiments. One is in neurophysiologic research, where the observation of the time course of the signal can shed new light on the mechanism of cortical activation, especially if the time course of the change in various MR-observable parameters (T2*, T2, T1, spin density ρ, etc.) is observed.

In neurocognitive research, time-resolved experiments can become important for the study of complex stimulation paradigms. The intrinsic time scale of cortical activation is known from electrophysiologic measurements to lie on the order of 20 to 400 ms. If the time scale of the MR-observable effect can be made short enough, this would allow the spatiotemporal evolution of brain activation, especially for complex paradigms.

The optimal measurement methods for following the time course of activation is not necessarily the same as that for localizing experiments. Whereas localization requires data acquisition in many voxels covering a sufficiently large part of the brain, time-resolved experiments can be performed in a few (or even only one) voxels at the site of activation, which can then be studied in great detail.

EPI certainly is fast enough for most time-resolved experiments. The high acquisition bandwidth leads, however, to a severe penalty in signal-to-noise ratio that makes EPI not necessarily the method of choice when the time course in one or a few voxels is to be observed. Localized single-voxel experiments measuring the water signal in a voxel defined by three slice-selective pulses under orthogonal gradients have been demonstrated to give very high effect-to-noise ratio (100). In addition, the measurement of the full signal yields important information about the nature of the observed effect, whereas imaging techniques are limited to the observation of a single value, the pixel intensity, per acquisition. An initial signal dip has been reported that shows some T2* effect according to an initial inverse BOLD effect (Fig. 100) (58, 104). Although an initial inverse BOLD effect would not be totally unexpected from optical measurements, the nature of the fast MR response seems not to exclusively follow a BOLD mechanism.

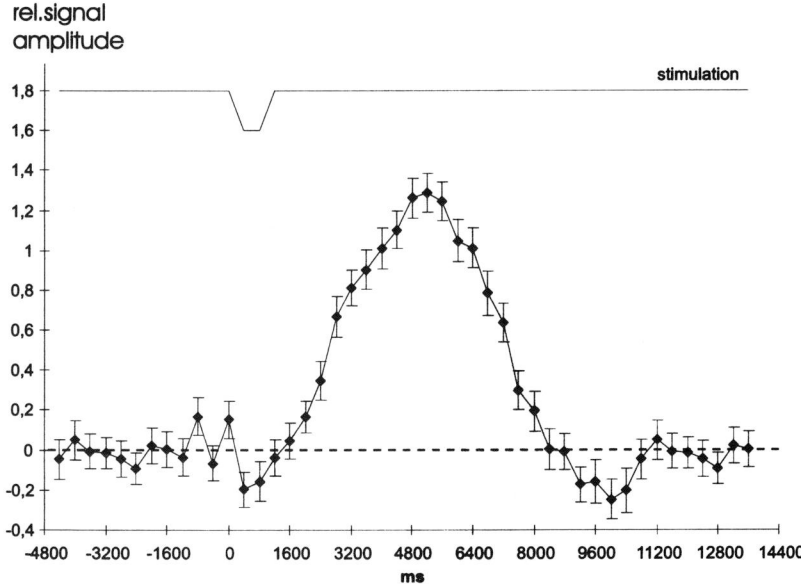

Figure 100. Result from a single-voxel study of the temporal evolution of the signal after excitation by a short light flash. The diagram shows the integral over the difference FIDs acquired at 400-ms time interval. Three different time regimes are demonstrated. An initial negative response is observed at $t = 400$ to 1600 ms after the onset of the stimulus, followed by the normal hemodynamic response with a maximum at about 4 to 5 s and an undershoot at $t = 8$ to 11 s.

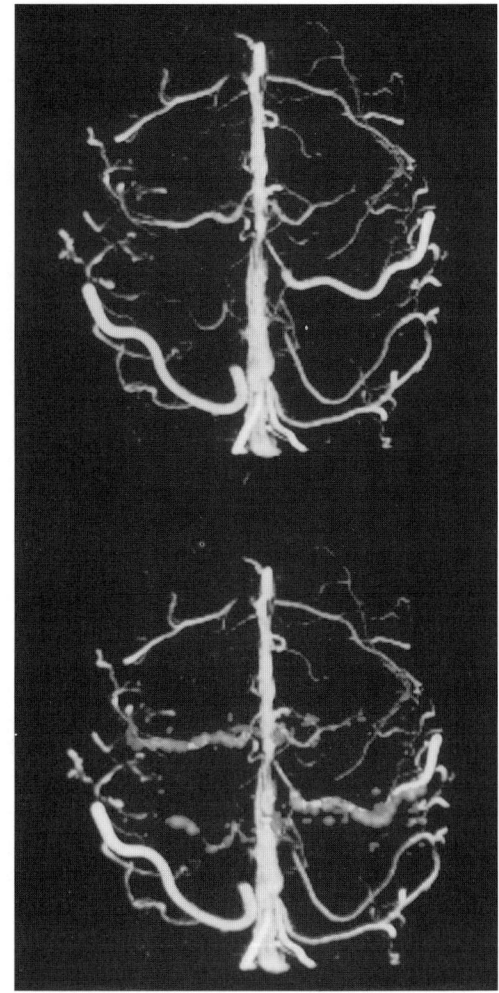

Figure 101. Changes in the signal intensities of draining veins as demonstrated by time-of-flight angiography in two volunteers using a paradigm for stimulation of the primary motor areas. The image at the top shows the MR angiogram prior to stimulation; at the bottom an overlay of the stimulation angiogram (*red*) is shown on the reference image. See Color Plate 40. (From Belle V, Delon-Martin C, Massarelli R, et al. Intracranial gradient-echo and spin-echo functional MR angiography in humans. *Radiology*, 195, 739–746 [1995].)

A negative short-term response also has been observed by MRI techniques (147). Just as in localization measurements, where hybrid experiments can be used in order to reach an optimal compromise between the single-shot (EPI) acquisition and the multishot (gradient-echo) approach, hybridization also can be used for time-resolved experiments in order to reach an optimal compromise between the number of observed voxels per unit time and the effect-to-noise ratio.

Artefacts

BOLD-type experiments have pitfalls that can give rise to false-positive as well as false-negative results. Some of the potential artefacts are as follows.

False-Positive Results. False-positive results can be a consequence of changes in flow in draining veins (51, 81, 89, 120, 186). This is not a false-positive result with respect to the stimulation effect per se. It can, however, lead to a severe mislocation of the activated site by several centimeters. Gradient-echo techniques can be more sensitive to this effect if large flip angles (<30°) are chosen, which lead to in-flow enhancement. TOF angiograms beautifully demonstrate the change in oxygenation even in larger veins several centimeters downstream from the site of activation (12) (Fig. 101 and Color Plate 40). Even at lower flip angles, vessels do not simply become invisible but rather become isointense with surrounding tissues. When gradient-echo images are acquired with sufficient spatial resolution, vascular stimulation can be identified by the vascular shape of the stimulated area and thus be identified and distinguished from more diffuse parenchymal effects.

EPI—especially spin-echo-based EPI—has a lower sensitivity to vascular blood but is by no means totally insensitive, especially when the flow velocities are not too high. Due to the intrinsic low spatial resolution of EPI and the nature of its flow artefacts, vascular effects will most often appear to be blurred and cannot be identified on EPI images as such.

Flow effects have been measured in draining veins using MR angiographic techniques. They can be reduced by using proper imaging parameters and totally avoided by saturating the adjacent slices. As long as care is taken that the vascular signal changes are confined to the activated areas, they are often welcome, since they give rise to much higher effects compared with the often minute ''proper'' parenchymal effects.

A second mechanism that has been discussed as a source of false-positive functional MRI is motion (88, 112, 195). Intrascan motion, especially if it is stimulus-related (as in a subtle startling motion at the onset of the stimulus) can lead to severe misinterpretation, especially if examinations are performed using small surface coils that reduce the volume of observation more or less to the area where the effect is expected to occur. For larger fields of view, it is hard to image a mechanism by which motion can lead to an artefact exactly at the supposed-to-be activation site but nowhere else, although some results along these lines have been published.

False-Negative Results. False-negative effects can arise from a much broader variety of conditions. The first is a low S/N ratio. Although this appears to be trivial, it needs to be mentioned. Parenchymal activation effects seldom produce signal changes above 2% to 4%, even for strongly activating paradigms, the detection of which can be a challenge due to the notoriously poor S/N ratio of strongly $T2^*$-weighted scans.

A second condition is low scan reproducibility. The detection of the small activation effects occurring on stimulation is restricted by the scan-to-scan reproducibility of the experiment rather than by the S/N ratio of each single scan for images with decent quality. The scan-to-scan reproducibility for a state-of-art MRI scanner rarely exceeds 0.5% to 1% and is often considerably lower, since this was not considered a very important engineering goal in the pre-functional MRI era.

A second and very serious cause of low scan reproducibility is patient motion. This will lead to nondetection of the proper effect by multiple motion-related artefacts that can appear all over the image. Artefacts can be produced either by motion between scans or by motion during scans. The latter effect can be minimized by fast image acquisition, but even with EPI such artefacts cannot be avoided altogether.

Extrinsic means to reduce motion artefacts are fixation of the head by an appropriate holder such as a bitebar. Correction for residual motion can be performed with various degrees of refinement. Navigator echo (55) approaches can be used to detect the actual motion status immediately prior to data acquisition. They use the acquisition of a 1D scan in order to detect the principal components (translation, rotation) of rigid-body motion. Position-tracking devices that register head motion throughout the examination also can be used.

By making some basic assumptions about the nature of the motion occurring, information about inter- and intrascan motion also can be derived directly from the acquisition data. Correction for intrascan motion requires the availability of the full complex *k*-space data set (or its real and imaginary part after Fourier transformation), which is normally discarded in conventional scans. Using these data, highly exact corrections for in-plane motion even by fractions of a pixel are feasible.

Through-the-plane motion leads to severe signal artefacts due to the change in the T1 contrast of sequential images. Since it also introduces new features in the image about which no prior knowledge can be assumed, they are much harder to correct for than in-plane motion effects. They are less conspicuous when sequences with very low T1 weighting are used. The best approach to correct for them uses 3D acquisitions in which they can be treated as in-plane motion in the respective direction of the data set.

The severity of motion artefacts strongly depends on the spatial resolution and intrinsic image contrast of the sequence used. Low-resolution scans are more tolerant to motion than high-resolution scans. Flat images that do not show much anatomic contrast also will be tolerant to motion, except at the edges. This type of contrast behavior is, of course, not very desirable for the identification of a detected area of activation to the anatomy of the brain.

At the current state of development of functional brain imaging, correction of motion artefacts seems to be the most critical step. A number of algorithms have been proposed and tested that considerably improve the reliability of the measured data. Even under optimized considerably improve the reliability of the measured data. Even under optimized conditions, however, the signal-to-noise ratio along the time curve of a functional MRI experiment caused by nonreproducibilities very often is appreciably higher than the in-plane signal-to-noise ratio of each signal image. Robust experiments will thus produce better functional data, even if they might yield images with lower signal-to-noise ratios.

Data Evaluation

Although the principles of data-evaluation techniques are covered elsewhere in this book (Chap. 3), some remarks seem to be appropriate about various options to extract the optimal information content from a functional MRI experiment. Practically all functional MRI experiments today are based on an on-off experimental design. Gradual designs that offer some advantages from a statistical point of view are not commonly used mainly because the observed signal change is expected to be strongly nonlinear, which means doubling the intensity of the stimulus cannot be expected to double the signal response.

Even for on-off designs, a huge number of possible postprocessing strategies exist. These can be roughly categorized into two groups: data-driven and model-driven algorithms.

Model-Driven Algorithms. Model-driven algorithms are based on some basic assumptions about the expected signal changes as a function of the stimulus. The most simple such algorithm is to assume that images acquired during the "on" period differ from those acquired during the "off" period. Data are thus put into two different groups and tested for differences using textbook statistical methods ranging from simple difference images to tests such as the t test, Wilcoxon test, and others (Fig. 102 and Color Plate 41).

A more refined model-driven method uses a correlation analysis, where the time course of the pixel intensities is compared with that from one (or a group of) pixels in an area known to be activated (11). The activated pixels used as reference are normally derived from difference images.

An advantage of model-driven algorithms, especially when applied on a pixel-to-pixel basis, is that they are abundantly available and easy to use. The resulting effect images immediately demonstrate the activated areas and allow a distinction at least of gross artefacts from proper effects. These tests can be further refined by using appropriate pre- and postprocessing steps. Filtering the data in the spatial domain as well as along the time axis (most commonly by median filter) and noise suppression by thresholding *or* clustering can be used to improve the effect-to-noise ratio. Very often the resulting images are presented as a color overlay on an appropriate anatomic image in order to make the best use of the available statistical and anatomic information. Such additional postprocessing steps lead to very condensed (and often aesthetically pleasing) results. They suffer, however, from the disadvantage compared with more pedestrian evaluation approaches that they do not transport any information about potential artefacts either during data acquisition or during evaluation.

Especially when various postprocessing algorithms are applied consecutively, it is not always evident how imperfections in the data will affect the result, especially if the spread of the experimental data follows a strong non-Gaussian distribution due to effects such as baseline drifts, motion, long-term system instabilities, etc.

Data-Driven Algorithms. Data-driven evaluation methods do not make any initial assumption about which category an acquired image belongs to. They rather use appropriate clustering algorithms that categorize the temporal evolution of the various pixel inten-

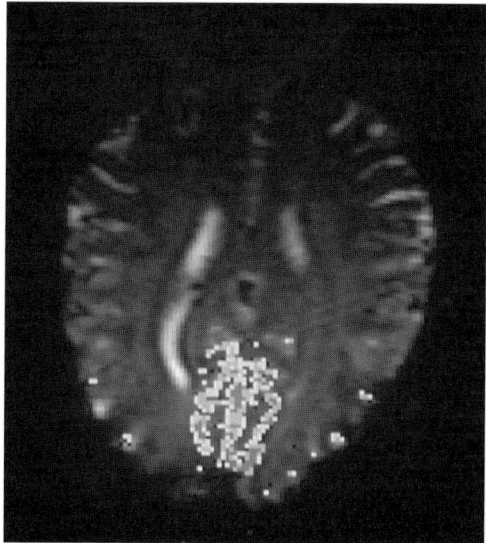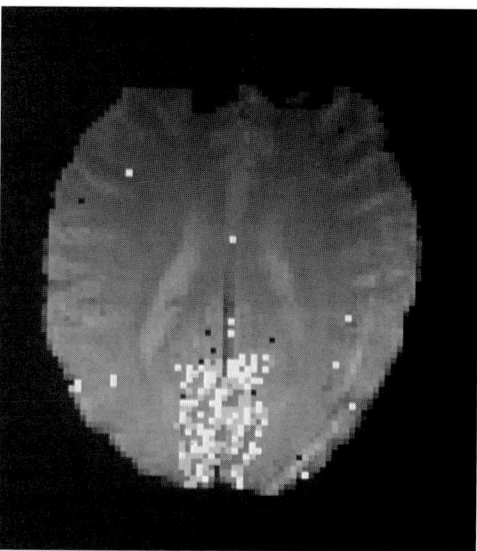

Figure 102. Stimulation images derived by cross-correlation on the time scores in regions of interest that appear bright in the difference images between stimulated and nonstimulated periods. For evaluation, the same data sets were used as those leading to the difference images shown in Figs. 96 and 97. The correlation maps are color encoded and superimposed on one image of the time series in order to show the anatomic correlation of activated areas. See Color Plate 41.

sities. The attribution of which of the so-defined categories corresponds to stimulation has then to be made in a second step.

The advantage of such an approach is that it does not require any initial assumption about the temporal change of the signal intensities as a function of the stimulation. Voxels that react in a similar way to the stimulus will show good correlation independent of the actual profile of the time course. Systematic effects like those discussed in the preceding section that lead to serious problems in model-driven algorithms are thus irrelevant as a source of artefacts as long as they affect all pixel intensities in the same way.

A crucial point in correlation analysis, of course, is finding the right set of voxels that really is representative of activation. If the preselected time function is in any way atypical for the proper stimulation effect, only pixels with a similar atypical signal behavior will ''light up.'' If—in the extreme case—pixels are chosen that for some reason do not show any activation-related effect at all, correlation analysis will identify all the wrong voxels. Correlation analysis can indeed be used not only to find areas of stimulation but also to identify systematic signal fluctuations due to other mechanisms (ECG-related or breathing effects, as well as system-dependent artefacts).

A disadvantage of correlation analysis is the fact that it does not allow one to find and distinguish voxels that show dissimilar but still activation-dependent signal changes. Finding areas with different response patterns by correlation analysis in principle requires correlation of the signal from each pixel with each other. For an image with n^2 pixels, this leads to n^4 calculation steps, which is impractical on a routine basis even for powerful workstations.

A much less cumbersome approach for this task of grouping pixels with similar time course together is to use cluster-analysis techniques (43, 67, 78, 117, 182, 183). Here, the time course of each signal in an experiment with m repetitions is represented as a point in an m-dimensional data space. Pixels with similar time courses are then identified by being adjacent. Various clustering algorithms have been demonstrated to reliably find activated areas without any initial assumption about the activation pattern (Fig. 103 and Color Plate 42).

Clustering algorithms are thus to be expected to be an efficient way to extract a maximum amount of information from the measured data without the necessity of a priori information, which is a steady source of potential fallacies in model-driven approaches.

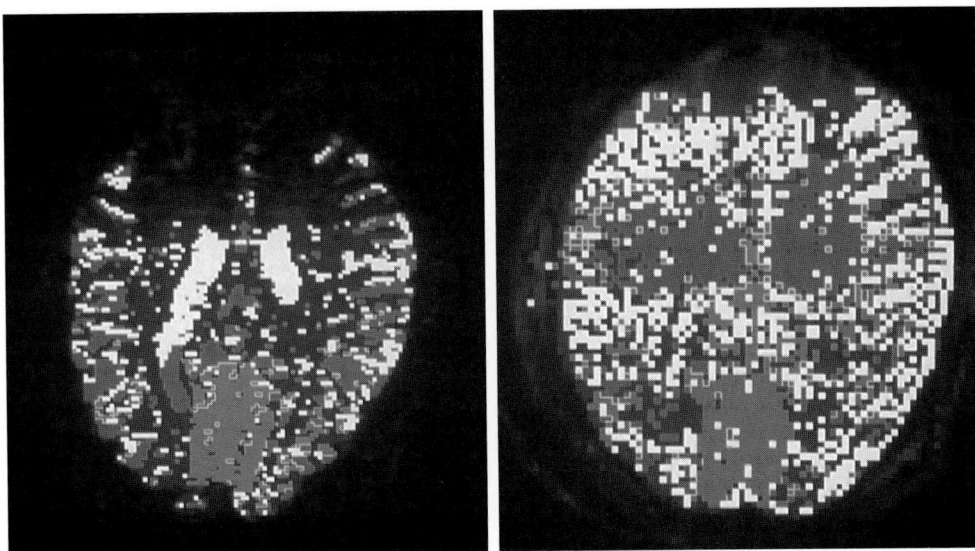

Figure 103. Results of cluster analysis of the data sets used for Fig. 102. Pixels are color encoded according to their membership in different classes found by the algorithm. Note that the activated areas (*red*) are identified, although the algorithm did not use any prior knowledge about the course of the stimulation. See Color Plate 42.

Other data-based approaches such as principal-component analysis (183) also have been applied successfully to functional MRI data.

Temperature Measurements

Temperature measurements are of interest in various clinical applications. The local temperature in inflamed tissue is known to be elevated; temperature also changes in a working muscle. Most interesting, noninvasive temperature measurements facilitate better control of temperature-based therapeutic methods.

A great number of parameters, such as relaxation rates (especially T1) (42, 162), spin density, diffusion coefficients (41, 153, 181, 210) and the chemical shift of various substances, show some temperature dependence (122) and thus can be used—at least in principle—to measure the local temperature inside the body (Table 2). A problem of all these approaches is the fact that the tissue itself undergoes some physiologic change with temperature. Even at mild elevations of a few degrees, changes in tissue perfusion have been reported that might severely affect the measured intensities in many of the sequences meant to measure temperature alone. Very drastic changes occur, of course, beyond 42°C, when proteins start to coagulate.

These physiologic changes are hard to predict, especially in pathologic tissue, and make the feasibility of exact absolute temperature measurements somewhat doubtful. The very good results of temperature measurements on phantoms are therefore hard to transfer to living tissues.

Table 2. *Methods for temperature mapping*

Spin-lattice relaxation time $T1$	(Self) diffusion coefficient D	Temperature-sensitive contrast agents	Static nuclear susceptibility χ_0 $$M = \frac{N\gamma^2\hbar^2 I(I+1)}{3\mu_0 kT} B_0$$ $= \chi_0 B_0$	Water resonance chemical shift $\Delta\nu_{H_2O}$
$\Delta T1 \cong 1.4\%/°C$ (Cline et al., 1994)	$\Delta D \cong 2.4\%/°C$ (Le Bihan et al., 1991)	$\Delta\nu \cong 0.12–0.15$ ppm/°C (Schering, 1994)	$\Delta\chi_0 \cong -0.32\%/°C$	$\Delta\nu_{H_2O} \cong 0.01$ ppm/°C
Tissue dependent	Tissue dependent	Tissue independent?	Tissue independent	Tissue independent

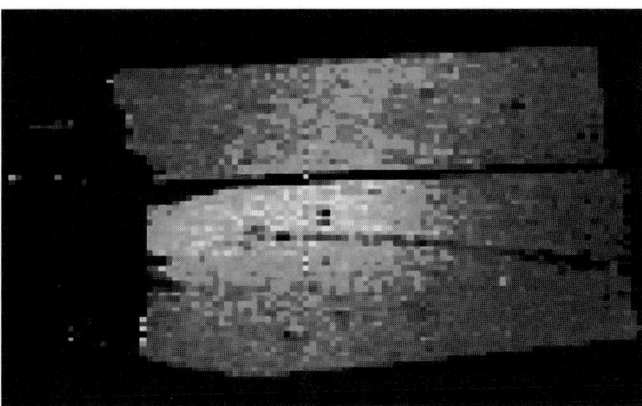

Figure 104. Color-coded image of the diffusion coefficient of a gel phantom heated by an rf probe shown as a curved dark line at the center of the phantom. The temperature gradient as measured with a thermocouple ranged from 45°C (*white*) to 25°C (*dark red*). See Color Plate 43.

There is some debate about whether the physical value of the temperature is really the relevant parameter to measure. For many applications, information about the temperature is required in order to then predict potential changes in the tissues. MRI has a very direct sensitivity to observe these physiologic changes. It thus needs to be questioned whether it would not be preferable to short circuit the temperature measurement by basing an assessment of the temperature effect on the directly observed physiologic effects rather than going the indirect way of first deriving a physical value from the observed effects and then trying to assess possible consequences of some physical temperature value on the tissues.

A semiquantitative approach to measure temperature is to use some method that has an intrinsic high sensitivity to subtle changes in any temperature-sensitive parameter. Especially for therapeutic intervention, some access to the region of interest already exists in order to place the heat applicator (laser or rf). This access also can be used to make a 1D measurement of temperature using a small thermocouple. Isotherms can then be generated and calibrated from the primarily qualitative temperature map (Fig. 104 and Color Plate 43).

Diffusion Methods. The most successful applications for direct temperature mapping have been produced using measurements of the diffusion coefficient (41, 153, 181, 210) which shows a comparatively high temperature sensitivity. A reliable measure of the diffusion coefficient requires several measurements with different gradient b values (see below), which necessitates the availability of very fast imaging techniques, especially for interventional applications.

For many thermal interventions, the required spatial resolution of the temperature map is not very high, since the applicator delivers a rather broad spatial temperature distribution. This helps in the fast and efficient acquisition of the necessary images.

An important exception is laser ablation of brain tumors, where exact measures have to be taken within a few millimeters around the focus of interest.

Chemical-Shift Methods. The chemical shift of many compounds is known to be temperature-sensitive (123). This even includes the shift of the water resonance, which is, however, very small. The 0.01 ppm per degree centigrade is much lower than local susceptibility effects so that even the possibility of detection of temporal temperature changes appears to be questionable.

Contrast agents exist that show a proton resonance with more pronounced chemical shift. Since the water signal is available to serve as a local reference, the temperature-dependent shift difference can be measured very exactly. Separating the comparatively small signal of the agent from the water resonance is not problematic due to the rather large chemical-shift difference between both substances.

Like all directly observed MRI contrast agents, the use of such an agent is severely hindered by the low signal-to-noise ratio due to the low applicable concentration. Future developments will show whether temperature maps with sufficient spatial and temporal resolution can be acquired by such an approach.

MR SPECTROSCOPY

MR spectroscopy (MRS) deals with the use of the already mentioned difference in the Larmor frequency of different chemical compounds as a consequence of the interaction of the molecular electrons with the outer magnetic field. The resulting MR spectrum is thus typical for a given substance, a fact that has led to the use of NMR spectroscopy to identify and analyze unknown substances. This application of the MR phenomenon is about 30 years older than MRI. Its implementation for looking at the chemical composition of living tissues, however, is severely hindered by a number of obstacles.

The most severe restriction for in vivo MRS is the signal-to-noise ratio. MRI measures signals from water protons, whose concentration is on the order of 100 mol/kg. Metabolites, whose signals can in principle be measured and distinguished by in vivo MRS, typically occur in concentrations in the micromolar range and are thus 5 to 8 orders of magnitude less abundant than water protons. The signal-to-noise ratio of the respective signals measured with a given MR sequence is thus smaller compared with what one gets with MRI. It is therefore clear that in MRS one has to make significant compromises in terms of the voxel size, the measurement time, and the signal-to-noise ratio in order to observe even the most abundant metabolites, whose concentration is on the order of a few millimoles. In order to measure the proton signal from creatine, which at roughly 5 mmol/kg is one of the most naturally abundant metabolites, the voxel size has to be made 20,000 times larger in order to get the same S/N ratio compared with water. Thus the typical voxel size of 1 mm^3 in MRI is supplemented by voxels in the range of several millimeters used for MRS. It is thus clear that the spatial resolution of MRS will always be several orders of magnitude lower than that of MRI.

The visibility problem becomes even worse when magnetic nuclei other than hydrogen are to be used for observation. The low concentration factor has then to be multiplied by the lower sensitivity of the observed nucleus. The worst case occurs when the most naturally abundant isotope of some element is nonmagnetic and MR observation has to rely on the observation of a more or less abundant tiny fraction of magnetic isotopes. As shown in Fig. 105, the order of in vivo visibility of the different elements is thus not only considerably different from their natural abundance, but the dynamic range of the scale is also vastly enlarged and covers nearly 10 orders of magnitude for the 10 most common elements.

Most biologically active molecules, such as enzymes, are macromolecules, which are characterized by very short T2 relaxation times. The measurement of signals with decay constants on the order of a few microseconds is not compatible with spatial selection, which even with very strong and fast gradients is hard to perform in much less than a millisecond. Localized MRS is thus restricted to the selective observation of highly abundant small molecules (MW < 1000).

For molecules that occur in useful concentrations (>0.1 mmol/kg) and which possess sufficiently long T2 values for observation, the final problem is the possibility of identifying the spectrum and distinguishing it from spectra of other substances. This problem is closely linked to the spread of the chemical shift, which is vastly different for different nuclei. This chemical-shift range depends on the variety of ways an atomic nucleus can be surrounded by the shielding electrons. As shown in Fig. 106, this chemical-shift range is vastly different for different nuclei.

A huge chemical-shift range is beneficial for the ability to distinguish different molecules. It will, however, also lead to chemical-shift misregistration problems in localized MRS experiments. Localization techniques that work sufficiently well for one type of nucleus might thus be inadequate for others.

In the following sections, first experimental techniques for localized spectroscopy are presented, followed by some brief remarks on some aspects of MRS on different nuclei.

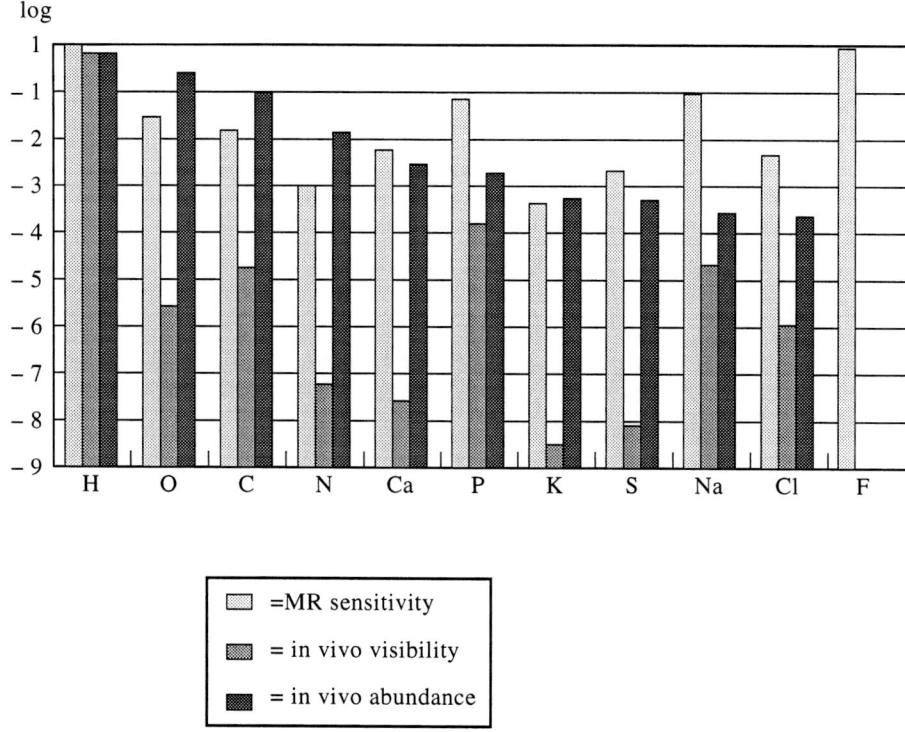

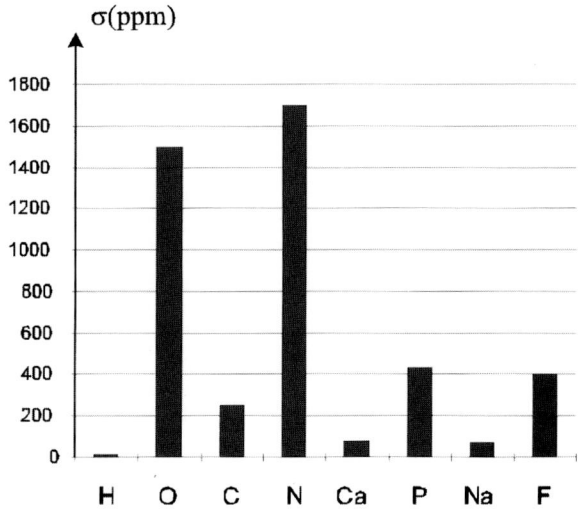

Figure 105. MR sensitivity of some physiologically relevant nuclei. The first 10 elements are listed according to their physiologic abundance in the body in terms of relative numbers of atoms (*gray area*). In order to establish their in vivo MR sensitivity, this number has to be multiplied by the relative MR sensitivity of each nucleus (*striped area*) and the in vivo abundance of the MR-sensitive isotope. The resulting in vivo visibility spans nearly 10 orders of magnitude. The diagram shows that phosphorous as the next sensitive element is already nearly, by a factor of 1:10,000, less sensitive than protons.

Localization Techniques

Basically all principles presented for spatial selection in MRI are also fully applicable to MRS. The magnetic nuclei have no way of knowing whether they are submitted to an experiment that is meant to measure their chemically dependent Larmor frequency or to a mere imaging experiment. The huge gap that seems to exist between MRI and MRS

Figure 106. Chemical-shift range of some elements of physiologic interest. Protons as the most MR-sensitive element have a very low chemical-shift range and will thus allow the distinction of different molecules only to a limited degree. The elements with the highest chemical-shift range and thus the best possibility for in vivo chemical analysis are very MR-insensitive.

thus has nothing to do with the physics involved but seems to be rather a reflection of the different range of scientific disciplines interested in one or the other.

As in MRI, spatial selection can be performed in MRS either during the excitation (with a slice selection gradient) or between the excitation and the data acquisition (with a phase-encoding gradient) or during acquisition (with a readout gradient). The first possibility will lead to volume-selective techniques, whereas the latter two will be described together as chemical-shift imaging.

Volume-Selective Techniques

This approach is based on the selection of a well-defined volume of interest by using one (or more) slice-selective pulses. A single selective pulse will select a planar section; with two successive pulses under orthogonal gradients, a spin echo from a column can be generated. A sequence of three pulses under mutually orthogonal gradients finally can be used to generate either a refocused (second) spin echo (PRESS = point-resolved spectroscopy) (17) or a stimulated echo (STEAM = stimulated echo acquisition) (69) from a voxel (Fig. 107).

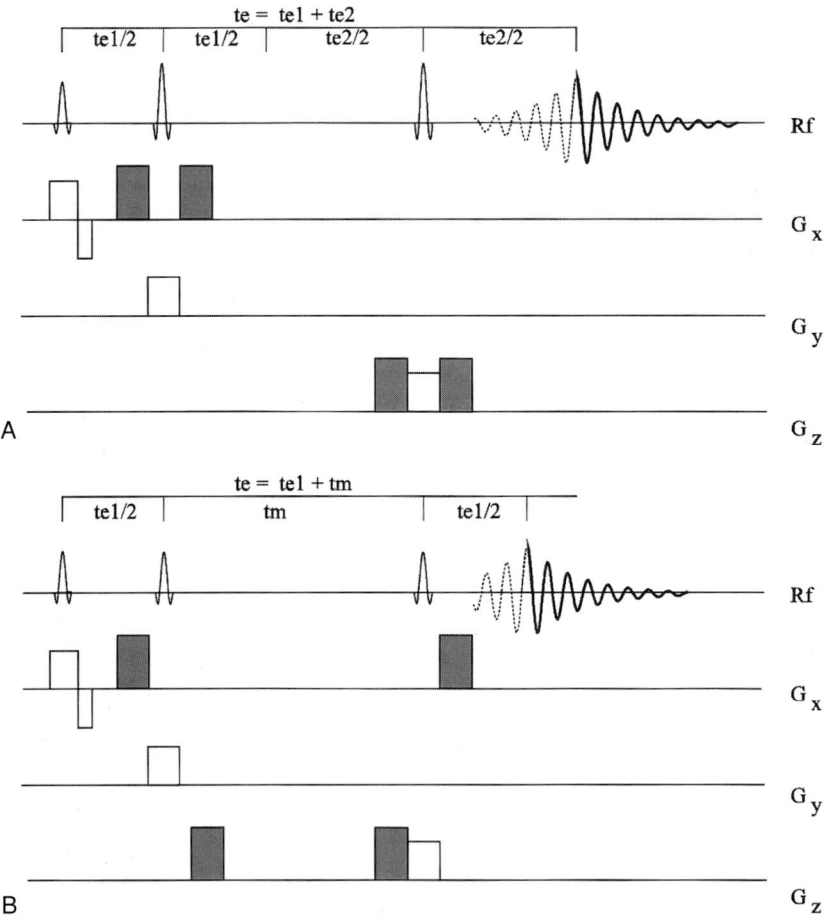

Figure 107. Diagrams of the PRESS (**A**) and STEAM (**B**) experiment used for volume-selective spectroscopy. Both sequences use three selective rf pulses under mutually orthogonal gradients for selecting a voxel inside the volume under observation. The PRESS sequence uses additional gradients (*shaded*) that select the refocused spin echo and destroy all other signals. This spin echo occurs at a time $t_e = t_{e1} + t_{e2}$ after excitation. In the STEAM experiment, selection gradients (*shaded*) are applied such that only the stimulated echo occurring at time $t_e = t_{e1} + t_m$ is observed. Note that the signal decay of the FID, which is applied without any magnetic field gradient, is very slow such that normally only the decaying half of the echoes is acquired.

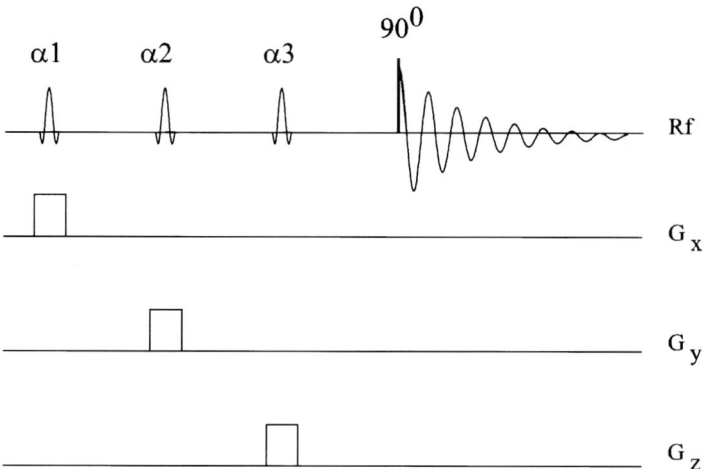

$\alpha 1$ $\alpha 2$ $\alpha 3$ 90^0

Rf

G_x

G_y

G_z

Figure 108. Volume selection by ISIS. The data acquisition is performed as an FID following a single excitation pulse. The sequence is preceded by three pulses with flip angles a_1, a_2, and a_3 that can assume values of 0° or 180°, respectively. After permutation of all flip angles through all three pulses, the signal from the selected voxel will be uniquely labeled and can be extracted by linear combination.

The shape of the voxel in both STEAM and PRESS is assumed to be a rectilinear box. In practice, this is not quite correct due to the imperfections of the slice profile, which lead to a rounding of the edges. Due to the interaction of three pulses at each point inside the voxel, this imperfection is more pronounced than in MRI applications with only 1D slice selection. Pulses with an improved excitation profile are thus required in order to ensure a tolerable agreement between theoretical and practical voxel shape. It should be noted that the use of pulses with Gaussian profile will select a spherical voxel.

For observations of metabolites with T2 values that are so short that the 10- to 20-ms minimum t_e for STEAM or PRESS is not acceptable, spatial selection can be performed

---

COMPARISON STEAM AND PRESS

A problem of both sequences is the fact that three pulses can in principle generate eight different signals (see Fig. 8): three free induction decays from each pulse, three spin echoes from any pair of pulses, plus one spin echo and one stimulated echo involving all three pulses. All except the proper signal are a source of potential artefacts and have to be removed from data acquisition. This is achieved by adding appropriate spoiler gradients that are chosen such that only the proper signal will be refocused at the time of data acquisition. The problem with removal of these unwanted signals is the fact that the voxels from which they originate are much larger than the voxel of interest, which yields the proper signal. Therefore, gradients with sufficient amplitude and duration have to be chosen in order to achieve proper spoiling. For STEAM, this is somewhat easier, since the desired signal is stored as z-magnetization in the t_m interval between the second and the third pulses. This time therefore can be made long enough to incorporate strong gradients that take care of all spurious signals except the FID from the last pulse. For a given gradient performance, STEAM thus allows one to realize shorter echo times t_e. The penalty for this is a signal loss by a factor of 2 due to the intrinsic properties of the stimulated echo mechanism. For strong and stable gradient systems, the achievable echo times t_e with PRESS are insignificantly longer compared with STEAM such that PRESS more or less replaces STEAM.

by using slice-selective pulses that prepare z-magnetization such that the signal from the desired voxel can be generated after one or a few appropriate cycles of the experiment. The earliest such technique was the ISIS sequence (167) which uses a combination of slice-selective inversion pulses (Fig. 108). Linear combination after eight cycles allows generation of the proper signal, whereas signal from outside the desired voxel is canceled. Signal is read out as an FID after a short and hard pulse, which allows measurement with a nominal t_e of zero.

A disadvantage of such an approach is the fact that cancellation relies on perfect reproducibility of the experiment, which is difficult to maintain under in vivo conditions. Volume selection is also compromised by T1 relaxation occurring during the spatial selection period. ISIS and its subsequent improvements (138) are thus limited to applications where an extremely short t_e is more important than any compromise in the quality of volume selection. This applies not only to the observation of nuclei with very short T2 values but also to signals showing very strong j-coupling, which can be shown to produce strong phase artefacts when acquired with nonzero t_e.

THE ISIS TECHNIQUE

Volume selection by ISIS uses three slice-selective inversion pulses under mutually orthogonal gradients followed by signal readout after a nonselective ("hard") excitation pulse. The inversion pulses divide the total volume into four compartments that can be categorized by (a) the outside volume, which is not covered by any of the pulses, (b) three orthogonal planes, where spins are covered by one of the three pulses, (c) three columns at the intersection of any two of these pulses, where spins experience two of the three pulses, and (d) one voxel, in which spins see all three pulses. Only (d) represents the desired voxel. Since z-magnetization in each compartment can take on two values (plus and minus), $2^3 = 8$ experiments are required to compensate for the unwanted signals in the other three compartments.

Multivoxel Techniques

The principle of multislicing, which is used in MRI to fill the T1-dependent recovery time with the acquisition of data from adjacent sections, also can be transferred to volume-selective spectroscopy. In the STABLE technique (59), spectra from two different voxels are acquired in an interleaved manner using either a PRESS or a STEAM experiment. A difficulty for transferring the concept of multislicing to volume-selective spectroscopy is the avoidance of cross-saturation effects, which can occur when one voxel lies in the plane of any of the three gradients used for selection of the other.

For cubic voxels maximum avoidance is ensured if the space diagonal of the two voxels is aligned along the line connecting their position. Another possibility to extend single-voxel techniques to data acquisition in several voxels is to use selection pulses with a profile that acts on more than one frequency bandwidth. Such pulses can be generated easily by superposition of two (or more) pulses with identical profile but different carrier frequencies.

Separation of the signals from several such simultaneously acquired voxels can be performed by linear combination using appropriate inversion cycles (Hadamard spectroscopy) (77, 160). Another possibility is to use phase cycles of each voxel profile with a constant and unique phase offset for each signal and subsequent Fourier transformation.

Since all voxel signals are excited simultaneously, these approaches do not allow interleaving as in STABLE. At least in principle they do allow, however, the acquisition of signals from many voxels in the same time and with identical signal-to-noise ratios as in single-voxel techniques.

Table 3. *Major metabolites*

Metabolite	Chemical shift (ppm)	Function
N-Acetylaspartate (NAA)	2.02	Neuronal marker
	2.6	
Creatine : phosphocreatine	3.04	Energy metabolism
(Cr/PCr)	3.93	
Choline-containing comp (Cho)	3.22	Membranes
Inositol (Ino)	3.56	Osmolyte/glia-marker
Glutamate : glutamine (Glu/Gln)	2.11–2.49	Neurotransmitter, fatty acid
	3.6–3.8	synthesis, precursor of GABA, regulation of ammonia
Lactate	1.3	Anaerobic metabolism
Taurin (weak)	3.4–3.5	Neurotransmitter?

A typical spectrum from a normal brain is shown in Fig. 109A. More or less characteristic changes in these metabolites have been reported in the literature for a variety of pathologic conditions (Fig. 109B). From the point of view of functional applications, the observation of signal variations of lactate and glucose on cortical stimulation has been demonstrated to yield new insight into the neurophysiology of neuronal activation (72), although the as yet unpublished scarce experimental data are still somewhat contradictory and inconclusive.

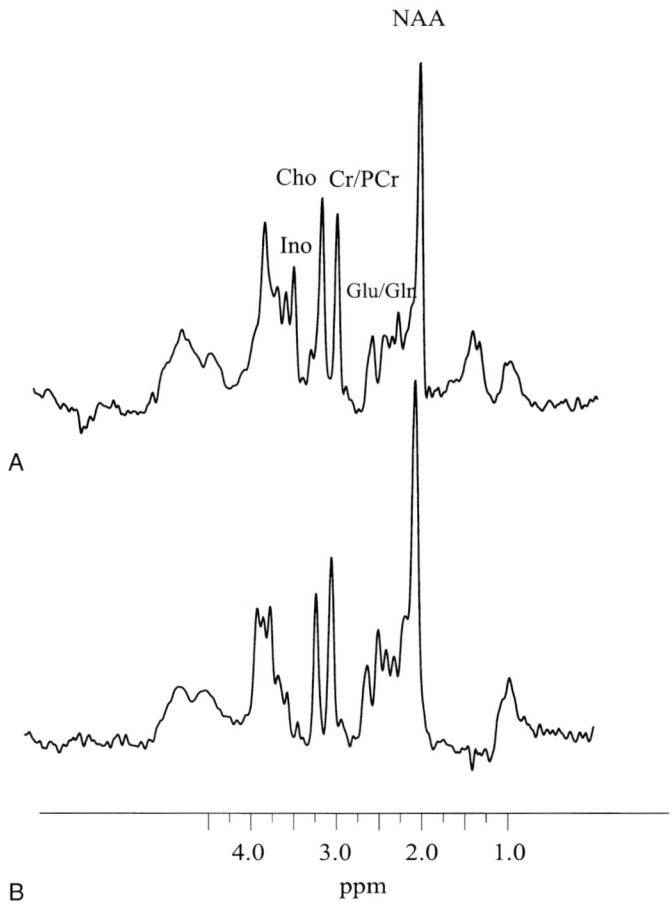

Figure 109. Proton spectra of a normal volunteer (**A**) and a spectrum of a patient with hepatic encephalopathy (**B**). For the identification of the various metabolites, see Table 3. Note the reduction of inositol and the increase of glutamate/glutamine in the patient spectrum.

Methodologically, proton MRS is performed as single-voxel acquisition as well as by chemical-shift imaging. Single-voxel techniques produce superior spectrum quality, which allows the observation of subtle changes in the range of ±5%, which is essential for many clinical and functional applications.

In terms of chemical-shift misregistration problems, proton MRS requires pulses with high bandwidth (and thus strong gradients for a given voxel size) in order to optimize the coincidence of the voxel location as a function of chemical shift. A misregistration by 20% to 30% between chemically different protons corresponds to 1 mm or more in MRI, which most often is of no concern. For MRS, where the voxel size is larger, this corresponds to a shift on the order of 1 cm, which is hardly acceptable, since it might mean that signals in different parts of the spectrum might be originating from different anatomic origins.

Metabolite mapping is much cruder in terms of spatial resolution and spectrum quantification. Its superior spatial information has proven to be useful, however, in the assessment of regional variations of the metabolic state of normal and pathologic tissue.

Phosphorous

MRS of ^{31}P was the earliest application of in vivo MR spectroscopy (174). Its advantages compared with the observation of other nuclei lie in the fact that only a few molecules in the body contain significant amounts of MR-visible phosphorous and that the metabolism of these molecules is known and very important. The main focus in early in vivo ^{31}P MRS (and still today) lies in the observation of the metabolism of high-energy phosphates (Fig. 110). The MR spectrum allows the observation of the metabolic shift of aerobic to anaerobic energy production by measuring the signal intensities of the high-energy phosphates involved. In addition, the pH of the cells can be monitored by looking at the pH-dependent chemical shift of inorganic phosphate. ^{31}P MRS has thus proven to be a valuable tool in functional examinations of energy metabolism.

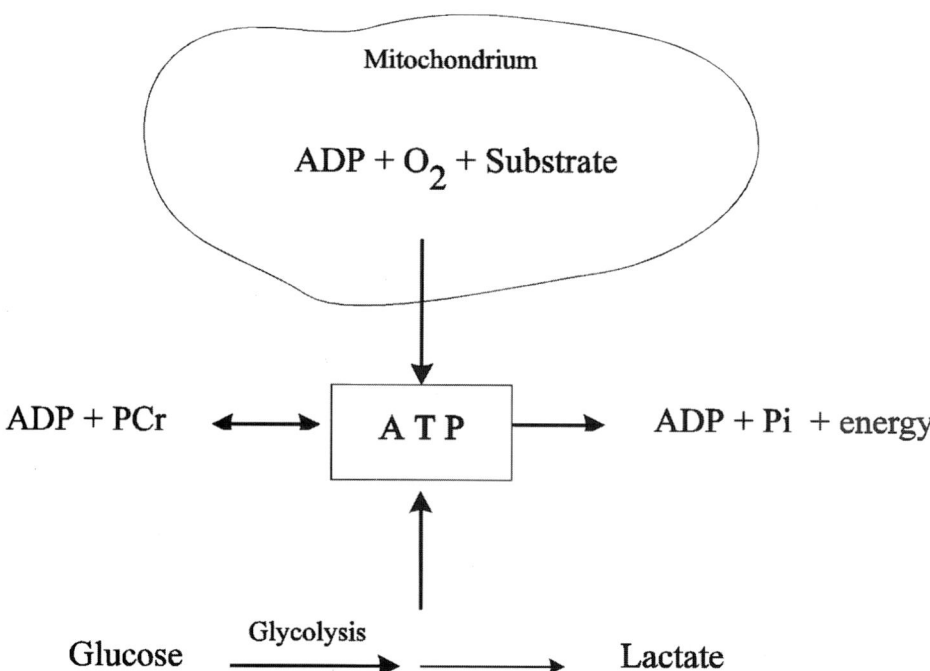

Figure 110. Scheme of high-energy phosphate metabolism. The direct source of energy is the conversion of ATP to ADP and inorganic phosphate. ATP is (slowly) restored by use of oxygen in the mitochondria or via glycolysis. Phosphocreatine (PCr) serves as an intermediate energy buffer for fast release of ATP for peak energy demand. All substances written in blue are observable by ^{31}P spectroscopy.

Experimentally, ^{31}P MRS requires somewhat different approaches compared with proton MRS. First, it should be noted that the chemical-shift range for ^{31}P is significantly larger than that for protons. Localization techniques based on selective pulses thus require pulses with very broad spectral bandwidth in order to avoid chemical-shift misregistration.

The relaxation rates of most compounds are also significantly shorter, which leads to significantly broader natural linewidths and thus to reduced sensitivity to susceptibility effects. ^{31}P is thus not limited to applications in homogeneous organs but can and has been applied successfully all over the body. The short T2-relaxation rates limit applications of PRESS and STEAM techniques, although such experiments have been reported in the literature.

Many early applications of ^{31}P MRS used either surface coil localization or ISIS. More recent applications mainly use chemical-shift imaging. In order to homogenize the spatial response for surface coil applications, adiabatic pulses are commonly used for slice selection (188).

The main use of ^{31}P MRS consists of functional applications in energy metabolism by observation of high-energy phosphates not only in peripheral muscle but also in the heart. More recently, the observation of the phosphomonoester and diester resonances has been put into the center of attention. Although these resonances consist of superpositions of signals from quite a variety of substances, they have been demonstrated to be markers for the metabolic validity of tissues with potential applications for noninvasive testing of transplant organs.

Finally, ^{31}P spectroscopy has been used as an important tool to demonstrate developmental changes in phosphorous metabolite concentrations (23).

Carbon 13

Carbon atoms possess a very large flexibility to arrange electrons in their vicinity. This flexibility is the reason for the great variety of chemical structures that can be based on a carbon backbone and is the reason for the fact that all known life forms are carbon-based. It also leads to a vast variety in the shielding effect and thus to a huge chemical-shift range. In terms of selectivity for different metabolites, ^{13}C spectroscopy thus offers the greatest information content. The severe disadvantage of ^{13}C spectroscopy is its exceedingly low sensitivity caused first by the low magnetic moment of ^{13}C compared with protons and second by its low natural abundance (Fig. 111). The number of papers reporting direct observations of in vivo ^{13}C spectra is thus extremely scarce; the voxel sizes used are on the order of liters in order to attain tolerable S/N ratios.

The problem of low natural abundance can—at least in principle—be overcome by introducing ^{13}C-enriched metabolites. Such examinations are, however, extremely costly due to the high cost and limited availability of appropriately labeled substances.

A further increase in signal-to-noise ratio can be achieved if the ^{13}C resonance is measured by observation of resonances of protons that are coupled to the carbon nuclei. In this case, the ^{13}C magnetization can be transferred to the protons and observed with the higher sensitivity of the proton signal. Even when both measures are combined, only metabolites occurring in high concentrations in the millimolar range can be observed in reasonably sized voxels and within reasonable measurement times.

A number of such experiments using ^{13}C glucose have been published for observation of glucose metabolism, most notably in patients with diabetes mellitus.

Other Nuclei

As shown in Fig. 111, the sensitivity of in vivo MRS for other nuclei is exceedingly low. Such applications are consequently still quite exotic, although some such measurements are of (potentially) high clinical interest. Examples include measurements of Li in psychiatric patients under lithium therapy, determination of F in patients using fluorine-

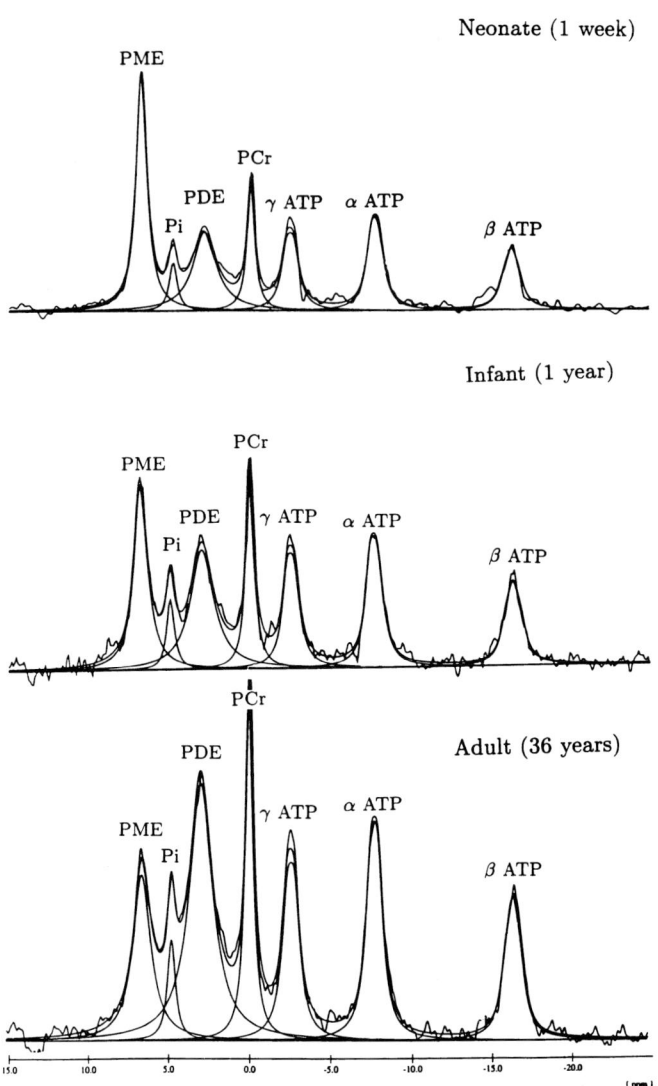

Figure 111. [31]P spectra of a neonate (*top*), a 1-year-old infant (*middle*), and an adult (*bottom*) showing the age-related shift in the concentration of various metabolites. (From Buchli R, Martin E, Boesiger P, Rumpel H. Developmental changes of phosphorous metabolite concentrations in the human brain: A 31P magnetic resonance spectroscopy study. *Pediatr Res*, 35, 431–435 [1994].)

containing neuroleptica, AI MRS (and MRI) after gastric application of aluminum-containing compounds, and hyperpolarized Xe, which was mentioned earlier as a possible means for perfusion studies.

REFERENCES

1. Abragam A. *Principles of nuclear magnetism.* Oxford Science Publication, Clarendon Press (1983).
2. Ahn CB, Kim JH, Cho ZH. High-speed spiral-scan echo planar NMR imaging. *IEEE Trans Med Imaging,* MI-5, 2–7 (1986).
3. Ahn CB, Lee SY, Nalcioglu O, Cho ZH. An improved nuclear magnetic resonance diffusion coefficient imaging method using an optimized pulse sequence. *Med Phys,* 13, 789–793 (1986).
4. Albert MS, Cates GD, Driehuys B et al. Biological magnetic resonance imaging using laser-polarized 129Xe. *Nature,* 370, 199–201 (1994).
5. Atlas SW, Grossman RI, Axel L et al. Orbital lesions: Proton spectroscopic phase-dependent contrast MR imaging. *Radiology,* 164, 510–514 (1987).
6. Axel L, Dougherty L. MR imaging of motion with spatially modulation of magnetization. *Radiology,* 172, 349 (1989).

7. Axel L, Shimakawa A, MacFall J. A time-of-flight method of measuring flow velocity by magnetic resonance imaging. *Magn Reson Imaging,* 4, 199–205 (1986).
8. Bailes DR, Bryant DJ, Bydder GM et al. Localised phosphorous-31 NMR spectroscopy of normal and pathological human organs in vivo using phase encoding techniques. *J Magn Reson,* 74, 158–170 (1987).
9. Bailes DR, Young IR, Thomas DJ et al. NMR imaging of the brain using spin-echo sequences. *Clin Radiol,* 33, 395–414 (1982).
10. Balaban RS, Chesnick S, Hedges K et al. Magnetization transfer contrast in MR imaging of the heart. *Radiology,* 180, 671–675 (1991).
11. Bandettini PA, Jesmanowicz A, Wong EC, Hyde JS. Processing strategies for time-course data sets in functional MRI of the human brain. *Magn Reson Med,* 30, 161–173 (1993).
12. Belle V, Delon-Martin C, Massarelli R et al. Intracranial gradient-echo and spin-echo functional MR angiography in humans. *Radiology,* 195, 739–746 (1995).
13. Bishop JE, Santyr GE, Kelcz F, Plewes DB. Accuracy of keyhole data acquisition in quantitative analysis of dynamic contrast-enhanced breast MRI. *Proc 3rd Ann Meeting SMR, Nice,* 639 (1995).
14. Bloch F, Hansen WW, Packard M. The nuclear induction experiment. *Phys Rev,* 70, 474–485 (1946).
15. Bloembergen N, Purrcell EM, Pound RV. Relaxation effects in nuclear magnetic resonance absorption. *Phys Rev,* 73, 679 (1948).
16. Bolster BD Jr, McVeigh ER, Zerhouni EA. Myocardial tagging in polar coordinates with use of striped tags. *Radiology,* 177, 769–772 (1990).
17. Bottomley PA. Spatial localization in NMR spectroscopy in vivo. *Ann NY Acad Sci,* 508, 333–348 (1987).
18. Bottomley PA, Foster TH, Leue WM. In vivo nuclear magnetic resonance chemical shift imaging by selective irradiation. *Proc Natl Acad Sci USA,* 81, 6856–6860 (1984).
19. Bracewell RM. *The Fourier transform and 1st applications.* New York: McGraw-Hill (1965).
20. Brant-Zawadzki M, Davis PL, Crooks LE et al. NMR demonstration of cerebral abnormalities: Comparison with CT, AJR. *Am J Roentgenol,* 140, 847–854 (1983).
21. Brown TR, Buchthal SD, Murphy-Boesch J et al. A multi-slice sequence for 31P in vivo spectroscopy. *J Magn Reson,* 82, 629–633 (1989).
22. Buchalter MB, Weiss JL, Rogers WJ et al. Noninvasive quantification of left ventricular rotational deformation in normal humans using magnetic resonance imaging myocardial tagging. *Circulation,* 81, 1236–1244 (1990).
23. Buchli R, Martin E, Boesiger P, Rumpel H. Developmental changes of phosphorous metabolite concentrations in the human brain: A 31P magnetic resonance spectroscopy study. *Pediatr Res,* 35, 431–435 (1994).
24. Burstein D, Taratuta E, Manning WJ. Factors in myocardial ''perfusion'' imaging with ultrafast MRI and Gd-DTPA administration. *Magn Reson Med,* 20, 299–305 (1991).
25. Butts K, Riederer SJ. Analysis of flow effects in echo-planar imaging. *J Magn Reson Imaging,* 2, 285–293 (1992).
26. Bydder GM, Pennock JM, Steiner RE et al. The short TI inversion recovery sequence: An approach to MR imaging of the abdomen. *Magn Reson Imaging,* 3, 251–254 (1985).
27. Chapman B, Turner R, Ordidge RJ et al. Real-time movie imaging from a single cardiac cycle by NMR. *Magn Reson Med,* 5, 246–254 (1987).
28. Chien D, Buxton RB, Kwong KK et al. MR diffusion imaging of the human brain. *J Comput Assist Tomogr,* 14, 514–520 (1990).
29. Chien D, Edelman RR. Ultrafast imaging using gradient echoes [Review]. *Magn Reson Q,* 7, 31–56 (1991).
30. Cho ZH, Ro YM. A DANTE fast MR imaging technique using frequency modulation. *Proc 3rd Ann Meeting SMR, Nice,* 485 (1995).
31. Cline HE, Lorensen WE, Herfkens RJ et al. Vascular morphology by three-dimensional magnetic resonance imaging. *Magn Reson Imaging,* 7, 45–54 (1989).
32. Constable RT, Anderson AW, Zhong J, Gore JC. Factors influencing contrast in fast spin-echo MR imaging [Review]. *Magn Reson Imaging,* 10, 497–511 (1992).
33. Constable RT, Gore JC. The loss of small objects in variable TE imaging: implications for FSE, RARE, and EPI. *Magn Reson Med,* 28, 9–24 (1992).
34. Cooley JW, Tukey JW. An alogorithm for the machine computation of complex Fourier series. *Math Comp,* 19, 297–315 (1965).
35. Crawley AP, Wood ML, Henkelman RM. Elimination of transverse coherences in FLASH MRI. *Magn Reson Med,* 8, 248–260 (1988).
36. Crooks L, Arakawa M, Hoenninger J et al. Nuclear magnetic resonance whole-body imager operating at 3.5 KGauss. *Radiology,* 143, 169–174 (1982).
37. Crooks LE, Mills CM, Davis PL et al. Visualization of cerebral and vascular abnormalities by NMR imaging: The effects of imaging parameters on contrast. *Radiology,* 144, 843–852 (1982).
38. Crooks LE, Ortendahl DA, Kaufman L et al. Clinical efficiency of nuclear magnetic resonance imaging. *Radiology,* 146, 123–128 (1983).
39. Czervionke LF, Daniels DL, Wehrli FW et al. Magnetic susceptibility artifacts in gradient-recalled echo MR imaging. *Am J Neuroradiol,* 9, 1149–1155 (1988).
40. Daskiewics OK, Hennel JW, Lubas B. Proton magnetic relaxation and protein hydration. *Nature,* 200, 1006 (1963).
41. Delannoy J, LeBihan D, Hoult DI, Levin RL. Hyperthermia system combined with a magnetic resonance imaging unit. *Med Phys,* 17, 855–860 (1990).
42. Dickinson RJ, Hall AS, Hind AJ, Young IR. Measurement of changes in tissue temperature using MR imaging. *J Comput Assist Tomogr,* 10, 468–472 (1986).
43. Ding X, Masaryk T, Ruggieri P, Tkach J. Detection of activation patterns in dynamic functional MRI with a clustering technique. *Proc 1st Ann Meeting ISMRM, New York,* 1798 (1996).
44. Dixon WT. Simple proton spectroscopic imaging. *Radiology,* 153, 189–194 (1984).

45. Dixon WT, Engels H, Castillo M, Sardashti M. Incidental magnetization transfer contrast in standard multislice imaging. *Magn Reson Imaging,* 8, 417–422 (1990).

46. Dumoulin CL. A method for chemical-shift-selective imaging. *Magn Reson Med,* 2, 583–585 (1985).

47. Dumoulin CL, Cline HE, Souza SP et al. Three-dimensional time-of-flight magnetic resonance angiography using spin saturation. *Magn Reson Med,* 11, 35–46 (1989).

48. Dumoulin CL, Souza SP, Darrow RD. Real-time positron monitoring of invasive devices using magnetic resonance. *Magn Reson Med,* 29, 411–415 (1993).

49. Dumoulin CL, Souza SP, Walker MF, Wagle W. Three-dimensional phase contrast angiography. *Magn Reson Med,* 9, 139–149 (1989).

50. Duyn JH, Frank JA, Ramsey NR et al. Effects of large vessels in functional magnetic resonance imaging at 1.5T. *Int J Imaging Sys Tech,* 6, 271–279 (1995).

51. Duyn JH, Moonen CTW, deBoer RW et al. Inflow versus deoxyhemoglobin effects in ''BOLD'' functional MRI using gradient echoes at 1.5T. *Proc XIIth Ann Meeting SMRM, New York,* 168 (1993).

52. Duyn JH, van Gelderen P, Liu G, Moonen CT. Fast volume scanning with frequency-shifted BURST MRI. *Magn Reson Med,* 32, 429–432 (1994).

53. Edelman RR, Buxton RB, Brady TJ. Rapid MR imaging [Review]. *Magn Reson Annu,* 189–216 (1988).

54. Edelman RR, Siewert B, Darby DG et al. Qualitative mapping of cerebral blood flow and functional localization with echo-planar MR imaging and signal targeting with alternating radio frequency. *Radiology,* 192, 513–520 (1994).

55. Ehman RL, Felmlee JP. Flow artifact reduction in MRI: A review of the roles of gradient moment nulling and spatial presaturation. *Magn Reson Med,* 14, 293–307 (1990).

56. Eng J, Ceckler TL, Balaban RS. Quantitative 1H magnetization transfer imaging in vivo. *Magn Reson Med,* 17, 304–314 (1991).

57. Ernst RR, Anderson WA. *Rev Sci Instrum,* 37, 93 (1966).

58. Ernst T, Hennig J. Observation of a fast response in functional MR. *Magn Reson Med,* 32, 146–149 (1994).

59. Ernst T, Hennig J. Double-volume 1H spectroscopy with interleaved acquisitions using tilted gradients. *Magn Reson Med,* 20, 27–35 (1991).

60. Feinberg DA, Hale JD, Watts JC et al. Halving MR imaging time by conjugation: Demonstration at 3.5 kg. *Radiology,* 161, 527–531 (1986).

61. Feinberg DA, Kiefer B, Litt AW. Dual contrast GRASE (gradient-spin echo) imaging using mixed bandwidth. *Magn Reson Med,* 31, 461–464 (1994).

62. Feinberg DA, Mark AS. Human brain motion and cerebrospinal fluid circulation demonstrated with MR velocity imaging. *Radiology,* 163, 793–799 (1987).

63. Feinberg DA, Mills CM, Posin JP et al. Multiple spin-echo magnetic resonance imaging. *Radiology,* 155, 437–442 (1985).

64. Felmlee JP, Ehman RL, Riederer SJ, Korin HW. Adaptive motion compensation in MRI: Accuracy of motion measurement. *Magn Reson Med,* 18, 207–213 (1991).

65. Firmin DN, Nayler GL, Kilner PJ, Longmore DB. The application of phase shifts in NMR for flow measurement. *Magn Reson Med,* 14, 230–241 (1990).

66. Firmin DN, Nayler GL, Klipstein RH et al. In vivo validation of MR velocity imaging. *J Comput Assist Tomogr,* 11, 751–756 (1987).

67. Fischer H, Hennig J. Clustering of functional MR data. *Proc 1st Ann Meeting ISMRM, New York,* 1779 (1996).

68. Fisher MR, von Schulthess GK, Higgins CB. Multiphasic cardiac magnetic resonance imaging: Normal regional left ventricular wall thickening. *Am J Roentgenol,* 145, 27–30 (1985).

69. Frahm J, Bruhn H, Gyngell ML et al. Localized high-resolution proton NMR spectroscopy using stimulated echoes: Initial applications to human brain in vivo. *Magn Reson Med,* 9, 79–93 (1989).

70. Frahm J, Haase A, Matthaei D. Rapid NMR imaging of dynamic processes using the FLASH technique. *Magn Reson Med,* 3, 321–327 (1986).

71. Frahm J, Haase A, Matthaei D. Rapid three-dimensional MR imaging using the FLASH technique. *J Comput Assist Tomogr,* 10, 363–368 (1986).

72. Frahm J, Krüger G, Merboldt KD, Kleinschmidt A. Dynamic uncoupling and recoupling of perfusion and oxidative metabolism during focal brain activation in man. *Magn Res Med,* 35, 143–149 (1996).

73. Frahm J, Merboldt KD, Hänicke W. Functional MRI of human brain activation at high spatial resolution. *Magn Reson Med,* 29, 139–144 (1993).

74. Friedburg H, Bockenheimer S. Clinical NMR tomography with sequential T_2 images: Carr-Purcell spin-echo sequences [German]. *Radiologe,* 23, 353–356 (1983).

75. Gamsu G, Webb WR, Sheldon P et al. Nuclear magnetic resonance imaging of the thorax. *Radiology,* 147, 473–480 (1983).

76. Gersonde K, Felsberg L, Tolxdorff T et al. Analysis of multiple T_2 proton relaxation processes in human head and imaging on the basis of selective and assigned T_2 values. *Magn Reson Med,* 1, 463–477 (1984).

77. Goelman G. Fast Hadamard spectroscopic imaging techniques. *J Magn Reson,* Series B 104, 212–218 (1994).

78. Golay X, Kollias S, Meier D, Boesiger P. Optimization of a fuzzy clustering techique and comparison with conventional post-processing methods in fMRI. *Proc 1st Ann Meeting ISMRM, New York,* 1787 (1996).

79. Graumann R, Oppelt A, Stetter E. Multiple-spin-echo imaging with a 2D Fourier method. *Magn Reson Med,* 3, 707–721 (1986).

80. Gyngell ML. The application of steady-state free precession in rapid 2DFT NMR imaging: FAST and CE-FAST sequences. *Magn Reson Imaging,* 6, 415–419 (1988).

81. Haacke EM, Hopkins AL, Lai S et al. 2D and 3D high-resolution gradient functional imaging of the brain: Venous contributions to signal in motor cortex studies. *NMR Biom,* 7, 54–62 (1994).

82. Haacke EM, Masaryk TJ, Wielopolski PA et al. Optimizing blood vessel contrast in fast three-dimensional MRI. *Magn Reson Med,* 14, 202–221 (1990).

83. Haacke EM, Tkach JA. Fast MR imaging: Techniques and clinical applications [Review]. *Am J Roentgenol,* 155, 951–964 (1990).

84. Haase A. Snapshot FLASH MRI: Applications to T_1, T_2, and chemical-shift imaging. *Magn Reson Med,* 13, 77–89 (1990).

85. Haase A, Frahm J, Hanicke W, Matthaei D. 1H NMR chemical shift selective (CHESS) imaging. *Phys Med Biol,* 30, 341–344 (1985).

86. Hahn EL. Spin echoes. *Physiol Rev,* 80, 580–594 (1950).

87. Hajnal JV, Bryant DJ, Kasuboski L et al. Use of fluid attenuated inversion recovery (FLAIR) pulse sequences in MRI of the brain. *J Comput Assist Tomogr,* 16, 841–844 (1992).

88. Hajnal JV, Myers R, Oatridge A et al. Artifacts due to stimulus correlated motion in functional imaging of the brain. *Magn Reson Med,* 31, 283–291 (1994).

89. Hajnal JV, Oatridge A, Schwieso J et al. Cautionary remarks on the role of veins in the variability of functional imaging experiments. *Proc XIIth Ann Meeting SMRM, New York,* 166 (1993).

90. Hawkes RC, Patz S. Rapid Fourier imaging using steady-state free precession. *Magn Reson Med,* 4, 9–23 (1987).

91. Healy DM Jr, Lu J, Weaver JB. Two applications of wavelets and related techniques in medical imaging. *Ann Biomed Eng,* 23, 637–665 (1995).

92. Heid O, Deimling M, Huk WJ. Ultra-rapid gradient echo imaging. *Magn Reson Med,* 33, 143–149 (1995).

93. Henkelman RM, Hardy PA, Bishop JE et al. Why fat is bright in RARE and fast spin-echo imaging. *J Magn Reson Imaging,* 2, 533–540 (1992).

94. Henkelman RM, Bronskill MJ. Artifacts in magnetic resonance imaging. *Rev Magn Reson Med,* 2, 1–126 (1987).

95. Hennel F, Nedelec JF. Interleaved asymmetric EPI with standard gradients. *Proc 3rd Ann Meeting SMR, Nice,* 631 (1995).

96. Hennig J. Echoes: How to generate, recognize, use or avoid them in MR-imaging sequences. *Concepts Magn Reson,* 3, 125–143, 179–192 (1991).

97. Hennig J. Generalized MR interferography. *Magn Reson Med,* 16, 390–402 (1990).

98. Hennig J. Multiecho imaging sequences with low refocusing flip angles. *J Magn Reson,* 78, 397–407 (1988).

99. Hennig J. Two-dimensional time-of-flight angiography using reduced object matrices: First results using triangulation and phase encoding methods. *Proc 12th Ann Meeting SMRM, New York,* 565 (1993).

100. Hennig J, Ernst TH, Speck O et al. Detection of brain activation using oxygenation sensitive functional spectroscopy. *Magn Reson Med,* 31, 85–90 (1994).

101. Hennig J, Friedburg H, Strobel B. Rapid nontomographic approach to MR myelography without contrast agents. *J Comput Assist Tomogr,* 10, 375–378 (1986).

102. Hennig J, Hennel F, Oesterle C et al. Fast and robust measurements of brain activation using modified RARE-sequence with variable contrast. *Proc Second Meeting Soc Magn Reson, San Francisco,* 660 (1994).

103. Hennig J, Hodapp M. Burst imaging. *Magn Reson Materials (MAGMA),* 1, 39–48 (1993).

104. Hennig J, Janz C, Speck O. The Ernst functional spectroscopy of brain activation following a single light pulse: Examinations of the mechanism of the fast initial response. *Int J Imaging Sys Tech,* 6, 203–208 (1995).

105. Hennig J, Mueri M. Fast imaging using burst excitation pulses. *Proc 7th Meeting SMRM, San Francisco,* 238 (1988).

106. Hennig J, Mueri M, Brunner P, Friedburg H. Quantitative flow measurement with the fast Fourier flow technique. *Radiology,* 166, 237–240 (1988).

107. Hennig J, Mueri M, Friedburg H, Brunner P. MR imaging of flow using the steady state selective saturation method. *J Comput Assist Tomogr,* 11, 872–877 (1987).

108. Hennig J, Nauerth A, Friedburg H. RARE imaging: A fast imaging method for clinical MR. *Magn Reson Med,* 3, 823–833 (1986).

109. Hoult DI. Rotating frame zeugmatography. *Philos Trans R Soc Lond [Biol],* 289, 543–547 (1980).

110. Howseman AM, Stehling MK, Chapman B et al. Improvements in snap-shot nuclear magnetic resonance imaging. *Br J Radiol,* 61, 822–828 (1988).

111. Hricak H, Crooks L, Sheldon P, Kaufman L. Nuclear magnetic resonance imaging of the kidney. *Radiology,* 146, 425–432 (1983).

112. Hu X, Le TH, Parrish T, Erhard P. Retrospective estimation and correction of physiological fluctuation in functional MRI. *Magn Reson Med,* 34, 201–212 (1995).

113. Huk W, Heindel W, Deimling M, Stetter E. Nuclear magnetic resonance (NMR) tomography of the central nervous system: Comparison of two imaging sequences. *J Comput Assist Tomogr,* 7, 468–475 (1983).

114. Hutchinson M, Rusinek H, Nenov VI et al. Specificity and sensitivity of functional MRI with RARE-sequences. *Proc 3rd Ann Meeting SMR, Nice,* 240 (1995).

115. Hyde JS, Jesmanowicz A, Froncesz W et al. Parallel image acquisition from noninteracting local coils. *J Magn Reson,* 70, 512–517 (1986).

116. Jones RA, Southon TE. A magnetization transfer preparation scheme for snapshot FLASH imaging. *Magn Reson Med,* 19, 483–488 (1991).

117. Khosla D, Singh M, Patel P. Principal component analysis to detect fMRI activity. *Proc 1st Ann Meeting ISMRM, New York,* 1797 (1996).

118. Kiefer B, Kolem H. Imaging the abdomen in a single breathhold with 2-shot HASTE. *Proc 2nd Meeting SMR, San Francisco,* 481 (1994).

119. Kim SG, Ashe J, Hendrich K et al. Functional magnetic resonance imaging of motor cortex: Hemispheric asymmetry and handedness. *Science,* 261, 615–617 (1993).

120. Kim SG, Hendrich K, Hu X et al. Potential pitfalls of functional MRI using conventional gradient-recalled echo techniques. *NMR Biomed,* 7, 69–74 (1994).

121. King KF, Foo TKF, Craford CR. Spiral scan gradient waveform design algorithm. *Proc 3rd Ann Meeting SMR, Nice,* 623 (1995).

122. Knuttel B, Juretschke HP. Temperature measurements by nuclear magnetic resonance and its possible use as a means of in vivo noninvasive temperature measurement and for hyperthermia treatment assessment. *Recent Results Cancer Res,* 101, 109–118 (1986).

123. Konstanczak P, Schründer S, Schaäfer A et al. Contrast media for localized temperature measurements using proton spectroscopy. *Proc 3rd Ann Meeting SMR, Nice,* 1110 (1995).

124. Kumar A, Welti D, Ernst RR. NMR Fourier zeugmatography. *J Magn Reson,* 18, 69–83 (1975).

125. Kwong KK, Belliveau JW, Chesler DA et al. Dynamic magnetic resonance imaging of human brain activity during primary sensory stimulation. *Proc Natl Acad Sci USA,* 89, 5675–5679 (1992).

126. Laub G. Displays for MR angiography. *Magn Reson Med,* 14, 222–229 (1990).

127. Laubenberger J, Buchert M, Schneider B et al. Breath-hold projection magnetic resonance-cholangio-pancreaticography (MRCP): A new method for the examination of the bile and pancreatic ducts. *Magn Reson Med,* 33, 18–23 (1995).

128. Lauterbur PC. Image formation by induced local interactions: Examples employing nuclear magnetic resonance. *Nature,* 242, 190–191 (1973).

129. Le Bihan D. Intravoxel incoherent motion imaging using steady-state free precession. *Magn Reson Med,* 7, 346–351 (1988).

130. Le Bihan D, Breton E, Lallemand D et al. MR imaging of intravoxel incoherent motions: Application to diffusion and perfusion in neurologic disorders. *Radiology,* 161, 401–407 (1986).

131. Le Bihan D, Breton E, Lallemand D et al. Separation of diffusion and perfusion in intravoxel incoherent motion MR imaging. *Radiology,* 168, 497–505 (1988).

132. Lenz GW, Haacke EM, Masaryk TJ, Laub G. In-plane vascular imaging: Pulse sequence design and strategy. *Radiology,* 166, 875–882 (1988).

133. Le Roux P, Pauly J, Macovski A. Burst excitation pulses. *Proc 10th Meeting SMRM, San Francisco,* 238 (1991).

134. Leung DA, Debatin JF, Wildermuth S et al. Real-time biplanar needle tracking for interventional MR imaging procedures. *Radiology,* 197, 485–488 (1995).

135. Liu G, Sobering G, Duyn J, Moonen CT. A functional MRI technique combining principles of echo-shifting with a train of observations (PRESTO). *Magn Reson Med,* 30, 764–768 (1993).

136. Loenneker T, Hennig J. MUSIC: A fast T_2-sensitive MRI technique with enhanced volume coverage. *Magn Reson Med,* (1996), in print.

137. Ludeke KM, Roschmann P, Tischler R. Susceptibility artefacts in NMR imaging. *Magn Reson Imaging,* 3, 329–343 (1985).

138. Luyten PR, Groen JP, Vermeulen JW, den Hollander JA. Experimental approaches to image localized human 31P NMR spectroscopy. *Magn Reson Med,* 11, 1–21 (1989).

139. Mansfield P. Real-time echo-planar imaging by NMR. *Br Med Bull,* 40, 187–190 (1984).

140. Mansfield P, Chapman B. Active magnetic screening of gradient coils in NMR imaging. *J Magn Reson,* 66, 573 (1986).

141. Mansfield P, Maudsley AA. Planar spin imaging by NMR. *J Magn Reson,* 27, 101–119 (1977).

142. McKinnon GC. Ultrafast interleaved gradient-echo-planar imaging on a standard scanner. *Magn Reson Med,* 30, 609–616 (1993).

143. McKinnon GC, Fischer SE, Maier SE. Noninvasive measurement of myocardial motion using magnetic resonance tagging. *Australas Phys Eng Sci Med,* 14, 189–196 (1991).

144. Meiboom S, Gill D. Modified spin-echo method for measuring nuclear relaxation times. *Rev Sci Instrum,* 29, 688–691 (1958).

145. Melki PS, Jolesz FA, Mulkern RV. Partial RF echo-planar imaging with the FAISE method: I. Experimental and theoretical assessment of artifact. *Magn Reson Med,* 26, 328–341 (1992).

146. Melki PS, Jolesz FA, Mulkern RV. Partial RF echo-planar imaging with the FAISE method: II. Contrast equivalence with spin-echo sequences. *Magn Reson Med,* 26, 342–354 (1992).

147. Menon RS, Ogawa S, Hu X et al. BOLD based functional MRI at 4 tesla includes a capillary bed contribution: Echo-planar imaging correlates with previous optical imaging using intrinsic signals. *Magn Reson Med,* 33, 453–459 (1995).

148. Menon RS, Ogawa S, Strupp JP, Ugurbil K. Evidence for human ocular dominance columns mapped using submillimeter resolution FLASH. *Proc 3rd Ann Meeting SMR, Nice,* 163 (1995).

149. Meyer CH, Hu BS, Nishimura DG, Macovski A. Fast spiral coronary artery imaging. *Magn Reson Med,* 28, 202–213 (1992).

150. Middleton H, Black RD, Saam B et al. MR imaging with hyperpolarized 3He gas. *Magn Reson Med,* 33, 271–275 (1995).

151. Moonen CT, van Zijl PC, Frank JA et al. Functional magnetic resonance imaging in medicine and physiology. [Review]. *Science,* 250, 53–61 (1990).

152. Moran PR, Moran RA, Karstaedt N. Verification and evaluation of internal flow and motion: True magnetic resonance imaging by the phase gradient modulation method. *Radiology,* 154, 433–441 (1985).

153. Morvan D, Leroy-Willig A, Jehenson P et al. Temperature changes induced in human muscle by radio-frequency H-1 decoupling: Measurement with an MR imaging diffusion technique: Work in progress. *Radiology,* 185, 871–874 (1992).

154. Moseley ME, Cohen Y, Kucharczyk J et al. Diffusion-weighted MR imaging of anisotropic water diffusion in cat central nervous system. *Radiology,* 176, 439–445 (1990).

155. Moseley ME, Sevick R, Wendland MF et al. Ultrafast magnetic resonance imaging: Diffusion and perfusion. *Can Assoc Radiol J,* 42, 31–38 (1991).

156. Mosher TJ, Smith MB. A DANTE tagging sequence for the evaluation of translational sample motion. *Magn Reson Med,* 15, 334–339 (1990).

157. Mugler JP 3rd. Brookeman JR. Three-dimensional magnetization-prepared rapid gradient-echo imaging (3D MP RAGE). *Magn Reson Med,* 15, 152–157 (1990).
158. Mulkern RV, Melki PS, Jakab P et al. Phase-encode order and its effect on contrast and artifact in single-shot RARE sequences. *Med Phys,* 18, 1032–1037 (1991).
159. Mulkern RV, Wong ST, Winalski C, Jolesz FA. Contrast manipulation and artifact assessment of 2D and 3D RARE sequences. *Magn Reson Imaging,* 8, 557–566 (1990).
160. Muller S, Hafner HP, Beckman N. Simultaneous multivolume spectroscopy (SIMUVOSP) using local techniques. *NMR Biomed,* 2, 209–215 (1989).
161. Nayler GL, Firmin DN, Longmore DB. Blood flow imaging by cine magnetic resonance. *J Comput Assist Tomogr,* 10, 715–722 (1986).
162. Nelson TR, Tung SM. Temperature dependence of proton relaxation times in vitro. *Magn Reson Imaging,* 5, 189–199 (1987).
163. Norman D, Mills CM, Brant-Zawadzki M et al. Magnetic resonance imaging of the spinal cord and canal: Potentials and limitations. *Am J Roentgenol,* 141, 1147–1152 (1983).
164. Norris DG. Ultrafast low-angle RARE: U-FLARE. *Magn Reson Med,* 17, 539–542 (1991).
165. Oesterle C, Hennig J. Improvement of spatial resolution of keyhole effect images. *Proc 1st Ann Meeting ISMRM, New York,* 1527 (1996).
166. Ogawa S, Lee T-M, Nayak AS, Glynn P. Oxygenation-sensitive contrast in magnetic resonance image of rodent brain at high magnetic fields. *Magn Res Med,* 14, 68–78 (1990).
167. Ordidge RG, Connelly A, Lohman JAB. Image selected in vivo spectroscopy (ISIS): A new method for spatially selective NMR spectroscopy. *J Magn Reson,* 66, 283–294 (1986).
168. Ordidge RJ, Knight RA, Helpern JA. Magnetization transfer contrast (MTC) in flash MR imaging. *Magn Reson Imaging,* 9, 889–893 (1991).
169. Oshio K, Feinberg DA. Single-shot GRASE imaging without fast gradients. *Magn Reson Med,* 26, 355–360 (1992).
170. Panych LP, Oesterle C, Zientara GP, Hennig J. Implementation of a fast gradient-echo SVD encoding technique for dynamic imaging. *Magn Reson Med,* 35, 554–562 (1996).
171. Park HW, Kim YH, Cho ZH. Fast gradient-echo chemical-shift imaging. *Magn Reson Med,* 7, 340–345 (1988).
172. Pettigrew RI, Avruch L, Dannels W et al. Fast-field-echo MR imaging with Gd-DTPA: Physiologic evaluation of the kidney and liver. *Radiology,* 160, 561–563 (1986).
173. Purrcell EM, Tottey HC, Pound RV. Resonance absorption by nuclear moments in a solid. *Phys Rev,* 69, 37–38 (1946).
174. Radda GK, Bore PJ, Gadian DG et al. 31P NMR examination of two patients with NADH-CoQ reductase deficiency. *Nature,* 295, 608–609 (1982).
175. Reese TG, Weisskoff RM, Rosen BR et al. Diffusion anisotropy of the beating heart. *Proc 3rd Meeting SMR, Nice,* 249 (1995).
176. Riederer SJ, Tasciyan T, Farzaneh F et al. MR fluoroscopy: Technical feasibility. *Magn Reson Med,* 8, 1–15 (1988).
177. Rosen BR, Belliveau JW, Chien D. Perfusion imaging by nuclear magnetic resonance [Review]. *Magn Reson Q,* 5, 263–281 (1989).
178. Rosen BR, Wedeen VJ, Brady TJ. Selective saturation NMR imaging. *J Comput Assist Tomogr,* 8, 813–818 (1984).
179. Runge VM, Wood ML. Fast imaging and other motion artifact reduction schemes: A pictorial overview [Review]. *Magn Reson Imaging,* 6, 595–607 (1988).
180. Russ JC. *The image processing handbook* (2nd ed.). Boca Raton: CRC Press (1995).
181. Samulski TV, MacFall J, Zhang Y et al. Noninvasive thermometry using magnetic resonance diffusion imaging: Potential for application in hyperthermic oncology. *Int J Hyperthermia,* 8, 819–829 (1992).
182. Scarth G, McIntyre M, Wowk B, Somorjai R. Detection of novelty in functional images using fuzzy clustering. *Proc 3rd Ann Meeting SMR, Nice,* 238 (1995).
183. Scarth G, Somorjai RL. Fuzzy clustering versus principal component analysis of fMRI. *Proc 1st Ann Meeting ISMRM, New York,* 1782 (1996).
184. Scheffler K, Hennig J. Regular and stochastic k-space trajectories: Methods and properties in fast MR imaging. *Proc 3rd Ann Meeting SMR, Nice,* 487 (1995).
185. Sechtem U, Pflugfelder P, Higgins CB. Quantification of cardiac function by conventional and cine magnetic resonance imaging. *Cardiovasc Intervent Radiol,* 10, 365–373 (1987).
186. Segebarth C, Belle V, Delon C et al. Functional MRI of the human brain: Predominance of signals from extracerebral veins. *Neuroreport,* 5, 813–816 (1994).
187. Sigmund G, Stoever B, Zimmerhackl LB et al. RARE-MR-urography in the diagnosis of upper urinary tract abnormalities in childern. *Pediatr Radiol,* 21, 416–420 (1991).
188. Silver MS, Joseph RI, Hoult DI. Highly selective p/2 and p pulse generation. *J Magn Reson,* 59, 347–351 (1984).
189. Simon JH, Foster TH, Ketonen L et al. Reduced-bandwidth MR imaging of the head at 1.5 T_1. *Radiology,* 172, 771–775 (1989).
190. Soila KP, Viamonte M Jr, Starewicz PM. Chemical shift misregistration effect in magnetic resonance imaging. *Radiology,* 153, 819–820 (1984).
191. Stejskal EO, Tanner JE. Spin diffusion measurements: Spin echoes in the presence of a time-dependent field gradient. *J Chem Phys,* 42, 288 (1965).
192. Stover B, Laubenberger J, Hennig J et al. Value of RARE-MRI sequences in the diagnosis of lymphangiomatosis in children. *Magn Reson Imaging,* 13, 481–488 (1995).
193. Thomsen C, Henriksen O, Ring P. In vivo measurement of water self-diffusion in the human brain by magnetic resonance imaging. *Acta Radiol,* 28, 353–361 (1987).
194. Thulborn KR, Waterton JC, Matthews PM, Radda GK. Oxygenation dependence of the transverse relation time of water protons in whole blood at high field. *Biochim Biophys Acta,* 714, 265–270 (1982).

195. Turner R, Friston KJ, Howard R et al. Automated registration and normalization of fMRI time course changes. *Proc 3rd Ann Meeting SMR, Nice,* 235 (1995).
196. Turner R, Jezzard P, Wen H et al. Functional mapping of the human visual cortex at 4 and 1.5 tesla using deoxygenation contrast EPI. *Magn Res Med,* 29, 277–279 (1993).
197. Twieg DB. The k-trajectory formulation of the NMR imaging process with applications in analysis and synthesis of imaging methods. *Med Phys,* 10, 610–621 (1983).
198. van der Meulen P, Groen JP, Tinus AM, Bruntink G. Fast field echo imaging: An overview and contrast calculations [Review]. *Magn Reson Imaging,* 6, 355–368 (1988).
199. van Gelderen P, Duyn JH, Moonen CT. Analytical solution for phase modulation in BURST imaging with optimum sensitivity. *J Magn Reson,* Series B 107, 78–82 (1995).
200. Van Vaals JJ, Brummer ME, Dixon WT et al. Keyhole method for accelerating imaging of contrast agent uptake. *J Magn Reson Imaging,* 3, 671–675 (1993).
201. Walker MF, Souza SP, Dumoulin CL. Quantitative flow measurement in phase contrast MR angiography. *J Comput Assist Tomogr,* 12, 304–313 (1988).
202. Waterton JC, Jenkins JP, Zhu XP et al. Magnetic resonance (MR) cine imaging of the human heart. *Br J Radiol,* 58, 711–716 (1985).
203. Wedeen VJ, Meuli RA, Edelman RR et al. Projective imaging of pulsatile flow with magnetic resonance. *Science,* 230, 946–948 (1985).
204. Wehrli FW, Shimakawa A, Gullberg GT, MacFall JR. Time-of-flight MR flow imaging: Selective saturation recovery with gradient refocusing. *Radiology,* 160, 781–785 (1986).
205. Wolff SD, Balaban RS. Magnetization transfer contrast (MTC) and tissue water proton relaxation in vivo. *Magn Reson Med,* 10, 135–144 (1989).
206. Wood ML, Silver M, Runge VM. Optimization of spoiler gradients in FLASH MRI. *Magn Reson Imaging,* 5, 455–463 (1987).
207. Young IR, Bailes DR, Burl M et al. Initial clinical evaluation of a whole body nuclear magnetic resonance (NMR) tomograph. *J Comp Assist Tomogr,* 6, 1–18 (1982).
208. Zerhouni EA. New directions in cardiac magnetic resonance imaging. *Top Magn Reson Imaging,* 2, 67–71 (1990).
209. Zha L, Lowe IJ. Optimized ultra-fast imaging sequence (OUFIS). *Magn Reson Med,* 33, 377–395 (1995).
210. Zhang Y, Samulski TV, Joines WT et al. On the accuracy of noninvasive thermometry using molecular diffusion magnetic resonance imaging. *Int J Hyperthermia,* 8, 263–274 (1992).
211. Zhuo WF, Yi W, Grimm RC, Rossman PJ et al. Orbital navigator echoes for motion measurements in magnetic resonance imaging. *Magn Reson Med,* 34, 746–753 (1996).
212. Zientara GP, Panych LP, Jolesz FA. Dynamically adaptive MRI with encoding by singular value decomposition. *Magn Reson Med,* 32, 268–274 (1994).
213. Zur Y, Wood ML, Neuringer LJ. Spoiling of transverse magnetization in steady-state sequences. *Magn Reson Med,* 21, 251–263 (1991).

Functional Imaging, edited by
Gustav von Schulthess and Jürgen Hennig.
Lippincott–Raven Publishers, Philadelphia, © 1998.

9

Electroencephalogram (EEG)

Michael Bach

The electroencephalogram (EEG) is a window to the function of the brain, if a cloudy one. The electroencephalograph graphically renders electric potentials from the brain. The EEG has had its ups and downs. Initially, it seemed to provide direct access to the workings of the brain; then it frustrated many researchers by its very complex nature and was nearly proclaimed obsolete—at least for localization—after the rise of many exciting imaging techniques. Driven by research on the magnetoencephalogram (MEG), improved analysis techniques rejuvenated the EEG as a means to study cortical function with moderate spatial resolution (centimeters) but with high temporal resolution (1 ms).

Even though the reader may be less than happy to learn that there is more to read on the EEG than this treatise, I would like to mention some sources that I consider especially valuable: Nunez (30) treats all technical aspects of the EEG, from Maxwell's equations to electrode properties, in a most comprehensive way. Regan (35), while stressing the field of visual evoked potentials, adds excellent neurobiologic background. As general textbooks on the EEG for technical aspects, Cooper (10) and for clinical applications Niedermeyer (29) should be considered. The present chapter only scratches the surface and stresses technical aspects.

Since 1929, when psychiatrist Hans Berger described human brain potentials for the first time, the EEG has developed into a powerful diagnostic instrument for the neurologist and brain scientist, since the EEG and its derivatives provide the easiest objective correlates of brain function. However, it also has been observed with some justice that measuring the EEG is like trying to understand the function of an automobile engine by analyzing its exhaust (G. Baumgartner, personally communicated by W. Berger). However, the latter view also is applicable to the functional MRI (Chap. 8) or PET (Chap. 5).

M. Bach: Division of Neuroophthalmology, University Hospital, Freiberg, Germany.

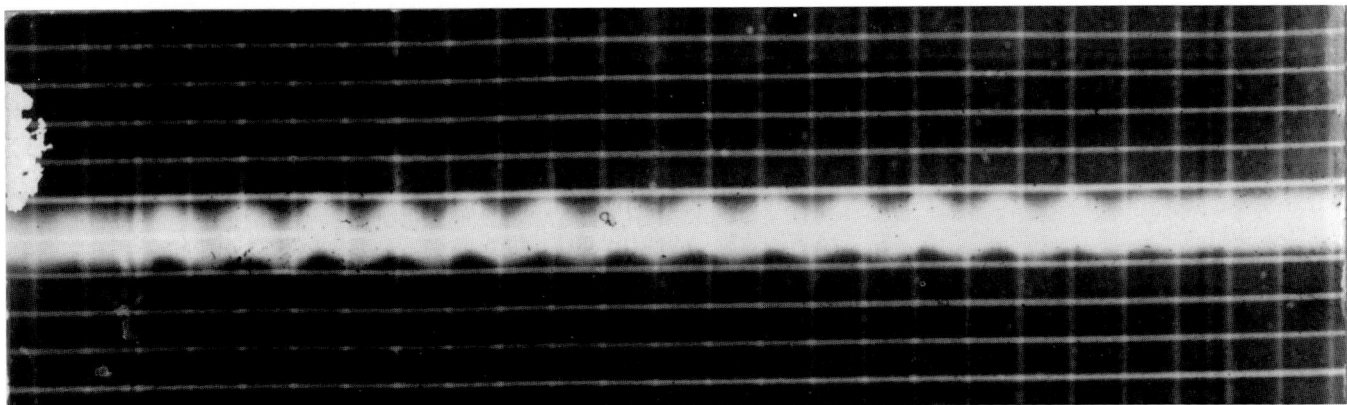

Figure 1. Historical recordings. The first alpha waves measured by H. Berger with a string galvanometer. (Reproduced from an original recording courtesy W. Berger.)

The popularized term *flatliners* derives from an EEG-based definition of being alive: Death is assumed when no EEG is recordable; its lines are flat (the clinical definition of "death" is more involved, of course). But to what degree is consciousness "nothing but" the cooperation of our neurones? This would be a monistic or, more specifically, the "emergent materialism" position in the ongoing mind-brain discussion. While this position is open to argument, there is a general tenet in current brain research, an agreement to see to what end this approach will lead us. In this respect, the EEG is an arena where interesting correlates between mental processes and electrophysiologic measures can be found and/or concepts refuted.

HISTORY

Brazier (7) compiled a number of excellent treatises on the history of the EEG. Here I mention only some highlights. In 1808, the French Academy refused to admit Gall (who had proposed the concept of localization of mental functions in the cortex) on the grounds that the cortex has nothing to do with thinking. In 1875, Caton (8) published observations of spontaneous and evoked electrical activity at the exposed cortex of rabbits and monkeys. Finally, in 1924, psychiatrist Berger recorded the first human EEG from the intact skull, and in 1929, Berger (6, 20) published the first report on the human EEG, describing and defining the alpha and beta rhythms (Fig. 1) that he recorded.

Initially, there were reservations in the scientific community as to the significance of these new and most remarkable findings. Even Berger's own observations cast doubt on the idea that these brain potentials were associated with the mind. In a mentally relaxed state with eyes closed, the EEG amplitude proved very large, showing mainly alpha waves with a dominant frequency of approximately 10 Hz. With mental activity, such as arithmetic calculation, the EEG amplitudes decreased markedly.

After considerable time, it finally became clear that mental activity corresponded with several ongoing forms of desynchronized cortical activity with consequently lower mass potentials (1). Grey Walter (41) was the first to localize a brain tumor with the EEG.

EEG SOURCES

What kinds of sources generate the EEG, and where are they? This important issue has received surprisingly little attention, and it is currently not an active research topic. The current understanding may be summarized as follows (11, 12, 21, 26): The EEG is a mass phenomenon, the net outcome of a great number of electrical processes adding constructively or destructively in space and time (Figs. 2 and 3). For a measurable scalp potential to occur, a degree of synchrony between a large number of sources is required.

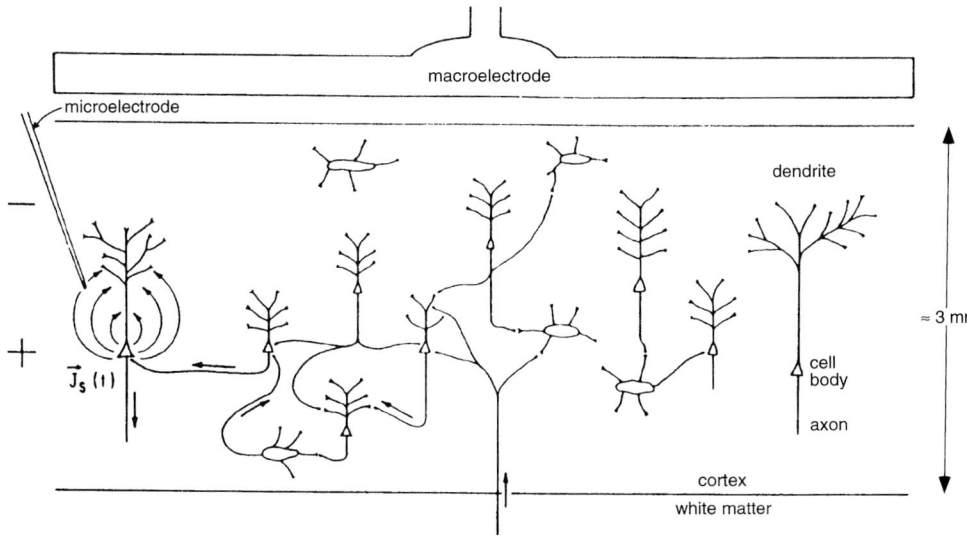

Figure 2. Micro- and macropotentials. Simplified diagram of the relations of white matter (*bottom*), cortex, EEG electrode (macrocelectrode), and some intracortical cells and connections. A scalp electrode averages the signals of millions of neurones. (From Nuñez PL, Katznelson RD. *Electric fields of the brain: the neurophysics of the EEG.* New York: Oxford University Press [1981].)

These sources are not the action potentials (spikes) themselves. The spikes are too brief and the probability too low for sufficient synchronization to add constructively. More likely candidates are the excitatory and inhibitory postsynaptic potentials (EPSPs/IPSPs) that can add up to a sizable scalp potential with their longer time constants and larger current loops. Probably the EEG is dominated by postsynaptic potentials in the large pyramidal cells (Fig. 4), since only currents in their elongated axial dendrites will build up sufficiently large uncompensated current loops. Over cortical areas that exhibit a convex fold (gyri), the following rule of thumb holds: IPSPs generate scalp surface positivity; EPSPs generate negativity (26). EPSPs from thalamic input (arriving in layer

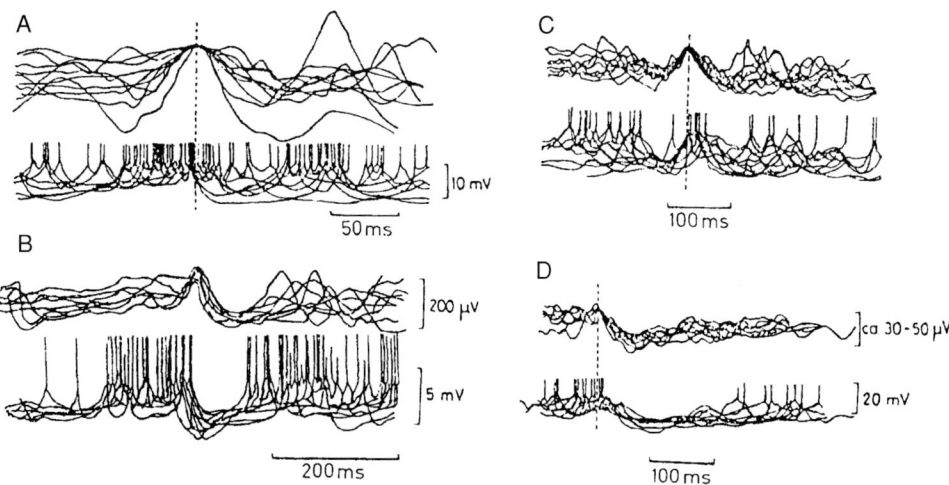

Figure 3. Spikes and EEG. Correlation of surface potential (*top traces*) and single-unit activity (*below*). (**A, B**) Recordings from the same neuron. (**C, D**) Likewise from another. (**A, C**) Correlation between surface negativity and higher spike frequency. (**D**) Surface negative-positive transition in parallel with high spike rates and inhibition. (From Kiloh LG, McComas AJ, Osselton JW. *Clinical electroencephalography.* London: Butterworths [1972].)

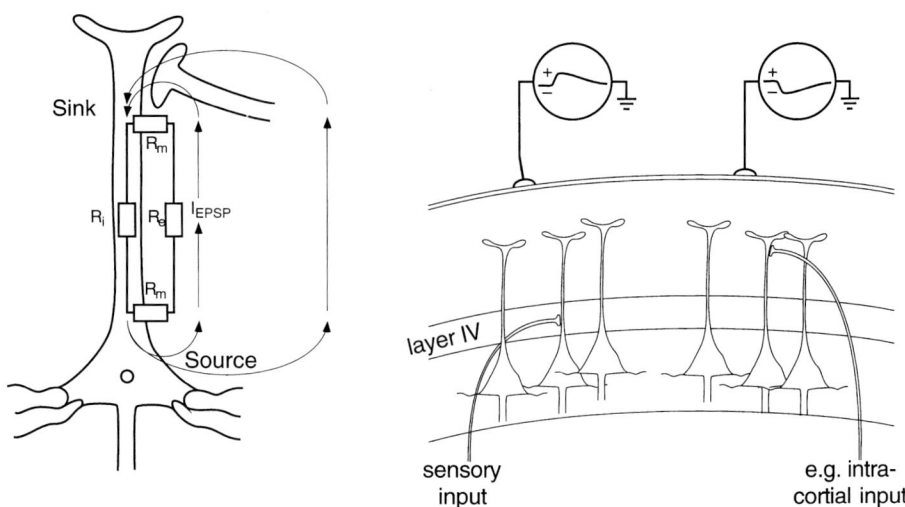

Figure 4. Cellular currents and EEG. Sketch of currents and polarities originating from EPSPs and IPSPs. Not only the type of postsynaptic potential (EPSP/IPSP) but also the vertical position of the synapse and hence cortical connectivity affect the surface polarity. (Modified from Martin JH. The collective electrical behavior of cortical neurons: The electroencephalogram and the mechanisms of epilepsy. In: ER Kandel, JH Schwartz, TM Jessel (Eds.). *Principles of neural science*, 777–791. New York: Elsevier [1991].)

IVc) evoke surface negativity; intracortical input arriving in layer II/III evokes surface positivity (25). However, given our incomplete understanding as well as the complexities of cortical topology, it is best not to draw too specific conclusions from the EEG polarity.

FROM GENERATOR TO SURFACE ELECTRODE

The EEG speads electronically. Thus the usual electrical cable equations apply to physiologic propagation from the generator to white matter, pia mater, liquor, dura mater, bone, and skin. The propagation time is very fast (<1 ms) compared with neuronal conduction times. The sequence of high and low resistances from the neuron to the scalp surface (Table 1) leads to a marked spatial spread of the local potential distribution even from narrow sources, making it difficult to reason backwards, i.e., to deduce the sources from surface potential distributions (see below). The MEG, in contrast to the EEG, does not suffer from this ''blurring'' of the sources. In a physical description of the relation between generators and their potential fields, one discerns the term *near field* (where the strength of a dipole field falls off in proportion to r^3) and *far field* (fall-off proportional to r). The EEG, however, always corresponds to the near field, regardless of the generating site. As Nunez (30) stated ironically, ''The use of the term 'far field' to describe potentials originating from 'far away' is a good illustration of very noisy communication between physics and the EEG.''

Table 1. *Approximate resistivities of some biologic materials at low frequencies*

Material	Resistivity [$\Omega \cdot m$]
White matter (average)	6.5
Cortex	3.5
Cerebrospinal fluid	0.64
Skull	200
For comparison	
Copper	2×10^{-8}
Seawater	0.2

Source: Modified from Nunez PL, Katznelson RD. *Electric fields of the brain: The neurophysics of the EEG.* New York: Oxford University Press (1981).

EEG MEASUREMENT

Electrical Matters

The EEG is an electrical signal ranging in amplitude from about 10 to 100 μV. With the current state of electronics, amplification and electronic noise are no longer a problem in EEG recording. Since the electrode leads are rarely shielded (otherwise they might loose flexibility), a preamplifier with a gain of about 100 is mounted near the subject's head (''headbox''), with wiring to the main amplifiers, where the signal is also appropriately filtered. Digitization for computer processing also has become easy with the current state of the art; e.g., 1-ms sampling rate with 12-bit resolution is readily achieved. However, the large number of channels coming en vogue for source analysis (up to 250) is somewhat unwieldy. Unwanted interference from outside sources is rejected, to a large degree, with current operation amplifiers that have a high common mode rejection ratio.

In most cases, of particular interest is the time course of brain potentials rather than their absolute values. Thus ac recording is quite adequate (and also much easier than dc recording). The interesting frequency range lies (arguably) between 1 and 40 Hz, possibly up to 100 Hz. An EEG test setup for clinical routine recording typically uses a time constant of 0.3 s [corresponding to a highpass filter with a cutoff frequency of $1/(2 \cdot \pi \cdot 0.3) = 0.5$ Hz] and a ''filter'' (lowpass is implied) of 30 to 70 Hz.

Electrodes and Drift

While present-day amplifiers pose few technical problems, electrodes still do, especially if dc recording with low drift is desired. It is mandatory that the active and the reference electrodes be of identical material. Otherwise, the electrode pair acts as a galvanic element with a voltage of up to 1 V (''offset voltage''). One could assume that this is of no consequence if rejected by ac recording, but two problems still remain:

1. *Pre*amplifiers are often dc coupled. With a gain of 100, an offset voltage of 100 mV would result in a preamplifier output of 10 V, overloading most amplifiers. After highpass filtering by the main amplifier, an overloaded preamplifier will lead to a constant zero output.
2. Any offset voltage will drift due to changes in the ionic composition of the metal-skin interface, which is affected by any residual debris on the surface of the electrode. The drift is roughly proportional to the offset voltage itself and consequently will contain intrusive noise power in the relevant frequency range of 1 to 30 Hz.

With these caveats, the use of silver–silver chloride or gold cup electrodes is fairly simple. It is a myth that low resistance results in a higher amplitude, since the electrode resistance of 1 to 10 kΩ is always low compared with the preamplifier's input impedance of 10 to 100 MΩ. A large resistance, however, is indicative of poor electrode-skin contact that can generate intrusive noise. The more important goal is similarity of electrode resistance among all electrodes; any differing resistance degrades the common-mode rejection of the preamplifiers, inviting mains interference (50 Hz in Europe, 60 Hz in the United States).

Derivation, Electrode Positions

The question of the ''ideal'' electrode position previously led to considerable debate. For a start, it must be realized that there is no absolute zero for potentials and that only potential *differences* are meaningful. ''Inactive'' or ''indifferent'' electrode positions on the body are only approximations to zero. An EEG channel represents the voltage difference between the two inputs of its differential input amplifiers connected to two electrodes.

Thus the electrode positions (the *montage*) should not be ruled by dogmatic beliefs but rather by the specific experimental or clinical question. Typically one wants to link

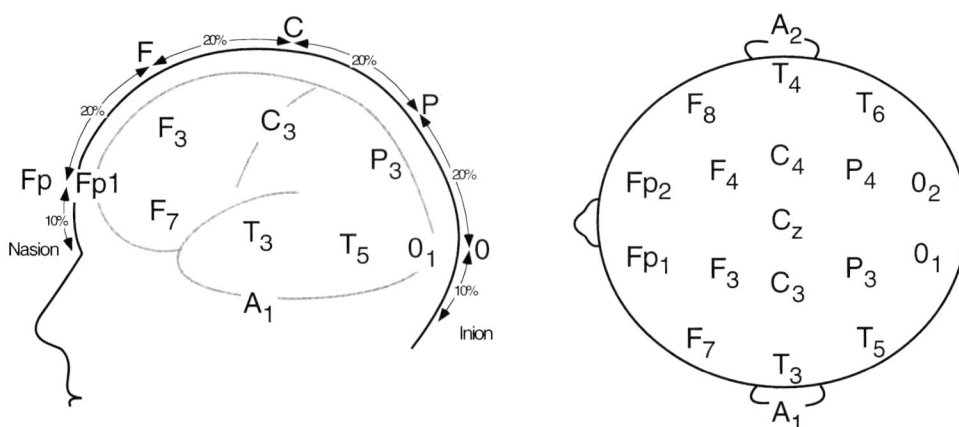

Figure 5. Electrode positions in the International 10/20 System. The distance between the electrodes is measured in relative units between landmarks on the scalp; the nomenclature is mnemonic (frontal, central, posterior); the numbers are odd for the left, even for the right hemisphere. (Modified from Jasper HH. Report of the Committee on methods of clinical examination in electroencephalography: The ten-twenty electrode system of the international federation. *Electroencephalogr Clin Neurophysiol*, 10, 370–375 [1958].)

electrode position to an underlying cortical area. Here, the International 10/20 System (18) has proven useful: Standard, easily detectable bony landmarks on the head (nasion and inion as front-back measures and the vertex and the preauricular points for lateral measures) serve as reference. The electrodes are positioned at relative distances of 10% or 20% between these landmarks, hence the name *10/20 System* (Fig. 5). This technique takes varying head size into account and has been shown to correlate with underlying brain morphology.

The number of electrodes varies from 2 to 128. For early evoked potentials, 2 may suffice. For clinical EEG interpretation, 12 to 16 channels are routinely used. For mapping and source derivation, 16 would be considered too low. Previously, there was debate as to whether a bipolar derivation (difference between equivalent positions on the two hemispheres) or a "linked ear" reference or an "average reference" is more advantageous. With current equipment, the debate has become nearly irrelevant, since any montage can be simulated by appropriate postprocessing. The main requirement is that the electrode(s) used for reference are noise-free and preferably carry little activity; a popular choice is the sum (not galvanic linkage!) of A_1 and A_2. In a bipolar montage, an epileptic focus may be most evident.

Unfortunately, there is some discrepancy on the choice of polarity for depicting electrophysiologic recordings. The history on the "correct" polarity may be illuminated by the following anecdote (G. F. A. Harding, personal communication):

> It was the congress on evoked potentials organised in April 1974 in Brussels. On the day before the meeting we were taken out to a chateau and all discussed various items related to standards. Desmedt conducted a vote as to which way would be up, would it be positive up as ophthalmologists and physicists wanted it or would it be negative up as electroencephalographers, physiologists and biologists wanted it. Having taken the vote on that he then asked for people to vote on whether if the vote went against their choice they would be prepared to change their convention in their laboratory. All this got progressively more confusing until David Ingvar from Sweden stood up and said that in his laboratory positive was to the right and negative was to the left! Amidst the general hilarity everybody of course went on exactly the way they had and we still have evoked potentials which can either be positive up or negative up.

All normal EEG systems are set up to give an upward deflection when the noninverting input becomes more negative than the inverting input. In contrast, traces of the electroretinogram (ERG) are always positive up, while evoked potentials (EPs) can be found both positive up and negative up. If in doubt, the polarity should be ascertained, and it is good practice to indicate it near the traces depicted.

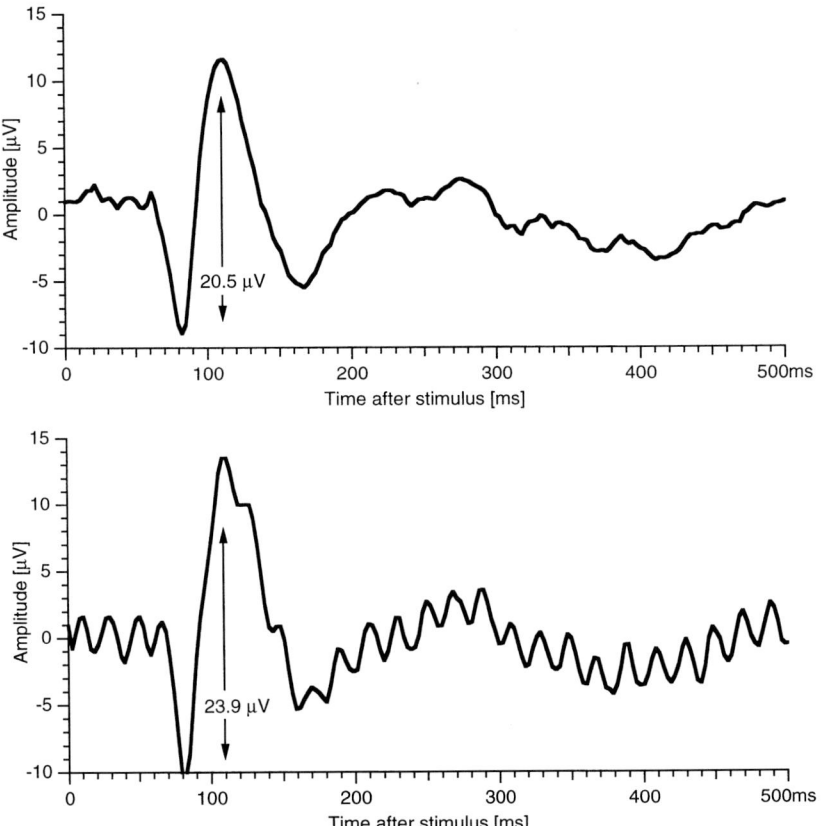

Figure 6. Example of artefact from mains interference. (*Top*) Normal visual evoked potential in response to a phase-reversing checkerboard, average of 160 repetitions. The main features are the trough at ~90 ms, the peak at ~110 ms, and the trough at ~180 ms. (*Bottom*) Repeat recording showing mains interference (the small sinusoidal excursions) after removing the ground electrode. It can be seen that mains interference, like noise, has a tendency to erroneously enhance the measured peak-trough amplitudes.

The subject, the electrodes, and the wiring are the most common sources for problems in EEG recording. Recordings in the operating theater, on convulsive patients, or from infants pose special problems. It is my experience that interference problems (Fig. 6) occasionally can present a sizable challenge even in a laboratory environment.

POTENTIAL MAPS

A powerful method to visualize the spatial pattern of EEG recordings is the construction of potential maps for a given instant in time (for a recent review, see Skrandies 1993 [38]). When potential surface maps are generated, the reference electrode is irrelevant; its choice does not change the intrinsic shape of the "mountainous" surface, only its absolute height (Fig. 7).

An interpretatory artefact may occur, though, if false-color mapping of the potential surface is used (a technique appealing to the naive observer) and the color scale is unwisely chosen. For example, if a gradual change in the voltage is transformed into a qualitative color change (e.g., from red to green), this may lead to striking (artefactual) contours. If the entire map is raised or lowered, an operation that should not affect the interpretation in ac recording, this contour will likely undergo remarkable changes.

In clinical routine, maps have not superseded visual inspection of long voltage-versus-time printouts. This need not reflect on the inertia of routine but rather on the implicit recognition that the EEG carries more information in the temporal domain as compared with the spatial domain.

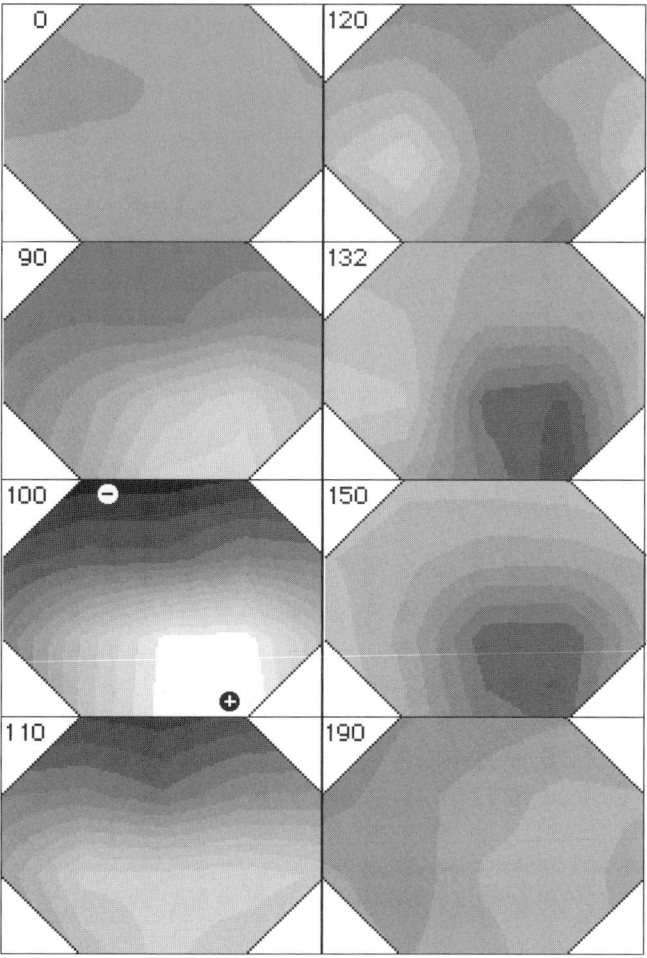

Figure 7. Potential maps. These examples were derived from a 24-channel recording seen from above the head; nose is top. The eight maps represent averaged evoked potentials at different times. The delay relative to the stimulus (a phase-reversing checkerboard) is given at top right of every map from 0 to 190 ms; negativity is black, positivity is white. At around 100 ms after the stimulus, a positivity peaks over the posterior pole changing into a negative peak at 132 ms (compare Fig. 6). The small excursions at 0 and 190 ms represent the noise level. (From Meigen, Skrandies, and Bach, unpublished observations.)

THE ELECTROOCULOGRAM (EOG)

Depending on the specific application, blink artefacts can be obnoxious because they intrude in all derivations with varying amplitude (see Figs. 9 and 10). The eye is a dipole resulting in a cornea-positive potential of about 0.1 V. Depending on eye position, the dipoles may project potentials all over the head. Measured by electrodes around the eye, these potentials are called an *electrooculogram* (EOG, Fig. 8). Thus simultaneous measurement of the EOG is mandatory, and by parametric models, the EOG may be adequately subtracted from the EEG (23).

THE SPONTANEOUS NORMAL EEG

The "normal" EEG (Fig. 9) is immensely variable. Some people present a dominant alpha rhythm, some do not, some are irregular, and some have a nearly flat EEG. An early problem for the EEG was the following finding that the EEG had the largest amplitude when there was little mental activity. The large alpha waves, with a frequency

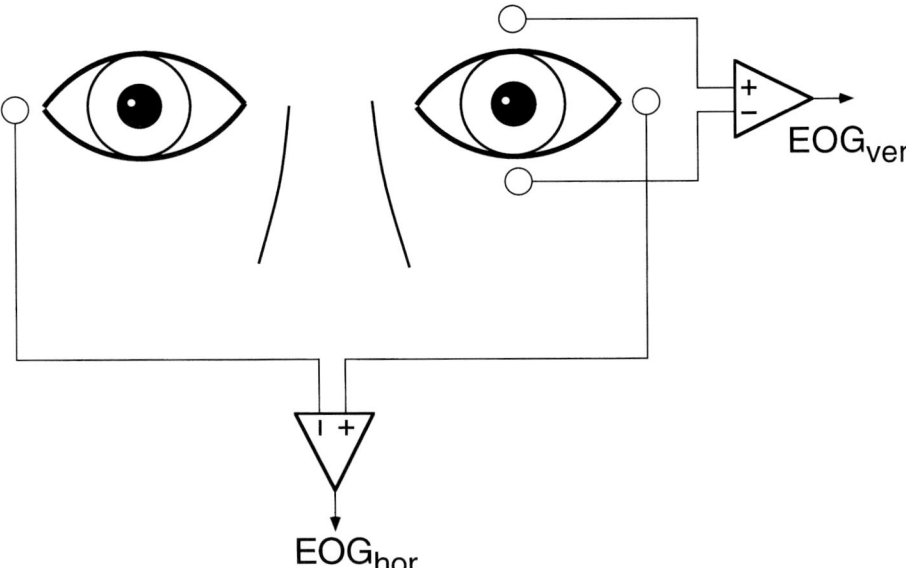

Figure 8. The EOG. The drawing shows, in a subject's frontal view, the schematized arrangement of skin electrodes for the binocular horizontal and vertical EOG. The projection of the eyes' dipoles on the electrodes will result in potential differences depending on eye position. For measurement of eye movements, this is advantageous; for measuring the EEG, the EOG is a major source of artefacts, eye blinks often resulting in markedly higher amplitude than the EEG itself. The intrusion of the EOG into the EEG depends on the specific montage's orientation and distance to the eyes.

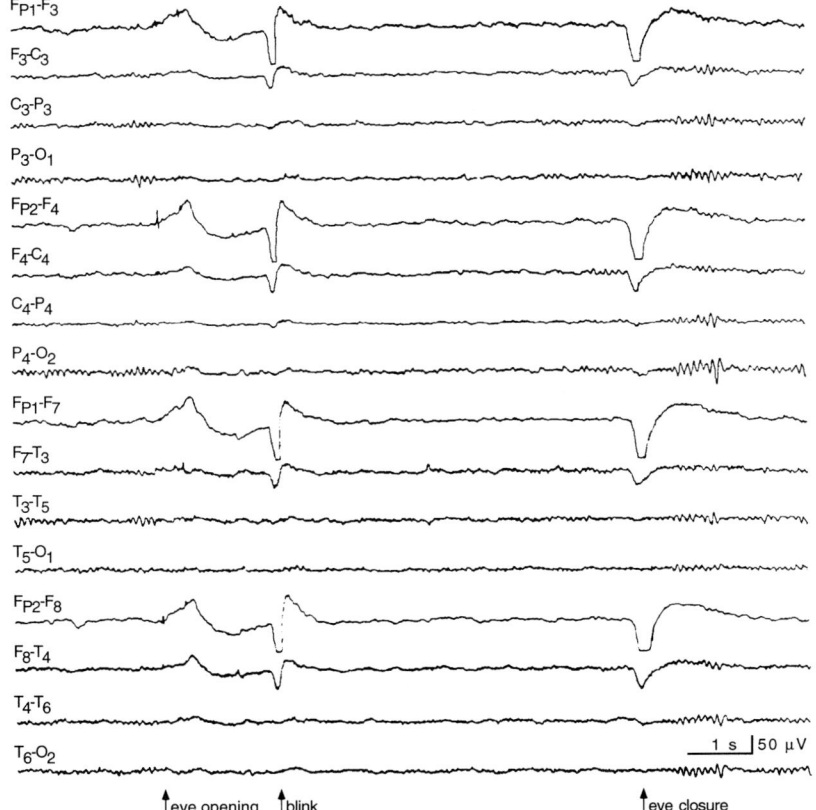

Figure 9. The normal EEG of the waking adult. (After Christian W. *Klinische Elektroenzephalographie: Lehrbuch und Atlas.* Thieme: Stuttgart, Germany [1968].)

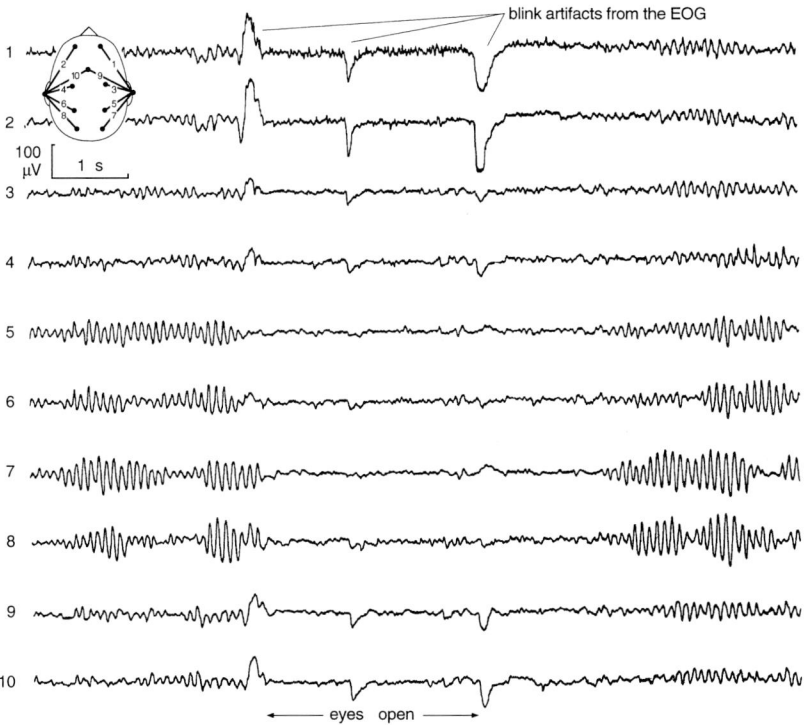

Figure 10. Alpha blocking. The eyes are initially closed. When the eyes are opened (notice the blink artefacts), the alpha rhythm that was most prominent in the occipital leads (5 to 7 from top) vanishes and recurs about 1 s after eye closure. (After Christian W. *Klinische Elektroenzephalographie: Lehrbuch und Atlas.* Thieme: Stuttgart, Germany [1968].)

of 8 to 12 Hz and an amplitude of 40 to 100 μV, dominating in occipital areas, occur in a relaxed state with eyes closed (Fig. 10). When mental activity increases (i.e., starting mental arithmetic), these waves disappear, and only irregular, small deflections remain (Fig. 10, *center*). This discrepancy, more mental activity leading to a smaller EEG, can be easily interpreted in terms of *desynchronization* (1); many cortical sources with different temporal sequences will sum up to smaller scalp potentials as opposed to synchronized activity throughout the brain, which seems to characterize the *alpha* state. Other rhythms have been termed *beta* (14 to 30 Hz, occurring in normal subjects preferentially in frontocentral leads with an amplitude much smaller than alpha), *theta* (4 to 7 Hz), and delta (0.5 to 3 Hz; Fig. 11). The phase of the alpha waves is identical in corresponding leads between the two hemispheres but inverts between occipital and frontal leads; the latter finding, however, may depend on the reference electrodes chosen. Normally, the EEG has a high degree of right-left symmetry.

PHYSIOLOGIC PARAMETERS AND PATHOPHYSIOLOGIC CONDITIONS

Age has a strong influence on the EEG. An infant's EEG would be considered abnormal for an adult. The alpha rhythm, for instance, develops between 1 and 5 years of age, increasing in frequency from 4 Hz at the age of 3 months to the adult value of 10 Hz at the age of 10 (though it may be arguable whether the initially low-frequency rhythm should be termed *alpha rhythm*). EEG changes ascribed to old age, however, are essentially due to cerebrovascular, degenerative, or metabolic disorders (27).

A dramatic change in the EEG occurs between waking and sleeping. Whereas the alpha peak frequency is typically 10 Hz, a sleep EEG generally is dominated by lower frequencies but of 3 to 10 times larger amplitude than the alpha rhythm. The EEG is often used to classify sleep stages (four categories) (34).

Clinical use of the EEG is a wide field that lies beyond the scope of this chapter. Briefly, the merit of the EEG is its relation to the function of the brain, while its local-

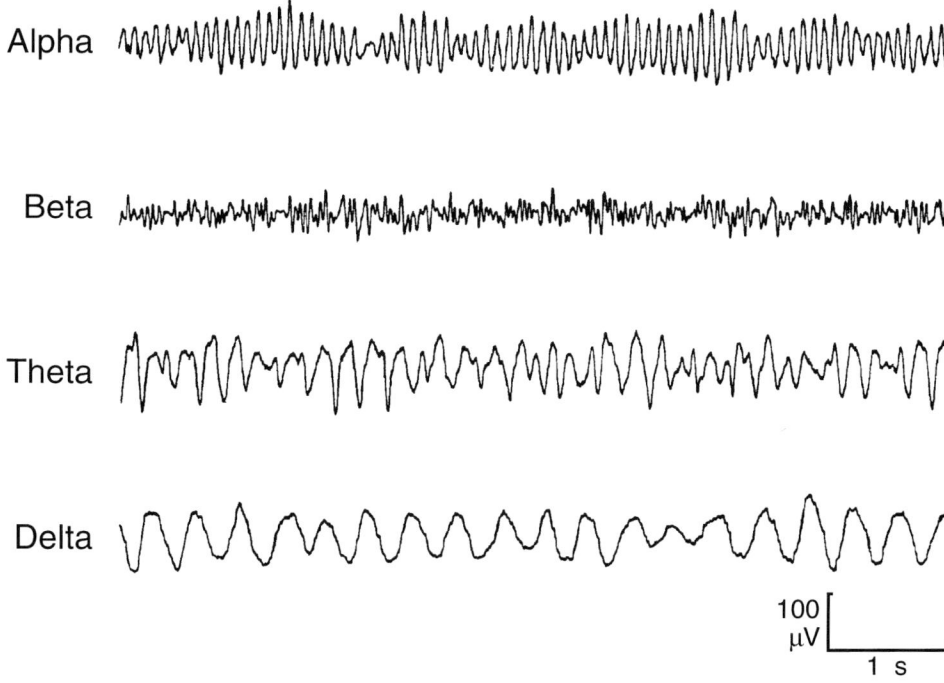

Alpha

Beta

Theta

Delta

100 µV

1 s

Figure 11. EEG rhythms. Alpha rhythm, 8 to 12 Hz; beta rhythm, 14 to 30 Hz; theta rhythm, 4 to 7 Hz; and delta rhythm, 0.5 to 3 Hz. (After Christian W. *Klinische Elektroenzephalographie: Lehrbuch und Atlas.* Thieme: Stuttgart, Germany [1968].)

ization power is low as compared with computed tomography (CT) or magnetic resonance imaging (MRI). In clinical routine, without intricate source-derivation methods, one should only rely on frontal, temporal, posterior, right or left. For the diagnosis of epilepsy, the EEG is indispensable (Fig. 12): "Clinical evaluation of a presumed epileptic individual without the use of the EEG is almost unthinkable (28)." Reading the EEG requires extensive training and must always take the background of the patient's history and other clinical findings into account.

EVENT-RELATED POTENTIALS: EVOKED, COGNITIVE, AND MOTOR POTENTIALS

The so-called spontaneous EEG will contain potentials both from endogenous processing (some of it prior to an efference, e.g., preparation of a movement) and from processing sensory input of endogenous sources. Normally, the latter are too small to be seen against the background EEG. With the technique of stimulus-synchronized averaging (13), the *evoked potentials* can be revealed, reflecting processing of afferent stimuli; the stimulus is repeated many (~100) times, and EEG pieces of, say, 1 second length after each stimulus are averaged. The background EEG will randomly have positive and negative excursions and tend to average out, but any recurrent waveform that is time-locked to the stimulus will emerge, i.e., the evoked potential (Fig. 13).

Depending on the stimulated modality, somatosensory, auditory, and visual evoked potentials can be discerned. Early potentials (not later than about 200 ms after the stimulus) depend mainly on physical parameters of the stimulus (e.g., which finger is stimulated, what is the loudness of the auditory stimulus click, etc.). Later potentials can be modulated by instruction to the subject and are called *cognitive potentials*.

By averaging backwards from motor actions, motor potentials and preparatory brain activity (contingent negative variation, CNV) (14, 22, 42) can be revealed from the prerolandic supplementary motor area (Fig. 14). The term *event-related potentials* (ERPs) encompasses both sensory and motor potentials, but in the literature on cognition it is mostly used in the sense of cognitive potentials, as defined above.

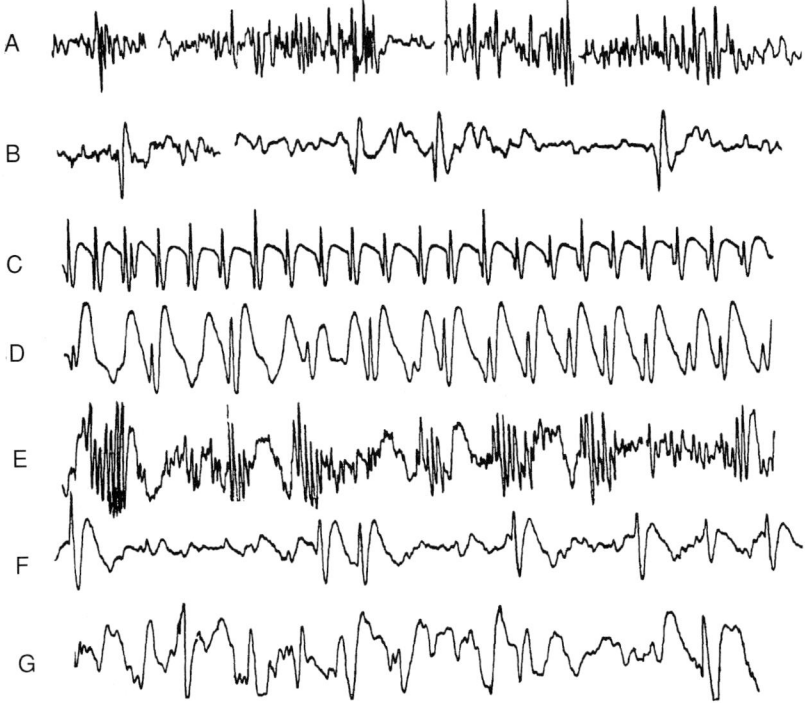

Figure 12. Seizure potentials. Various seizure potentials; trace (**D**) shows a typical spike-wave combination. (After Christian W. *Klinische Elektroenzephalographie: Lehrbuch und Atlas.* Thieme: Stuttgart, Germany [1968].)

Event-related potentials utilize the high temporal resolution of the EEG. ERP analysis profits from advances in our understanding of the anatomic pathways, since this narrows down the cortical sources (see ''Source Analysis'' below). In turn, ERPs can provide valuable insights into the workings of the brain, especially by linking information from animal experiments and psychophysical findings in humans.

THE EEG FROM A SIGNAL-ANALYSIS PERSPECTIVE

Generally, the amplitude of the EEG can be regarded as normally (Gaussian) distributed, even though no physiologic signal can be distributed completely normally. However, there can be a marked asymmetry between negative and positive excursions, as is obvious in seizures (see Fig. 12) and evoked potentials (see Fig. 13). The amplitude spectrum of a typical normal subject on occipital leads is depicted in Fig. 15. It shows a marked peak around 10 Hz and a sizable drop in amplitude density above 20 Hz.

The EEG has always been a playground for new signal-analysis theories. A recent example is the application of chaos theories to the EEG. If the EEG were not due to a stochastic but rather a deterministic process, its fractal dimension might be estimated from EEG time series. This dimension might be an indicator of brain state, pathology, or whatever. Several authors have indeed communicated measures of the fractal dimension of the EEG, with values ranging from 2 to 11 (2, 4, 15). However, many fallacies exist in estimating the fractal dimension reliably (19, 31, 33). Specifically, too many data points are necessary to obtain a representative sample of the entire invariant set (in a chaotic case this set would be an attractor). To estimate a dimension of D, the number of data points to be sampled should exceed $10 \cdot 50^{D/2}$ (15). For a dimension of 6, this results in an EEG interval of 9 hours (assuming $\tau = 25$ ms for independent data points). Over this period of time, stationarity (i.e., a steady state) cannot be expected in a biologic system. Thus, while the chaos approach to the EEG is very tempting, it does not seem to yield reliable insights to date.

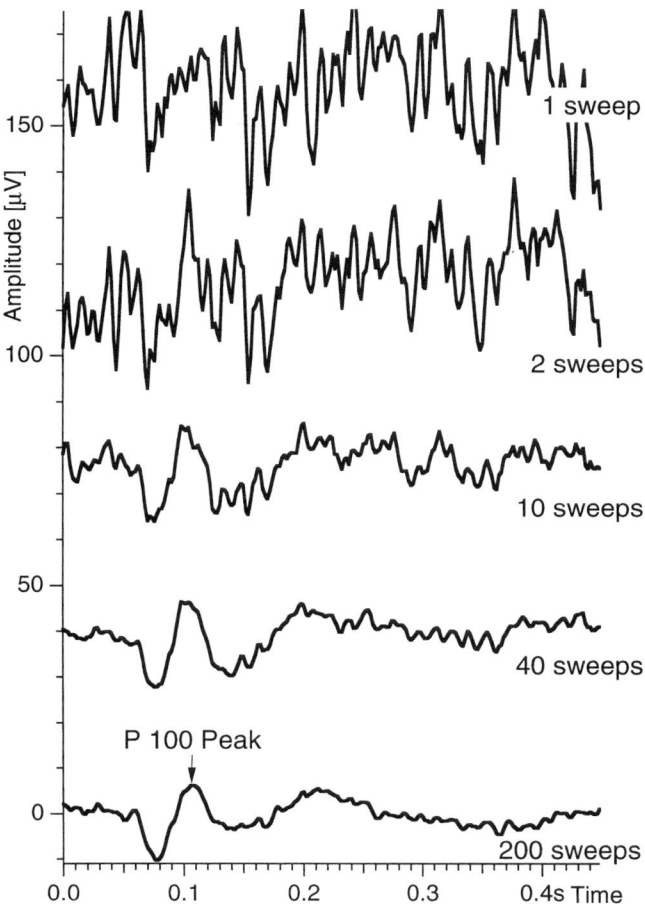

Figure 13. Averaging. Visual evoked potentials in response to a phase-reversing check-erboard with a varying number of averaged sweeps (positive up). The dominant structure (the positivity at 100 ms) becomes clearer, while noise gradually disappears.

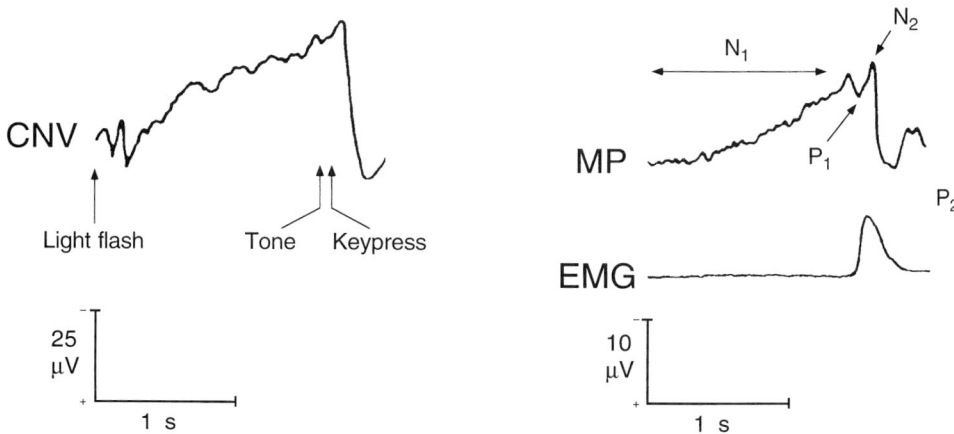

Figure 14. CNV and Bereitschaftspotential. The contingent negative variation (CNV) is a low-frequency negative wave preceding an expected stimulus (here, tone). It varies during stages of conditioned learning, with motivation, attention, distraction, and other cognitive variables. The Bereitschaftspotential (readiness potential N_1) precedes conscious motor actions, here indicated by the electromyogram of a finger movement. Surprisingly, it is of similar size on both hemispheres.

SOURCE ANALYSIS: FROM THE SURFACE MAP BACK
TO THE CORTICAL GENERATOR

The Inverse Problem

The spatial information of the EEG is initially contained in the surface potential map at the skull. This in itself directly provides important information, but it is mostly interpreted in terms of underlying generators. To infer the spatial distribution of generators (*source analysis*) from the potential map is a very difficult problem. Widely differing source distributions can yield identical surface maps. Furthermore, superficial inspection of the potential map can even lead one to localize a source in the wrong hemisphere (3). In theoretical terms, source analysis is an "ill-posed inverse problem"; the path from a given source distribution to the resulting surface map is well understood, at least in principle (see "Forward Problem" below). The inverse problem, from the potential map to the source distribution, however does not have a unique solution; i.e., a single potential map can be generated by an infinite number of different source distributions. Any solution to the inverse problem requires that the forward problem be solved in an explicit and numerically fast way. To achieve this, additional assumptions are necessary. These include constraints on the source distribution (a single dipole or a finite small number of dipoles and/or their position), assumptions on temporal and/or spatial coherence (moving dipole or stationary dipoles amplitude modulated in time), and assumptions on the cortical topography (e.g., shape of sulci) and the distribution of resistivity. These approaches have graduated from simple ones (spheres to model the skull and a single dipole source) to complete MRI-derived numerical models of the head with associated three-dimensional resistivity distributions, whereby the contribution from any source in the head to any pair of surface points can be modelled (see 'Leadfield', below).

The Forward Problem

The canonical form of the forward problem is $\vec{y} = \mathbf{K} \cdot \vec{x}$, where the vector $\vec{y}$ represents the measurements, which are derived from the state vector $\vec{x}$ via the operator $\mathbf{K}$. To solve the inverse problem, deriving $\vec{x}$ from $\vec{y}$, first the forward problem, deriving $\vec{y}$ from $\vec{x}$, must be solved in a way that allows convenient numerical treatment of the inverse problem.

Potentials generated by distributed current densities in a conducting medium are described by Maxwell's equations. Their solution, while in the general case nontrivial, can be approximated by a quasi-stationary solution for the purposes of EEG analysis. This approximation holds if

$$1 >> \omega \frac{e_0}{s} \approx 2 \times 10^{-3}$$

where e_0 is the dielectricity constant (~100 for the brain) (16), s is conductivity ($s = 0.3\ \Omega/m$), and ω is the highest relevant frequency (~100 Hz for the EEG, ~1 kHz for action potentials).

Still, even with this approximation, the quasi-stationary solution leads to an integral equation for the potential surface that does not fit the canonical form of the inverse problem above. Two types of models have been used herein: (a) the *dipole model* makes enough simplifying physiologic assumptions to eventually solve the nonlinear inverse problem, and (b) the *leadfield model* makes few, if any, physiologic assumptions and requires as much geometric and electrical information from the subject's head as possible (from which the dipole model also profits). Still, the leadfield model remains underdetermined and requires additional heuristics.

Head models can vary from very simple to very complicated. In order of increasing complexity, one can assume a single sphere, a sequence of spheres with varying resistivities (5), add holes for neck and eyes, up to using a complete MRI scan, where the cortex is separately identified from skull and white matter (*segmentation*).

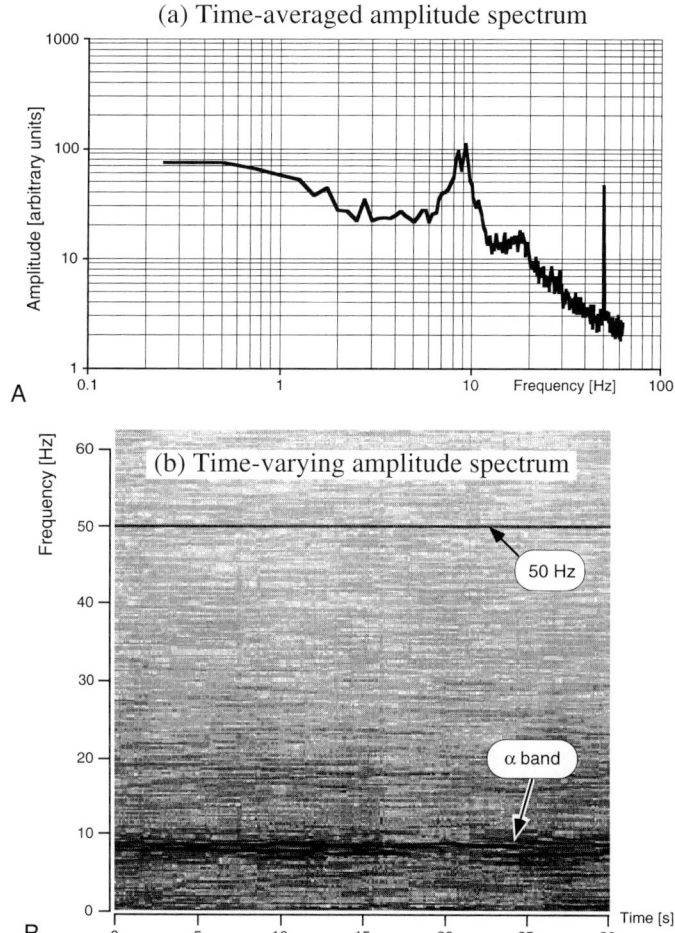

Figure 15. Amplitude spectrum. (**A**) The time-averaged amplitude spectrum of a normal subject shows a marked peak around 10 Hz and a sizable drop of amplitude density above 20 Hz (note the logarithmic scales). The peak at 50 Hz is an obvious mains interference artefact. (**B**) The same data as **A**, without averaging over time. The alpha band is present to varying degrees and with slightly varying frequency between 8 and 10 Hz.

The Dipole Model

In the analysis developed by Scherg and colleagues (36, 37) the basic assumptions are that only a small number of relatively narrow sources is active at any given time. This assumption probably holds for seizure loci and ''early'' (<150 ms) evoked potentials but less so for later ones and even less for the spontaneous EEG. The dipole assumption largely simplifies the equation linking the surface potential to the current density, and the surface potential distribution from a linear combination of an (arbitrary) number of dipoles with any orientation and strength can be computed, still using as much information on the distribution of conductivity by an appropriate head model as possible.

Further simplification can be achieved by assuming either that (a) the dipoles are stationary in the cortex but modulated in time or (b) dipole sources change over time both in intensity and in localization but ''slowly'' (''moving dipole'' analysis, a model of little physiologic attractiveness).

The dipole analysis, while physiologically somewhat restrictive, is numerically more easily tractable than the leadfield approach (see below) but has two major mathematical drawbacks: It is overdetermined, since generally the number of degrees of freedom in the data (electrodes $\times$ sample points) is greater than the number of free parameters, and it is nonlinear, since the unknown distance of the dipole enters as $1/r$.

The Leadfield Approach

The *leadfield* (17) is a field that describes the contribution to the surface potential from any given dipole (with location, strength, and orientation) in the brain. It contains the entire geometry of the problem and should be computed on a head model that is as realistic as possible. For rapid computation, the leadfield is often precomputed and stored as a huge matrix, the size of which can exceed hundreds of megabytes.

The leadfield approach leads to an underdetermined problem. There is a huge number of variables, depending on the discretization scale of the spatial sampling of the head for all dipole locations. Hence further assumptions are needed to arrive at a unique solution. A popular form of this regularization is to assume the *minimum norm*. In simple terms, this means that among the infinite number of solutions, the one with the smallest amplitude of all dipoles is chosen (a typical application of Occam's razor, but physiologically sound?).

The situation is even more complicated because the inverse problem is typically ill posed. The Eigenvalues of the characteristic matrix differ widely in magnitude. Consequently, small changes in the data (noise) will drastically affect the solution.

Currently, there is a swing from the dipole model to the leadfield approach, which was pioneered by Hämäläinen (16); implementations of this approach are now commercially available (32) (Fig. 16 and Color Plate 44). Time will tell how successful this technique will be, particularly in terms of the substantial numerical problems mentioned above.

COMPARISON OF EEG AND MEG

Historically, the MEG field was dominated by physicists and engineers, who, after having developed sophisticated SQUIDs for basic research interests, were searching for applications for their new technology. In contrast, during the 1980s, the vast majority of electroencephalographers were neurologists who performed routine clinical examinations with less than 20 channels and with visual inspection of traces after decades of training (43). This led to the impression that the localization capabilities of the MEG were much higher than those of the EEG. When the same amount of analysis from the MEG was applied to the EEG, though, its localization capabilities turned out to be better than previously assumed. Currently, the main advantage of MEG is the absence of spatial "blurring" when the magnetic fields pass through layers of widely varying resistivity from source to scalp; its main disadvantages are that the subject cannot move during recording and that the technical installations are formidable, including a massively shielded room. Conversely, the main advantage of the EEG is that the cost of equipment is more than a magnitude lower than that of the MEG; it also may be better suited for recording signals from deep subcortical sources. Its major disadvantage is that substantial information on the geometric and electrical properties of the subject's head is necessary to compute the source distribution.

CONCLUSIONS AND OUTLOOK

During the last few decades, imaging techniques seemed to displace the EEG. Surprisingly, however, since the early 1990s, a renaissance of the EEG has occurred, driven by a number of factors including (a) a deeper mathematical understanding of the source localization problem, (b) the use of many electrodes (64 to 200, vastly beyond the 10/20 system), (c) improvement in number-crunching power at lower cost with advanced computer technology, and (d) the use of individual morphologic data from MRI in source localization. The EEG is a relatively inexpensive tool to study the function of the brain on a time scale from milliseconds to days. It supplements and relies on both morphologic and functional imaging techniques. In a speculatory vein, I venture the following predictions:

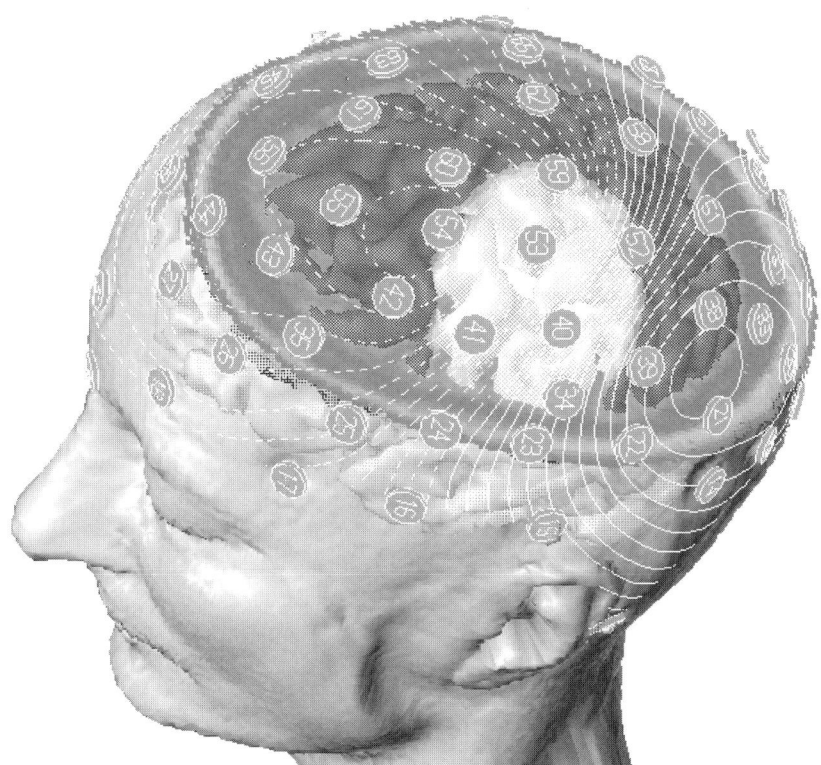

Figure 16. Source reconstruction. Somatosensory evoked potential after electric stimulation of the right hand's median nerve, measured with 65 electrodes. Skin and cortex surface were segmented from T1-weighted MRI data. The dashed blue and red lines represent equipotential lines at 20 ms after the stimulus (N_{20}); the yellow arrow underneath electrode 53 represents the fit of a single equivalent moving dipole (see also Color Plate 44). (From CURRY, Philips Research, Hamburg.)

- Source analysis will mature and become inexpensive and widespread.
- CT, MRI, functional MRI, EEG, and MEG will remain complementary tools.
- Evoked or event-related potentials as a research tool will rely on advanced experimental paradigms inspired by single-unit data to selectively analyze specific cortical functions/modules.
- Temporal information has gained little interest thus far. However, the "high-frequency" region above 30 Hz might contain correlates of neuronal ensemble activity (24, 39).
- The EEG will be utilized as brain output for articulation and/or manipulation by handicapped people.

ACKNOWLEDGMENTS

I drew much material from M. Wagner's thesis (40); J. Timmer advised me on source analysis; and W. Berger helped me with her vast clinical EEG experience. W. Spatz advised me on neuroanatomic matters. A. Jedynak, W. Skrandies, D. Ullrich, and P. Apkarian gave valuable criticism of the manuscript.

REFERENCES

1. Adrian ED, Matthews BHC. The Berger rhythm. Potential changes from the occipital lobes in man. *Brain*, 57, 356–385 (1934).
2. Babloyantz A. Evidence of chaotic dynamics of brain activity during the sleep cycle. In: G Mayer-Kress. *Dimensions and entropies in chaotic systems: Quantification of complex behavior. Springer series in synergetics,* Vol 32, 241–245. New York: Springer Verlag (1986).

3. Barret G, Blumhardt L, Halliday AM et al. A paradox in the lateralisation of the visual evoked response. *Nature*, 261, 253–255 (1976).
4. Basar E. *Chaos in brain function.* Berlin: Springer (1990).
5. Berg P, Scherg M. A multiple source approach to the correction of eye artifacts. *Electroencephalogr Clin Neurophysiol*, 90, 229–241 (1994).
6. Berger H. Über das Elektroenkephalogramm des Menschen. *Arch Psychiatr Nervenkr*, 87, 527–570 (1929).
7. Brazier MAB. *A history of the electrical activity of the brain.* London: Pitman (1961).
8. Caton R. The electric currents of the brain. *Br Med J*, 2, 278 (1875).
9. Christian W. *Klinische Elektroenzephalographie: Lehrbuch und Atlas.* Thieme: Stuttgart, Germany (1968).
10. Cooper R, Osselton JW, Shaw J. *EEG technology.* London: Butterworth (1974).
11. Creutzfeld OD, Watanabe S, Lux HD. Relation between EEG phenomena and potentials of single cortical cells: I. Evoked responses after thalamic and epicortical stimulation. *Electroencephalogr Clin Neurophysiol*, 20, 1–18 (1966a).
12. Creutzfeld OD, Watanabe S, Lux HD. Relation between EEG phenomena and potentials of single cortical cells: II. Spontaneous and convulsoid activity. *Electroencephalogr Clin Neurophysiol*, 20, 19–37 (1966b).
13. Dawson GD. A summation technique for the detection of small evoked potentials. *Electroencephalogr Clin Neurophysiol*, 6, 65–84 (1954).
14. Deecke L, Scheid P, Kornhuber HH. Distribution of readiness potential, pre-motion positivity and motor potential of the human cerebral cortex. *Exp Brain Res*, 7, 158–168 (1969).
15. Graf KE, Elbert T. Dimensional analysis of the waking EEG. In: E Basar (Ed.). *Chaos in brain function*, 134–152. Berlin: Springer (1990).
16. Hämäläinen MS, Hari R, Ilmoniemi RJ et al. Magnetoencephalography: Theory, instrumentation and applications to noninvasive studies of the working human brain. *Rev Mod Phys*, 413, 413–497 (1993).
17. Hämäläinen MS, Ilmoniemi RJ. Interpreting measured magnetic fields of the brain: Estimates of current distributions. Report TKK-F-A559 (1984).
18. Jasper HH. Report of the Committee on methods of clinical examination in electroencephalography: The ten-twenty electrode system of the international federation. *Electroencephalogr Clin Neurophysiol*, 10, 370–375 (1958).
19. Jedynak A, Bach M, Timmer J. Failure of dimension analysis in a simple five-dimensional system. *Physical Rev Lett*, 50, 1770–1780 (1994).
20. Jung R, Berger W. Fünfzig Jahre EEG. *Arch Psychiatr Nervenkr*, 227, 279–300 (1979).
21. Kiloh LG, McComas AJ, Osselton JW. *Clinical electroencephalography.* London: Butterworths (1972).
22. Kornhuber HH, Deecke L. Hirnpotentialänderungen bei Willkürbewegungen und passiven Bewegungen des Menschen: Bereitschaftspotential und reafferente Potentiale. *Pflügers Arch Gesamte Physiol Menschen Tierre*, 284, 1–17 (1965).
23. Krieger S, Timmer J, Lis S, Olbrich HM. Some considerations on estimating event-related brain signals. *J Neural Transm Gen Sect*, 99, 103–129 (1995).
24. Malsburg C v.d., Buhmann J. Sensory segmentation with coupled neural oscillators. *Biol Cybern*, 67, 233–242 (1992).
25. Martin JH. The collective electrical behavior of cortical neurons: The electroencephalogram and the mechanisms of epilepsy. In: ER Kandel, JH Schwartz, TM Jessel (Eds.). *Principles of neural science*, 777–791. New York: Elsevier (1991).
26. Mitzdorf U. Evoked potentials and their physiological causes: An access to delocalized cortical activity. In: E Basar (Ed.). *Springer Series in Brain Dynamics*, New York, Springer Verlag 140–153 (1988).
27. Niedermeyer E. EEG and old age. In: E Niedermeyer, F Lopes da Silva. *Electroencephalography*. Baltimore: Urban & Schwarzenberg (1987a).
28. Niedermeyer E. Epileptic seizure disorders. In: E Niedermeyer, F Lopes da Silva. *Electroencephalography*. Baltimore: Urban & Schwarzenberg (1987b).
29. Niedermeyer E, Lopes da Silva F. *Electroencephalography*. Baltimore: Urban & Schwarzenberg (1987).
30. Nuñez PL, Katznelson RD. *Electric fields of the brain: The neurophysics of the EEG*, New York: Oxford University Press (1981).
31. Nuñez PL. *Neocortical dynamics and human EEG rhythms.* New York: Oxford University Press (1995).
32. Philips Electronics N.V. Tutorial Curry. Multi-model neuroimaging (1995).
33. Rapp PE, Albano AM, Schmah TI, Farwell LA. Filtered noise can mimic low-dimensional chaotic attractors. *Phys Rev E*, xx2289–2297 (1993).
34. Rechtschaffen A, Kales A. *A manual of standardized terminology, techniques and scoring systems for sleep stages of human subjects*, NIH publication No. 204. Washington, DC: U.S. Department of Health and Human Services (1968).
35. Regan D. *Human brain electrophysiology: Evoked potentials and evoked magnetic fields in science and medicine.* New York: Elsevier (1989).
36. Scherg M. From EEG source localization to source imaging. *Acta Neurol Scand Suppl*, 152, 29–30 (1994).
37. Scherg M, Berg P. Use of prior knowledge in brain electromagnetic source analysis. *Brain Topogr*, 4, 143–150 (1991).
38. Skrandies W. EEG/EP: New techniques [Review]. *Brain Topogr*, 5, 347–350 (1993).
39. Tallon C, Bertrand O, Bouchet P, Pernier J. Gamma-range activity evoked by coherent visual stimuli in humans. *Eur J Neurosci*, 7, 1285–1291 (1995).
40. Wagner M. Grenzen der Quellenlokalisation bei EEG und MEG. Diploma Thesis, Fakultät für Physik, Albert-Ludwigs-Universität Freiburg (1995).
41. Walter WG. The location of the cerebral tumours by electroencephalography. *Lancet*, 2, 305–312 (1936).
42. Walter WG, Cooper R, Aldrige V et al. Contingent negative variation: An electrical sign of sensorimotor association and expectancy in the human brain. *Nature*, 203, 380–384 (1964).
43. Wikswo JP Jr, Gevins A, Williamson SJ. The future of the EEG and MEG. *Electroencephalogr Clin Neurophysiol* 87, 1–9 (1993).

Functional Imaging, edited by
Gustav von Schulthess and Jürgen Hennig.
Lippincott–Raven Publishers, Philadelphia, © 1998.

10

Methods and Applications of Magnetoencephalography

R. Beisteiner, J. Vrba, and L. Deecke

HISTORY

When Hans Berger discovered the electroencephalogram (EEG) using string galvanometers, he certainly did not anticipate that it would be possible one day to also record the minute magnetic fields that are generated by the human brain, even though he and his contemporaries already knew that there must exist relationship between electric and magnetic fields. It was not until some 40 years later that the Berger rhythm was first recorded magnetically (31) using the conventional coil technique at room temperature and the term *magnetoencephalography* coined. Magnetocardiography (MCG) had been introduced only a few years earlier (14).

In order to magnetically record the more subtle EEG equivalents such as event-related potentials, considerably higher sensitivity was needed. This leap in sensitivity was made possible by advances in both theoretical and applied physics. In 1973, the Nobel prize in physics was awarded to Brian David Josephson for theoretical work he carried out on the properties of two superconducting metals separated by a thin insulating oxide layer (75). The Josephson effect, Josephson junction, Josephson weak link were the fundamental prerequisites for realizing an extremely sensitive magnetic recording principle called the *superconducting quantum interference device* (SQUID) (175). The SQUID had been used in numerous applications (geographic, paleomagnetic, basic research, military, etc.) before it was widely employed in medicine and life sciences. It was the SQUID that started what could be called a "revolution" and what is now called *biomagnetism.*

R Beisteiner and L Deecke: University Clinic of Neurology, Vienna, Austria.
J Vrba: CTF Systems, Port Coquitlam, B.C., Canada.

Table 1. *Development of magnetoencephalography systems*

First generation (1978–1985)	One-channel systems	$N = 1$
Second generation (1986–1988)	Oligochannel systems	$N = 5–7$ Some bilateral (e.g., Gemini)
Third generation (1989–1992)	Polychannel systems	$N = 28–37$ Some bilateral (e.g., Magnes)
Fourth generation (1993–present)	Whole-head systems covering entire neurocranium	$N = 65, 122–143$ (e.g., Neuromag, CTF143)

Our focus will be on recordings from the organ brain (MEG), which is only one of the biomagnetic applications.

The MEG and EEG detect identical electrical sources. In the years following the initial recordings, practically all graphoelements that are classically seen in the EEG also have been demonstrated in the MEG, such as, for example, epileptic interictal spikes. These were recorded by Barth et al. (11, 12), Ricci et al. (128), Baumgartner et al. (17), and others. Epilepsy is a condition where the MEG method is most likely to have a useful clinical application. In the past, it was difficult to localize foci using oligochannel systems (Table 1).

Repeated recordings with numerous repositioning of the dewar require a certain degree of stability of the phenomenon under investigation, which is surely lacking in epilepsy. However, thanks to technical progress, the number of channels per MEG system and area coverage rapidly increased. A few examples of more recent systems are (the list is not intended to be exhaustive) a 19-channel system developed at the University of Twente (152), a double 14-channel system developed by Dornier (18, 46), a 19-channel system built by a Russian company Cryoton (104), an 83-channel system developed at PTB Berlin (48), a double 31-channel system built by Philips (47), a double 37-channel system commercially produced by BT (21), and a 256-channel system being developed by Superconducting Sensor Laboratory in Japan (173). Only the fourth generation of MEG systems (see Table 1), the "whole-head systems" (more precisely, helmet devices covering the entire neurocranium) now offer a true chance for the MEG to firmly join the family of tools for functional brain topography in clinical neurology, which includes EEG, PET, SPECT, and functional MRI.

Somatosensory evoked fields (SEFs) are a good example for successful joint application of EEG and MEG; MEG was helpful in localizing the neural generators of the SEF. In conjunction with surface EEG and ECoG (electrocorticogram), it was shown that the SEFs stem from two generators, whereby one produces the N_{20}–P_{30} component, the other the P_{25}–N_{35} component (15, 171). The two components are spatially and temporally superimposed in a complex manner: N_{20}–P_{30} is generated by activity in the posterior wall of the central sulcus corresponding to area 3b of Brodmann, i.e., representing a tangential electric dipole. A tangential dipole can be seen in the MEG; a radial one cannot. By means of the MEG it was thus possible to differentiate between activity in the posterior wall of the central sulcus (tangential dipole) and the one in pre- and postcentral gyri (two radial dipoles), which was not possible using EEG and ECoG alone (171). P_{25}–N_{35} is produced by activity in the anterior portion of the postcentral gyrus corresponding to area 1 of Brodmann, i.e., by a radial dipole. Thus the MEG signal due to this component is either absent or has only a small amplitude.

Since Hughlings Jackson carefully observed epileptic patients, and since Wilder Penfield used electrical cortical stimulation, we know that the primary somatosensory area (SI) is organized in the form of a topographic representation of the body periphery (somatotopic representation, sensory homunculus) (120). Penfield's classic results—although obtained by unphysiologic electrical stimulation mapping in epileptic patients—are still valid to the present. However, experiments in primates have shown that the functional organization of the SI is very complicated and that there exist at least four different representations of the body periphery in SI (76). The somatotopic representation of the body surface in SI has been confirmed by noninvasive recordings (MEG) and using electrical stimulation of the median nerve rather than of the cortex. Stimulation of individual fingers, for example, revealed that the projection of the thumb is 1 to 2 cm more lateral than that of the little finger (111). The late components of the SEF in contrast to the early ones are bilaterally represented—probably in SII—and do not show pure somatotopic representation (71, 112). Painful stimulation of the teeth and nasal mucosa revealed SEFs in the MEG (67). Furthermore, functional properties of SI were revealed by MEG; it has been shown that different somatosensory qualities are represented in different cytoarchitectonic areas of the cortex (81). An important clinical significance of SEFs in MEG rests in the possibility of noninvasive localization of the central sulcus in the human brain (151), which can be identified intraoperatively only in 50% of patients (172).

Auditory evoked fields (AEFs) were recorded early by MEG. Similar to the somatosensory system, a topographic distribution also exists in the auditory system. The tonotopic representation, i.e., that the cortical projection of pitch—the frequency band of audible tones—is spread over a few millimeters of suprasylvian cortex (Heschl's gyrus, AI) in an orderly manner. Functional imaging methods that can demonstrate tonotopicity must have a fine spatial resolution. Thus the AI was a particular challenge to the MEG. Romani et al. (133) were the first to demonstrate its tonotopic organization by noninvasive means in humans, showing that high tones are localized deeper than are low tones. Later this was substantiated by Pantev et al. (117). In contrast to the cochlea, where single frequencies are represented, the representation in AI is organized in terms of pitch of the perceived tone. Thus on the way from the cochlea to AI there is a recoding of the acoustic information (117). The supratemporal region of the human auditory cortex consists of several cytoarchitectonic structures with different thalamic afferents that process acoustic information in parallel and sequentially. Acoustic information is cortically represented in a bilateral fashion, and this is why small cortical lesions escape clinical observation. Furthermore, auditory stimuli evoke widespread responses in the EEG. AEP therefore are of little help in detecting small lesions in auditory cortex. Great expectations were thus directed toward the MEG. By means of latency, three categories of AEPs can be distinguished: early, middle, and late latency AEPs. While early AEPs or AEFs are generated in the brain stem (BAEP), middle and late latency AEPs are generated in the cortex. N_{19}, P_{30m}, and P_{50m} are the main components of the middle latency AEP. MEG was able to demonstrate that different generators are responsible for P_{19m}–N_{30m} than for P_{50m} (141). Late AEPs/AEFs are characterized by N_{100m}, P_{200m}, SF (sustained negativity), and off-response (63). The magnetic fields of these components show a dipole structure with phase reversal between the anterior and posterior ends of the Sylvian fissure and were attributed to the activity of neuronal populations in the Sylvian fissure at a depth of 2 to 3 cm. Dipole localizations showed that N_{100m}, P_{200m}, and SF are generated by different neuronal populations, whereby the generator of N_{100m} is localized approximately 2 cm posterior to the P_{200m} generator (168). The SF generator is located anteriorly to the N_{100m} generator (97). Generators of middle AEPs are separated from those of the late AEPs; the P_{30m} generator is located approximately 12 to 15 mm anterior to the N_{100m} generator. The special component of the mismatch negativity recorded under certain experimental conditions according to Näätänen has been shown by MEG to be generated in auditory association cortex rather than in AI (6). Even later AEF components in the P_{300} range related to cognition and memory have been localized in MEG. Using a verbal short-term memory task (Sternberg paradigm) with spoken numbers, Starr et al. (145) were able to localize the memory-related P_{300} component; it was bilaterally represented in the hippocampal region.

Movement-related fields (MRFs) have been recorded early in the MEG (45). Human voluntary movements are accompanied by complex activity in several brain regions that are responsible for planning, preparation, and execution of voluntary movement (40, 85). These are recorded in the EEG in form of the Bereitschaftspotentials (BPs) or readiness potentials (RPs). Their magnetic equivalents have been recorded as Bereitschaftsfelds (BFs) or readiness fields (RFs) preceding finger movement (45) and foot and toe movements (42, 64). BPs/BFs start early (1 to 2 s prior to the onset of movement in the EMG). In the EEG they start with bilateral symmetry even prior to unilateral movements and maintain bilateral symmetry during the early component BP_1 or BF_1 (1.5 to 0.5 s prior to movement). There has been evidence provided in the MEG that the generator for BF_1 is in the supplementary motor area (SMA, the mesial area 6a* after Brodmann) (89). This area seems to be involved in the planning and control of complex serial movements and actions (for a recent review, see Deecke and Lang) (44). The late BP component (BP_2, 0.5 to 0 s prior to movement onset, or NS') is asymmetric with unilateral movement. It is stronger over the contralateral hemisphere. MEG has provided evidence that the BF_2 generator is the primary motor area (MI), since this part of the BF faithfully models the motor homunculus. The generator is probably area 4 itself (24, 25). After the onset of movement, there are several components that were termed in the EEG *reafferent potentials* (40, 43, 85). The MEG helped clarify these components; in the MEG the term *movement-evoked fields* (MEFs I–III) was coined (24). It was of particular interest whether they are unilateral or bilateral accompanying unilateral movement. This was investigated by comparing unilateral with bilateral finger movements (87), where bilateral MEFs for unilateral movements could be shown. Since the first report (85), we have emphasized the bilateral nature of voluntary movement organization. Recently it was reported that MEF components thought to be unilateral (only contralateral) for unilateral movements also have an ipsilateral equivalent (135). It is clear, though, that usually MEF components are much stronger contralaterally than ipsilaterally for unilateral movements. For MEF I and III components, mainly contralateral generators in the postcentral gyrus, i.e., in SI, were found, which could be indicative of sensory feedback processes from more peripheral motor centers (reafferents), which are surely necessary for precise motor control. A neuronal population in the motor cortex responsible for MEF II may be different from the one generating the RFs and MFs.

This short historical survey may have shown that MEG has a unique analytical power and in combination with EEG provides better analysis of information processing in the functioning human brain. As a consequence of the MEG challenge, the EEG mathematical modeling and localization accuracy also have improved recently. Let us now have a deeper look into the methodology of this interesting new tool of functional brain topography.

METHODOLOGY

General Physical Principles

Various parts of the human body produce magnetic fields, which have been detected successfully from the heart (MCG), the brain (MEG), the eye (the magnetooculogram and the magnetoretinogram), the stomach (magnetogastrogram), skeletal muscles (magnetomyogram), etc. Even though magnetic fields are detectable from many parts of the human body, the most scientifically and commercially developed application is MEG (168).

The magnetic fields due to the electrical activity of the brain are in the range from tens of femtoteslas (fT) to about 1 pT and in the frequency range from about 0.1 Hz to several hundred hertz. To detect such weak and relatively broadband fields, it is necessary to use high-sensitivity SQUID magnetometers. Such devices are superconducting and operate on principles of quantum mechanics (30).

The magnetic fields of the brain are much smaller than the magnetic fields present in a typical environment—the environmental fields are approximately 5 to 8 orders of magnitude stronger than the brain fields. To illustrate this point, consider, for example, fields evoked by auditory stimulation. The magnitude of such fields is normally about 300 fT. A typical passenger car at a distance of about 50 m will produce a magnetic field of approximately 3,000,000 fT (162), which is about 10,000 times stronger. Even a single transistor or an IC chip at a distance of about 2 m will produce fields of approximately 1000 fT, or about 3 times stronger than the AEF. To make the measurement of the brain fields possible, the magnetic interference from the environment must be reduced. This interference elimination can be accomplished either by shielding or by some noise-cancellation method or by a combination of both.

Shielding is most often accomplished by means of μ-metal-shielded rooms. Roughly speaking, two types of μ-metal rooms are in use: rooms with a modest low-frequency shielding factor (less than 100) (7, 150, 155, 156) and rooms with large low-frequency shielding factor (Å 10^4) (52, 82). Sometimes, the shielding is accomplished by eddy currents using a thick layer of high-conductivity metal (149). An example of extremely good shielding is a high-temperature superconducting whole-body shield already in operation (58, 101), that provides a shielding factor of approximately 10^7 to 10^8 at all operating frequencies.

The noise-cancellation methods are usually implemented in software or firmware and are based on spatial filtering by high-order gradiometers (46, 162), adaptive noise cancellation (169, 170), or filtering in the sensor space (130).

Comparison of MEG and EEG

The electrical activity of the brain is manifested not only by magnetic fields, measured by MEG, but also by electric potentials on the surface of the scalp, which can be detected electrically (electroencephalography or EEG). Both MEG and EEG measure the same sources (at least at higher frequencies; at very low frequencies the EEG is affected by drifts in skin potentials), and both exhibit excellent temporal resolution (on the order of milliseconds). However, the MEG signals are generated by intracellular currents and are not strongly affected by the conductivity in the surrounding tissues, while the EEG signals correspond to extracellular (volume) currents and are strongly affected by the conductivity in various parts of the measured structure (e.g., skin, skull, brain, etc.). Furthermore, MEG is sensitive to tangential currents relative to the brain surface, while the EEG is sensitive to both radial and tangential currents. The MEG measurements are noncontacting and only require that the subject's head be brought to the vicinity of the detector, while the EEG measurements require attachment of electrodes and assurance of good contact between the electrodes and the skin, which is somewhat more difficult, especially if large numbers of electrodes are used.

The MEG and EEG should be viewed as complementary rather than competing technologies. Simultaneous use of both methods has the potential for improving the accuracy of the source analysis.

Techniques Used for Magnetic Recordings

Detection of small MEG fields requires the use of high-sensitivity SQUID magnetometers. The SQUID is a ring (inductor) of superconducting material interrupted by one or two Josephson junctions. The Josephson junctions are special quantum mechanical devices that can support supercurrent when the current is below some critical value. The characteristics of the Josephson junctions cause the impedance of the SQUID inductor to be modulated by application of an external magnetic field (30). When the SQUID loop impedance is measured by rf methods, the SQUID is called an rf SQUID and employs one Josephson junction; when the SQUID loop impedance is measured by dc methods, the SQUID is called a dc SQUID and employs two Josephson junctions. In either case, the SQUID output is connected to readout electronics that convert the signal flux sensed by the SQUID to a measurable voltage. Generally, dc SQUIDs are more sensitive and are used in the majority of research or commercial applications.

The geometry of the SQUID sensors is not suitable for direct detection of biomagnetic fields, and the SQUIDs are matched to the measured fields using flux transformers. The flux transformer is a superconducting circuit consisting of field coils that are exposed to the measured field and a coupling coil that is inductively coupled to the SQUID ring. Since the flux transformer is superconducting, it provides noiseless gain, and its fre-

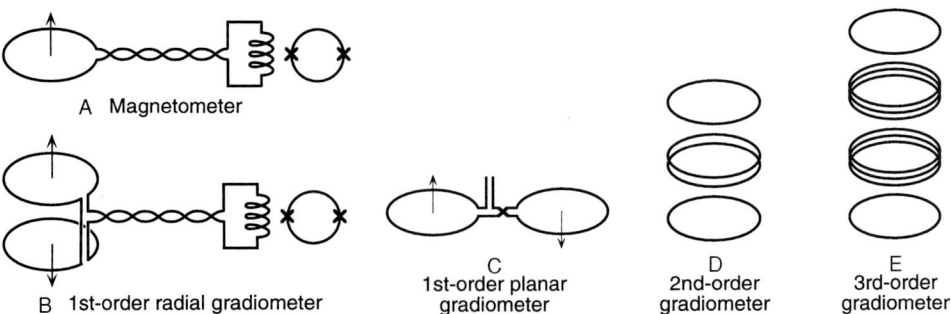

Figure 1. Examples of flux transformers: **(A)** magnetometer; **(B)** first-order radial gradiometer; **(C)** first-order planar gradiometer; **(D)** second-order radial gradiometer; **(E)** third-order radial gradiometer.

quency response is flat in the frequency range from dc up to the maximum operating frequency. An example of a magnetometer flux transformer is shown in Fig. 1A. In this case the field coil is a simple loop of one or several turns of superconducting wire. The current in the loop is proportional to the projection of the magnetic field to the loop normal. The SQUID ring in Fig. 1A is shown in a circle with two crosses representing Josephson junctions.

Magnetometers are extremely sensitive to environmental noise fields and must be operated in reasonably well shielded rooms or in conjunction with some noise-cancellation method. To reduce the noise sensitivity, the flux transformers can be configured into various forms of gradiometers. The simplest gradiometer is a first-order gradiometer, which typically consists of two magnetometer coils separated by some distance called the *baseline*. The coils are wound in opposing directions and are connected by a common superconducting wire to the SQUID coupling coil. The first-order gradiometer can be configured either as a radial (Fig. 1B) or a planar (Fig. 1C) device. When a gradiometer is exposed to a uniform magnetic field, the currents generated in its coils have the same magnitude, they cancel and no signal is detected. The gradiometers are sensitive only to the variations in magnetic fields over the gradiometer baseline.

The capability of gradiometers to reject the environmental noise increases with increasing gradiometer order, and second- and third-order hardware gradiometers have been used for biomagnetic detection. Similar to the extension of a magnetometer to a first-order gradiometer, a second-order gradiometer can be realized by separating two oppositely wound first-order gradiometers by some distance (the second-order gradiometer baseline) and connecting them by a common wire to a SQUID sensor (a schematic example of such a gradiometer is shown in Fig. 1D). Such a second-order gradiometer is insensitive to uniform magnetic fields and uniform first gradients and is sensitive only to the spatial variation of the first gradient. Similarly, a third-order gradiometer can be constructed by connecting two second-order gradiometers in an opposing sense to a SQUID sensor. A schematic example of a third-order hardware gradiometer is shown in Fig. 1E.

Hardware gradiometers are relatively complex, difficult to produce, and physically large. Therefore, they have been used only in systems with a small number of channels. In larger systems, only magnetometers or first-order hardware gradiometers have been used, often in combination with some software noise cancellation. The noise-cancellation methods usually utilize a reference system to detect the environmental noise, which is then subtracted from the sensor outputs. The noise cancellation is accomplished either by software formation of higher-order gradiometers or by adaptive procedures. The software formation of high-order gradiometers is preferable, because the coefficients of the procedure are stable, independent of time, noise character, or dewar orientation. In contrast, the adaptive procedures are dependent on various system and noise characteristics and require frequent redetermination of the noise-cancellation coefficients.

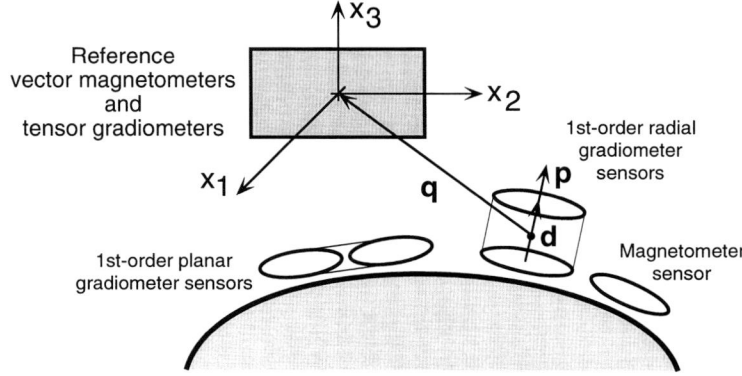

Figure 2. General method of software formation of high-order gradiometer.

A general method of software higher-order gradiometer formation is shown in Fig. 2. The software higher-order gradiometers consist of the sensors (which are usually magnetometers or first-order gradiometers), a reference system, and a set of coefficients. The reference system contains a sufficient number of magnetometers and first-order gradiometers to characterize the vector fields and tensor gradients. The coefficients are determined such that after the subtraction of the reference outputs from the sensor outputs, the results are equivalent to high-order gradiometers. Thus it is possible to have a software (or firmware) selectable gradiometer order (first, second, or third).

Noise cancellation by high-order gradiometers can be explained using an example of a dipole source (the explanation for other source types is similar). The magnetic field generated by a dipole source depends on the distance R from the source as R^{-3}. The spatial gradients are obtained from the magnetic field by spatial differentiation, which means that increasing the gradient order by 1 increases the distance decay exponent also by 1. As a result, the distance dependence of a kth-order gradient is proportional to R^{-3-k}, and the signal decay is faster for larger k values. Therefore, the higher-order gradiometers are less sensitive to distant noise sources than are the lower-order gradiometers (162). Noise elimination by high-order gradiometers can be termed *spatial filtering* (23), and it works by assuming that the noise sources are distant while the signal sources are near.

So far the gradiometers have been discussed assuming that their construction is perfect and the gradiometers detect only the gradient tensor component for which they have been designed. However, real devices are subject to numerous constructional errors and external disturbances: Gradiometer coils may not have equal areas, coils may be tilted, or there may be superconducting or normal metal objects in their vicinity. All these effects collude to make a gradiometer sensitive not only to the intended gradient component but also to field, lower gradients, and gradient tensor components for which the gradiometer has not been designed. Also, the gradiometers may be sensitive to time derivatives of various fields and gradients. Thus, for example, a third-order gradiometer output may contain components of field, first, and second gradients. This unwanted gradiometer sensitivity to the components for which the gradiometers have not been designed is usually described by common-mode and eddy-current vectors.

The gradiometer sensitivity to various unwanted field and gradient components is usually minimized by the system design and further reduced by the common-mode and eddy-current balancing. The balancing procedures can be executed either in hardware, electronically, or in software. The three methods are shown in Fig. 3.

In the hardware method (Fig. 3A, B), only the common-mode vector is usually balanced. The balancing can be carried out either by bringing small pieces of superconductor (e.g., superconducting loops) to the gradiometer vicinity, or the gradiometer flux-transformer leads can be made to contain small auxiliary axial gradiometers and movable shields that allow variable exposure to the environmental fields (22, 139). In electronic

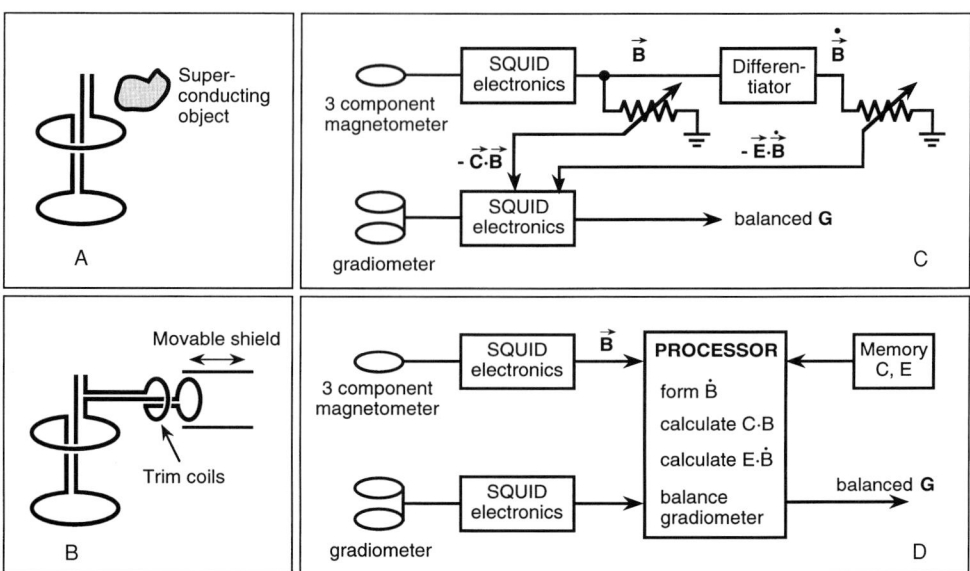

Figure 3. Methods of gradiometer balancing: hardware balancing by (**A**) superconducting vanes, (**B**) trim coils, (**C**) electronic method, (**D**) software method.

balancing (99, 169) (Fig. 3C), the gradiometer signal is measured together with three components of magnetic field. The measured magnetic field and its time derivatives are then combined with the gradiometer signal to yield a balanced gradiometer output. Software balancing (163) (Fig. 3D) is similar to electronic balancing, except that the subtraction of the common-mode and eddy-current terms is done in software.

Environmental noise also can be removed using adaptive noise-cancellation methods. Similar to the software gradiometer formation, the adaptive methods also utilize a reference system to remove environmental noise from the sensor outputs. To determine the adaptive coefficients, a system of sensors and references is observed during the application of some unwanted signals (or noise), and the subtraction coefficients are adjusted to minimize the effect of such signals (169, 170). The adaptive subtraction can be frequency-dependent or frequency-independent. Adaptive noise cancellation is a useful tool only when the noise has a time-independent character; adaptive methods do not perform well when the character of the noise is rapidly changing because the optimal adaptive coefficients also change (in contrast, the coefficients for gradiometer formation are independent of the noise character). For noise sources with variable character, continuous readaptation methods could be used.

The SQUID sensor and its associated flux transformers must be operated at superconducting temperatures. The majority of the present-day SQUIDs are made from niobium or its compounds, and their operation requires cooling to temperatures close to the boiling point of liquid helium (about 4.2 K). The cooling is usually accomplished by directly immersing the SQUID devices into a liquid helium bath or in some cases by cooling the devices indirectly by providing a heat link between the liquid helium bath and the SQUID. In either case, the liquid helium, SQUID detectors, and the flux transformers are contained in a special cryogenic vessel called a *dewar*. The dewar is a vacuum-insulated "Thermos flask," and it contains various heat reflectors and heat shields in the vacuum space.

Presently, all commercial MEG systems are based on low-temperature SQUIDs, which are cooled by liquid helium. However, SQUIDs based on high-temperature superconductors are also being developed. Even though the present high-temperature SQUIDs are not as sensitive as their low-temperature counterparts, their intrinsic performance is steadily being improved, and they might already be suitable for applications where the magnetic fields are larger.

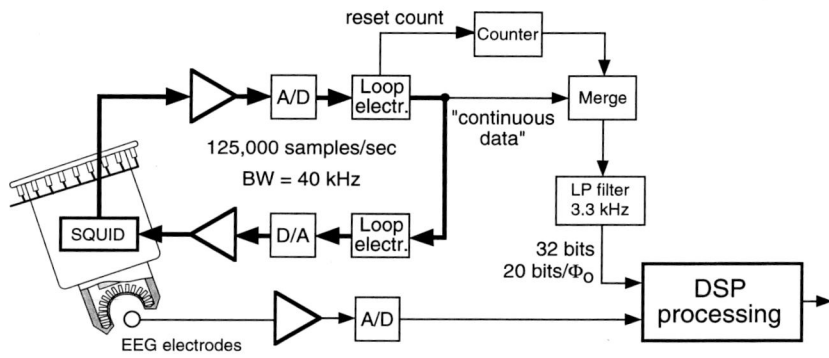

Figure 4. A schematic diagram of the digital SQUID electronics loop and incorporation of EEG into the data-collection system.

The high-temperature superconducting devices are usually cooled by liquid nitrogen. The main advantage of liquid nitrogen over liquid helium, apart from being simpler and cheaper to handle, is that the heat of evaporation of liquid nitrogen is approximately 60 times larger than that of liquid helium. As a consequence, liquid nitrogen dewars are expected to have significantly longer time between refills when compared with the corresponding liquid helium dewars.

The SQUID sensors with their associated flux transformers are connected to control and readout electronics, which can be either analog or digital. For SQUID sensor operation in an unshielded environment, or for various advanced noise-cancellation methods, it is necessary to have electronics with large dynamic ranges and good linearity. Such stringent requirements can be met by digital SQUID electronics (163). In such electronics (Fig. 4), the SQUID outputs are transmitted from the cryogenic dewar to room temperature, amplified, and digitized, and the feedback loop is closed digitally using a DSP processor (103). The system utilizes the inherent quantization of the SQUID output and the associated periodic character of the SQUID transfer function. The feedback loop is locked at a certain minimum of the transfer function and maintains lock for SQUID signals in the range of $\pm 1\ F_0$ around the lock point. When the applied signal exceeds this range, the loop lock is released, the loop relocks in an adjacent minimum of the transfer function, and the electronics registers an up or down count. The signal from within the $\pm 1\ F_0$ range is then combined with the counter to yield a 32-bit data word.

In MEG systems that are also equipped with EEG, it is important to have both MEG and EEG signals measured simultaneously and subjected to as similar transfer functions as possible. A schematic diagram of such a system is shown in the lower part of Fig. 4. The EEG signals are amplified and digitized (with the sample and hold triggered by an MEG trigger), and both EEG and MEG signals are subjected to common DSP processing to ensure essentially identical transfer functions.

The complete SQUID MEG system, i.e., the dewar, SQUID sensors, flux transformers, SQUID electronics, and various signal conditioning and processing procedures, results in white noise levels typically in the rnage from 1 fT rms/*Hz up to 10 fT rms/*Hz. For many applications it is desirable to have the white noise extended to as low frequency as possible, and in practical systems, onset frequencies of low-frequency noise in the range 0.1 to 0.5 Hz have been achieved (161).

The preceding principles integrated into whole-cortex MEG systems with large numbers of channels were pioneered by CTF Systems, Inc. (35), and by Neuromag, Ltd. (109), and first released as commercial products in 1992. In such systems, the dewar tail has a helmet shape, and the flux transformers are positioned on the helmet surface to cover a large area of the cortex. A schematic diagram of such a system is shown in Fig. 5.

The operation of high-order gradiometers will be illustrated using examples obtained with a whole-cortex MEG system in an unshielded environment (26, 160, 163) (the performance of MEG systems with smaller number of channels or in shielded environments has been described elsewhere) (1, 48, 101, 107, 108, 127).

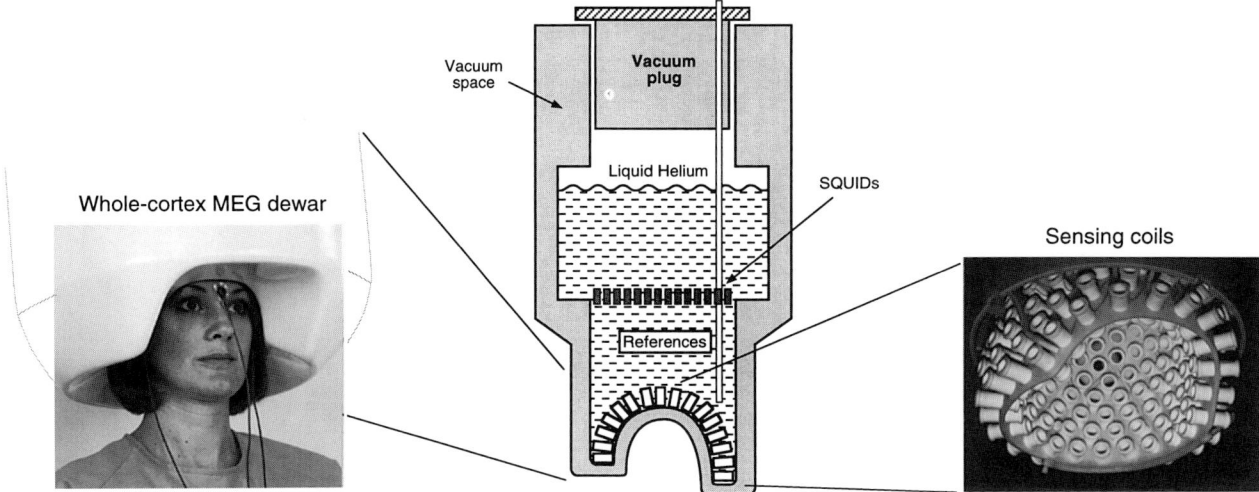

Figure 5. Schematic diagram of a whole-cortex MEG system.

An auditory evoked field (AEF) experiment performed with a 143-channel system (35) is shown in Fig. 6. The stimulus was a 1-kHz tone of 50-ms duration applied to both ears, and the results correspond to 100 averages plotted in the bandwidth from dc to 40 Hz. The AEF signals in the ''as collected'' data are difficult to see; however, when the third-order gradients are formed, the environmental noise is removed and the AEF signals become clearly visible.

To further test the noise cancellation by high-order gradiometers, the AEF experiment was repeated while strong magnets (eight magnets with dipole moments ranging from 10^{13} to 10^{15} fTácm^3) were randomly moved at a distance of Å 7 m from the MEG system (26). The data were recorded in the bandwidth from dc to 70 Hz (powerline signals were notched out), and only 10 averages were used. One of the channels, corresponding to a strong AEF signal, is shown in Fig. 7. In the first-order gradiometer mode, the noise is an order of magnitude larger than the AEF signal, and similarly, the AEF signal would not be discernible in the second-order gradiometer mode. Only when the third-order gradiometer is formed does the environmental noise become sufficiently suppressed and the AEF signal is clearly observed, despite the use of only 10 trial averaging.

Data Analysis

The magnetic fields have their origin in the electrical activity of the brain cells. The magnetic fields due to the currents in individual cells are weak and not detectable; how-

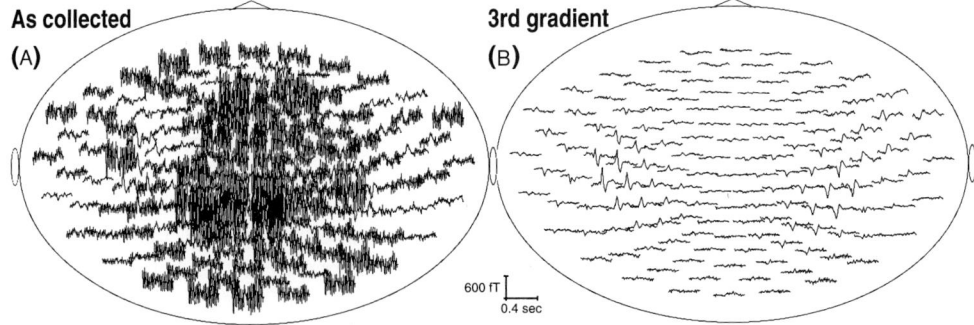

Figure 6. AEF experiments in an unshielded environment of CTF laboratories using a 143-channel MEG system; f_s = 1250 samples per second, duration = 0.7 s, bandwidth = dc to 40 Hz, 100 averages, subject ER, file: Dec 13/95:24. The stimulus was a 1-kHz tone of 50-ms duration into both ears. (**A**) As collected data with first-order gradiometer sensors. (**B**) After formation of third-order gradiometers in software.

Channel: SR44-6

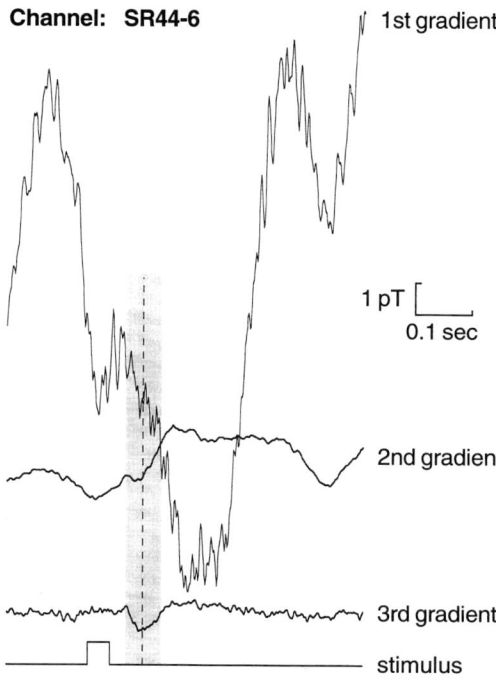

1st gradient

1 pT

0.1 sec

2nd gradient

3rd gradient

stimulus

Figure 7. AEF experiment in an unshielded environment with randomly moving magnets at a distance of 7 m from the MEG system; 1-kHz tone, 50-ms duration, right ear, f_s = 625 samples per second, duration 0.82 s, bandwidth = dc to 50 Hz, 10 averages.

ever, a collective depolarization of a large number of dendrites (10^4 to 10^5) results in sufficiently strong tangential currents in certain regions of the cortex that the resulting magnetic fields are observable outside the head.

However, the magnetic fields themselves are not the final goal of the MEG measurements; rather, it is the underlying current distribution in the head that caused the magnetic fields in the first place. Therefore, it is desirable to invert the measured magnetic fields and to deduce the current distribution in the head. However, it is well known that the inversion of biomagnetic fields has no unique solution (due to the existence of "magnetically silent" sources), and to make the inversion problem tractable, additional simplifying assumptions and/or constraints must be added.

For well-localized sources, a current dipole model can be used, where the current dipole can be thought of as a miniature biologic battery embedded in the conducting medium of the head. The simplest mathematical model of such a system is a current dipole in a spherical medium, for which closed solutions exist (62, 138). In a spherical medium, the MEG is sensitive only to tangential dipoles, and if only radial magnetic fields are of interest, they can be calculated simply using a Biot-Savart law. The current dipole solutions also were extended to prolate and oblate spheroidal conducting media (37). In all cases the magnetic fields due to the current dipole models are nonlinear in dipole position coordinates.

A number of inversion methods were developed that effectively remove the nonlinear dependence on the position. In these methods, a collection of dipoles is assumed to be located at fixed points in space, typically on some regular grid. The system is usually undetermined, and additional assumptions must be made to select a unique solution out of many possible. The problem can be solved by a linear estimation, and a number of different techniques have been proposed. Here, only a few examples of such methods are cited: the minimum norm estimation (72), which minimizes the euclidean norm of the current vectors subject to the condition that the measured fields are given by the projection of the current vector to the leadfields; LORETA (low resolution brain electromagnetic tomography) (118), which is a weighted minimum norm method subject to a neurophysiologic assumption of maximally smooth current distribution; and spatially selective filters (130), where the spatial selectivity is maximized subject to unity source gain constraint. It is shown that in the derivation of the optimal noise-reduction coefficients for the spatially selective filters, the covariance matrix (the statistical measure of the signal) can be used instead of the inner product of the leadfields.

Generally, the accuracy of all inversion techniques is significantly improved if the real shape of physiologically meaningful tissue is considered instead of a simple spherical or spheroidal medium.

Current Technical State of the Art

Biomagnetic measurements, and especially MEG, are currently pursued at many laboratories, and MEG instruments are being constructed at noncommercial and commercial institutions. Recently, whole-cortex helmet-type SQUID MEG systems have been developed commercially. At the time of this writing, the helmet-type systems have been produced and installed at various customer sites by two commercial vendors: CTF Systems, Inc., and Neuromag, Ltd.

CTF's MEG system (35) has been produced either with 64 or 143 channels. The sensors are radial first-order gradiometers, uniformly distributed over the head surface. The gradiometers have a 5-cm baseline and 2-cm coil diameters, are connected to dc SQUIDs, and the system noise is typically about 5 fT/ÃHz (in shielded rooms). The system is housed in a helmet-shaped dewar, where two helmet shapes are available: Caucasian helmet shape, based on the average of 20,000 North American male heads (123), and a Japanese helmet shape, which has been modified to account for differences between the Japanese and North American heads. The distance from the liquid helium surface to the room temperature surface in the helmet region is about 1.6 cm. The readout electronics, after the initial analog amplification, is completely digital, based on DSP processors, and has a large dynamic range (32 bits). The system is equipped with noise cancellation by up to third-order gradiometers and allows operation in unshielded environments if the magnetic noise is not too harsh; if used in combination with a modestly shielded room, it provides noise cancellation equivalent to that of high quality μ-metal rooms.

The Neuromag's MEG system (109) uses 122 planar first-order gradiometers located at 61 sites. The planar gradiometers have a 1.65-cm baseline, the effective total area of each oppositely wound gradiometer coil is 5.3 cm^2, and the intrinsic gradient sensitivity of each gradiometer component is less than 5 fT/(cm ÃHz) in the white noise frequency range. At each site there is a plug-in unit, each containing two orthogonal planar gradiometer flux transformers and two dc SQUIDs. The system is housed in a helmet-shaped dewar, where the helmet consists of two spherical sections with the centers 41 mm apart; in the room temperature shell, the front, against the forehead, has a radius of curvature of 83 mm, whereas the curvature of the back part is 91 mm. The distance from the liquid helium surface to the room temperature surface against the subject's head is 16 mm. The dc SQUID readout electronics use a positive feedback configuration with a flux-locked feedback control loop and a separate integrating feedback control circuit to eliminate drifts, maintaining the output voltage close to zero. The highpass cutoff caused by this slow integrator can be adjusted over the range from dc to 4 Hz. The system is operated inside a shielded room.

Current Directions of Methodologic Research

Recent studies dedicated to methodologic issues indicate possible future developments of MEG methodology as well as current demands for further knowledge. For example, Lü et al. investigated principles of magnetic field generation and found that coherent neuronal activity over 40 to 400 mm^2 of cortex is necessary for generation of a somatosensory evoked potential. Cuffin et al. (36) investigated effects of local variations in skull and scalp thickness on MEG. A variety of authors tested MEG localization accuracy in vitro (61) and in vivo (8, 33, 60, 106, 144), including localization reproducibility (116). In vitro localization error was below 2 mm, in vivo most studies showed errors below 10 mm, and for reproducibility an error below 4 mm was reported (116). Other investigations concern data-analysis strategies. Vieth et al. (159) developed a dipole density plot, Wang et al. (165) use the minimum norm least-squares (MNLS) inverse solution, and Freeman et al. (57), Kowalik et al. (86), and Muhlnickel et al. (105) apply chaos theory to MEG data analysis. Akhtari et al. (2) describe a method for SSEP localization using the actual cortical surface as spatial constraint. Concerning pure brain research, the following section will review current applications.

APPLICATION OF MEG

General Overview of MEG Research

MEG has been applied increasingly to a growing variety of issues within the last 10 years. These comprise fundamental research on somatosensory, motor, auditory, visual, and cognitive tasks, as well as clinical applications. Most of the recent studies use MEG for brain mapping and apply dipole models to localize brain activity. To give an impression about the diversity of questions that can be technically addressed by MEG, an overview of the subjects of very recent publications is given now.

Investigations of the somatosensory system include processing of pain stimuli (78), gating of SSEP during active finger movement (78), localization of somatosensory evoked 600-Hz brain activity (38), interhemispheric asymmetries of somatosensory evoked magnetic fields to right and left median nerve stimulation (134), differences in SSEP localization to airpuffs and electric stimuli (56), superadditive combination of MEG and EEG for SSEP localizations (16), noninvasive somatosensory homunculus mapping using a large-array biomagnetometer (174), and functional organization of the human first and second somatosensory cortices (66). Application of MEG to the peripheral somatosensory system (nerve, plexus, spinal cord, e.g., for monitoring injury currents) also has been described (39).

Within the motor system there are recent studies on prediction of the side of movement from premovement fields using neural networks and dipole and analysis (27), homuncular organization of the human sensorimotor cortex (24, 164), EEG/MEG and SPECT results of premovement activity (41), topography and analysis of cortical sources with unilateral and bilateral voluntary movements (87), three-dimensional localization of supplementary motor area activity preceding voluntary movements in a patient with infarction of the right supplementary motor area (89), and localization of primary sensorimotor areas (19).

The auditory system is one of the most studied. Recent examples comprise tone-duration discrimination (84), analysis of cortical reorganization taking place within 1 year after abrupt unilateral deafness (157), processing of syllables (88), processing of tones and pseudowords (113), processing of tones and vowels (53), cortical mechanisms of sound lateralization (91), influence of interaural time difference of sound on acoustically evoked potentials (102), tonotopic organizations of different areas of the human auditory cortex (115, 125, 158), processing of rare interruptions of a steady rhythm of tones (65), investigation of the memory trace of a complex sound in the supratemporal auditory cortex, auditory magnetic source localization in twins (126), sustained fields of tones and glides, activation of parietal brain regions by auditory stimuli (90), and demonstration of differing lifetimes for activation traces of the human auditory primary and association cortex (93).

Concerning cerebral processing of visual information, MEG was used to investigate the brain's various capabilities to recognize objects (124). Here, brain responses to luminance-defined form of object recognition, motion-defined form, color-defined form, texture-defined form, and disparity-defined form were compared. In other studies (131) it was found that not only the visual cortex but also the superior temporal sulcus contributes to visual evoked magnetic fields and that seeing faces activates three separate areas outside the occipital visual cortex (94). With simultaneous presentation of speech sound and speech video—the video either fitting or nonfitting—Sams et al. (137) found that visual information modified auditory cortex activity.

Sophisticated studies exist concerning cognitive tasks. Investigations comprise processing of unattended stimuli (4), MEG and PET during a verb-generation task (54), relation of 40-Hz spontaneous brain activity to the processing of time between two auditory stimuli (138) (it could be shown that below the 12- to 15-ms interstimulus interval, only the first stimulus provokes this 40-Hz activity), preattentive sensory memory governs the capability of humans to detect novel events (154), identification of the cortical area responsible for passive sensory storage of information about loudness of a tone (echoic memory) (95), during memory scan for tones auditory cortex contributes to spontaneous alpha activity suppression (79), activation sequence of discrete brain areas during cognitive processes (73), late magnetic fields following infrequent and unpredictable omissions of visual stimuli (132), dynamics of brain activation during picture naming (136) (see below), visual recognition tasks (13), studies of sensory functions and mental imagery (80), and localization of brain activity during auditory verbal short-term memory (145).

Recent clinical applications of MEG comprise pediatric neurologic diseases (28, 29, 104), evaluation of candidates for epilepsy surgery, presurgical brain mapping (59, 60, 98, 129, 143), location of epileptic focus (3, 15, 114, 140, 142, 143, 146–148, 163, 166), investigation of trigeminally triggered epileptic hemifacial convulsions (55), psychiatric disorders (122), cortical reorganization after nervous system injury (51), hypometabolism (PET) and dipole localization in hemimegalencephaly (110), investigations on the restitutional effects of the potassium channel blocker 4-aminopyridine on demyelinated nerve fibers after spinal cord injury (69), localizing of noninfarcted tissue in stroke patients (96), and investigations on migraine (9, 10, 167).

Selected Examples of MEG Application

To give an insight into methodologic details and current state of the art of performing MEG investigations, recent MEG work of different groups is described more exhaustively in the following examples. Every example thereby illustrates different aspects of data-recording and data-analysis methodology.

Motor System

Cheyne et al. (27) published a study on left- and right-sided finger movements, where they used artificial neural networks for data analysis and showed that these networks can predict the side of an intended movement even from single trials instead of averages. In addition, this study used a dipole model for data analysis—a very common procedure for locating brain activity with MEG—which will be exemplified here.

A 64-channel whole-head MEG system with coils (first-order gradiometers) of 5-cm baseline and 2-cm diameter was used to record movement-related magnetic fields simultaneously over both hemispheres. Instead of a shielding room, software-constructed third-order spatial gradients were used for noise reduction. Two right-handed subjects performing voluntarily started rapid extensions of the right or the left index finger, which interrupted an optical switch. By interrupting the switch, data recording was started in a way that the magnetic fields of all 64 channels could be saved from 2 s before the movement to 0.4 s after the movement. Magnetic fields were lowpass filtered (dc to 40 Hz) and sampled with 125 data points per second. For every finger, data of 100 movements were recorded, and after exclusion of artefacts (usually arising from eye blinks or muscle activity), these records were averaged (arithmetic mean for every data point). Averaging is usually done with MEG experiments, since the signal-to-noise ratio of one single record is too low for visual detection of task-related signal changes. On average, left- and right-sided movements were preceded by slow magnetic fields (Bereitschaftsmagnetfeld) beginning around 600 ms prior to movement onset in the average waveforms over the left and right lateral scalp. For data analysis, a two-dipole model was established that represented somatomotor cortex activity ipsi- and contralateral to the side of movement. The initial spatial positions of those dipoles within the brain were set by the experimenter using a priori neurophysiologic knowledge about possible locations of brain activity with this task. Using a simplex-based least-squares minimization algorithm, the initial dipole positions were then systematically varied until the theoretical magnetic field distribution of the two dipoles showed maximum correspondence to the measured field distribution over the brain. This procedure was done repetitively for small time windows of 48 ms, starting 1040 ms before movement onset (− 1040 ms) and ending 80 ms before movement onset (− 80 ms). Results show that the dipole locations for the various 48-ms periods showed much variations up to − 300 ms. Then they converged to consistent locations over the somatomotor cortex of both hemispheres. Different dipole analysis procedures furthermore showed that beginning with − 300 ms, there was a faster increase of dipole strength over the contralateral hemisphere, indicating a lateralization of brain activity there.

A second data-analysis approach used a three-layer neural network trained with single trials (single records of one movement) to be able to predict the side of the forthcoming movement. Training was done using only 24 MEG channels and data of 96-ms time windows taken every 32 ms. The training procedure used a standard backpropagation algorithm until an error level of 0.1 or less was achieved, and it was repeated four times with randomly chosen subsets of single trials. The results showed a success rate of 60% between − 950 to − 250 ms before movement onset. Afterwards, a rapid increase of the success rate to over 95% correct determinations at movement onset was achieved. Therefore, the optimal time for prediction was consistent with lateralization of brain activity. This result shows that neural networks can be applied successfully to analysis of humans' intentions to move. Furthermore, it is shown that MEG offers a unique possibility to monitor rapidly changing weights of involved cortical areas, e.g., to detect lateralization of already ongoing symmetric activity within milliseconds. Thus MEG can be used to localize brain activity but also to investigate rapidly changing relations between those localizations.

Auditory System

Pantev et al. (115) tried to localize a consistently observed electrophysiologic brain response to short tones arising around 30 ms after stimulus onset. This distinctly positive EEG wave (referenced to the mastoids) was called the P_a *wave* in the electroencephalogram and the P_{am} wave with MEG. To draw maximum information, simultaneous MEG (sensitive only to intracellular currents with tangential orientation) and EEG (sensitive to extracellular currents of all orientations) measurements were performed. The goal was to localize P_a/P_{am} as response to different tone frequencies. Twelve subjects were presented 50-ms tone bursts (either 400, 1000, or 4000 Hz) to their right ear. Each frequency was presented 1500 times, and a 37-channel MEG system (first-order gradiometers, 5-cm baseline, 2-cm coil diameter) was placed over the left temporal skull. Recordings were performed within a magnetically shielded room to improve signal-to-noise ratio. Data were recorded from 100 ms before to 200 ms after start of a tone using a bandpass of 1 to 100 Hz and a sampling rate of 520.8 data points per second. For simultaneous EEG recordings, 26 electrodes placed over the whole scalp and referenced to the nose were used. To exclude records with artefacts, those records containing signal variations of more than 3 pT (MEG) per 100 μV (EEG), i.e., magnitudes that are not expected to be produced by the brain, were automatically excluded from further analysis. The non-contaminated records were averaged for every subject individually. For EEG data, two dipoles were used as representing the centers of bilateral temporal cortex activity for the P_a wave. To calculate the dipole positions, a short time period around the P_a peak was taken, and an iterative algorithm (based on dipoles having a stationary location and orientation but changing magnitude over time) minimized the differences between the theoretical dipole fields and the actually measured magnetic fields. This was done using a grand average over all subjects to further improve signal-to-noise ratio. In contrast to EEG, only one left temporal dipole was fitted to represent the magnetic P_{am}, since right temporal magnetic fields should be negligible at the left temporal recording position. In addition, no grand average was used, but locations were calculated for every subject independently. This can be done because MEG—due to low sensitivity to deep sources, lack of sensitivity to radial magnetic field components, and negligible distortion of magnetic fields on their way through the head—shows a much better signal-to-noise ratio than EEG. The model for fitting the dipole to the measured MEG data was that of a single moving equivalent current dipole in a spherical volume conductor. Anatomic as well as statistical constraints were used to obtain the final results. To visualize the anatomic locations of the sources (dipoles) found, anatomic MRI images were recorded and dipole positions integrated there. For both EEG and MEG, additional statistics were applied to analyze changes of field topography over the scalp with EEG or changes of signal amplitude, dipole location, dipole strength, and quality of dipole fit (i.e., differences between dipole field pattern and measured field pattern) with MEG when applying the different tone frequencies. Results show agreement between EEG and MEG data concerning general localization differences between P_{am} and a later auditory evoked field component occurring around 100 ms after stimulus onset, the N_1/N_{1m}. P_a/P_{am} was consistently located anterior to N_1/N_{1m} for all three tone frequencies. EEG data showed a mean difference of 10 mm, MEG of 5 mm. Analysis of the anatomic location of P_{am} and N_{1m} using MRI images showed P_a/P_{am} most likely to be generated by the primary auditory cortex and N_1/N_{1m} by secondary auditory cortex areas. However, due to the poor EEG signal-to-noise ratio, an interesting additional result could only be elucidated by MEG. The center of neuronal activation shifted laterally with higher frequencies for the P_{am}. The opposite was true for the N_{1m}, which shifted medially with higher tones. Thus tonotopic processing of tones taking place at functionally different brain areas, separated by a few millimeters in space and functionally by a few milliseconds in time, was analyzed successfully. Pantev et al. demonstrate what will probably soon be the methodologic standard, namely, integrating MEG, EEG, and anatomic MRI, with a clear predominance of the first.

Visual System and Cognitive Information Processing

Salmelin et al. (136) observed processing of visual information from seeing to naming an object, thereby using an interesting data-analysis methodology. Six right-handed subjects were presented line drawings of everyday objects (e.g., vase, book, cat). The objects were presented for 100 ms and only to the lower quadrant of the left or right visual field. Three different tasks were employed: passive viewing, covert naming (silent speech), and overt naming. Magnetic fields were recorded using a whole-head neuromagnetometer with 122 channels distributed over the whole scalp. Data were recorded from shortly before to 1500 ms after picture onset using a lowpass filter of 100 Hz and a sampling rate of 300 data points per second. For every task, 80 to 100 stimuli were presented, and the corresponding artefact-free records were averaged, time locked either to the appearance of the visual stimulus or to the onset of speech. For being able to find temporally and spatially distinct brain activation related to seeing, recognizing, and naming, subsets of channels corresponding to local activated brain areas were visually defined. In a second step, the location, strength, and direction of an equivalent current dipole were determined that should represent the local brain activity. Only dipoles representing more than 85% of the measured field variance were accepted. After repeating this procedure for every channel subset, all resulting dipoles were introduced simultaneously into a multidipole model. Using all 122 channels, the validity of the found source (=dipole) distribution was tested by allowing the strengths of the dipoles to vary over time but not the locations and orientations. The capability of the multidipole model to explain the field variance over the whole scalp during the 1500-ms data records was then evaluated. For visualization, the final sources were projected into a three-dimensional MRI rendering of the subject's brain. Results for overt naming show the earliest activation to occur in the posterior occipital cortex (visual area), contralateral to the stimulated visual field. Within the following 200 ms, cortex close to the temporoparieto-occipital junction (including sensory speech area and others) became active, but in both hemispheres. Around the same time, the left auditory area also became active, and 100 to 200 ms later, the right auditory cortex became active too. Further, 100 to 200 ms later, motor areas representing face muscles, motor preparation, and active speech were activated bilaterally. Immediately following was activity within the somatomotor area (motor coordination area coordinating muscle activity). Comparing passive viewing with the speech tasks showed naming-specific signals in the left auditory cortex and the motor areas. A different analysis showed that motor preparation and motor coordination areas seem not to be related to visual processing, although their activation was triggered by the visual input. This study shows that MEG offers the opportunity to map human brain activity in three dimensions over the whole brain and to disentangle activations related to viewing, language, and vocalization.

FUTURE DEVELOPMENTS: MULTIMETHODOLOGIC REGISTRATIONS (MEG +, PET, SPECT, FUNCTIONAL MRI, EEG)

As shown earlier, MEG offers the possibility to investigate a large variety of questions concerning activity of the healthy and diseased human brain. However, there is also a disadvantage when compared with other brain mapping methods, namely, the so-called inverse problem. Therefore, modeling the brain activity, e.g., by using dipole models, relies partly on extrinsic constraints such as a priori neurophysiologic assumptions of possible activation sources. It seems desirable, therefore, to achieve such constraints by direct measurements on the same subjects using an independent methodology such as SPECT, PET, functional MRI, or some of the various optical methods. Most of these methods measure localized blood flow changes, thereby using the correlation of local neuronal activation with local blood flow increase. This may provide independent evidence of areas active with a given task and thus tranfer MEG constraints from a theoretical to an experimental basis. In addition, there are good reasons to expect a multimethodologic approach to yield overadditive experimental results. More than other combinations, future combinations of MEG and functional MRI seem promising due to the high spatial resolution and noninvasiveness of the latter. Recent studies applying combined methodology concern preparation of movements (41), three-dimensional localization of SMA activity preceding voluntary movements in a patient with infarction of the right supplementary motor area (89), localization of motor activity using functional MRI and MEG (19), analysis of the sensorimotor cortex (54, 153, 164), investigation of epilepsy (55, 142, 146, 147), and other clinical issues (50, 83, 121).

Selected Examples of Multimethodologic Approaches

To exemplify the methodology of such approaches, a recently published first investigation combining MEG and functional MRI will be described in more detail. Beisteiner et al. tried to compare localization of somatomotor activity with MEG and functional MRI. Eight subjects were investigated during tapping of the right index finger. Magnetic fields were recorded using a 7-channel Biomagnetometer that was placed at four different positions over the left central hemisphere. Field maps thus were constructed from 28 sensor locations. Two left-central dipoles, representing the primary motor and primary sensory cortex, were fitted according to the criteria "goodness of fit" and "physiologic dipole positions." The timepoint for the dipole fit was chosen somewhere within -200 to $+100$ ms from onset of the electromyogram attached over the active muscles. For comparison with functional MRI, the point midway on the line connecting both the motor and the sensory dipole ($=$ middle between both dipoles) was taken as neuronal center. MEG head reference points were marked with a tiny oil ball for the functional MRI measurements. Functional MRI measurements were performed using a flow-compensated gradient-echo FLASH sequence on a conventional Siemens Magnetom 1.5 T ($t_r = 91$ ms, $t_e = 60$ ms, flip angle $= 40°$, slice thickness $= 3$ mm, FOV $= 230$, matrix $=$

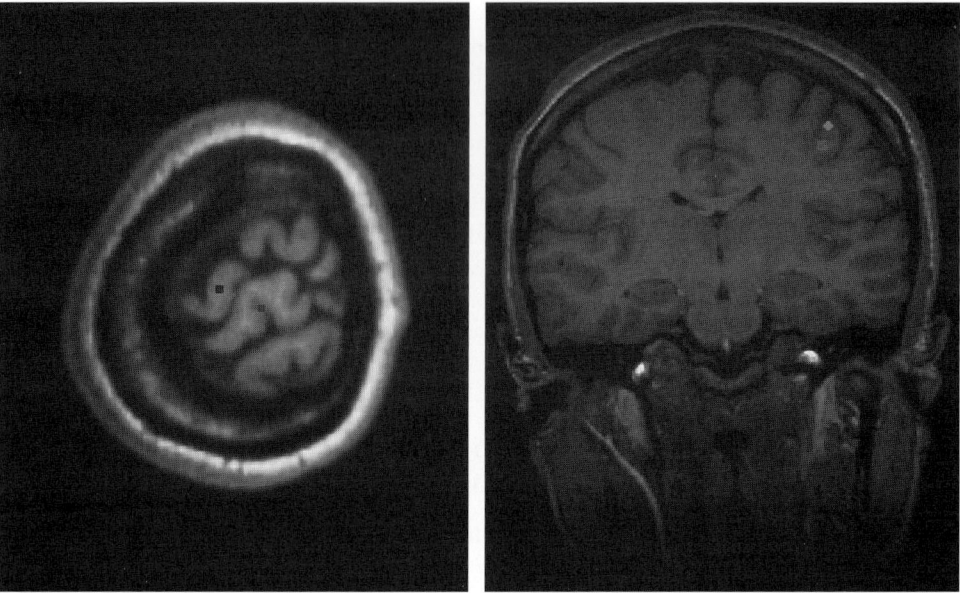

Figure 8. (**A**) Laterally tilted transverse slice of the left hemisphere of one subject of the MEG–functional MRI comparison. Anterior is up, left is medial. The blue square shows the location of the motor cortex dipole; the green square shows the position of the sensory cortex dipole. The red cross shows the location of the functional MRI center, lying directly within the central sulcus. See also Color Plate 45. (**B**) Coronal section of the same subject. Up is up, left is right. Here the mean MEG localization (calculated as the mean of the motor and sensory cortex dipole locations) is shown (*green square*). The center of the functional MRI response is shown by the red cross. See also Color Plate 46.

256 × 256). Three resting phases and two finger-tapping phases were applied, and five images were recorded in each phase. To mimic the MEG tapping procedure, a tapping phase during functional MRI was defined as cycling 3-s finger tapping per 3-s rest. Each tapping and resting phase lasted about 3 minutes and was started by a light signal. According to cortex anatomy, laterally tilted transversal functional MRI slices were recorded. Data analysis was performed by correlating the signal course of each pixel relative to a step function representing 0 for the resting phase and 1 for tapping: Only pixels with a correlation >0.6 were further processed. A second criterion was introduced to reduce signals resulting from large vessels, which could lead to mislocalizations: Only pixels with signal increases below 10% were accepted. The average position of all accepted pixels was defined as the functional MRI center. The mean distance between both centers was then calculated (Fig. 8 and Color Plates 45 and 46). Taking the average over all subjects, results showed a mean MEG–functional MRI localization difference of 16.7 mm, ranging from 8.5 to 27.8 mm. With every subject, the main discrepancies resulted from variations in the radial axis. The distance here sometimes was twice that along the other axes. The study shows that—using an oligochannel MEG system and a 1.5-T clinical MRI unit—localization of sensorimotor activity differs considerably yet. However, major improvements may be expected when using whole-head MEG systems and high-field MRI units as developed recently.

ACKNOWLEDGMENTS

The work on combined MEG–functional MRI methodology was supported by the Austrian National Bank (Jubiläumsfonds No. 5111) and the Ludwig Boltzmann Institut für Radiologisch-Physikalische Tumordiagnostik. R. Beisteiner and L. Deecke would like to thank Dr. Vinod Edward for proofreading and important scientific comments. J. Vrba would like to express his thanks to Drs. A. A. Fife and M. B. Burbank for reviewing the manuscript and for their constructive comments and to Drs. A. Ahonen and J. Hämäläinen of Neuromag, Ltd., for kindly providing information on their MEG systems. The work was supported in part by the Canadian Departments of National Defense, Supply and Services, Transport Canada, and the BC Science Council.

REFERENCES

1. Ahlfors SP, Illmoniemi RJ, Kajola MJ et al. Whole-head distribution of visual evoked magnetic fields. In: C Baumgartner, L Deecke, G Stroink, S Williamson (Eds.). *Biomagnetism: Fundamental research and clinical applications.* Amsterdam: Elsevier/IOS-Press (1995).
2. Akhtari M, McNay D, Mandelkern M et al. Somatosensory evoked response source localization using actual cortical surface as the spatial constraint. *Brain Topogr* 7(1), 63–69 (1994).
3. Alarcon G, Guy CN, Binnie CD et al. Intracerebral propagation of interictal activity in partial epilepsy: Implications for source localisation. *J Neurol Neurosurg Psychiatry* 57(4), 435–449 (1994).
4. Alho K. Cerebral generators of mismatch negativity (MMN) and its magnetic counterpart (MMNm) elicited by sound changes. *Ear Hear* 16(1), 38–51 (1995).
5. Alho K, Huotilainen M, Tiitinen H et al. Memory related processing of complex sound patterns in human auditory cortex: A MEG study. *Neuroreport* 4(4), 391–394 (1993).
6. Alho K, Tervaniemi M, Huotilainen M et al. Mismatch responses to frequency changes in simple and complex sounds: Whole-head MEG recordings. In: C Baumgartner, L Deecke, G Stroink, SJ Williamson (Eds.). *Biomagnetism: Fundamental research and clinical applications. Vol 7, Studies in applied electromagnetics and mechanics.* Amsterdam: Elsevier/IOS-Press (1995).
7. Amuneal Manufacturing Corp., 4737 Darrah Street, Philadelphia, PA 19124, USA.
8. Balish M, Sato S, Connaughton P, Kufta C. Localization of implanted dipoles by magnetoencephalography. *Neurology* 41, 1072–1076 (1991).
9. Barkley GL, Tepley N, Nagel-Leiby S et al. Magnetoencephalographic studies of migraine. *Headache* 30(7), 428–434 (1990).
10. Barkley GL, Tepley N, Simkins R et al. Neuromagnetic fields in migraine: Preliminary findings. *Cephalalgia* 10(4), 171–176 (1990).
11. Barth DS, Baumgartner C, Sutherling WW. Neuromagnetic field modeling of multiple brain regions producing interictal spikes in human epilepsy. *Electroencephalogr Clin Neurophysiol* 73, 389–402 (1989).
12. Barth DS, Sutherling WW, Engel J, Beatty J. Neuromagnetic localization of epileptiform spike activity in the human brain. *Science* 218, 891–894 (1982).
13. Basile LF, Rogers RL, Bourbon WT, Papanicolaou AC. Slow magnetic flux from human frontal cortex. *Electroencephalogr Clin Neurophysiol* 90(2), 157–165 (1994).
14. Baule GM, McFee R. Detection of the magnetic field of the heart. *Am Heart J* 66, 95–96 (1963).
15. Baumgartner C, Deecke L. Magnetoencephalography in clinical epileptology and epilepsy research. *Brain Topogr* 2, 203–219 (1990).
16. Baumgartner C, Doppelbauer A, Sutherling WW et al. Human somatosensory cortical finger representation as studied by combined neuromagnetic and neuroelectric measurements. *Neurosci Lett* 134, 103–108 (1991).
17. Baumgartner C, Sutherling WW, Di S, Barth DS. Multiple source modeling of the human epileptic spike complex in the magnetoencephalogram. In: SJ Williamson, M Hoke, G Stroink, M Kotani (Eds.). *Advances in biomagnetism: Proceedings of the seventh international conference on biomagnetism,* August 1989, New York. New York: Plenum Press, 299–306 (1989).
18. Becker W, Dickmann V, Jurgens R, Kornhuber C. First experiences with a multichannel software gradiometer recording normal and tangential components of MEG. *Physiol Meas* 14, A45–A50 (1993).
19. Beisteiner R, Gomiscek G, Erdler M et al. Comparing localization of conventional functional magnetic resonance imaging and magnetoencephalography. *Eur J Neurosci* 7, 1121–1124 (1995).
20. Berger H. Über das elektrenkephalogramm des Menschen. *Arch Psychiatr Nervenkr* 7, 527 (1929).
21. Biomagnetic Technologies, Inc., 9727 Pacific Heights Blvd., San Diego, CA 92121-3719, USA.
22. Brenner D, Kaufman L, Williamson SJ. Applications of a SQUID for monitoring magnetic response of the human brain. *IEEE Trans Magn*, MAG-13, 365–368 (1977).
23. Bruno AC, Dolce CS, Soares SD, Ribeiro PC. Spatial Fourier technique for calibrating gradiometers. In: SJ Williamson, M Hoke, G Stroink, M Kotani (Eds.). *Advances in biomagnetism: Proceedings of the seventh international conference on biomagnetism,* August 1989, New York. New York: Plenum Press, 709–712 (1989).
24. Cheyne D, Kristeva R, Deecke L. Homuncular organization of human motor cortex as indicated by neuromagnetic recording. *Neurosci Lett* 122, 17–20 (1991).
25. Cheyne D, Kristeva R, Lang W et al. Neuromagnetic localisation of sensorimotor cortex sources associated with voluntary movements in humans. In: SJ Williamson, M Hoke, G Stroink, M Kotani (Eds.). *Advances in biomagnetism: Proceedings of the seventh international conference on biomagnetism,* August 1989, New York. New York: Plenum Press, 177–180 (1989).
26. Cheyne D, Vrba J, Crisp D et al. Use of an unshielded 64 channel whole-cortex MEG system in the study of normal and pathological brain function. *Fourteenth annual international conference of the IEEE Engineering in Medicine and Biology Society: Proceedings of the satellite symposium on neuroscience and technology,* Lyon, France, 46–50 (November 1992).
27. Cheyne D, Weinberg H, Gaetz W, Jantzen KJ. Motor cortex activity and predicting side of movement: Neural network and dipole analysis of pre-movement magnetic fields. *Neurosci Lett* 188(2), 81–84 (1995).
28. Chiron C, Syrota A. L'imagerie fonctionnelle cerebrale chez l'enfant: Progres et perspectives. *Arch Pediatr* 2(2), 111–115 (1995).

29. Chuang SH, Otsubo H, Hwang P et al. Pediatric magnetic source imaging. *Neuroimaging Clin North Am* 5(2), 289–303 (1995).

30. Clarke J. Low-frequency applications of superconducting quantum interference devices. *Proc IEEE* 61, 8–19 (1973).

31. Cohen D. Magnetoencephalography: Evidence of magnetic fields produced by alpha-rhythm currents. *Science* 161, 784–786 (1968).

32. Cohen D. Magnetoencephalography: Detection of the brain's electrical activity with a superconducting magnetometer. *Science* 175, 664–666 (1972).

33. Cohen D, Cuffin BN, Yunokuchi K et al. MEG versus EEG localization test using implanted sources in the human brain. *Ann Neurol* 30(2), 222–224 (1991).

34. Cohen D, Edelsack EA, Zimmerman JE. Magnetocardiograms taken inside a shielded room with a superconducting point-contact magnetometer. *Appl Phys Lett* 16, 278–280 (1970).

35. CTF Systems Inc., 15–1750 McLean Ave, Port Coquitlam, B.C., Canada, V3C 1M9.

36. Cuffin BN. Effects of local variations in skull and scalp thickness on EEGs and MEGs. *IEEE Trans Biomed Eng* 40(1), 42–48 (1993).

37. Cuffin BN, Cohen D. Magnetic fields of a dipole in special volume conductor shapes. *IEEE Trans Biomed Eng* BME-24, 372–381 (1977).

38. Curio G, Mackert BM, Burghoff M et al. Localization of evoked neuromagnetic 600 Hz activity in the cerebral somatosensory system. *Electroencephalogr Clin Neurophysiol* 91(6), 483–487 (1994).

39. Curio G, Reill L, Sandfort J et al. Nerve, plexus and spinal cord: Possible targets for non-invasive neuromagnetic measurements in man. *Physiol Meas* 14 (Suppl 4A), A91–A94 (1993).

40. Deecke L. Bereitschaftspotential as an indicator of movement preparation in supplementary motor area and motor cortex. In: R Porter (Chairman). *Motor areas of the cerebral cortex* (Ciba Foundation Symposium 132). Chichester: Wiley, 231–250 (1987).

41. Deecke L. Electrophysiological correlates of movement initiation. *Rev Neurol (Paris)* 146(10), 612–619 (1990).

42. Deecke L, Boschert J, Weinberg H, Brickett P. Magnetic fields of the human brain (Bereitschaftsmagnetfeld) preceding voluntary foot and toe movements. *Exp Brain Res* 52, 81–86 (1983).

43. Deecke L, Grözinger B, Kornhuber HH. Voluntary finger movement in man: Cerebral potentials and theory. *Biol Cybern* 23, 99–119 (1976).

44. Deecke L, Lang W. Generation of movement-related potentials and fields in the supplementary sensorimotor area and the primary motor area. In: HO Lüders (Ed.). *Advances in neurology. Vol 70, Supplementary sensorimotor area.* 127–146 (1996).

45. Deecke L, Weinberg H, Brickett P. Magnetic fields of the human brain accompanying voluntary movement: Bereitschaftsmagnetfeld. *Exp Brain Res* 48, 144–148 (1982).

46. Dieckmann V, Jurgens R, Becker W et al. *RF- to DC-SQUID upgrade of a 28-channel magnetoencephalography (MEG) system.* Manuscript submitted for publication (1995).

47. Dossel O, David B, Fuchs M et al. A 31-channel SQUID system for biomagnetic imaging. *IEEE Trans Appl Supercond* 3, 1813–1825 (1993).

48. Drung D, Absmann, Curio G et al. The PTB 83-SQUID system for biomagnetic applications in a clinic. *IEEE Trans Appl Supercond* 5, 2112–2117 (1995).

49. Ebersole JS, Squires KC, Eliashiv SD, Smith JR. Applications of magnetic source imaging in evaluation of candidates for epilepsy surgery. *Neuroimaging Clin North Am* 5(2), 267–288 (1995).

50. Eckardt MJ, Rohrbaugh JW, Rio D et al. Brain imaging in alcoholic patients. *Adv Alcohol Subst Abuse* 7(3–4), 59–71 (1988).

51. Elbert T, Flor H, Birbaumer N et al. Extensive reorganization of the somatosensory cortex in adult humans after nervous system injury. *Neuroreport* 5(18), 2593–2597 (1994).

52. Erne SN, Hahlbohm H-D, Scheer H, Trontelj Z. The Berlin Magnetically Shielded Room (BMSR). Section B: Performances. In: SN Erne, H-D Hahlbohm, H Lubbig (Eds.). *Biomagnetism: Proceedings of the third international workshop on biomagnetism,* May 1980, Berlin. Berlin: Walter de Gruyter (1981).

53. Eulitz C, Diesch E, Pantev C et al. Magnetic and electric brain activity evoked by the processing of tone and vowel stimuli. *J Neurosci* 15(4), 2748–2755 (1995).

54. Eulitz C, Elbert T, Bartenstein P. Comparison of magnetic and metabolic brain activity during a verb generation task. *Neuroreport* 6(1), 97–100 (1994).

55. Forss N, Makela JP, Keranen T, Hari R. Trigeminally triggered epileptic hemifacial convulsions. *Neuroreport* 6(6), 918–920 (1995).

56. Forss N, Salmelin R, Hari R. Comparison of somatosensory evoked fields to airpuff and electric stimuli. *Electroencephalogr Clin Neurophysiol* 92(6), 510–517 (1994).

57. Freeman WJ. Characterization of state transitions in spatially distributed, chaotic, nonlinear, dynamical systems in cerebral cortex. *Integr Physiol Behav Sci* 29(3), 294–306 (1994).

58. Furukawa Electric Co., Ltd., 2-4-3 Okano, Nishi-ku, Yokohama 220, Japan.

59. Gallen CC, Bucholz R, Sobel DF. Intracranial neurosurgery guided by functional imaging. *Surg Neurol* 42(6), 523–530 (1994).

60. Gallen CC, Schwartz BJ, Bucholz RD et al. Presurgical localization of functional cortex using magnetic source imaging. *J Neurosurg* 82(6), 988–989 ( ).

61. Gharib S, Sutherling WW, Nakasato N et al. MEG and ECoG localization accuracy test. *Electroencephalogr Clin Neurophysiol* 94(2), 109–114 (1995).

62. Grynszpan F, Geselowitz DB. Model studies of the magnetocardiogram. *Biophys J* 13, 911–925 (1973).

63. Hari R. Neuromagnetic studies of the human auditory cortex: Recent results. In: K Atsumi, M Kotani, S Ueno et al. (Eds.). *Biomagnetism '87: Proceedings of the sixth international conference on biomagnetism,* August 1987, Tokyo. Tokyo: Tokyo Denki University Press, 34–41 (1988).

64. Hari R, Antervo A, Katila T et al. Cerebral magnetic fields associated with voluntary limb movements. *Nuovo Cimento* 2D, 484–494 (1983).

65. Hari R, Joutsiniemi SL, Hämäläinen M, Vilkman V. Neuromagnetic responses of human auditory cortex to interruptions in a steady rhythm. *Neurosci Lett* 99, 164–168 (1989).
66. Hari R, Karhu J, Hämäläinen M et al. Functional organization of the human first and second somatosensory cortices: A neuromagnetic study. *Eur J Neurosci* 5, 724–734 (1993).
67. Hari R, Kaukoranta E. Neuromagnetic studies of somatosensory system: Principles and examples. *Prog Neurobiol* 24, 233–256 (1985).
68. Hari R, Pellizoni M, Mäkelä JP et al. Neuromagnetic responses of the human auditory cortex to on- and off-sets of noise bursts. *Audiology* 26, 31–43 (1987).
69. Hayes KC, Potter PJ, Wolfe DL et al. 4-Aminopyridine-sensitive neurologic deficits in patients with spinal cord injury. *J Neurotrauma* 11(4), 433–446 (1994).
70. Huotilainen M, Tiitinen H, Lavikainen J et al. Sustained fields of tones and glides reflect tonotopy of the auditory cortex. *Neuroreport* 6(6), 841–844 (1995).
71. Huttunen J, Hari R, Leinonen L. Cerebral magnetic responses to stimulation of ulnar and median nerves. *Electroencephalogr Clin Neurophysiol* 66, 391–400 (1987).
72. Illmoniemi RJ, Hämäläinen MS. *Interpreting measured magnetic fields of the brain: Estimates of current distributions.* Report TKK-F-A559. Helsinki, Finland: Helsinki University of Technology (1984).
73. Ioannides AA, Fenwick PBC, Lumsden J et al. Activation sequence of discrete brain areas during cognitive processes: Results from magnetic field tomography. *Electroencephalogr Clin Neurophysiol* 91, 399–402 (1994).
74. Joliot M, Ribary U, Llinas R. Human oscillatory brain activity near 40 Hz coexists with cognitive temporal binding. *Proc Natl Acad Sci USA* 91(24), 11748–11751 (1994).
75. Josephson BD. Possible new effects in superconductive tunneling. *Phys Lett* 1, 251–253 (1962).
76. Kaas JH, Nelson RJ, Sur M et al. Multiple representations of the body within primary somatosensory cortex of primates. *Science* 204, 521–523 (1979).
77. Kakigi R, Koyama S, Hoshiyama M et al. Gating of somatosensory evoked responses during active finger movements: Magnetoencephalographic studies. *J Neurol Sci* 128(2), 195–204 (1995a).
78. Kakigi R, Koyama S, Hoshiyama M et al. Pain-related magnetic fields following painful CO_2 laser stimulation in man. *Neurosci Lett* 192(1), 45–48 (1995b).
79. Kaufman L, Curtis S, Wang JZ, Williamson SJ. Changes in cortical activity when subjects scan memory for tones. *Electroencephalogr Clin Neurophysiol* 82, 266–284 (1991).
80. Kaufman L, Williamson SJ. Neuromagnetic studies of sensory functions and mental imagery. *Electroencephalogr Clin Neurophysiol* 42, Suppl 13–23 (1991).
81. Kaukoranta E, Hämäläinen M, Sarvas J, Hari R. Mixed and sensory nerve stimulations activate different cytoarchitectonic areas in the human primary somatosensory cortex SI. *Exp Brain Res* 63, 60–66 (1986).
82. Kelha VO. Construction and performance of the Otaniemi magnetically shielded room. In: SN Erne, HD Hahlbohm, H Lubbig (Eds.). *Biomagnetism: Proceedings of the Third International Workshop on Biomagnetism*, May 1980, Berlin. Berlin: Walter de Gruyter (1981).
83. Khan N, Wieser HG. Limbic encephalitis: A case report. *Epilepsy Res* 17(2), 175–181 (1994).
84. Kofoed B, Bak CK, Rahn E, Saermark K. Auditory event-related magnetic fields in a tone-duration discrimination task. Source localization for the mismatch field and for a new component M2". *Acta Neurol Scand* 91(5), 362–371 (1995).
85. Kornhuber HH, Deecke L. Hirnpotentialänderungen bei Willkürbewegungen und passiven Bewegungen des Menschen: Bereitschaftspotential und reafferente Potentiale. *Pflügers Arch* 284, 1–17 (1965).
86. Kowalik ZJ, Elbert T. Changes of chaoticness in spontaneous EEG/MEG. *Integr Physiol Behav Sci* 29(3), 270–282 (1994).
87. Kristeva R, Cheyne D, Deecke L. Neuromagnetic fields accompanying unilateral and bilateral voluntary movements: Topography and analysis of cortical sources. *Electroencephalogr Clin Neurophysiol* 81, 284–298 (1991).
88. Kuriki S, Okita Y, Hirata Y. Source analysis of magnetic field responses from the human auditory cortex elicited by short speech sounds. *Exp Brain Res* 104(1), 144–152 (1995).
89. Lang W, Cheyne D, Kristeva R et al. Three-dimensional localization of SMA activity preceding voluntary movement. A study of electric and magnetic fields in a patient with infarction of the right supplementary motor area. *Exp Brain Res* 87, 688–695 (1991).
90. Lavikainen J, Huotilainen M, Pekkonen E et al. Auditory stimuli activate parietal brain regions: A whole-head MEG study. *Neuroreport* 6(1), 182–184 (1994).
91. Loveless N, Vasama JP, Makela J, Hari R. Human auditory cortical mechanisms of sound lateralisation: III. Monaural and binaural shift responses. *Hear Res* 81(1–2), 91–99 (1994).
92. Lu ZL, Williamson SJ. Spatial extent of coherent sensory-evoked cortical activity. *Exp Brain Res* 84, 411–416 (1991).
93. Lu ZL, Williamson SJ, Kaufman L. Human auditory primary and association cortex having differing lifetimes for activation traces. *Brain Res* 572(1–2), 236–241 (1992).
94. Lu ST, Hämäläinen MS, Hari R et al. Seeing faces activates three separate areas outside the occipital visual cortex in man. *Neuroscience* 43(2–3), 287–290 (1991).
95. Lu ZL, Williamson SJ, Kaufman L. Behavioral lifetime of human auditory sensory memory predicted by physiological measures. *Science* 258, 1668–1670 (1992).
96. Maclin EL, Rose DF, Knight JE et al. Somatosensory evoked magnetic fields in patients with stroke. *Electroencephalogr Clin Neurophysiol* 91(6), 468–475 (1994).
97. Mäkelä JP, Hari R. Evidence for cortical origin of the 40 Hz auditory evoked response in man. *Electroencephalogr Clin Neurophysiol* 539–546 (1987).
98. Martin NA, Beatty J, Johnson RA et al. Magnetoencephalographic localization of a language processing cortical area adjacent to a cerebral arteriovenous malformation. Case report. *J Neurosurg* 79(4), 584–588 (1993).
99. Matlashov A, Zhuravlev YU, Lipovich A et al. Electronic noise suppression in a multichannel neuromagnetic system. In: SJ Williamson, M Hoke, G Stroink, M Kotani (Eds.). *Advances in biomagnetism:*

Proceedings of the seventh international conference on biomagnetism, August 1989, New York. New York: Plenum Press, 725–728 (1989).

100. Matlashov A, Slobodchikov VY, Bakharev AA et al. A biomagnetic multichannel system built with 19 cryogenic probes. In: C Baumgartner, L Deecke, G Stroink, S Williamson (Eds.). *Biomagnetism: Fundamental research and clinical applications.* Amsterdam: Elsevier Science/IOS-Press, 493–496 (1995).

101. Matsuba H, Shintomi K, Yahara A et al. Superconducting shield enclosing a human body for biomagnetism measurement. In: C Baumgartner, L Deecke, G Stroink, S Williamson (Eds.). *Biomagnetism: Fundamental research and clinical applications.* Amsterdam: Elsevier Science/IOS-Press (1995).

102. McEvoy L, Makela JP, Hämäläinen M, Hari R. Effect of interaural time differences on middle-latency and late auditory evoked magnetic fields. *Hear Res* 78(2), 249–257 (1994).

103. McKay J, Vrba J, Betts K et al. *Implementation of a multichannel biomagnetic measurement system using DSP technology: Proceedings of the 1993 Canadian conference on electrical and computer engineering.* Vol II, 1090–1093 (September 1993).

104. Minami T. Clinical application of magnetoencephalography in pediatric neurologic diseases. *No To Hattatsu* 27(2), 132–137 (1995).

105. Muhlnickel W, Rendtorff N, Kowalik ZJ et al. Testing the determinism of EEG and MEG. *Integr Physiol Behav Sci* 29(3), 262–269 (1994).

106. Nakasota N, Levesque MF, Barth DS et al. Comparisons of MEG, EEG, and ECoG source localization in neocortical partial epilepsy in humans. *Electroencephalogr Clin Neurophysiol* 171, 171–178 (1994).

107. Nakasato N, Fujita S, Matani A et al. Clinical application of the whole-head MEG: Auditory evoked response in patients with intracranial structural lesions. In: C Baumgartner, L Deecke, G Stroink, S Williamson (Eds.). *Biomagnetism: Fundamental research and clinical applications.* Amsterdam: Elsevier Science/IOS-Press (1995).

108. Nakasato N, Fujita S, Seki K et al. Functional localization of bilateral auditory cortices using an MRI-linked whole head magnetoencephalography (MEG) system. *Electroencephalogr Clin Neurophysiol* 94, 183–190 (1995).

109. Neuromag Ltd., P.O. Box 68, FIN-00511, Elimaenkaru 22 A, Helsinki, Finland.

110. Ohta Y, Hiraiwa M, Murayama K et al. Hypometabolism and dipole localization in hemimegalencephaly: A case report. *Neuropediatrics* 25(5), 255–258 (1994).

111. Okada YC, Tanenbaum R, Williamson SJ, Kaufman L. Somatotopic organization of the human somatosensory cortex as revealed by neuromagnetic measurements. *Exp Brain Res* 56, 197–205 (1984).

112. Okada YC, Williamson SJ, Kaufman L. Magnetic fields of the human sensorimotor cortex. *Int J Neurosci* 17, 33–38 (1982).

113. Paetau R, Ahonen A, Salonen O, Sams M. Auditory evoked magnetic fields to tones and pseudowords in healthy children and adults. *J Clin Neurophysiol* 12(2), 177–185 (1995).

114. Paetau R, Hämäläinen M, Hari R et al. Magnetoencephalographic evaluation of children and adolescents with intractable epilepsy. *Epilepsia* 35(2), 275–284 (1994).

115. Pantev C, Bertrand O, Eulitz C et al. Specific tonotopic organizations of different areas of the human auditory cortex as revealed by simultaneous magnetic and electric recordings. *Electroencephalogr Clin Neurophysiol* 94, 26–40 (1995).

116. Pantev C, Gallen C, Hampson S et al. Reproducibility and validity of neuromagnetic source localization using a large array biomagnetometer. *Am J EEG Technol* 31, 83–101 (1991).

117. Pantev C, Hoke M, Lehnertz K et al. Tonotopic organization of the human auditory cortex as revealed by transient auditory evoked magnetic fields. *Electroencephalogr Clin Neurophysiol* 69, 160–170 (1988).

118. Pascual-Marqui RD, Michel ChM. LORETA (Low resolution brain electromagnetic tomography): New authentic 3D functional images of the brain. *ISBET Newsletter.* No. 5, 4–8 (1994).

119. Pellizoni M, Hari R, Mäkelä J et al. Cortical origin of middle-latency auditory evoked responses in man. *Neurosci Lett* 82, 303–307 (1987).

120. Penfield W, Jasper J. *Epilepsy and the functional anatomy of the brain.* Boston: Little, Brown (1954).

121. Perrine K. Future directions of functional mapping. *Epilepsia* 35 (Suppl 6), S90–S102 (1994).

122. Pfefferbaum A, Roth WT, Ford JM. Event-related potentials in the study of psychiatric disorders. *Arch Gen Psychiatry* 52(7), 559–563 (1995).

123. Racansky D. Loan of the human headform shaped on the basis of the survey of North American males. University of Toronto, Institute of Biomedical Engineering.

124. Regan D. Spatial vision in adults and infants: A tribute to Russell Harter. *Int J Neurosci* 80(1–4), 153–172 (1995).

125. Reite M, Adams M, Simon J et al. Auditory M100 component 1: Relationship to Heschl's gyri. *Brain Res Cogn Brain Res* 2(1), 13–20 (1994).

126. Reite M, Scheuneman D, Gilger JW et al. Auditory magnetic source localization in twins. *Brain Res Bull* 28(4), 641–644 (1992).

127. Ribary U, Llinas R, Lado F et al. The spatial and temporal organization of the 40 Hz response in the human brain. In: M Hoke, SN Erne, YC Okada, GL Romani (Eds.). *Biomagnetism: Clinical aspects. Proceedings of the eighth international conference on biomagnetism,* August 1991, Munster, Amsterdam: Excerpta Medica, 159–163 (1992).

128. Ricci GB, Leoni R, Romani GL et al. 3-D neuromagnetic localization of sources of interictal activity in cases of focal epilepsy. In: H Weinberg, G Stroink, T Katila (Eds.). *Biomagnetism: Applications and theory.* New York: Pergamon Press, 304–310 (1985).

129. Roberts T, Rowley H, Kucharczyk J. Applications of magnetic source imaging to presurgical brain mapping. *Neuroimaging Clin North Am* 5(2), 251–266 (1995).

130. Robinson SE, Rose DF. Current source image estimation by spatially filtered MEG. In: M Hoke, SN Erne, YC Okada, GL Romani (Eds.). *Biomagnetism: Clinical aspects. Proceedings of the eighth international conference on biomagnetism,* August 1991, Munster. Amsterdam: Excerpta Medica, 761–765 (1992).

131. Rogers RL, Basile LF, Papanicolaou AC et al. Visual evoked magnetic fields reveal activity in the superior temporal sulcus. *Electroencephalogr Clin Neurophysiol* 86(5), 344–347 (1993).
132. Rogers RL, Papanicolaou AC, Baumann SB, Eisenberg HM. Late magnetic fields and positive evoked potentials following infrequent and unpredictable omissions of visual stimuli. *Electroencephalogr Clin Neurophysiol* 83(2), 146–152 (1992).
133. Romani GL, Williamson SJ, Kaufman L. Tonotopic organization of the human auditory cortex. *Science* 216, 1339–1340 (1982).
134. Rossini PM, Narici L, Martino G et al. Analysis of interhemispheric asymmetries of somatosensory evoked magnetic fields to right and left median nerve stimulation. *Electroencephalogr Clin Neurophysiol* 91(6), 476–482 (1994).
135. Salmelin R, Forss N, Knuutila J, Hari R. Bilateral activation of the human somatomotor cortex by distal hand movements. *Electroencephalogr Clin Neurophysiol* 95, 444–452 (1995).
136. Salmelin R, Hari R, Lounasmaa OV, Sams M. Dynamics of brain activation during picture naming. *Nature* 368(6470), 463–465 (1994).
137. Sams M, Aulanko R, Hämäläinen M et al. Seeing speech: Visual information from lip movements modifies activity in the human auditory cortex. *Neurosci Lett* 127(1), 141–145 (1991).
138. Sarvas J. Basic mathematical and electromagnetic concepts of the biomagnetic inverse problem. *Phys Med Biol* 32, 11–22 (1987).
139. Sarwinski RE. Superconducting instruments. *Cryogenics* 17, 671–679 (1977).
140. Sato S, Malow BA. Electroencephalography and magnetoencephalography in epilepsy and nonepileptic disorders. *Curr Opin Neurol* 6(5), 708–714 (1993).
141. Scherg M, Hari R, Hämäläinen M. Frequency-specific sources of the auditory N19.P30–P50 response detected by a multiple source analysis of evoked magnetic field and potentials. In: SJ Williamson, M Hoke, G Stroink, M Kotani (Eds.). *Advances in biomagnetism: Proceedings of the seventh international conference on biomagnetism,* August 1989, New York. New York: Plenum Press, 97–100 (1989).
142. Shibasaki H, Ikeda A. Intractable epilepsy—neurophysiological evaluation and indication for surgical treatment. *Rinsho Shinkeigaku* 34(12), 1234–1236 (1994).
143. Smith JR, Gallen C, Orrison W et al. Role of multichannel magnetoencephalography in the evaluation of ablative seizure surgery candidates. *Stereotact Funct Neurosurg* 62(1–4), 238–244 (1994).
144. Smith JR, Gallen CC, Schwartz BJ. Multichannel magnetoencephalographic mapping of sensorimotor cortex for epilepsy surgery. *Stereotact Funct Neurosurg* 62(1–4), 245–251 (1994).
145. Starr A, Kristeva R, Cheyne D et al. Localization of brain activity during auditory verbal short-term memory derived from magnetic recordings. *Brain Res* 558, 181–190 (1991).
146. Stefan H, Quesney LF, Feistel HK et al. Presurgical evaluation in frontal lobe epilepsy. A multimethodological approach. *Adv Neurol* 66, 213–220 (1995).
147. Stefan H, Schneider S, Feistel H et al. Ictal and interictal activity in partial epilepsy recorded with multichannel magnetoelectroencephalography: Correlation of electroencephalography/electrocorticography, magnetic resonance imaging, single photon emission computed tomography, and positron emission tomography findings. *Epilepsia* 33(5), 874–887 (1992).
148. Stefan H, Schuler P, Abraham-Fuchs K et al. Magnetic source localization and morphological changes in temporal lobe epilepsy: Comparison of MEG/EEG, ECoG and volumetric MRI in presurgical evaluation of operated patients. *Acta Neurol Scand Suppl* 152, 83–88 (1994).
149. Stroink G, Blackford B, Brown B, Horacek M. Aluminum shielded room for biomagnetic measurements. *Rev Sci Instrum* 52(3), 463–468 (1981).
150. Sullivan GW, Flynn ER. Performance of the Los Alamos Shielded Room. In: K Atsumi, M Kotani, S Ueno et al. (Eds.). *Biomagnetism '87: Proceedings of the sixth international conference on biomagnetism,* August 1987, Tokyo. Tokyo: Tokyo Denki University Press, 486–489 (1988).
151. Sutherling WW, Crandall PH, Darcey TM et al. The magnetic and electric fields agree with intracranial localizations of somatosensory cortex. *Neurology* 38, 1705–1714 (1988).
152. ter Brake HJM, Flokstra J, Jaszczuk W et al. The UT 19-channel dcSQUID based neuromagnetometer. *Clin Phys Physiol Meas* 12B, 45–50 (1991).
153. Thatcher RW. Tomographic electroencephalography/magnetoencephalography. Dynamics of human neural network switching. *J Neuroimaging* 5(1), 35–45 (1995).
154. Tiitinen H, May P, Reinikainen K, Naatanen R. Attentive novelty detection in humans is governed by pre-attentive sensory memory. *Nature* 372(6501), 90–92 (1994).
155. Tokin Corporation, 6-7-1 Koriyama Tihakuku, Sendai-City, Miyagi-pref, 982, Japan.
156. Vacuumschmelze GmbH, Hanau, Germany; Shielded Room model AK-3.
157. Vasama JP, Makela JP, Pyykko I, Hari R. Abrupt unilateral deafness modifies function of human auditory pathways. *Neuroreport* 6(7), 961–964 (1995).
158. Verkindt C, Bertrand O, Perrin F et al. Tonotopic organization of the human auditory cortex: N100 topography and multiple dipole model analysis. *Electroencephalogr Clin Neurophysiol* 96(2), 143–156 (1995).
159. Vieth J, Sack G, Kober H et al. The dipole density plot (DDP), a technique to show concentrations of dipoles. *Physiol Meas* 14 (Suppl 4A), A41–A44 (1993).
160. Vrba J, Betts K, Burbank M et al. Whole cortex, 64 channel SQUID biomagnetometer system. *IEEE Trans Appl Supercond* 3, 1878–1882 (1993).
161. Vrba J, Betts K, Burbank MB et al. Whole cortex 64 channel system for shielded and unshielded environments. In: C Baumgartner, L Deecke, G Stroink, S Williamson (Eds.). *Biomagnetism: Fundamental research and clinical applications.* Amsterdam: Elsevier Science/IOS-Press (1995).
162. Vrba J, Haid G, Lee S et al. Biomagnetometers for unshielded and well shielded environments. *Clin Phys Physiol Meas* 12 (Suppl B), 81–86 (1991).
163. Vrba J, Taylor B, Cheung T et al. Noise cancellation by whole-cortex SQUID MEG System. *IEEE Trans Appl Supercond* 5, 2118–2123 (1995).

164. Walter H, Kristeva R, Knorr U et al. Individual somatotopy of primary sensorimotor cortex revealed by intermodal matching of MEG, PET, and MRI. *Brain Topogr* 5(2), 183–187 (1992).

165. Wang JZ, Williamson SJ, Kaufman L. Kinetic images of neuronal activity of the human brain based on the spatio-temporal MNLS inverse: A theoretical study. *Brain Topogr* 7(3), 193–200 (1995).

166. Watanabe Y, Sato S, Nakamura F et al. The practical benefits of magnetoencephalography in comparison with electroencephalography in a patient with epilepsia partialis continua. *No To Shinkei* 47(4), 357–362 (1995).

167. Welch KM, Barkley GL, Ramadan NM, D'Andrea G. NMR spectroscopic and magnetoencephalographic studies in migraine with aura: Support for the spreading depression hypothesis. *Pathol Biol Paris* 40(4), 349–354 (1992).

168. Wikswo JP Jr. SQUID magnetometers for biomagnetism and nondestructive testing: Important questions and initial answers. *IEEE Trans Appl Supercond* 5, 74–120 (1995).

169. Williamson SJ, Pelizzone M, Okada Y et al. Magnetoencephalography with an array of SQUID sensors. In: H Collan, P Berglund, M Kresius (Eds.). *Proceedings of the tenth international cryogenic engineering conference.* Guilford: Butterworth, 339–348 (1984).

170. Williamson SJ, Robinson SE, Kaufman L. Methods and instrumentation for biomagnetism. In: K Atsumi, M Kotani, S Ueno et al. (Eds.). *Biomagnetism '87: Proceedings of the sixth international conference on biomagnetism,* August 1987, Tokyo. Tokyo: Tokyo Denki University Press (1988).

171. Wood CC, Cohen D, Cuffin BN et al. Electrical sources in human somatosensory cortex: Identification by combined magnetic and potential recordings. *Science* 227, 1051–1053 (1985).

172. Wood CC, Spencer DD, Allison T et al. Localization of human sensorimotor cortex during surgery by cortical surface recording of somatosensory evoked potentials. *J Neurosurg* 68, 99–111 (1988).

173. Yamasaki S, Morooka T, Matsuda N et al. Design and fabrication of multichannel dc SQUIDs for biomagnetic applications. *IEEE Trans Appl Supercond* 3, 1887–1889 (1993).

174. Yang TT, Gallen CC, Schwartz BJ, Bloom FE. Noninvasive somatosensory homunculus mapping in humans using a large-array biomagnetometer. *Proc Natl Acad Sci USA* 90, 3098–3102 (1993).

175. Zimmerman JE, Silver AH. Quantum effects in type II superconductors. *Phys Lett* 10, 47–48 (1964).

Functional Imaging, edited by
Gustav von Schulthess and Jürgen Hennig.
Lippincott–Raven Publishers, Philadelphia, © 1998.

11

Sound Waves: Ultrasonography

Peter N.T. Wells

Mechanical vibrations with frequencies above the range of human hearing are known as *ultrasound*. Ultrasonic waves differ from electromagnetic waves in many fundamental respects; for example, a medium is required for their propagation, since they cannot travel in a vacuum. In some respects, however, the physics of ultrasound is similar to the physics of electromagnetic waves, both being forms of radiation. In any system using radiation to form an image, the wavelength is one of the factors that determines the spatial resolution; the shorter the wavelength, the better is the resolution.

The use of ultrasound to obtain diagnostic information is called *ultrasonography*. The information can be anatomic or physiologic or a combination of the two. Thus, although ultrasonography is usually thought of as a radiologic technique, it actually provides a surprising amount of functional information.

PROPAGATION OF ULTRASOUND IN BIOLOGIC TISSUES

General Considerations

Biologic tissues can support the propagation of ultrasonic waves. As the waves propagate through tissue, the tissue affects the waves and the waves affect the tissue. The effects of ultrasonic waves on tissue are relevant to the safety of ultrasonic diagnosis. The subject is both important and complicated (39).

Here, it is sufficient to note a few salient points. Ultrasound is known to affect biologic tissues by both thermal and mechanical effects. Thresholds below which no damaging effects occur seem to be associated with both mechanisms. Although the exposure levels

PNT Wells: Department of Medical Physics and Bioengineering, Bristol General Hospital, Bristol, UK.

used in contemporary techniques appear to be safe, it is prudent to apply the ALARA (as low as reasonably achievable) principle and not to use ultrasound for trivial purposes.

It is the effects of tissue on ultrasound that provide diagnostic information (8, 38). More precisely, it is generally the differences in the ultrasonic properties of different tissues, and within the tissues themselves, that are the relevant factors.

Speech and Wavelength

The speed of ultrasound in the soft tissues is about 1500 m/s, similar to that in water. The speed ranges from about 1480 m/s in fat to about 1600 m/s in muscle; an average value of 1540 m/s is generally assumed.

The speed c, the frequency f, and the wavelength λ of ultrasound are related by the equation

$$\lambda = \frac{c}{f} \tag{1}$$

Thus, at a frequency of 1 MHz (1,000,000 cycles per second), the wavelength in soft tissue is about 1.5 mm. This explains why megahertz-frequency ultrasound is used in ultrasonography: In order to obtain a resolution of a millimeter or better, frequencies of 1.5 MHz and above are needed.

Reflection and Scattering

When an ultrasonic wave meets an interface between two media that differ in characteristic impedance, some of the incident wave energy is reflected or scattered. The characteristic impedance Z of a medium is equal to the product of its density ρ and the speed at which ultrasound propagates within it. Thus

$$Z = \rho c \tag{2}$$

The different soft tissues of the body and the constituents that make up different types of soft tissues differ slightly in both respects. Consequently, echoes arise by reflection and scattering from within the tissues as ultrasound travels through them. This means that it is possible to estimate the depths of structures from measurements of time using the well-known pulse-echo technique. The information thus obtained can be displayed in a variety of ways, including real-time two-dimensional images. These images can further be analyzed in terms of tissue movement and three-dimensional relationships.

Absorption and Attenuation

Ultrasonic waves are attenuated as they travel through a medium. Attenuation is due to the combined effects of absorption (the process of conversion of ultrasonic energy to heat) and other mechanisms such as reflection and scattering. The half-power thickness in biologic soft tissue is about 6 cm at a frequency of 1 MHz. Expressed in this way, it is easy to get an idea of what is happening physically to the ultrasonic energy as it propagates through the tissue. When ultrasound is used for diagnosis, however, it is usually more convenient to think of the strength of the ultrasonic wave not in absolute terms but relative to some arbitrarily chosen reference level. This allows signal levels to be compared, and this is most conveniently done in logarithmic units of decibels (dB); thus, for example, halving the power of an ultrasonic wave means that the two waves differ by 3 dB. Expressed mathematically,

$$dB = 10 \log(P_1/P_2) \tag{3}$$

where the relative level of two waves carrying powers of P_1 and P_2, respectively, are described in decibels.

The attenuation of ultrasound in soft tissue is generally about 0.5 dB/cm at 1 MHz, and it increases roughly linearly with frequency. In gases and relatively uncomplicated liquids, the absorption is less at low frequencies than that in soft tissue, but it increases with the square of the frequency.

Because attenuation increases with frequency, there is a practical limit to the maximum frequency that can be used to penetrate any particular distance into the patient. This explains why the resolution of ultrasonography cannot be improved indefinitely simply by increasing the frequency to operate at shorter and shorter wavelengths.

GENERATION AND DETECTION OF ULTRASOUND

Transducers

In ultrasonography, a transducer is required to convert electrical energy into ultrasound for transmission and vice versa for reception. The most commonly used transducer for this purpose is lead zirconate titanate, which is a synthetic ferroelectric ceramic material polarized to give it piezoelectric properties. Although it is an efficient transducer material, lead zirconate titanate has the disadvantage that its characteristic impedance is much greater than that of soft tissues, so much of the ultrasonic energy is reflected at the transducer surface. This effect can be reduced by a suitable matching layer, usually a quarter-wavelength thick, with an intermediate value of characteristic impedance. Even better performance can be obtained if a composite transducer material is used, in which tiny pillars of ferroelectric ceramic are embedded in plastic. The result is a better match between the transducer and the tissue and a wider frequency response, which is an advantage in pulse-echo applications.

Beam Formation

Figure 1 shows a disk transducer and the geometry of the beam that it produces. The near-field length z_N is given by

$$z_N = \frac{a^2}{\lambda} \tag{4}$$

where a is the radius of the transducer. In the far field, the beam diverges at a half-angle ϕ given by

$$\phi = \sin^{-1}(0.61\lambda/a) \tag{5}$$

Consider, for example, a disk with diameter $2a = 10$ mm operating at a frequency of 5 MHz (corresponding to $\lambda = 0.3$); the near-field length is 83 mm, and the half-angle of divergence in the far field is 2.1°.

This description of the beam geometry is rather simplistic. The beam does not really have a sharp edge; in the far field it actually has a roughly Gaussian profile, and in the near field it becomes increasingly inhomogeneous closer to the transducer.

DISK TRANSDUCER

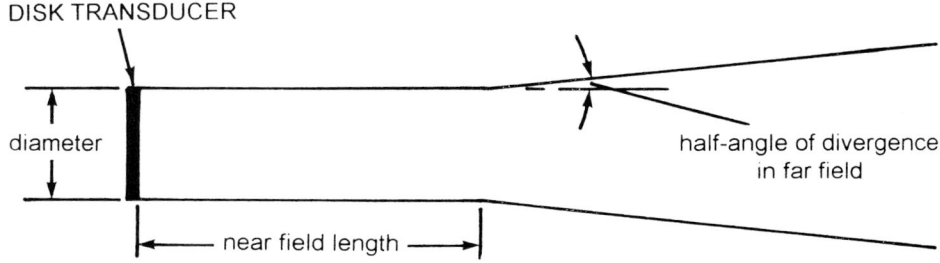

Figure 1. The geometry of the beam produced by a disk transducer. The beam is roughly cylindrical in the near field and diverges in the far field. The dimensions depend on the aperture of the disk in relation to the wavelength.

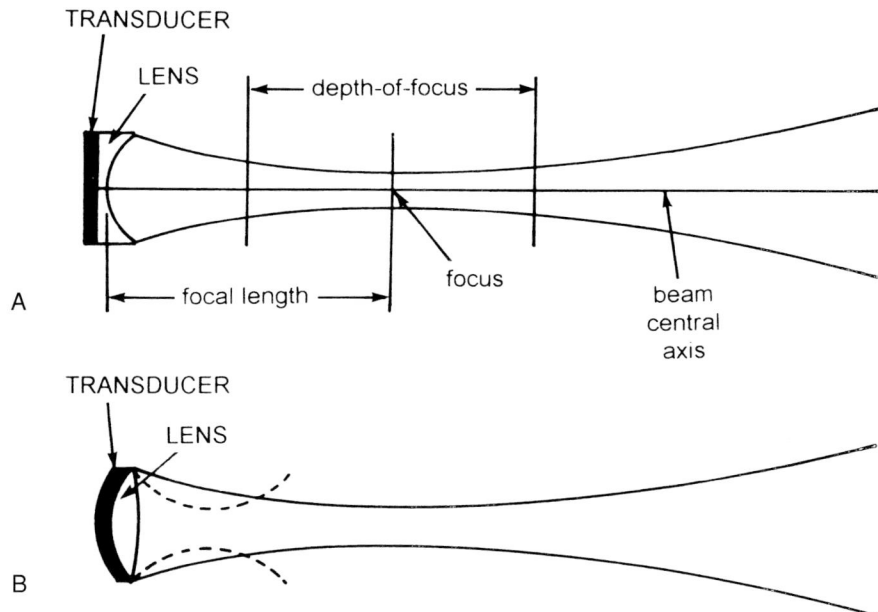

Figure 2. Beam focusing. (**A**) Flat transducer with concave plastic lens. The speed of ultrasound in the lens is higher than that beyond the lens. (**B**) Concave transducer, which by itself produces a strongly focused beam, combined with a convex plastic lens, to form a weakly focused probe with a convex surface.

The beam geometry is the same whether the transducer is operating as a transmitter or as a receiver. When the same transducer is operating both as a transmitter and as a receiver, the transmitting and receiving beams have to be multiplied together to form the combined beam.

Focusing

The width of the beam can be made narrower by focusing. Focused beams are used to provide better resolution.

In the near field of the beam, focusing can be accomplished by means of a lens, as shown in Fig. 2A. The lens works by refraction. When a beam is incident at an angle θ_i on the interface between two media,

$$\frac{\sin \theta_i}{\sin \theta_t} = \frac{c_i}{c_t} \tag{6}$$

where θ_t is the angle of transmission beyond the interface, and c_i and c_t are the speeds on the incident and transmission sides, respectively. With a flat transducer, the lens has to be concave if, as is usually the case, the speed in the lens is greater than that in tissue.

Because a concave surface is difficult to maintain in contact with skin, the approach illustrated in Fig. 2B is often used. A concave transducer, which would produce the strongly focused beam shown by the dashed lines, is combined with a convex plastic lens. The surface of the probe is convex, and the resulting beam is weakly focused as required for ultrasonography.

Note that the focal length with a lens is at a fixed distance from the transducer and that focusing narrows the beam only over a limited depth of focus.

Transducer Arrays

Although the focusing action of a lens can be explained by considering the refraction of rays originating from every point on the transducer surface, there is an equivalent

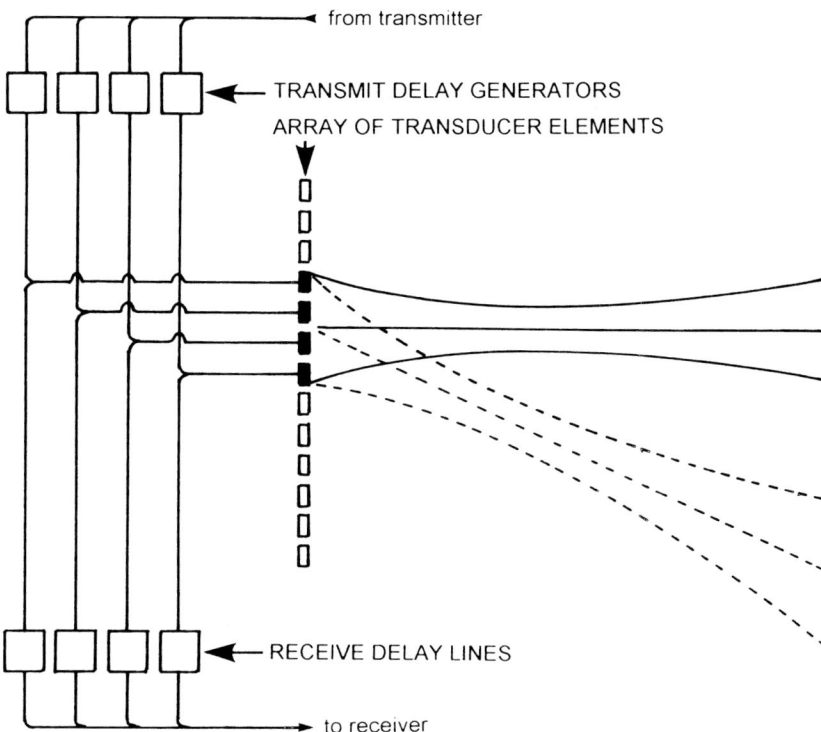

from transmitter

TRANSMIT DELAY GENERATORS

ARRAY OF TRANSDUCER ELEMENTS

RECEIVE DELAY LINES

to receiver

Figure 3. Beam formation with an array of transducer elements. A focused beam can be produced with fixed focal length on transmission and with the focus swept along the beam on reception. The beam can be perpendicular to the array (*solid lines*) or steered through an angle (*dashed lines*).

explanation that provides some additional insight. Every ray that passes through the focus is in phase at the focus. This means that a disturbance that occurs on the surface of the transducer (which can be considered to behave like a piston) arrives at the focus and is delayed by exactly the same time interval along every ray passing through the focus. Thus in Fig. 2A the path length from the transducer to the focus increases as the distance from the beam central axis increases, but the correspondingly increasing thickness of the lens, in which the speed is higher, means that the time for a disturbance to travel from any point on the surface of the transducer to the focus is the same.

With this explanation it should be easy to understand how an array of small transducer elements can be used to focus and steer an ultrasonic beam. Figure 3 shows a section through an array of small transducer elements. Typically, each element in the array has a width of about half a wavelength and a length of 10 wavelengths. At any particular time, a group of transducer elements (such as that shown by solid black in Fig. 3) is in operation. This means that the transducer aperture can be large enough to produce a narrow ultrasonic beam. The signal from the transmitter excites all the transmit delay generators simultaneously. By grading the time delays across the transducer elements in the active aperture, the transmitted beam can be focused (shown by continuous lines in Fig. 3) or steered through an angle as well as being focused (shown by dashed lines). Likewise, on reception, appropriate adjustment of the receive delay lines can focus and steer the beam. Although the beam geometry is necessarily fixed on transmission according to the selected transmit delay generators, on reception, the position of the focus can be driven dynamically along the central axis by continuous variation of the receive delay lines.

The arrangement shown in Fig. 3 is called a *linear array.* The position of the aperture from which the beam originates can be stepped in small intervals along the array, one element at a time. By alternately using even and odd numbers of elements to form the aperture, the step distance can be half the spacing between adjacent elements. If the array is given a convex profile (a curvilinear transducer array), the beam directions along the array trace out a sector pattern. If beam steering is used, with no stepping along the array, a sector scan is produced; this is *phased-array operation.*

PULSE-ECHO TECHNIQUES

General Principles

The time delay τ between the transmission of a pulse of ultrasound into a patient and the reception of its echo from a reflecting or scattering target is a direct measure of the distance d between the transducer and the target. Thus

$$d = 2\tau c \tag{7}$$

because the ultrasound has to travel twice the distance in order to complete the go-and-return round trip.

There are two other pieces of information that can be obtained. First, because the ultrasound travels along a beam, the position of the target within the patient can be determined. Second, the amplitude and structure of the echo signal provide some insight into the characteristics of the target and the attenuation in the overlying tissue.

In a pulse-echo system, the volume of tissue within which the physical interaction occurs that provides the echo signal is called the *resolution cell* or the *sample volume.* Its dimensions depend on the local geometry of the beam and the duration of the ultrasonic pulse, as well as on the dynamic range of the system. Within this dynamic range, changes in echo amplitude produce changes in the appearance of the information that is displayed.

> Typically, the dynamic range is set at about 100 dB. This is determined by the noise arising from the electrical circuitry of the receiver (which limits the detection of weak echoes) and by the maximum ultrasonic intensity that can be transmitted into the patient. The choice of the maximum intensity is likely to be influenced by safety considerations (including the problem of transducer heating and the risk of burning the patient's skin) and by the nonlinearity that occurs in the propagation of finite-amplitude waves. This nonlinearity results in the formation of shock waves that have a sawtooth shape and which are attenuated more rapidly than sine waves, thus limiting any potential gain in penetration at a given frequency.

The A-Scope

Figure 4 is a block diagram of the simplest kind of ultrasonic diagnostic instrument. It is called an *A-scope,* using the terminology of radar and sonar. The clock produces a continuous sequence of regularly-spaced pulses at the pulse repetition rate (PRF) of the system. Each pulse from the clock triggers the transmitter to produce a brief electrical impulse that causes the transducer in the probe to emit an ultrasonic pulse into the patient. As this pulse travels through the patient, changes in characteristic impedance along the beam give rise to echoes that return to the transducer, where they are converted into electrical signals that are amplified and rectified in the receiver. Simultaneously with the transmission of the ultrasonic pulse into the patient, the clock also triggers the timebase generator that is connected to the horizontal deflection plates of the cathode-ray tube. The output from the receiver is connected to the vertical deflection plates. As shown in Fig. 4, vertical deflections of the horizontal timebase trace corresponding to the echo-producing targets lying along the ultrasound beam. Because of the attenuation of ultrasound as it travels through tissue, echoes from deeper structures are increasingly attenuated. Correction for this is provided by the swept gain generator, which, after triggering by the clock, progressively increases the gain of the receiver with time.

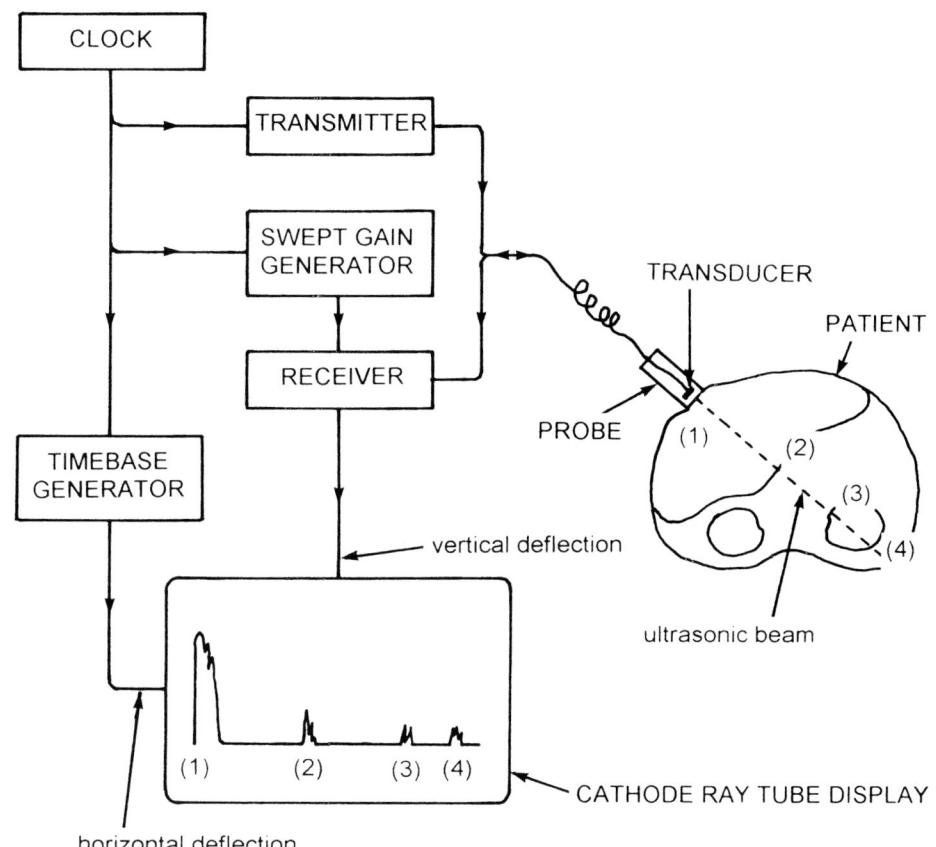

Figure 4. The A-scope. The ultrasonic beam intercepts numbered interfaces in the patient, and the same numbers indicate the corresponding echoes on the display.

The maximum PRF falls as the depth of penetration increases. This is a necessary constraint to avoid the ambiguity that could be caused by echoes resulting from the previous ultrasonic pulse being displayed erroneously during the reception of echoes from the current pulse. Consider, for example, a penetration of 150 mm. The time delay from the transmission of an ultrasonic pulse to the reception of the echo from a target at this range is 200 μs. To avoid ambiguity, the corresponding maximum PRF is 5000 Hz. Such a high PRF is, of course, well above the 16 Hz or so necessary for the persistence of vision to ensure a flicker-free display of an A-scan.

Time-Position Recording

In the preceding section, the description of the A-scope makes no mention of what happens if target structures move along the ultrasonic beam. It should be obvious that such movement is evident as change in the positions of corresponding registrations on the horizontal timebase.

As an alternative to arranging for echo signals to deflect the timebase trace, the brightness of the timebase can be controlled so that spots of light appear on an invisible line whenever echoes are received. In this kind of display, there is no deflection of the timebase. Just as the positions of deflections can change on an A-scan, so these bright spots move on the timebase to correspond to structure motion along the ultrasonic beam.

This kind of brightness-modulated display forms the basis of the time-position (M-mode) recording system shown in Fig. 5. The ultrasonic timebase is connected to the vertical deflection plates of the cathode-ray tube. Bright spots appear on the display, spaced vertically downward with increasing depth of penetration into the patient. A slow timebase generator, which may be free-running or triggered, for example, from the ECG,

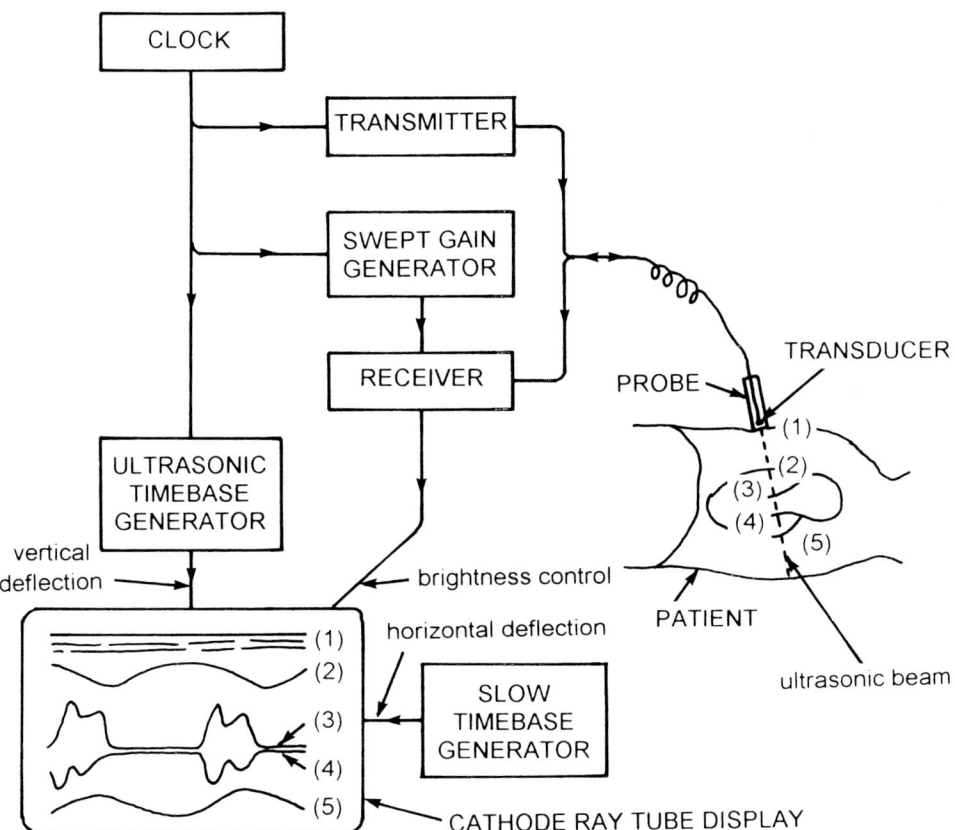

Figure 5. Time-position (M-mode) recording system. The ultrasonic beam intercepts numbered interfaces in the patient, and the same numbers indicate the corresponding echoes on the display.

drives the vertical timebase from left to right across the display; typically, a single sweep occupies 4 or 5 s. As shown in Fig. 5, time-position waveforms appear on the display, tracing out the motion of anatomic structures along the ultrasonic beam.

Although (as explained in the preceding section) the maximum PRF for unambiguous display is quite high (typically 5000 Hz), a higher PRF may be desirable if the fine details of motion of a high-velocity target are to be studied. It may then be acceptable to operate at a higher PRF, since echoes spuriously placed on the display often can be identified as being anatomically unreal.

Two-Dimensional Scanning

A two-dimensional image can be produced by scanning an ultrasonic beam through a tissue plane within the patient and displaying the received echoes on a brightness-modulated timebase that is linked spatially to the position and direction of the beam. An example of how this can be done with a curvilinear transducer array is illustrated in Fig. 6. The ultrasonic pulse-echo system consists of the clock, the transmitter, the transducer, the swept-gain-controlled receiver, and the cathode-ray-tube display. The switching circuits sequentially select groups of transducer elements along the array and produce beams in a sector-scan format. These switching circuits also control the amplitudes of the vertical and horizontal timebase generators so that the resulting timebase is appropriately positioned on the display.

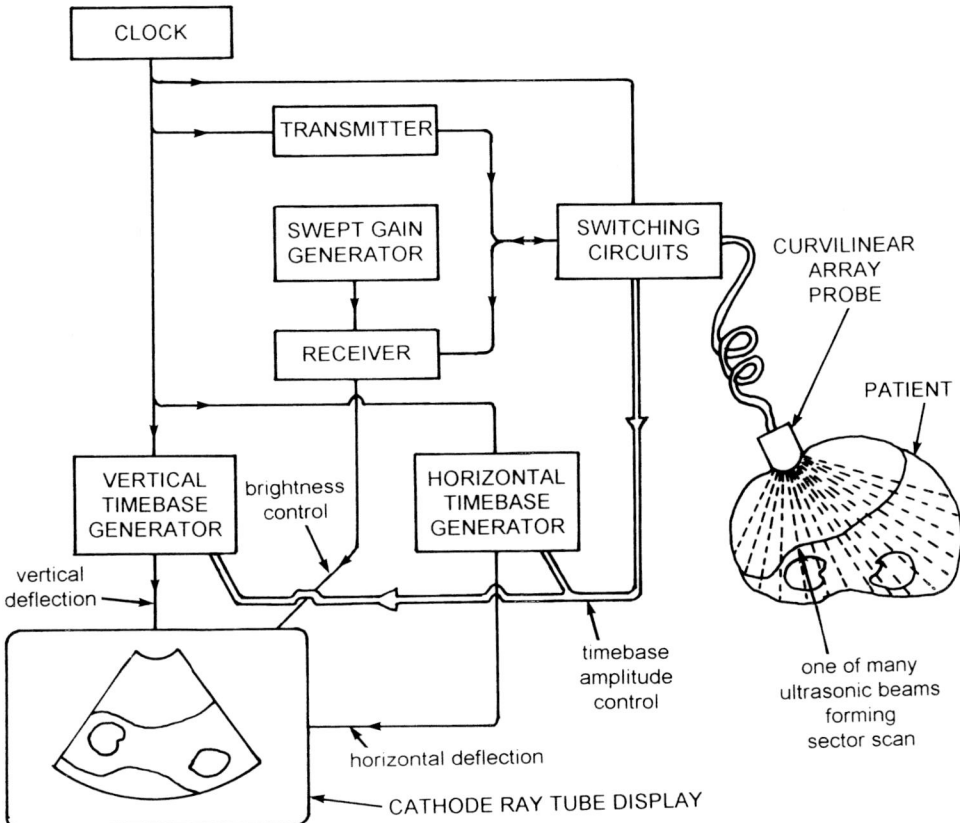

Figure 6. Two-dimensional B-scanning. In this typical arrangement, a curvilinear transducer produces a real-time sector scan.

There are numerous other methods by which the ultrasonic beam can be scanned in the two-dimensional plane. For example, a single-disk transducer can be oscillated mechanically to form a sector scan, or several disk transducers can be mounted on the rim of a wheel that is rotated continuously so that each transducer in turn sweeps across the same sector. Other possibilities are to use a linear-array transducer to produce a scan with a rectangular format or a phased-array transducer with beam steering in a sector format. With very small probes, for example, for intravascular use, radial scanning can be achieved either by the continuous rotation of a tiny disk transducer or by electronic control of a minute cylindrical array.

The maximum PRF is controlled by the required penetration, as explained earlier. In principle, a separate line of image information can be acquired with the transmission of each ultrasonic pulse. This is the situation if the beam is moved to a new position in the scan plane following the acquisition of each pulse-echo wave train. If the maximum PRF is 5000 Hz (corresponding to a penetration of 150 mm), and if, for example, 100 lines of pulse-echo information are used to form an image, images can be displayed at a frame rate of 50 per second. There are more lines per frame at lower frame rates, and vice versa.

DOPPLER TECHNIQUES

The Doppler Effect

Ultrasound reflected or scattered by a stationary target has the same frequency as that of the incident ultrasound. If the target is moving toward the source of ultrasound, however, the reflected waves have to be compressed into a decreasing space. Consequently, the wavelength is shortened and the frequency is shifted upward. The opposite occurs if the target is moving away from the source. The phenomenon is called the *Doppler effect*. The difference f_D between the transmitted frequency f and the received frequency is given by

$$f_D = 2v(\cos \theta)f/c \tag{8}$$

where v is the speed at which the target is moving, and θ is the angle between the directions of the target motion and the ultrasonic beam.

> Equation (8) is only an approximation. It is applicable provided that $v^2 \ll c^2$, which is generally the case with targets moving at physiologic velocities within the body.

It turns out that the Doppler shift frequency generally lies in the audible range when low-megahertz-frequency ultrasound is used to study motion and flow within the body. For example, if the ultrasonic frequency is 3 MHz and the target velocity is 1 m/s along the direction of the ultrasonic beam, $f_D = 4$ kHz. This is a very fortunate eventuality, since it means that the investigator can listen to the Doppler signals and thereby gain a good deal of useful information.

Continuous-Wave Doppler Techniques

The description of the Doppler effect given in the preceding section is directly applicable to continuously transmitted or interrupted ultrasonic waves. Figure 7 shows how

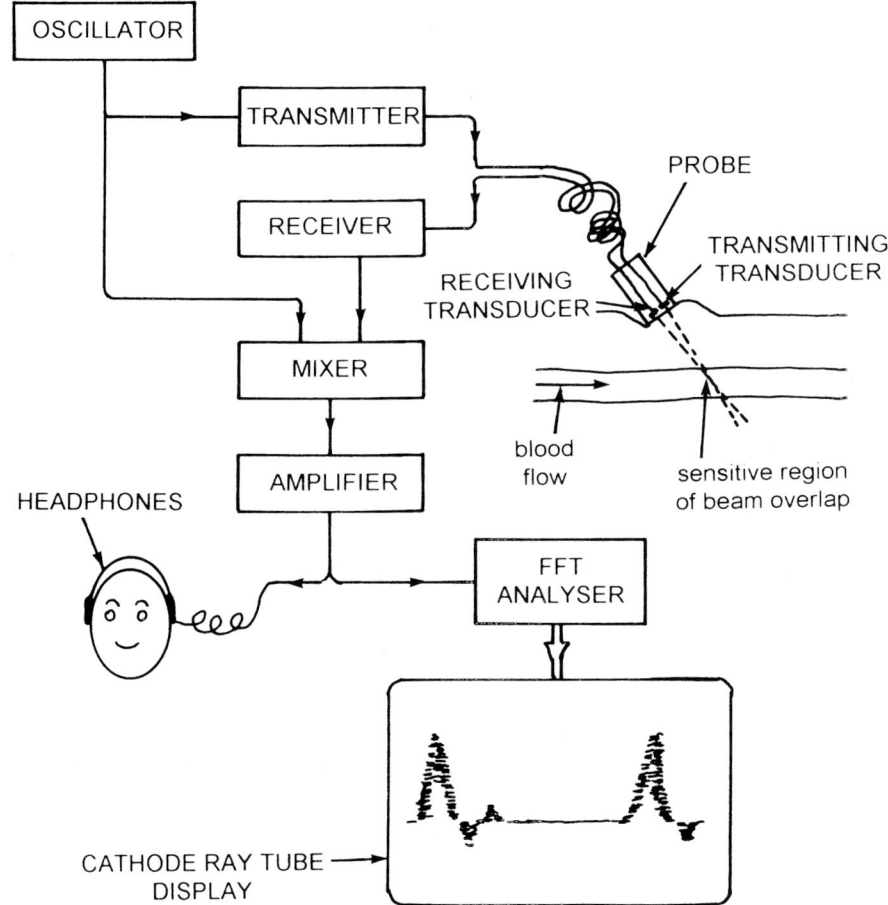

Figure 7. Continuous-wave Doppler system. The output from the amplifier consists of the audible Doppler signals, which also can be subjected to fast Fourier transform (FFT) analysis and displayed on the cathode-ray tube as a frequency spectrogram.

the Doppler effect is used in a simple ultrasonic instrument to give information about, for example, the velocity of blood flow.

The oscillator produces a continuous sine wave at the required ultrasonic frequency. The output from the oscillator is amplified by the transmitter and applied to the transmitting transducer, which is one of two transducers mounted side by side within the probe. The beams of these two transducers cross over at some appropriate distance within the patient. Targets lying in the region where the beams overlap give rise to echoes that are detected by the receiving transducer, the electrical output from which is amplified by the receiver. The mixer is a circuit that produces an output the amplitude of which corresponds to the strength of the echoes received from moving structures in the beam and the frequency of which is the corresponding Doppler shift frequency. This signal is amplified and fed to headphones worn by the investigator. Figure 7 shows how this signal can be subjected to fast Fourier transform analysis to provide a display of the frequency spectrum of the Doppler signal.

Separate transducers are usually used for the transmission and reception of ultrasound. Because ultrasound is transmitted without interruption, the transmitting signal would swamp the receiver if the same transducer were used for both functions. The circuit illustrated in Fig. 7 actually includes a technique for detecting the direction of the target motion (e.g., of the blood flow). In the interests of clarity, however, details of this technique are not shown. If the motion of the target is toward the probe, the received frequency is greater than that of the transmitter, whereas it is lower if the motion is in the reverse direction. Whether the received frequency is more or less than the transmitted frequency can be determined by the process of phase-quadrature detection. A fuller version of Fig. 7 would show this process in advance of the amplifier. That the system does have directional detection is evident from the forward and reverse flow that can be seen on the display of the frequency spectrum.

It is quite easy to understand how the Doppler effect gives rise to a detectable signal when the target is a simple reflector intercepted by the ultrasonic beam. When blood is the target, however, the situation is more complicated. This is so because blood can be considered to consist of numerous small scattering targets, each of which scatters ultrasound isotropically, that are randomly oriented. The ultrasound backscattered by blood and detected by the receiving transducer is the result of interference between the multiplicity of coherently scattered spherical wavelets, having a maximum value when the interference is constructive and a minimum value when it is destructive. Therefore, the received signal can be thought of as originating from an ensemble of red cells that happen to be oriented with respect to each other and to the ultrasonic beam in such a way that they interfere constructively. Because of the dynamic conditions, such ensemble-produced signals are subject to fading at a frequency related to the rate of rearrangement of cells within the sample volume of the ultrasonic beam.

The scattering power of a target that is very small in relation to the wavelength of the ultrasound satisfies the Rayleigh condition. It increases with the fourth power of the frequency. This is roughly the situation with an isolated red cell (diameter about 8 μm) with low-megahertz-frequency ultrasound (wavelength around 500 μm). When considering the ultrasonic frequency that gives rise to the strongest Doppler signal from blood, however, the situation is complicated by the attenuation of ultrasound in overlying tissue. This increases with frequency, eventually mitigating against the increase in the scattering power of blood. In practice, the best results are usually obtained when the ultrasonic frequency selected for Doppler studies is somewhat less than that which gives optimal imaging performance at the same depth of penetration.

Pulsed Doppler Techniques

It is only because the ultrasonic beam of a continuous-wave Doppler probe is directional that it can be used to obtain clinically useful information. The investigator knows through what anatomic structures the beam is likely to be passing and the nature of the Doppler signals to which they are likely to give rise. There is no depth selectivity, however, except for that due to the effects of attenuation and the geometry of the beam crossover region.

Depth selectivity can be obtained with a pulsed Doppler system, which combines the pulse-echo method for distance measurement with the Doppler method for velocity measurement. The principles are illustrated in Fig. 8. As in a pulse-echo system (see above), the clock determines the PRF. The oscillator runs continuously, and the transmitter gate, which allows the oscillator to excite the transducer, is opened by sequential clock pulses but only for an interval controlled by the transmit sample length generator. The echo wave train is detected by the same transducer and amplified to produce a signal that is

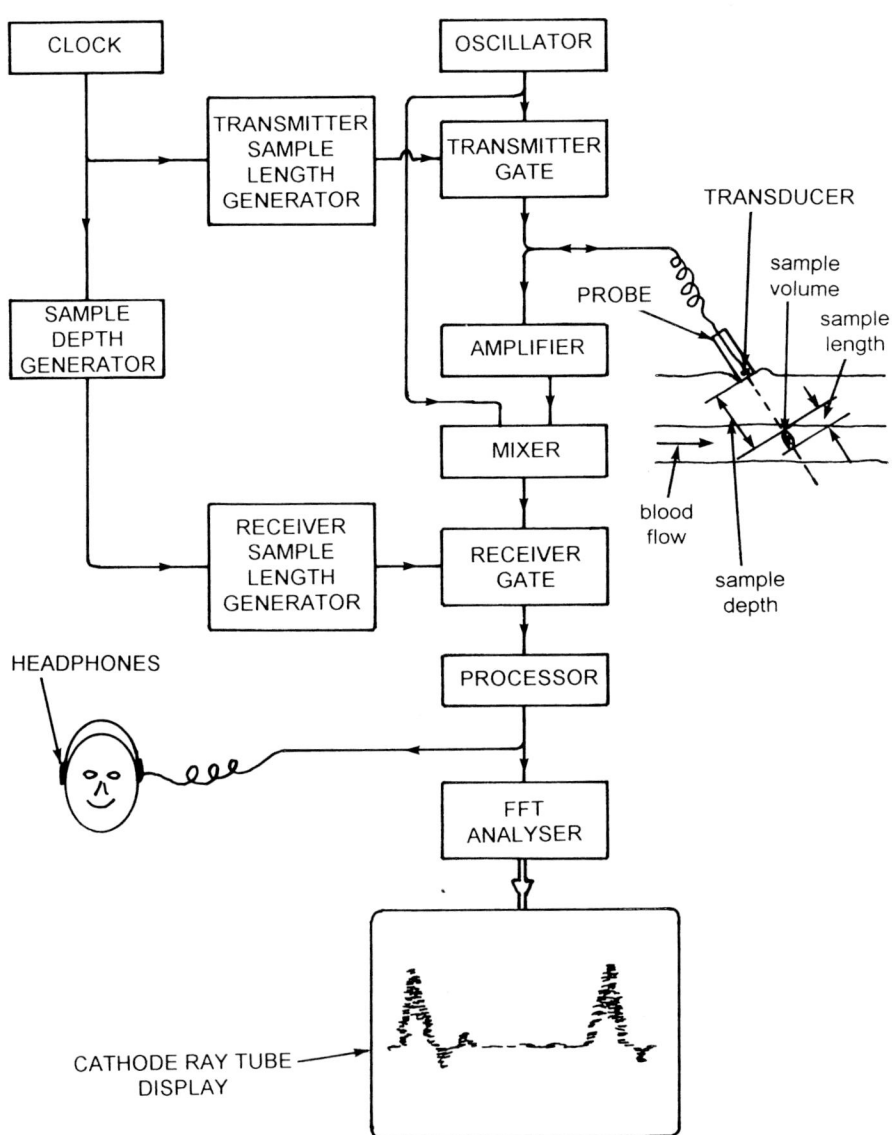

Figure 8. Pulsed Doppler system. The depth and length of the sample volume are under the control of the operator. In a multigated pulsed Doppler system, multiple receiver gates are triggered sequentially to acquire Doppler signals from a series of contiguous samples to display, for example, the flow velocity profile across the blood vessel.

mixed with another signal derived directly from the oscillator and, consequently, equal in frequency to that of the transmitter pulse of ultrasound. Therefore, the output from the mixer is a wave train that is identical in successive wave trains where it corresponds to echoes from stationary structures but changing according to the Doppler effect where it originates from moving targets. It now only remains to extract the Doppler signals from the chosen region of interest. This is done by the sample depth generator, which causes the receiver sample length generator to open the receiver gate for an interval equal to the ultrasonic pulse length, after a delay corresponding to the desired sample length. The processor samples consecutive outputs from the receiver gate and is updated with the reception of each successive echo wave train. Thus the output from the processor is the Doppler signal from the sample volume. Phase-quadrature detection (not shown in Fig. 8 but explained earlier) separates forward- and reverse-flow signals, either for the investigator to hear or for fast Fourier transform analysis and display as a frequency spectrum.

> Because it samples the Doppler shift frequency at a rate equal to the system PRF, a pulsed Doppler instrument can unambiguously estimate the target velocity only if the Doppler shift frequency is less than half the PRF. This result is an example of the application of the Nyquist criterion. The problem can be ameliorated by increasing the angle between the directions of motion and of the ultrasonic beam (not a desirable solution because of the difficulty of estimating the angle with a diverging or converging beam) or by reducing the ultrasonic frequency. Sometimes, however, it is acceptable to use a PRF that is less than twice the Doppler frequency. This is the case when any resulting ambiguity is easily recognized.

COMBINED IMAGING AND PULSED DOPPLER STUDIES

Duplex Scanning

By combining real-time two-dimensional scanning for structure visualization with the pulsed Doppler technique for motion and flow studies within a spatially controllable sample volume, an instrument known as a *duplex scanner* is realized. The principles are illustrated in Fig. 9. In the interest of clarity, the timing circuitry is omitted from this diagram; suffice it to say that there is a clock that controls the PRF and which provides synchronizing signals for the beam-steering, pulsed Doppler, and two-dimensional imaging subsystems.

As shown in Fig. 10 and Color Plate 47, the display consists of a real-time two-dimensional scan superimposed on which is an electronically generated marker that shows the position and extent of the Doppler sample volume on the scan line selected by the operator. With electronic beam steering, it is easy to arrange the switching circuitry to share the available time between imaging and Doppler signal acquisition so that both appear to proceed simultaneously. With mechanical beam steering, this may be more difficult (because of the mechanical inertia of the scanning transducer assembly, which may make it hard to stop and to start the scanning motion sufficiently rapidly). Note that it may be possible, as illustrated in Fig. 9, to adjust another marker on the display so that it is aligned, for example, with the direction of blood flow. By this means, the cosine correction factor in Eq. (8) may be automatically taken into account. In this way, the display of the Doppler frequency spectrum can be in units of velocity rather than frequency.

Color-Flow Imaging

It should be obvious that the flow conditions could be studied at every point (or sample volume) in a two-dimensional image by systematic control of a duplex scanner. The procedure, however, would be both slow and tedious.

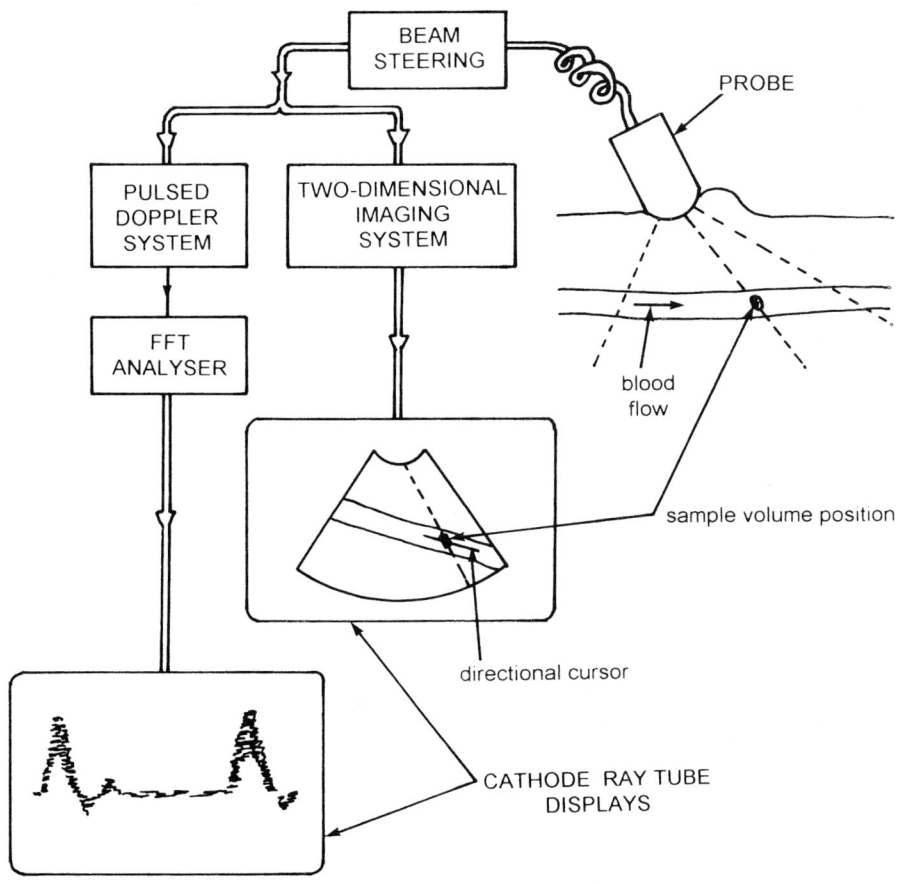

Figure 9. Duplex system for combined real-time two-dimensional imaging and pulsed Doppler flow detection. The operator can position the Doppler sample volume anywhere within the scanned area, which, in this example, has a sector format.

Figure 10. Display of information obtained by duplex scanning. In this example, a color-flow image of a normal common carotid artery (coded according to velocity) is shown in the upper part of the display; the dotted line shows the beam direction for acquisition of Doppler signals from the sample volume, the position and size of which are indicated by the superimposed yellow box. The lower part of the display shows the Doppler frequency spectrum over about six cardiac cycles. See also Color Plate 47. (Courtesy of M. Halliwell.)

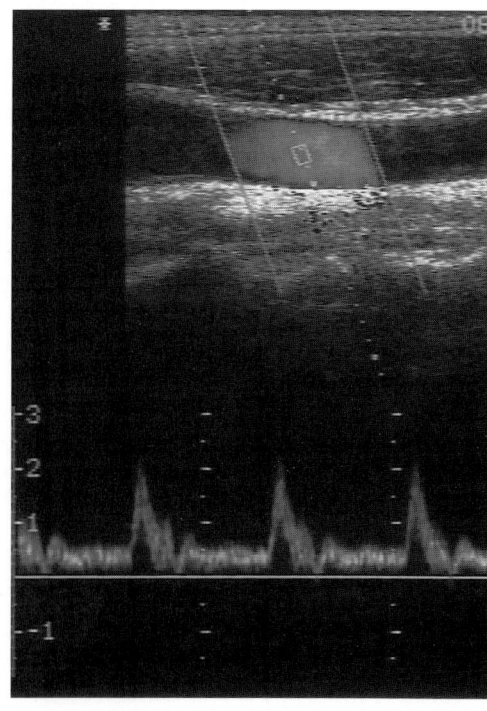

The real-time flow imaging system can employ any one of several detection schemes, two of which are described below.

Frequency-Domain Processing

The most commonly used scheme is the *autocorrelation detector*. This closely resembles the traditional Doppler approach, and processing can be considered to be in the frequency (or phase) domain. In brief, the signal from the receiver amplifier is split into two paths. One path leads directly to one input to a multiplying circuit. The other path is fed through a delay line that introduces a delay exactly equal to the interval between consecutively transmitted ultrasonic pulses. The output from this delay line leads to the other input to the multiplier. By this means, consecutive echo wave trains are multiplied together. Where these two wave trains are identical, there is no change in the output from the multiplier from pulse to pulse. When the waveforms differ because of motion along the ultrasonic beam, however, there is a phase change so that the output from the multiplier corresponds to the Doppler shift frequency. The values of Doppler shift frequency along each ultrasonic beam are discretely sampled to control the color assigned to the pixels in the image.

Frequency-domain processing is a narrow-band technique. The sensitivity is high, the ultrasonic intensity during the pulse is not particularly high, and the axial (or range) resolution is correspondingly poor.

In order to estimate the Doppler frequencies along any line in the image, the ultrasonic beam has to dwell for long enough to allow the lowest frequency to be sampled for at least a substantial part of a cycle. Moreover, each single estimate requires three ultrasonic pulses to be transmitted; strictly speaking, the detection scheme measures the pulse-pair covariance.

As far as higher Doppler frequencies are concerned, the detection scheme is subject to aliasing whenever the Nyquist limit is exceeded.

Time-Domain Processing

Time-domain processing for motion and flow detection resembles the approach adopted for time-position recording (see above). Successive echo wave trains are cross-correlated to extract information about the changing time delays between the transmission of individual ultrasonic pulses and the reception of echoes from diagnostic targets lying along the ultrasonic beam. If the targets are stationary, the corresponding time differences are equal to zero. The time difference increases with the velocities of the targets.

Time-domain processing is a broad-band technique. This means that in order to obtain adequate sensitivity, the ultrasonic pulse intensity has to be high, but the axial resolution is correspondingly good.

Comparison Between Frequency- and Time-Domain Processing

The protagonists of the different approaches to processing for color-flow imaging are inclined to adopt polarized positions concerning the merits of their method and the disadvantages of the method of their competitors. A fundamental difference between the two approaches is that frequency-domain processing is a narrow-band technique, whereas time-domain processing is a broad-band technique.

The conditions under which aliasing can occur and the relative sensitivities and exposures with the two methods were mentioned earlier in this box. Another important characteristic of performance is the image frame rate that can be obtained when low-velocity flow is being examined. With frequency-domain processing, the ultrasonic beam has to dwell in each position in the scan plane for long enough to allow the Doppler frequency to be estimated. For example, if the flow velocity is, say, 10 mm/s and the ultrasonic frequency is 3 MHz, the corresponding Doppler frequency is 40 Hz. This means that a single cycle of Doppler signal occupies 2.5 ms and that is likely to be about the minimum satisfactory beam dwell time. Thus, if there are 128 lines in the image (which, again, is about the minimum likely to be acceptable), the image frame time is 320 ms, which is equivalent to an image frame rate of just over 3 per second. This hardly merits the eulogy of real time! With time-domain processing, however, there is no fundamental limit on the lowest velocity that can be estimated by transmitting two separate pulses. Allowing for a penetration of, for example, 150 mm, the maximum PRF is 5000 Hz (see above). This means that the beam has only to dwell for 0.4 ms and, with 128 lines in the image, the corresponding frame rate is nearly 20 per second. Although this seems to be much better than can be achieved with frequency-domain processing, the performance of time-domain processing deteriorates rapidly in the presence of increasing noise in the signal, and in practice, this severely affects the detection of low velocities.

Figure 11 shows how the two-dimensional distribution of flow can be mapped and superimposed on a two-dimensional anatomic image (40). Because the flow imaging system is fast, the display can be in real time, at least when the flow velocities are moderately high. The two-dimensional anatomic image is displayed in gray scale. The flow image, however, is coded in color.

Color-Coding Schemes

The output from the color-flow imaging system contains information about the velocity of blood flow (or structure motion), the direction of flow, and the strength of the flow signal (which is at least related to the amount of flowing blood). In modern color-flow

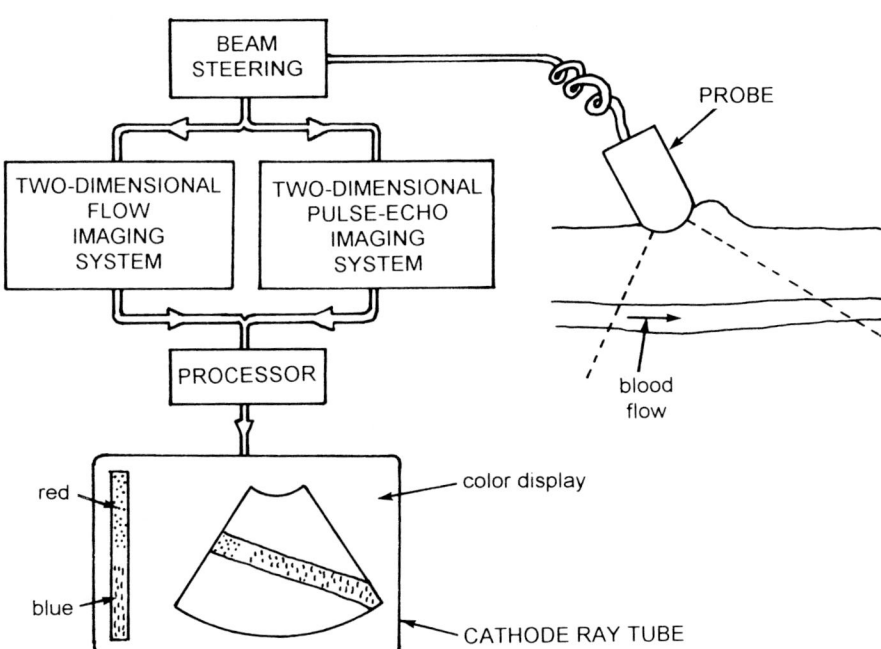

Figure 11. Color-flow imaging system. In this general diagram, the flow imaging system is typically based either on frequency- (phase) or time-domain processing. An image color coded according to velocity is illustrated. An alternative coding scheme is based on the power (or strength) of the flow signal.

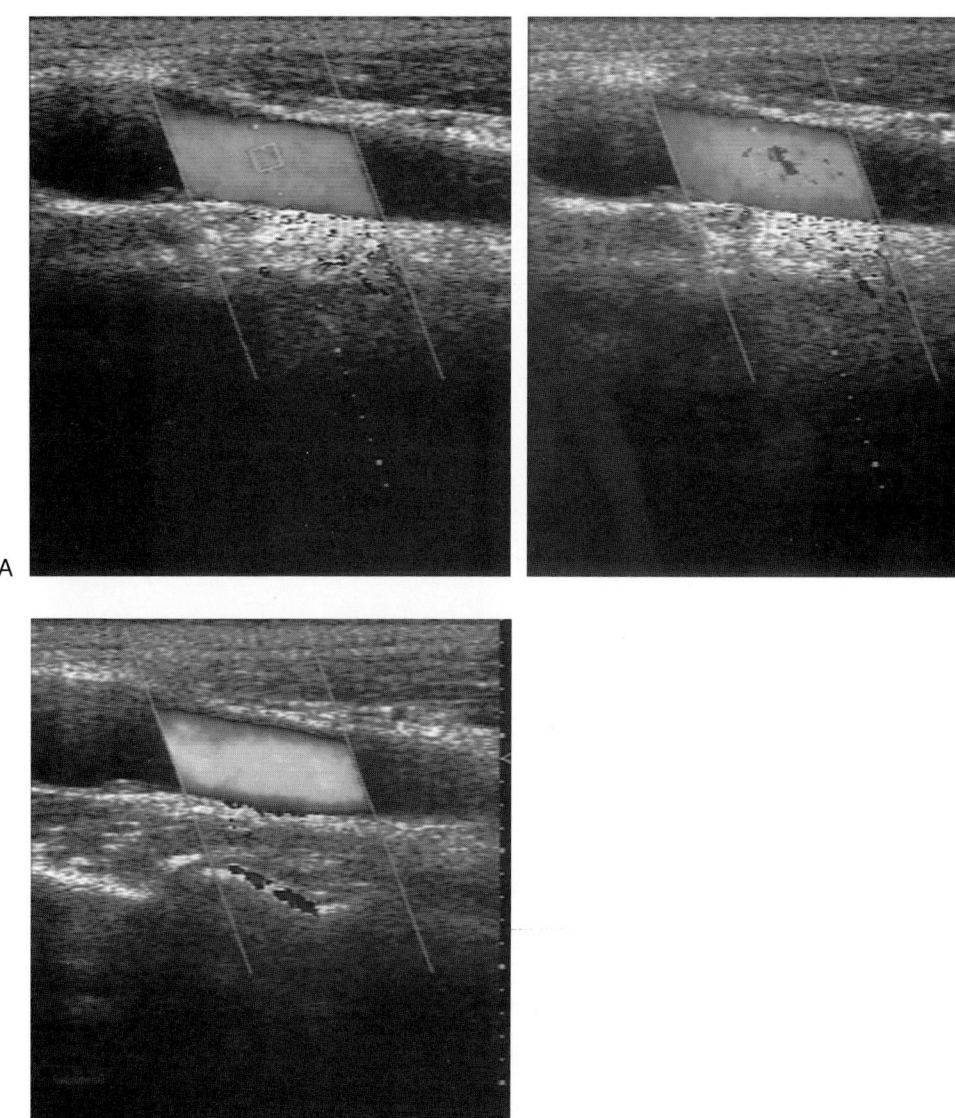

Figure 12. Examples of Doppler color-flow scans of a normal common carotid artery. A linear-array scanner was used, with the beam directed at an angle of about 65° to the flow direction. Blood flow was toward the probe. (**A**) Velocity-flow image. The thin black line that can be seen between the color-coded area and the vessel wall, particularly closer to the probe, is due to the highpass filter that suppresses artefacts due to the large-amplitude, low-frequency Doppler signals from the vessel wall. See Color Plate 48. (**B**) Velocity-flow image at a time during the cardiac cycle when high-velocity blood flow components produced Doppler shift frequencies exceeding the Nyquist limit. This is apparent as the green area in the image, the origin of which is confirmed by the absence of a black line that would be present around the green if it was due to flow reversal. See Color Plate 49. (**C**) Power-flow image, in which flow direction information is absent but which has fewer artefacts and higher sensitivity than the corresponding velocity flow image. See Color Plate 50. (Courtesy of M. Halliwell.)

scanners, information can be selected and displayed in two different ways, as illustrated in Fig. 12 and Color Plates 48, 49, and 50.

First, the velocity and direction of flow can be displayed. This is demonstrated in Fig. 12A. Usually, increasing velocity of flow toward the probe is coded on a scale extending from dark red through bright red to yellow and white. For flow in the reverse direction, the colors are dark blue, light blue, and white. In interpreting color-flow velocity images displayed in this way, it is essential to take into account the relative directions of the ultrasonic beam and the blood flow. This is so because, according to Eq. (8), the Doppler shift frequency depends on the angle between these two directions, besides being determined by the flow velocity itself.

Green is a color that contrasts well with both red and blue. Because of this contrast, green is sometimes used to tag isovelocity lines in the image or to identify regions where there is an unusually large value of velocity variance. Velocity variance is related to flow disturbance or to the presence of turbulence. Green also may be used to display the highest reverse velocities, and the matter is further complicated when the Nyquist limit is exceeded, as shown in Fig. 12B.

The second of the kinds of displays in common use is one in which flow is displayed independent of velocity and direction but with brightness increasing with the strength of the flow signal (29). This is called *power*, or *amplitude*, *flow imaging*, to distinguish it from velocity-flow imaging. It is illustrated in Fig. 12C. Although color lends itself to such a display, monochrome is used, and in fact, gray scale is perfectly satisfactory, since the coded region of the image is obvious because of its relatively poor resolution and lack of fine texture.

Because the low frame rate of practical color-flow imaging systems would be so discouraging if it was self-evident, instrument manufacturers use various strategies to disguise the problem. Color coding only part of the image is an obvious and straightforward scheme. Less obvious to the user and potentially misleading, although commonly used, is the acquisition of widely spaced lines with computer-calculated interpolation to fill the gaps in the image.

EXTRACTION OF FUNCTIONAL INFORMATION

In this section, various approaches to the extraction of functional information from data acquired by ultrasonography are introduced. Emphasis is given to the analytical methods; clinical applications are mentioned only by way of illustration.

Structure Motion

Essentially, there are two approaches to the ultrasonographic study of structure motion. These are described in the following subsections.

Time-Position Recording

The method of time-position recording was described earlier. It is most applicable to the study of the motion of structures that give rise to well-defined echoes, such as the cusps of the cardiac valves or the walls of blood vessels.

Figure 13A is an example showing how functional information can be extracted from a time-position recording. The normal mitral valve opens rapidly at the beginning of ventricular diastole, after which it begins to close, but with a transient increase in opening in atrial systole, until it closes completely in ventricular systole. Timing can be derived from the ECG in Fig. 13B. Both the amplitude of the excursion of the studied valve cusp and its acceleration can be measured at significant parts of the cardiac cycle. Figure 13A also shows how these two quantities are modified when the function of the valve is affected by disease such as stenosis.

Tissue Doppler Imaging

The time-position recording method is a good way of studying the motion of structures that have well-defined surfaces. The method is not suitable, however, for study of the motion of solid tissues. This is probably best done by the Doppler method (24), although

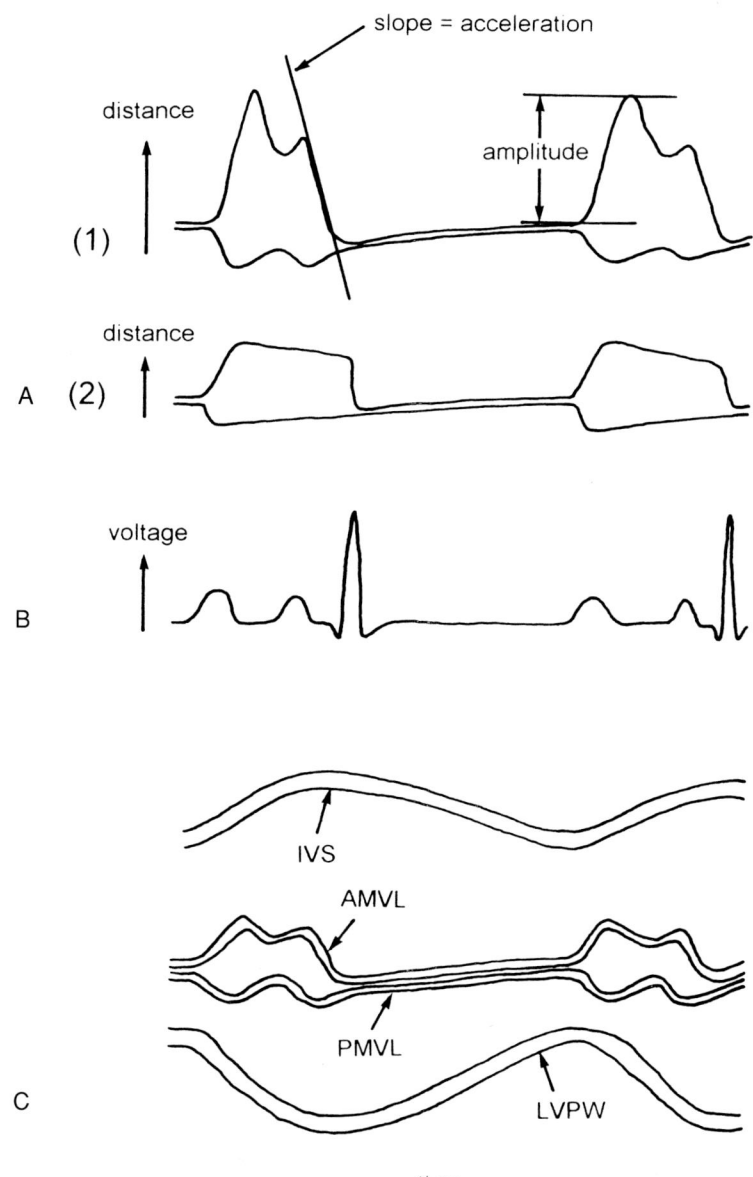

Figure 13. Examples of studies of structure motion. (**A**) Time-position recording of mitral valve motion: (1) normal valve, (2) stenotic valve. (**B**) ECG (for time reference). (**C**) Tissue Doppler imaging of normal heart (*IVS*, interventricular septum; *AMVL*, anterior mitral valve leaflet; *PMVL*, posterior mitral valve leaflet; *LVPW*, left ventricular posterior wall).

some quite encouraging results have been obtained with the alternative technique based on the measurement of the integrated backscatter from tissue (28, 42).

> Color-flow imaging as described earlier is prone to artefacts due to the relatively much higher amplitude of the echoes from solid tissues than those from blood. For blood flow imaging, circuits are built into the instrument to suppress the high-amplitude but relatively stationary echoes from the solid tissues that surround blood vessels. Indeed, it is the performance of these circuits that to a large extent determines how well one instrument compares with another.

Figure 13C represents a tissue Doppler image display like an M-mode recording and emphasizes how this approach allows the motion of the solid tissues of, for example, the interventricular septum and the myocardium to be studied. Moreoever, although not shown in Fig. 13C, the display is color coded according to the velocities of the tissues. Consequently, the instantaneous velocities can be measured in the region of interest by the green tagging method mentioned earlier. It is worth noting in particular that the motion of the myocardium, which reflects this function, may be modified both by regional ischemia due to coronary artery disease and by disturbances in electrical conduction.

Arterial Blood Flow

Blood flow is usually most conveniently studied by ultrasonography using either the continuous-wave (see Fig. 7) or the pulsed technique (see Fig. 8). For superficial arteries and for those in well-established anatomic situations, satisfactory results often can be obtained without the need for imaging guidance. Where this is not possible, however, either duplex (see Fig. 9) or color-flow imaging (see Fig. 11) can be used for vessel localization.

The characteristics of arterial blood flow can be related to normal function and to function modified by local, distal, proximal, or generalized disease. In general, the starting point for analysis is the Doppler frequency spectrum.

Figure 14 represents the arterial trees of the lower limbs; one side is normal, but the other has an artery occluded by atheroma that is bypassed by collaterals. The Doppler signals acquired at points along the arteries can be analyzed in several different ways, the most important of which are discussed in the following subsections.

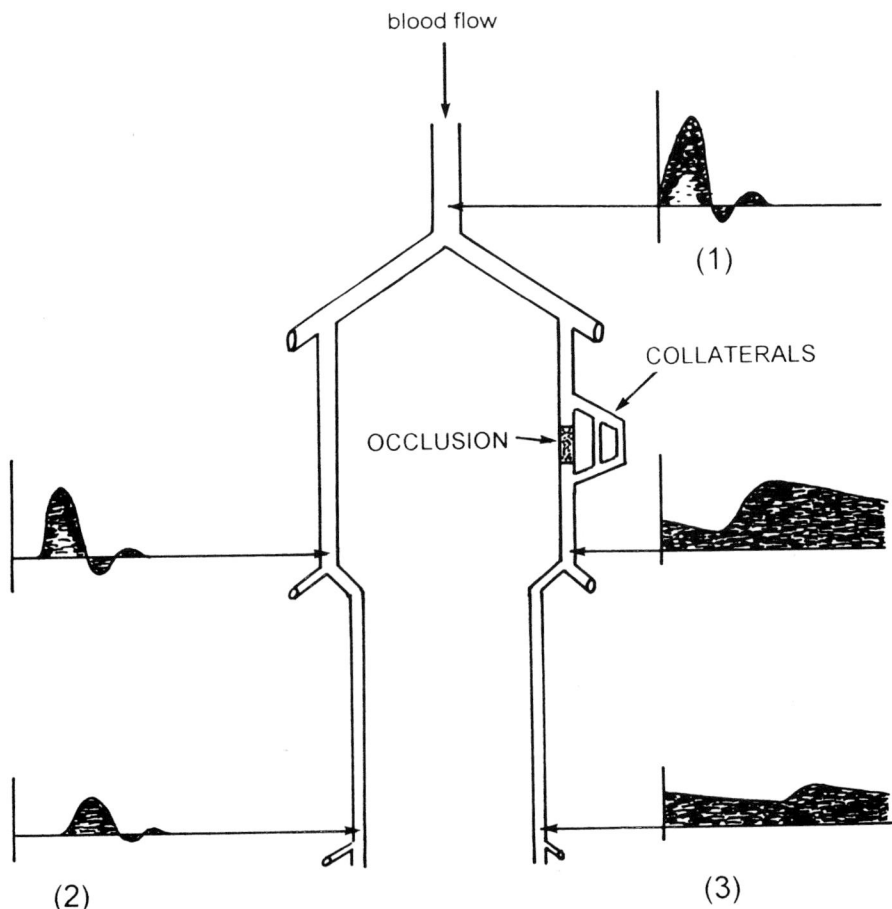

Figure 14. Examples of Doppler spectra acquired at points along typical normal and diseased arterial segments. Numbers against some of the spectra are for identification with the waveforms illustrated in Fig. 15.

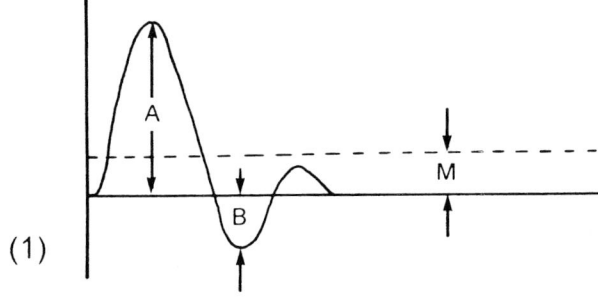

(1)

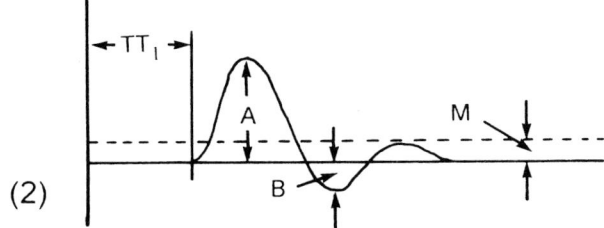

(2)

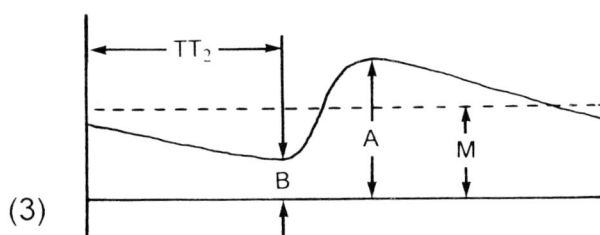

(3)

Figure 15. Examples of maximum (or instantaneous mean) blood flow velocity waveforms acquired at points along typical normal and diseased arterial segments. Numbers against the waveforms are for identification with the spectra illustrated in Fig. 14. Mean flow velocities are indicated by dashed lines.

Pulsatility Indices

The spectra illustrated in Fig. 14 can be processed to provide waveforms of either the maximum or the mean frequencies in the spectra. The maximum frequency is relatively uncontroversial, since it can be extracted by a maximum-frequency follower with a threshold set somewhat above the noise level (17, 33). It does not depend on the geometry of the ultrasonic beam (or the sample volume, if a pulsed Doppler system is used), provided that the beam intercepts the blood that flows at the maximum velocity. This is usually at the center of the vessel, although the situation may be complicated during flow deceleration in larger vessels. The beam geometry does affect the estimate of the mean Doppler frequency, however, if it results in nonuniform insonation of the flowing blood. The mean frequency is likely to be overestimated, since the contribution of the slower-moving blood closer to the vessel wall is then most probably under-represented in the frequency spectrum.

Typical flow velocity waveforms are illustrated in Fig. 15. These waveforms are numbered to correspond to the spectra in Fig. 14. On each of these waveforms, the mean flow velocity is indicated by a dashed line. Several indices are commonly used to describe waveforms like these, as follows:

$$\text{Pulsatility index } (PI) = (A - B)/M \qquad (9)$$

$$\text{Resistance index } (RI) = (A - B)/A \qquad (10)$$

$$\text{Systolic-to-diastolic ratio} = A/B \qquad (11)$$

$$\text{B/A ratio} = B/A \qquad (12)$$

Note that B has negative values in waveforms (1) and (2) in Fig. 15 so that $(A - B)$ is in all cases equal to the magnitude of the peak-to-peak amplitude of the waveform. Also note that calculation of the resistance index (sometimes called the *Pourcelot index*) from

Eq. (10) does not require knowledge of the mean blood flow velocity, which is very convenient.

Transit Time and Damping Factor

In situations where the blood flow velocity pulse can be observed at separate sites along an artery, the transit time TT between the two sites (which may be at the input and output of an arterial segment) can be measured. This is illustrated in Fig. 15, where it can be seen that waveform (2) is associated with a shorter transit time than waveform (3) because the latter has to travel through the collateral pathway. The transit time difference is $(TT_2 - TT_1)$.

Traveling through the collateral pathway also reduces the pulsatility of the waveform. This can be expressed quantitatively as follows:

$$\text{Damping factor } DF = \frac{PI_{input}}{PI_{output}} \qquad (13)$$

where PI_{input} is the pulsatility index at the input to the segment, and PI_{output} is that at the output. Similarly, for transit times,

$$\text{Transit time ratio TTR} = \frac{TT_2}{TT_2 - TT_1} \qquad (14)$$

Principal Components Analysis

Waveform shapes can be fully described most economically in terms of their principal components (23). This approach resembles Fourier analysis, but instead of using series of sine and cosine waves, the set of coefficients is selected to describe the corresponding waveforms most efficiently, i.e., with the minimum number of terms to give the required goodness of fit. The coefficients that result from this analysis cannot be interpreted in terms of physiologic or functional properties of the flow or of the vessels. They merely provide a mathematical description of the flow-velocity waveforms so that differences between waveforms can be quantitated. The relevance of such differences has to be established by correlation with measurement of relevant function made by other methods.

Laplace Transform Analysis

Developing an idea introduced earlier, the time-velocity waveform can indeed be transferred into the frequency domain by Fourier analysis. Once in the frequency domain, waveforms such as those illustrated in Fig. 15 have been found to fit quite well to a third-order Laplace equation (34). This is simply a mathematical tool, but it has the advantage over principal components analysis that the three coefficients of the Laplace transform do relate respectively to the arterial stiffness, distal impedance, and proximal lumen size.

Doppler Spectral Analysis

Examination of the Doppler frequency spectrum can give some insight into the characteristics of the blood flow at the observed site. An example of this is illustrated in Fig. 16. The Doppler spectrum from a normal carotid artery does not exhibit a large spread of velocities coexisting simultaneously, and the dichrotic notch is clearly visible. In the region of a stenosis, however, the frequency spectrum is modified (35). Minor degrees of stenosis result in broadening of the spectrum. As the stenosis becomes tighter, the degree of broadening increases with the increasing flow disturbance, and the systolic

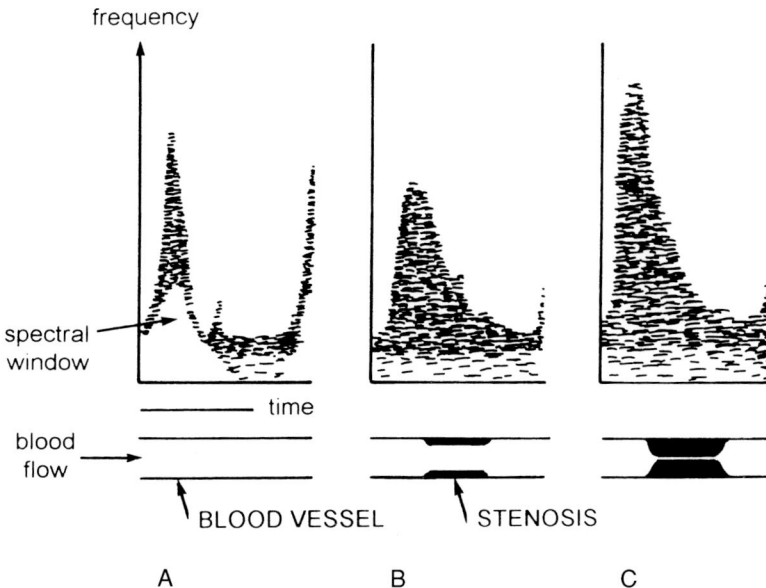

Figure 16. Examples of Doppler frequency spectra obtained from the carotid artery. (**A**) Normal. (**B**) In the region of a 30% stenosis. (**C**) In the region of a 70% stenosis.

velocity through the orifice increases markedly. This is a response that is presumably aimed at maintaining the blood flow volume rate.

If a simple descriptor of spectra such as those illustrated in Fig. 16 is needed, the so-called spectral window often can provide it. The extent of the spectral window relates to the complexity of the flow situation; as the flow becomes more disturbed, the spectral window becomes smaller.

There are numerous clinical applications based on examination of the Doppler spectrum. One of the more important functional studies of this kind in transcranial Doppler (1, 19). The method works well because, somewhat unexpectedly, there are several ultrasonic windows through the skull. The most important of these are the transtemporal, transorbital, suboccipital, and submandibular windows. When the transtemporal approach is used, it is often convenient to stabilize the ultrasonic probe position by means of a headband.

Venous Blood Flow

Blood flow in the veins, except those close to the heart, is characterized by lack of fast pulsatility and relatively low velocity. Ultrasonography is now the favored way to investigate veins in the upper and lower limbs (27). The examination is fast and accurate when carried out with color-flow imaging. The presence of thrombus can be inferred both from the local resistance of the vessel to collapse under applied pressure and from the lack of augmentation of flow due to distal compression. Venous valvular incompetence can be established by flow resulting from a Valsalva maneuver.

Flow in the inferior vena cava is modulated by respiration. The pulsatility of flow in the jugular vein is modified by incompetence of the tricuspid valve.

Wall Compliance and Shear Rate

The principal mechanical forces that act on the wall of a blood vessel are the blood pressure and the wall shear stress, which is equal to the product of the blood viscosity and the wall shear rate.

Arterial wall compliance determines the distensibility of an artery in response to the blood pressure, the force of which acts normal to the blood vessel wall. There are two approaches to the measurement of wall compliance C by ultrasonography (22). The first method is a direct application of the following definition:

$$C = \frac{\Delta D/D}{\Delta P} \qquad (15)$$

where ΔD is the change in diameter of the artery (diameter D) in response to a change in pressure ΔP. This method works well if the vessel is anatomically accessible so that its diameter can be accurately tracked by ultrasound and if the instantaneous blood pressure can be measured. The latter is, unfortunately, usually impracticable. The second method, however, is often easily applied. In order to estimate the compliance of a segment of artery, it is only necessary to measure the blood pulse wave velocity and to assume a value for the density ρ of blood. Then

$$C = (T/L)^2 2\rho \qquad (16)$$

where L is the length of the arterial segment and T is the time required for a blood pulse wave to travel across the segment in the absence of pressure wave reflections.

The wall shear stress is an important factor affecting the structural and functional behavior of the endothelial cells. Ultrasonography provides a method to estimate the wall shear rate in terms of the rate of change of blood flow velocity at the vessel wall (4, 15). This is done by differentiating the blood flow velocity profile, determined by a multigated pulsed Doppler system or some similar technique.

Pressure Gradients

When blood flows through an orifice, such as a stenosed cardiac valve, a simplified version of the Bernoulli equation can be used to estimate the pressure gradient across the orifice (16). Thus, by using the Doppler method to measure the flow velocity V through the orifice,

$$P_1 - P_2 = 4V^2 \qquad (17)$$

where P_1 and P_2 are the pressures on the input and output sides of the orifice, respectively, and provided that V is much greater than the velocity on the input side of the orifice.

Blood Flow Volume Rate

There are three main approaches to the measurement of blood flow volume rate. They are described, together with their advantages and disadvantages, in the following subsections.

Blood Velocity and Vessel Area

Figure 17A shows how the mean blood flow velocity $\overline{V}$ averaged over an appropriate time (e.g., the cardiac cycle) can be estimated from the Doppler frequency spectrum obtained with uniform insonation of the flowing blood. The importance of uniform insonation was explained earlier. The diameter D of the vessel can be measured from either an A-scan or a two-dimensional B-scan. It is usually assumed that the vessel is circular in cross section and that its diameter does not change over the cardiac cycle. It is then a simple matter to calculate the blood flow volume rate $\overline{Q}$ from the following equation, using data obtained by duplex scanning:

$$\overline{Q} = \overline{V}\pi D^2/4 \qquad (18)$$

The method is subject to numerous sources of error (13). Of the assumptions made, that the vessel has a circular cross section is most likely to be incorrect, particularly in the

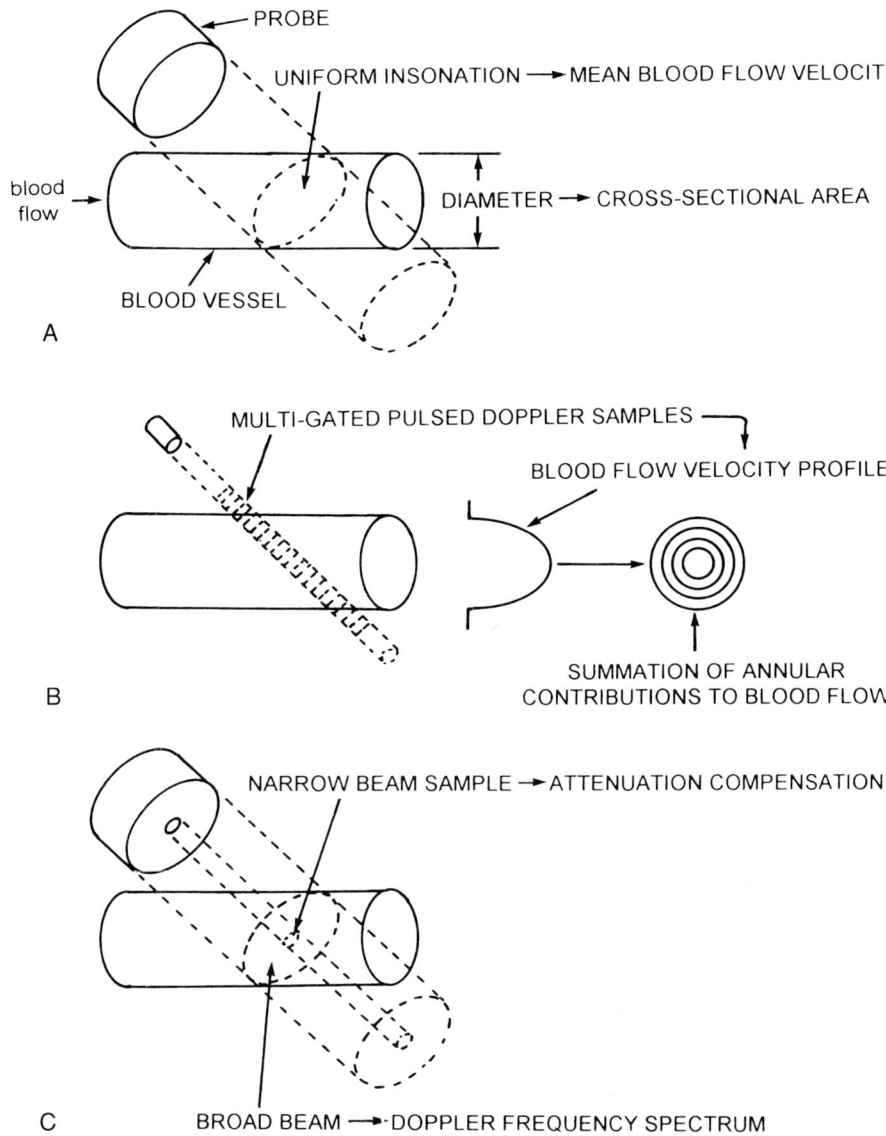

Figure 17. Methods for the measurement of blood flow volume rate. (**A**) Blood velocity and vessel area. (**B**) Velocity profile. (**C**) Attenuation-compensated volume flowmeter.

case of a vein. It may then be necessary, in order to obtain an accurate estimate, to measure the cross-sectional area from a two-dimensional B-scan orthogonal to the vessel axis.

Another important source of error is nonuniform insonation of the flowing blood. If a parabolic flow-velocity profile can be assumed, the average velocity $\overline{V}$ is half the maximum velocity $\hat{V}$, which is relatively easy to measure. The velocity profile is usually somewhere between plug and parabolic flow, however, and the pragmatic assumption is often made that $\overline{V} = 0.57\hat{V}$ (26). The other source of error that needs to be mentioned is that arising in the measurement of the Doppler signal itself, due to the cosine term in Eq. (8). Because of the shape of the cosine function, the errors in angle measurement introduce progressively larger errors in velocity estimation as the angle θ increases. For this reason, it is well worthwhile to try to keep θ below about 60°.

Intraoperative blood flow volume rate measurement provides a useful indication of the function of reconstructive arterial surgery. For this purpose, a clamp can be attached to the vessel or the graft to define both the diameter of the lumen and the angle of the ultrasonic beam (6).

Velocity Profile

The velocity profile can be measured along a diameter D of the blood vessel by means of a multigated pulsed Doppler system, as illustrated in Fig. 17B. By assuming that the velocity profile is circularly symmetric, the profile can be divided into a series of annular elements, within each of which all the blood moves at the same velocity (11). The blood flow volume rate is then given by

$$\overline{Q} = \pi t \sum_{d=0}^{d=D} d\overline{V}_d \qquad (19)$$

where d is the diameter of the annulus and $\overline{V}_d$ is the average velocity of blood flow through it.

It is worth noting that this approach has been engineered to quite an advanced stage using time-domain processing to obtain the flow-velocity profile (12).

Attenuation-Compensated Volume Flowmeter

The ultrasonic broad beam illustrated in Fig. 17C uniformly insonates all the blood flowing in the vessel. Intuitively, the power-frequency spectrum carries all the information necessary to estimate the blood flow volume rate through the vessel, provided that compensation is provided for attenuation of ultrasound in the overlying tissue. This compensation can be derived by measuring the power of ultrasound backscattered by a small-volume element lying entirely within the flowing blood by means of the narrow beam.

The attenuation-compensated volume flowmeter (9, 18) performs these functions. The method is independent of the angle between the flow direction and the ultrasonic beam (provided it is not too large) and the cross-sectional area of the vessel (provided that it is small enough to experience uniform insonation and large enough to accommodate the attenuation-compensating sample volume). It is assumed that the backscattering efficiency of blood is constant, independent of its velocity. This is known not always to be true (32), but the order of magnitude of the related error has not been established.

Tumor Blood Flow

The fact that blood flow associated with the neovascularization that accompanies malignant tumor growth has some quite well-defined characteristics was first observed many years ago (41). Since then, the phenomenon has been quite extensively studied, particularly in breast (3, 5), liver (36), and kidney (20) tumors, using both spectral Doppler and color-flow imaging.

The origin of the Doppler frequency spectrum from a malignant tumor is illustrated in Fig. 18. Typically, the spectrum is characterized by continuous flow in both forward and reverse (not shown in Fig. 18) directions, with high power at low velocities but also with some high-velocity low-power signals. Examples of Doppler frequency spectra obtained from a patient with breast cancer are shown in Fig. 19 and Color Plates 51 and 52.

Tissue Perfusion

Color-flow images of small vessels are illustrated in Fig. 20 and Color Plates 53 and 54. The strength of the ultrasonic blood flow signal detected from tissue must be at least related to the perfusion of the tissue. The microvascular bed is randomly oriented, and the flow velocities, particularly in the capillaries, which are where oxygen and metabolite

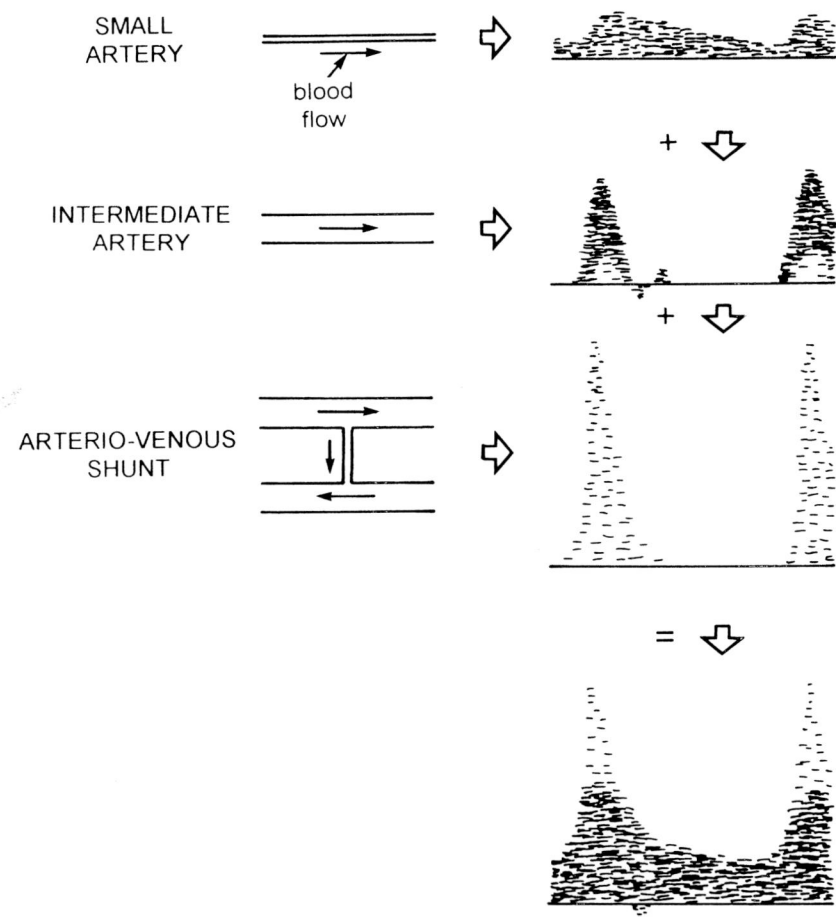

Figure 18. Origin of the Doppler frequency spectrum associated with malignant tumor neovascularization. The neovascular bed consists of small and intermediate-sized vessels, and arteriovenous shunting occurs. The vessels are also quite randomly orientated. The observed spectrum contains contributions from all these sources.

exchanges occur, are relatively very low. Because the tissue itself also moves, separation of the perfusion signals from the tissue signals is a formidable challenge.

There has been some research into this problem (7) using spectral Doppler analysis. This straightforward approach has not produced very encouraging results. Currently, there is interest in the fact that the echoes from solid tissues are deterministic, even though they vary as the tissues move as a whole; echoes from blood decorrelate with motion, however, and this may provide a sound basis for perfusion measurement (2).

Contrast Agents

Contrast agents, particularly those based on microbubbles, promise significantly to expand the clinical usefulness of ultrasonography in functional studies (14). The principle is simple. Because gas has a relatively low characteristic impedance, ultrasound is strongly scattered by inclusions of gas in soft tissue or blood. Moreover, the scattering is amplified if the size of the bubble is such that it resonates at the frequency of the incident ultrasound.

The resonance frequency f_0 of a gas bubble immersed in a liquid of density ρ and at pressure P is given by

$$f_0 \cong \tfrac{1}{2}\pi r \sqrt{3\gamma P/\rho} \qquad (20)$$

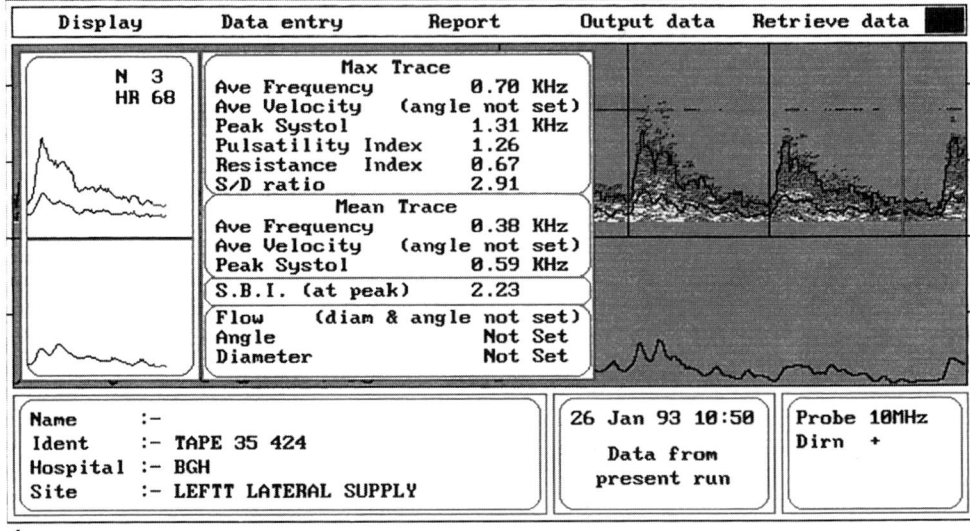

A

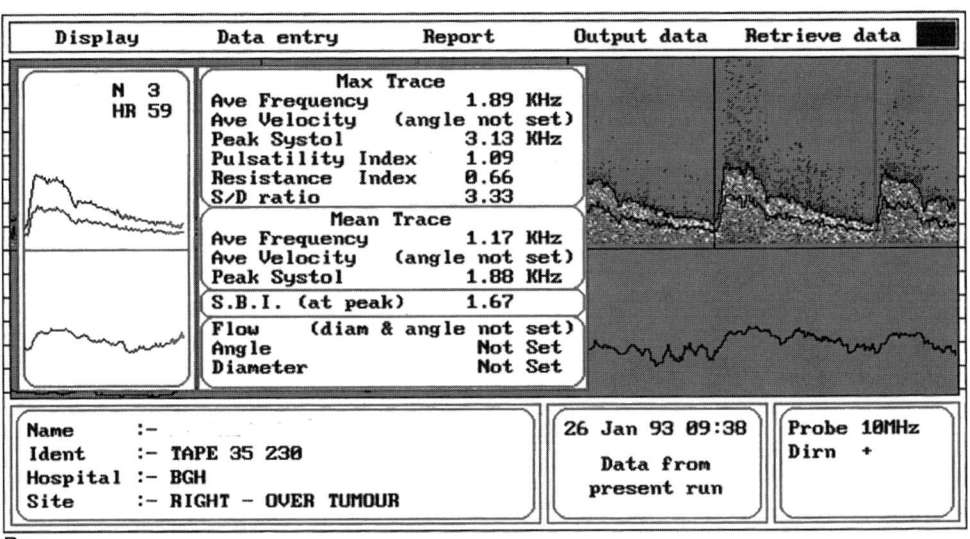

B

Figure 19. Examples of Doppler frequency spectra obtained from (**A**) a breast tumor and (**B**) the contralateral site in the same patient. The results of typical calculations performed by the Doppler frequency analyzer are presented on the display. Note the different frequency scales on the two panels; the markers on the right-hand side of each display are at intervals of 1 kHz. See also Color Plates 51 and 52. (Courtesy of M. Halliwell.)

where r is the bubble and γ is the adiabatic ideal gas constant. This means that a bubble with a diameter of 5 μm (comparable with that of a red blood cell) resonates at a frequency of between 1 and 10 MHz. The actual frequency depends partly on the nature of the shell that encapsulates the bubble. Commercially available contrast agents are encapsulated in a variety of substances, such as albumin, lipid, and palmitic acid, to stabilize the bubbles and thus to extend their life after injection into the blood. Because of the small sizes of the bubbles of some contrast agents, they can be injected into a vein, cross over the pulmonary capillary bed, and enter the systemic circulation. This is a less invasive approach than intraarterial injection.

Contrast agents can enhance the capability of ultrasonography to detect tumor vascularity, delineate areas of ischemia, and improve the visualization of vascular stenosis. They also can be used for clutter rejection (with consequential improvement in signal-to-noise ratio) by the process of second harmonic detection (30). The method depends on the fact that bubbles, because of their nonlinear properties, strongly scatter ultrasound

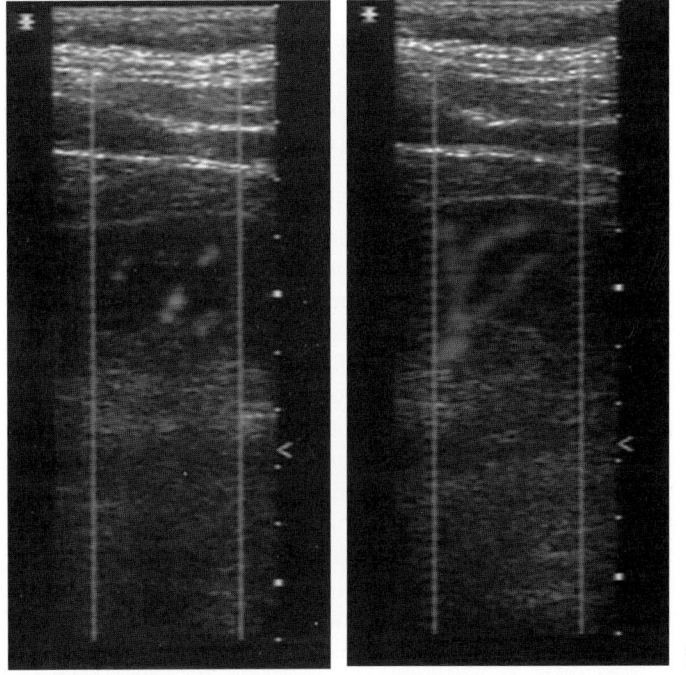

A   B

Figure 20. Examples of color-flow scans of small vessels in the kidney. **(A)** Velocity-flow image. **(B)** Power-flow image demonstrating greater sensitivity of this method for visualizing low-velocity, low-volume flow. See also Color Plates 53 and 54. (Courtesy of M. Halliwell.)

not only at the same frequency as that of the incident ultrasound but also at twice this frequency—at the second harmonic frequency. This hardly happens at all with scattering from solid tissues and blood in the absence of microbubble contrast agents.

The availability of suitable contrast agents raises the prospect that ultrasonography may be able to be substituted for some functional tests currently undertaken with radionuclides. Examples include wash-out studies (31) and, as already mentioned, myocardial blood flow (25).

An attractive but as yet undeveloped idea (10) may become practical with the development of contrast agents. In Eq. (20) it can be seen that the resonance frequency of the bubble is proportional to the square root of the ambient pressure. The idea is that if the sizes of the bubbles could be controlled in manufacture to a narrow range, the ambient pressure could be determined by measuring the resonance frequency. Even if suitable bubbles could be produced, however, the damping effects of their shells and the surrounding blood (or tissue) might broaden the frequency response to an extent that could make the pressure measurement too imprecise to be of any practical value. These matters remain to be explored.

CONCLUSIONS

Although ultrasonography is commonly considered to be a radiologic technique, with the emphasis on imaging anatomy and pathology, it is actually also a powerful tool for studying many aspects of physiologic function in health and disease. Ultrasonography is excellent for the investigation and quantitation of tissue motion and blood flow. The exposures used in contemporary ultrasonic diagnostic techniques appear to be safe. The method is limited, however, by certain physical constraints. First, ultrasound is strongly reflected at interfaces between soft tissue and bone or gas. Examination of or beyond gas-containing structures and bones is often impractical. Second, the attenuation of ultrasound increases with the frequency. This means that the maximum obtainable spatial resolution reduces as the penetration into the patient is increased. Third, the rate at which information can be obtained is limited by the speed of ultrasound in tissues. Although real-time two-dimensional imaging is possible, the time required to obtain information about structure movement and blood flow increases as the velocity of interest is decreased to the point that true real-time operation may become unobtainable. Fourth, even biologic soft tissues are sufficiently disparate to result in inhomogeneities that can distort ultrasonic wave propagation to the extent that image degradation may become significant. Finally, ultrasonography is associated with numerous artefacts, the origins of which lie in both the physics of the techniques and the properties of tissues.

No investigative method is without its problems, however, and it is appropriate to end on high notes for ultrasonography. It is a relatively inexpensive technology. It is already the method of choice for numerous functional studies. Although gas and bone are obstacles, they often can be circumvented by simple and sometimes ingenious protocols. There is tremendous scope for further developments. Ultrasonic contrast agents are in their infancy. Equipment needs to be specially designed to exploit their properties and for other novel approaches to functional imaging and measurement. It is also interesting to note that ultrasound can be used to produce trackless lesions within the body (37), which, under some circumstances, may be reversible. Thus, in animal experiments and perhaps also in research on humans, nervous pathways can be interrupted to elucidate brain function (21), and doubtless there are many other applications for techniques of this kind. Ultrasonography surely deserves to be ranked highly alongside all the other functional imaging methods.

REFERENCES

1. Aaslid R, Markwalder TM, Normes H. Noninvasive transcranial Doppler ultrasound recording of flow velocity in basal cerebral arteries. *J Neurosurg,* 57, 769 (1982).
2. Adler RS, Rubin JM, Fowlkes JB et al. Ultrasonic estimation of tissue perfusion: A stochastic approach. *Ultrasound Med Biol,* 21, 493 (1995).
3. Bell DS, Bamber-JC, Eckersley RJ. Segmentation and analysis of colour Doppler images of tumour vasculature. *Ultrasound Med Biol,* 21, 635 (1995).
4. Brands PJ, Hoeks APG, Hofstra L, Reneman RS. A noninvasive method to estimate wall shear rate using ultrasound. *Ultrasound Med Biol,* 21, 171 (1995).
5. Burns PN, Halliwell M, Webb AJ, Wells PNT. Ultrasonic Doppler studies of the breast. *Ultrasound Med Biol,* 8, 127 (1982).
6. Davies AH, Magee TR, Baird RN, Horrocks M. Intraoperative measurement of vascular graft resistance as a predictor of early outcome. *Br J Surg,* 80, 854 (1993).
7. Dymling SO, Persson HW, Hertz CH. Measurement of blood perfusion in tissue using Doppler ultrasound. *Ultrasound Med Biol,* 17, 433 (1991).
8. Evans DH, McDicken WN, Skidmore R, Woodcock JP. *Doppler ultrasound.* Chichester: Wiley (1989).
9. Evans JM, Skidmore R, Baker JD, Wells PNT. A new approach to the noninvasive measurement of cardiac output using an annular array Doppler technique: II: Practical implementation and results. *Ultrasound Med Biol,* 15, 179 (1989).
10. Fairbank WM, Scully MO. A new noninvasive technique for cardiac pressure measurement: Resonant scattering of ultrasound from bubbles. *IEEE Trans Biomed Eng,* 24, 107 (1977).
11. Fish PJ. A method of transcutaneous blood flow measurement—accuracy considerations. In: A Kurjak, A Kratochwil (Eds.). *Recent advances in ultrasonic diagnosis,* Vol 3, 110. Amsterdam: Elsevier (1981).
12. Forsberg F, Liu JB, Russel KM et al. Volume flow estimation using time domain correlation and ultrasonic flowmetry. *Ultrasound Med Biol,* 21, 1037 (1995).
13. Gill RW. Measurement of blood flow by ultrasound: Accuracy and sources of error. *Ultrasound Med Biol,* 11, 625 (1985).
14. Goldberg BB, Liu JB, Forsberg F. Ultrasound contrast agents: A review. *Ultrasound Med Biol,* 20, 319 (1994).
15. Hoeks APG, Samijo SK, Brands PJ, Reneman RS. Assessment of wall shear rate in humans: An ultrasound study. *J Vasc Invest,* 1, 108 (1995).
16. Holen J, Aaslid R, Landmark K, Simonsen S. Determination of pressure gradient in mitral stenosis with a non-invasive Doppler technique. *Acta Med Scand,* 199, 455 (1976).
17. Hoskins PR. Accuracy of maximum velocity estimates made using Doppler ultrasound systems. *Br J Radiol,* 69, 172 (1996).
18. Hottinger CF, Meindl JD. Blood flow measurement using the attenuation-compensated volume flowmeter. *Ultrason Imag,* 1, 1 (1979).
19. Katz ML, Comerota AJ. Transcranial Doppler: A review of technique, interpretation, and clinical applications. *Ultrasound Q,* 8, 241 (1991).

20. Kier R, Taylor KJW, Feyock AL, Ramos IM. Renal masses: Characterization with Doppler US. *Radiology,* 176, 703 (1990).
21. Lee AJ, Taberner PV, Halliwell M. Severing the corpus callosum in rats using ultrasound: Theoretical and experimental correlations. *J Acoust Soc Am,* 66, 1292 (1979).
22. Lehmann ED, Hopkins KD, Gosling RG. Aortic compliance measurements using Doppler ultrasound: In vivo biochemical correlates. *Ultrasound Med Biol,* 19, 683 (1993).
23. MacPherson DS, Evans DH, Bell PRF. Common femoral artery Doppler waveforms: A comparison of three methods of objective analysis with direct pressure measurements. *Br J Surg,* 71, 46 (1984).
24. McDicken WN, Sutherland GR, Moran CM, Gordon L. Colour Doppler velocity imaging of the myocardium. *Ultrasound Med Biol,* 18, 651 (1992).
25. Mor-Avi V, David D, Akselrod S et al. Myocardial regional blood flow: Quantitative measurement by computer analysis of contrast enhanced echocardiographic images. *Ultrasound Med Biol,* 19, 619 (1993).
26. Moriyasu F, Ban N, Nishida O et al. Clinical application of an ultrasonic duplex system in the quantitative measurement of portal blood flow. *J Clin Ultrasound,* 14, 579 (1986).
27. Pellerito JS, Hammers LW. Venous imaging. In: KJW Taylor, PN Burns, PNT Wells (Eds.). *Clinical applications of Doppler ultrasound,* 2nd ed, 263. New York: Raven Press (1995).
28. Rijsterborgh H, van der Steen AFW, Krams R et al. The relationship between myocardial integrated backscatter, perfusion pressure and wall thickness during isovolumic contraction: An isolated pig heart study. *Ultrasound Med Biol,* 22, 43 (1996).
29. Rubin JM, Bude RO, Carson PL et al. Power Doppler US: A potentially useful alternative to mean frequency-based color Doppler US. *Radiology,* 190, 853 (1994).
30. Schrope BA, Newhouse VL. Second harmonic blood perfusion measurements. *Ultrasound Med Biol,* 19, 567 (1993).
31. Schwarz KQ, Bezante GP, Chen X et al. Volumetric arterial flow quantification using echo contrast. An in vitro comparison of three ultrasonic intensity methods: Radio frequency, video and Doppler. *Ultrasound Med Biol,* 19, 447 (1993).
32. Shung KK, Cloutier G, Lim CC. The effects of hematocrit, shear rate and turbulence on ultrasonic Doppler spectrum from blood. *IEEE Trans Biomed Eng,* 39, 462 (1992).
33. Skidmore R, Follett DH. Maximum frequency follower for the processing of ultrasonic Doppler shift signals. *Ultrasound Med Biol,* 4, 145 (1978).
34. Skidmore R, Woodcock JP. Physiological interpretation of Doppler-shift waveforms: II. Validation of the Laplace transform method for characterisation of the common femoral blood-velocity/time waveform. *Ultrasound Med Biol,* 6, 219 (1980).
35. Sumner DS, Moore DJ, Miles RD. Doppler ultrasonic arteriography and flow velocity analysis in carotid artery disease. In: EF Bernstein (Ed.). *Noninvasive diagnostic techniques in vascular disease,* 349. St. Louis: Mosby (1985).
36. Taylor KJW, Ramos I, Morse SS et al. Focal liver masses: Differential diagnosis with pulsed Doppler US. *Radiology,* 164, 643 (1987).
37. ter Haar G. Ultrasound focal beam surgery. *Ultrasound Med Biol,* 21, 1089 (1995).
38. Wells PNT. *Biomedical ultrasonics.* London: Academic Press (1977).
39. Wells PNT. The prudent use of diagnostic ultrasound. *Br J Radiol,* 59, 1143 (1986).
40. Wells PNT. Ultrasonic colour flow imaging. *Phys Med Biol,* 39, 2113 (1994).
41. Wells PNT, Halliwell M, Skidmore R et al. Tumour detection by ultrasonic Doppler blood flow signals. *Ultrasonics,* 15, 231 (1977).
42. Wickline SA, Thomas LJ, Miller JG et al. A relationship between ultrasonic integrated backscatter and myocardial contractile function. *J Clin Invest,* 76, 2151 (1985).

Index

Numbers followed by the letter *f* indicate figures; numbers followed by the letter *t* indicate tables.